Type 2 Diabetes Mellitus

Type 2 Diabetes Mellitus

Exploring Immunogenetic Pathways

Edited by

Haamid Bashir

Department of Biochemistry, Government Medical College, Srinagar, Jammu & Kashmir, India

Shafat Ali

Department of Zoology, Hassan Khoyihami Memorial Degree College, Bandipora, Jammu & Kashmir, India

Yahya F. Jamous

Wellness and Preventive Medicine Institute, Health Sector, King Abdulaziz City for Science and Technology, Riyadh, Saudi Arabia

ELSEVIER

Elsevier
Radarweg 29, PO Box 211, 1000 AE Amsterdam, Netherlands
125 London Wall, London EC2Y 5AS, United Kingdom
50 Hampshire Street, 5th Floor, Cambridge, MA 02139, United States

ISBN: 978-0-443-33590-7

For information on all Elsevier publications visit our website at https://www.elsevier.com/books-and-journals

Publisher: Megan Ball
Acquisitions Editor: Patricia Osborn
Editorial Project Manager: Priyamvada Jha
Production Project Manager: Vijayaraj Purushothaman
Cover Designer: Miles Hitchen

Typeset by TNQ Tech

Contents

Contributors

Kripamoy Aguan Molecular Biology Laboratory, Department of Biotechnology and Bioinformatics, North Eastern Hill University, Shillong, Meghalaya, India

Hilal Ahmed Department of Zoology, HKM Degree College Bandipora, Jammu and Kashmir, India

Imtiaz Ahmed Fish Nutrition Research Laboratory, Department of Zoology, University of Kashmir, Srinagar, Jammu and Kashmir, India

Salman Akhtar Department of Bioengineering, Integral University, Lucknow, Uttar Pradesh, India; Novel Global Community Educational Foundation, Hebersham, NSW, Australia

Shafat Ali Department of Zoology, Hassan Khoyihami Memorial Degree College, Bandipora, Jammu & Kashmir, India

Annanya Antal Department of Biotechnology, Jaypee Institute of Information Technology, Noida, Uttar Pradesh, India

Shweta Arya Department of Biotechnology, Jaypee Institute of Information Technology, Noida, Uttar Pradesh, India

Rishikesh Shankar Bachhav Department of Pharmacology, R. G. Sapkal College of Pharmacy, Savitribai Phule Pune University, Nashik, Maharashtra, India

Dhanusmita Barman Department of Zoology, Auxilium College, Udalguri, Assam, India

Binty Centre for Emerging Diseases, Department of Biotechnology, Jaypee Institute of Information Technology, Noida, Uttar Pradesh, India

Prachi Chauhan Department of Biotechnology, Jaypee Institute of Information Technology, Noida, Uttar Pradesh, India

Pritee Chunarkar-Patil Department of Bioinformatics, Rajiv Gandhi Institute of IT and Biotechnology, Bharati Vidyapeeth (Deemed to be University), Pune, Maharashtra, India

Ghulam Mehdi Dar Central Molecular Lab, Govind Ballabh Pant Institute of Medical Education and Research, Delhi, New Delhi, India

Taief Ahmad Dar Department of Biochemistry, Government Degree College Kulgam, Kulgam Jammu & Kashmir, India

Harshit Devtalla Department of Biochemistry, Post Graduate Institute of Medical Education and Research, Chandigarh, India

Shazia Haider Department of Biosciences, Faculty of Natural Sciences, Jamia Millia University, Delhi, New Delhi, India

Showkat Hussain Faculty of Allied and HealthCare, Guru Kashi University, Bathinda, Punjab, India

Mohd Rizwan Jameel Centre for Interdisciplinary Research in Basic Science, Jamia Milia Islamia, Delhi, New Delhi, India

Yahya F. Jamous Wellness and Preventive Medicine Institute, Health Sector, King Abdulaziz City for Science and Technology, Riyadh, Saudi Arabia

Mohmmad Kaleem Department of Pharmacology, R. G. Sapkal College of Pharmacy, Savitribai Phule Pune University, Nashik, Maharashtra, India

Asaad Kayali Department of Health Sciences, Higher Colleges of Technology, Abu Dhabi, United Arab Emirates

Abdullah Khan C.G. Bhakta Institute of Biotechnology, Uka Tarsadia University, Bardoli, Surat, India

Fariya Khan Department of Biotechnology, Kanpur Institute of Technology (KIT), Kanpur, Uttar Pradesh, India

Rahul Kumar Faculty of Pharmacy, Vidya University, Meerut, Uttar Pradesh, India; Faculty of Pharmacy, Swami Vivekanand Subharti University, Meerut, Uttar Pradesh, India

Ajay Kumar Department of Biotechnology, Faculty of Engineering and Technology Rama University, Mandhana, Kanpur, Uttar Pradesh, India

Aryan Kumar Faculty of Pharmacy, Vidya University, Meerut, Uttar Pradesh, India

Puja Kumari Department of Biotechnology and Bioinformatics, North Eastern Hill University, Shillong, Meghalaya, India

Shivanshi Madeshiya Interdisciplinary Biotechnology Unit, Faculty of Life Sciences, Aligarh Muslim University, Aligarh, Uttar Pradesh, India

Bhawna Mahajan Central Molecular Lab, Govind Ballabh Pant Institute of Medical Education and Research, Delhi, New Delhi, India; Department of Biochemistry, Govind Ballabh Pant Institute of Medical Education and Research, Delhi, New Delhi, India

Shalini Mani Centre for Emerging Diseases, Department of Biotechnology, Jaypee Institute of Information Technology, Noida, Uttar Pradesh, India

Prem Shankar Mishra Faculty of Pharmacy, Vidya University, Meerut, Uttar Pradesh, India

Rakhi Mishra Noida Institute of Engg. & Technology (Pharmacy Institute), Noida, Uttar Pradesh, India

Rudrank Moharana C.G. Bhakta Institute of Biotechnology, Uka Tarsadia University, Bardoli, Surat, India

Khushi Negi Department of Biotechnology, Jaypee Institute of Information Technology, Noida, Uttar Pradesh, India

Sakshi Patel Faculty of Pharmacy, Vidya University, Meerut, Uttar Pradesh, India; Faculty of Pharmacy, Swami Vivekanand Subharti University, Meerut, Uttar Pradesh, India

Rituparna Paul Molecular Biology Laboratory, Department of Biotechnology and Bioinformatics, North Eastern Hill University, Shillong, Meghalaya, India

R. Rachana Centre for Emerging Diseases, Department of Biotechnology, Jaypee Institute of Information Technology, Noida, Uttar Pradesh, India

SK Abdul Rahman Department of Pharmaceutical Sciences, Vignan's Foundation for Science, Technology and Research, Guntur, Andhra Pradesh, India

Neha Raj Interdisciplinary Biotechnology Unit, Faculty of Life Sciences, Aligarh Muslim University, Aligarh, Uttar Pradesh, India

Roaf Ahmad Rather Department of Agricultural Technology, Government Degree College Kulgam, Kulgam Jammu & Kashmir, India

Abhishek Sharma Interdisciplinary Biotechnology Unit, Faculty of Life Sciences, Aligarh Muslim University, Aligarh, Uttar Pradesh, India

Abid Ali Sheikh National Institute of Biologicals, Noida, Uttar Pradesh, India

Unnati Shukla Centre for Emerging Diseases, Department of Biotechnology, Jaypee Institute of Information Technology, Noida, Uttar Pradesh, India

Waseem Ahmad Siddiqui Interdisciplinary Biotechnology Unit, Faculty of Life Sciences, Aligarh Muslim University, Aligarh, Uttar Pradesh, India

Manisha Singh Centre for Emerging Diseases, Department of Biotechnology, Jaypee Institute of Information Technology, Noida, Uttar Pradesh, India

Shriram Sisodia Faculty of Pharmacy, Vidya University, Meerut, Uttar Pradesh, India

Lyticia Philabet Sohtun Molecular Biology Laboratory, Department of Biotechnology and Bioinformatics, North Eastern Hill University, Shillong, Meghalaya, India

Sahar Surve Department of Bioinformatics, Rajiv Gandhi Institute of IT and Biotechnology, Bharati Vidyapeeth (Deemed to be University), Pune, Maharashtra, India

Jai Vardhan Faculty of Pharmacy, Vidya University, Meerut, Uttar Pradesh, India

Priyanka Yadav Department of Biotechnology, Jaypee Institute of Information Technology, Noida, Uttar Pradesh, India

Short biographies of editors

Dr. Haamid Bashir

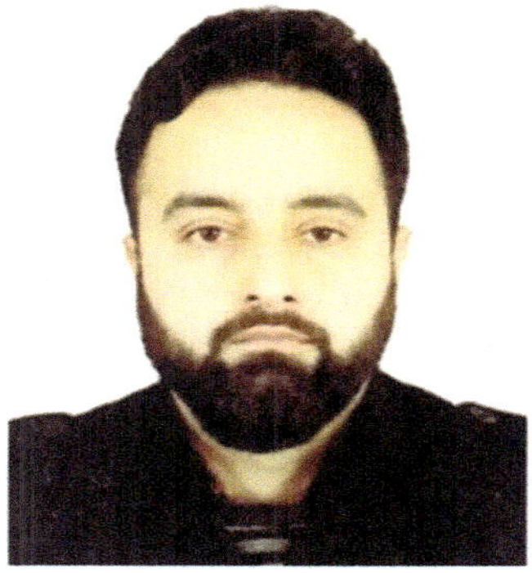

Dr. Haamid Bashir is an academician and researcher in the Department of Biochemistry at Government Medical College, Srinagar. He holds a PhD in Biochemistry and specializes in molecular and clinical aspects of metabolic disorders, particularly Type 2 Diabetes Mellitus (T2DM). His research focuses on immunogenetic and inflammatory pathways, including cytokine-mediated mechanisms in insulin resistance. Dr. Bashir has authored several research publications in reputed journals and is dedicated to advancing biomedical research, teaching, and the understanding of chronic diseases.

Dr. Shafat Ali

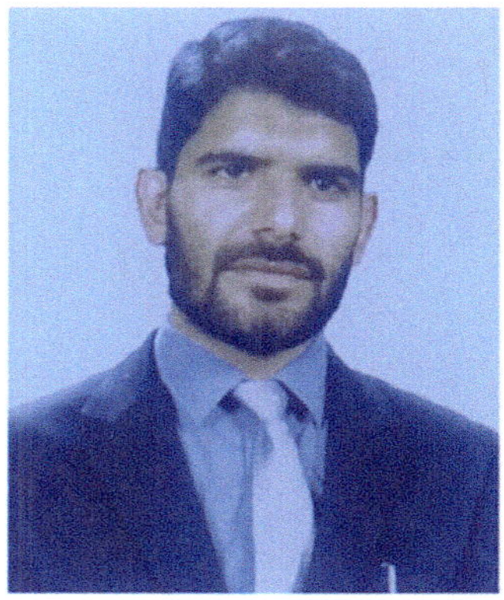

Dr. Shafat Ali earned his BSc from the University of Kashmir and his MSc in Zoology from Barkatullah Vishwavidyalaya, India. He has over 6 years of research experience and more than 6 years of teaching experience. Currently, he is engaged in teaching at Hassan Khoyihami Memorial Degree College, Bandipora, Jammu and Kashmir, India.

His research interests include reproductive immunogenetics, cytokine biology, molecular biology, and cancer biology. Dr. Ali has authored over 30 book chapters, edited 8 books, and published around 30 peer-reviewed international research articles. He has also contributed to the academic community by serving as a reviewer and associate editor for several reputed international journals.

Dr. Yahya F. Jamous

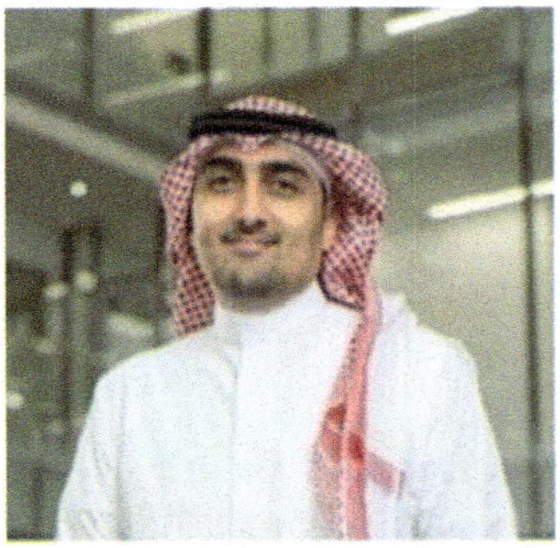

Dr. Yahya F. Jamous is a Saudi pharmaceutical scientist at the Wellness and Preventive Medicine Institute, Health Sector, King Abdulaziz City for Science and Technology (KACST), Riyadh, Saudi Arabia, with over 15 years of research and teaching experience and publications in pharmaceutical biotechnology, nanotechnology, and molecular pharmacology.

He has held several senior roles at KACST, including Associate Research Professor, Acting Director for National Partnerships, and former Director of the National Vaccines and Bioprocessing Centre (NVBC), contributing to initiatives aligned with Saudi Vision 2030.

He earned his PhD in Molecular Pharmacology from ETH Zurich and holds MSc and BSc degrees in Pharmaceutical Sciences from King Saud University. He is also a licensed Consultant of Pharmaceutical Sciences and a certified PMP and PMI-RMP.

Preface

Type 2 diabetes mellitus (T2DM) has emerged as one of the most significant global health challenges of the 21st century. Traditionally viewed as a metabolic disorder characterized by insulin resistance and impaired insulin secretion, T2DM is now increasingly recognized as a complex, multifactorial disease involving intricate interactions among genetic predisposition, environmental influences, metabolic disturbances, and immune system dysregulation. In recent years, advances in molecular biology, genomics, and immunology have revealed that immune-mediated mechanisms and immunogenetic factors play critical roles in the development, progression, and complications of T2DM.

This book, *Type 2 Diabetes Mellitus: Exploring Immunogenetic Pathways*, aims to provide a comprehensive overview of the evolving understanding of the immunogenetic basis of T2DM. The book brings together current scientific knowledge on how genetic variations, immune responses, and inflammatory processes interact to influence disease susceptibility, pathogenesis, and therapeutic outcomes. By integrating insights from genetics, immunology, and clinical research, this work seeks to bridge gaps between fundamental research and translational applications in diabetes care.

The opening chapters introduce the fundamental concepts of T2DM and outline the genetic landscape associated with the disease. Subsequent chapters explore the role of the immune system, highlighting the involvement of immune cells, cytokines, and inflammatory mediators in shaping insulin sensitivity and metabolic regulation. Special emphasis is given to genetic variations that influence immune responses, including gene–environment interactions and human leukocyte antigen (HLA) associations that may contribute to disease susceptibility.

Further sections of the book focus on immune-mediated complications of T2DM and emerging therapeutic strategies that target immune and inflammatory pathways. Discussions on antibody-based therapies, immunomodulatory interventions, and novel treatment approaches illustrate the growing potential of immunogenetics in shaping future diabetes therapies. In addition, chapters dedicated to personalized medicine emphasize how immunogenetic profiling may enable more precise and individualized treatment strategies for patients with T2DM.

The final chapters address emerging trends, unresolved questions, and ongoing challenges in immunogenetic research, while also emphasizing the importance of integrating immunogenetic insights into broader T2DM research and clinical practice. As scientific understanding continues to evolve, it is hoped that the knowledge compiled in this volume will stimulate further research, encourage interdisciplinary collaboration, and contribute to improved prevention, diagnosis, and management of type 2 diabetes mellitus.

This book is intended for researchers, clinicians, academicians, and students working in the fields of endocrinology, immunology, genetics, molecular biology, and biomedical sciences. We hope that this volume will serve as a valuable resource for understanding the complex interplay between genetics and immunity in T2DM and inspire new avenues of investigation in this rapidly advancing field.

Editors

1

Introduction to type 2 diabetes mellitus (T2DM)

Hilal Ahmed[1] and Imtiaz Ahmed[2]

[1]DEPARTMENT OF ZOOLOGY, HKM DEGREE COLLEGE BANDIPORA, JAMMU AND KASHMIR, INDIA; [2]FISH NUTRITION RESEARCH LABORATORY, DEPARTMENT OF ZOOLOGY, UNIVERSITY OF KASHMIR, SRINAGAR, JAMMU AND KASHMIR, INDIA

1. Introduction

Type 2 diabetes mellitus (T2DM) is a chronic metabolic disorder characterized by sustained hyperglycemia arising from the combined effects of peripheral insulin resistance and progressive pancreatic β-cell dysfunction. It accounts for approximately 90%–95% of all diabetes cases worldwide (IDF, 2025; WHO, 2023). Insulin resistance in skeletal muscle, liver, and adipose tissue impairs glucose uptake and enhances hepatic gluconeogenesis, while declining β-cell secretory capacity fails to compensate for rising metabolic demands (DeFronzo et al., 2015). This dual defect drives chronic hyperglycemia, predisposing individuals to microvascular and macrovascular complications, including nephropathy, retinopathy, neuropathy, and cardiovascular disease.

T2DM is one of the fastest-growing global health challenges of the 21st century. In 2021, more than 500 million adults were living with diabetes worldwide, a figure projected to exceed 780 million by 2045, with the steepest increases in low- and middle-income countries (IDF, 2021; Liu et al., 2020). Over the past 3 decades, diabetes-related incidence, mortality, and disability-adjusted life years have more than doubled, reflecting demographic aging, urbanization, obesity, and physical inactivity (Zimmet et al., 2016). The economic burden is profound, with global healthcare expenditures reaching hundreds of billions of USD annually.

Diabetes mellitus has transitioned from a relatively rare metabolic condition to a global epidemic within a single generation. Contemporary estimates indicate that T2DM constitutes nearly 95% of diagnosed diabetes cases, with prevalence increasing disproportionately in low- and middle-income nations undergoing rapid nutritional and lifestyle transitions (WHO, 2023; Zimmet et al., 2016). Alarmingly, T2DM is increasingly diagnosed in adolescents and young adults, reflecting early exposure to obesogenic

Type 2 Diabetes Mellitus. https://doi.org/10.1016/B978-0-443-33590-7.00002-2

environments interacting with genetic susceptibility (Narayan et al., 2021). These trends signify a shift in disease demography, amplifying the risk of lifetime complication and long-term strain on the health system.

The clinical syndrome now recognized as diabetes mellitus has been documented for over three millennia. The Ebers Papyrus (c.1550 BCE) described a wasting disease marked by excessive urination, while ancient Indian Ayurvedic texts identified *Madhumeha*, or "honey urine disease," explicitly recognizing glycosuria (Carpenter et al., 2006; Mishra & Adra, 2003). Notably, Ayurvedic scholars distinguished lean, early-onset forms from obesity-associated adult disease, presaging the modern classification of Type 1 and Type 2 diabetes. These early observations underscore the long-standing recognition of diabetes as a heterogeneous metabolic disorder (Table 1.1).

Between the 17th and 19th centuries, diabetes research entered an experimental phase that transformed descriptive medicine into mechanistic science. Thomas Willis formally coined the term *diabetes mellitus* in 1675, distinguishing it from diabetes insipidus (Afrin, 2016). Matthew Dobson later demonstrated the presence of glucose in the blood and urine, establishing its biochemical basis (Eknoyan, 2019). The identification of pancreatic islets by Langerhans and the induction of diabetes following pancreatectomy by Von Mering & Minkowski (1889) conclusively linked the pancreas to glucose regulation, laying the foundation for endocrine pathophysiology (Ornellas et al., 2020).

The isolation of insulin in 1921 revolutionized diabetes treatment and exposed fundamental disease heterogeneity. While insulin was lifesaving for some patients, others, typically adults, exhibited insulin resistance rather than absolute deficiency (Lewis and Brubaker, 2021). Harold Himsworth's 1936 distinction between insulin-sensitive and insulin-insensitive diabetes formalized the conceptual separation of Type 1 and Type 2 diabetes (Kim, 2011). Subsequent development of oral hypoglycemic agents, including sulfonylureas and metformin, further reinforced T2DM as a disorder of insulin action rather than insulin absence (Corremans, 2023) (Table 1.2).

Advances during the late twentieth century refined diabetes classification by standardizing diagnostic criteria that incorporated fasting plasma glucose, oral glucose tolerance testing, and HbA1c measurements (WHO; ADA, 1999–2010). Landmark trials such as the UKPDS established the clinical value of intensive glycemic and blood pressure control in T2DM (Rodríguez-Gutiérrez & Montori, 2016). In recent decades, genome-wide association studies have identified susceptibility loci such as *TCF7L2*, clarifying the genetic architecture, while novel agents including SGLT2 inhibitors have demonstrated cardio-renal benefits independent of glycemic control (Caruso & Giorgino, 2022). These developments reframed T2DM as a multisystem disease.

2. Epidemiology of type 2 diabetes mellitus

The global epidemiology of T2DM reflects a complex interplay among demographic transitions, urbanization, lifestyle changes, genetic susceptibility, and environmental

Table 1.1 Chronological milestones in the discovery, classification, and therapeutic evolution of diabetes mellitus.

Date/Period	Event	References
1550 BCE	Ebers Papyrus (Egypt) describes excessive urination, marking the earliest record of a diabetes-like condition.	Carpenter et al. (2006)
5th-2nd century BCE	Ayurvedic texts (Charaka, Sushruta) and Greco-Roman medicine describe "honey urine" and wasting, linking diabetes to glycosuria and emaciation.	Mishra and Adra (2003)
2nd century CE	Aretaeus of Cappadocia coins the term "diabetes" (meaning siphon), emphasizing polyuria and wasting.	Laios et al. (2012)
1025 CE	Avicenna's Canon of Medicine details diabetes symptoms and complications, systematizing chronicity and progression.	Dushenkov (2017)
1675	Thomas Willis notes the sweet taste of urine, reinforcing the link between diabetes and sugar metabolism.	Afrin (2016)
1776	Matthew Dobson demonstrates sugar in urine and blood, establishing the biochemical basis of diabetes.	Eknoyan (2019)
1850s	Claude Bernard elucidates glycogenesis and internal secretion, laying the foundation for understanding glucose regulation and insulin resistance.	Clarkson (1926)
1869	Paul Langerhans describes pancreatic islets, identifying the anatomical basis of endocrine pancreatic control.	Ornellas et al. (2020)
1889	Minkowski & von Mering induce diabetes in dogs via pancreatectomy, proving the pancreas' role in diabetes.	Jörgens (2020)
1909–10	Jean de Meyer and Sharpey-Schafer propose insulin as the antidiabetic substance, conceptualizing hormonal regulation.	Ayan and DeMirci (2023)
1921–22	Banting, Best, Macleod, Collip isolate and clinically apply insulin, revolutionizing diabetes treatment and distinguishing insulin deficiency from resistance.	Lewis and Brubaker (2021)
1936	Harold Himsworth distinguishes insulin-sensitive versus insulin-insensitive diabetes, laying the foundation for type 1 versus type 2 classification.	Kim (2011)
1940–50	Sulfonylureas introduced as the first oral hypoglycemics, enhancing insulin secretion for T2DM management.	Tomlinson et al. (2022)
1957	Metformin reported in French literature; later adopted globally as a cornerstone insulin-sensitizing therapy.	Corremans (2023)
1960–70	Discovery of insulin receptor and signaling pathways, clarifying molecular basis of insulin resistance in T2DM.	Saini (2010)
1979–80	National Diabetes Data Group/WHO classification frameworks formalize categories and diagnostic criteria, standardizing type-based classification.	Brigham (2025)
1985–99	WHO and ADA refine diagnostic thresholds (FPG, OGTT, HbA1c), improving global comparability of T2DM epidemiology.	Pragati and Paolo (2025)
1990s	UKPDS trial demonstrates benefits of glycemic and blood pressure control in T2DM, shaping evidence-based management.	Rodríguez-Gutiérrez and Montori (2016)
Late 1980–2000s	Incretin biology (GLP-1, GIP, DPP-4) clarified, leading to incretin-based therapies.	Nauck (2016)
1997–2008	Thiazolidinediones (TZDs) and DPP-4 inhibitors introduced, expanding therapeutic options for insulin resistance and incretin modulation.	Tan et al. (2022)
2013-Present	SGLT2 inhibitors adopted, showing cardio-renal protective benefits beyond glucose lowering.	Caruso and Giorgino (2022)
2007-Present	Genome-wide association studies (GWAS) identify T2DM risk loci (e.g., TCF7L2), clarifying genetic architecture.	Grant (2019)
2010–2020	HbA1c formalized as diagnostic criterion; precision medicine approaches emerge for stratified care.	Stranieri et al. (2015)

Continued

Table 1.1 Chronological milestones in the discovery, classification, and therapeutic evolution of diabetes mellitus.—cont'd

Date/Period	Event	References
2020s	Cardiometabolic framing integrates obesity, NAFLD, and cardiovascular risk, redefining T2DM as a multisystem disease.	Dongiovanni et al. (2021)
2024–25	Ongoing updates to global guidelines emphasize outcome-driven algorithms prioritizing cardio-renal protection in T2DM.	Weiskirchen and Lonardo (2025)

Table 1.2 Comparative features of Type 1 diabetes mellitus, Type 2 diabetes mellitus, and other major forms of diabetes mellitus.

Feature	Type 1 diabetes mellitus	Type 2 diabetes mellitus	Gestational diabetes mellitus	Other specific types	References
Typical age at onset	Childhood or adolescence	Adulthood (increasingly youth due to obesity epidemic)	Pregnancy (2nd-3rd trimester)	Variable (depends on etiology, e.g., MODY in youth, secondary diabetes at any age)	Seshiah et al. (2014); Athanasiadou and Paschou (2025); Ahamd (2022)
Primary etiology	Autoimmune β-cell destruction	Insulin resistance with relative insulin deficiency	Pregnancy-induced insulin resistance mediated by placental hormones	Genetic (MODY), endocrine (Cushing's, acromegaly), pancreatic disease, or drug-induced	Seshiah et al. (2014); Ahamd (2022)
Insulin secretion	Absent or near absent	Initially normal or elevated, declines progressively	Initially preserved, may decline if β-cell reserve insufficient	Variable depending on cause	Ahamd (2022); Jadon et al. (2024)
Insulin resistance	Minimal	Marked	Marked (physiological, pregnancy-related)	Variable	Jadon et al. (2024)
Autoantibodies	Present (GAD, IA-2, ZnT8, ICA)	Absent	Absent	Usually absent	Pihoker et al. (2005)
Body habitus	Often lean	Often overweight or obese	Variable (depends on maternal BMI)	Variable	Jae et al. (2016)
Immune involvement	Adaptive autoimmunity (T-cell mediated)	Chronic low-grade inflammation (innate immune pathways, adipokines)	Mild inflammatory state	Etiology-dependent	Thomas and Philipson (2015); Athanasiadou and Paschou (2025)
Core treatment	Lifelong insulin therapy	Lifestyle modification, oral pharmacotherapy ± insulin	Diet modification ± insulin if needed	Etiology-specific (e.g., sulfonylureas for MODY, surgery for endocrine causes)	Brennan et al. (2008); Ahamd (2022); Seshiah et al. (2014)

exposures. Data from the Global Burden of Disease Study 2021 indicate a dramatic rise in T2DM prevalence from approximately 135 million individuals in 1990 to over 530 million in 2021, with projections exceeding 700 million by 2050 (GBD, 2021; Huang et al., 2025). This increase spans all sociodemographic index strata, with age-standardized incidence rising globally, underscoring that T2DM is no longer confined to specific regions or income groups (He et al., 2024).

T2DM has evolved from a regionally concentrated metabolic disorder into a global pandemic, disproportionately affecting populations with limited access to preventive care and early diagnosis. Ethnic disparities are pronounced, with South Asians, Pacific Islanders, Indigenous populations, and certain African ancestries exhibiting higher prevalence, earlier onset, and greater complication risk compared with European populations (Huang et al., 2025). These differences reflect interactions between genetic architecture, epigenetic programming, and social determinants of health rather than genetics alone. Recognition of these epidemiological inequities is essential for informing culturally responsive prevention strategies and equitable health policy development (He et al., 2024).

Over the past 5 decades, the global distribution of T2DM has shifted markedly from high-income countries to low- and middle-income countries (LMICs). While T2DM was historically more prevalent in North America and Western Europe, the fastest growth now occurs in South Asia, East Asia, the Middle East, and sub-Saharan Africa (IDF, 2024). The International Diabetes Federation estimates a global adult prevalence of 10.5% in 2024, with LMICs accounting for nearly 80% of affected individuals (Gregg et al., 2018; WHO, 2023). This transition reflects rapid urbanization, dietary change, and constrained health system capacity.

In many high-income countries, T2DM prevalence has stabilized or increased modestly, largely due to improved screening, public health interventions, and risk factor modification. Nevertheless, absolute case numbers remain high because of population aging and increased survival (Gregg et al., 2018). In contrast, developing economies are experiencing steep increases in both prevalence and incidence, driven by urban migration, reduced physical activity, and nutrition transitions toward energy-dense diets. Limited access to preventive services and delayed diagnosis further amplify complication rates in these regions, intensifying the health and economic consequences of T2DM (IDF, 2024) (Table 1.3).

Traditionally regarded as a disease of middle and older age, T2DM is increasingly diagnosed in adolescents and young adults. Rising childhood obesity, physical inactivity, and early-life metabolic programming have contributed to a substantial rise in youth-onset T2DM over the past 2 decades (Gregg et al., 2018; Mayer-Davis et al., 2017). Early onset is associated with more aggressive disease progression and earlier onset of complications, substantially increasing lifetime morbidity and healthcare burden. These trends necessitate age-stratified surveillance and early preventive interventions for high-risk youth populations.

Table 1.3 Comparative prevalence of T2DM in developed and developing regions worldwide (Adults aged 20–79 years, 2024 estimates) (IDF Diabetes Atlas, 2025).

Region/Country group	Income category	Prevalence of T2DM (%)
North America & Caribbean	High-income (Developed)	13.6
Western Europe	High-income (Developed)	9.0
Japan	High-income (Developed)	8.3
South Asia (India, Pakistan, Bangladesh)	LMIC	11.4–13.1
East Asia (China, Indonesia)	LMIC/UMIC	11.0–12.4
Middle East & North Africa (Saudi Arabia, Egypt)	UMIC/LMIC	16.7–18.3
Sub-Saharan Africa	LMIC	4.5–6.0
Latin America	UMIC/LMIC	9.5–11.0

Sex-specific patterns in T2DM prevalence reflect biological, behavioral, and sociocultural influences. Men typically exhibit higher prevalence at younger ages, possibly due to greater visceral adiposity and hepatic insulin resistance. In contrast, women experience rising risk after menopause, associated with hormonal changes, weight gain, and reduced estrogen-mediated metabolic protection (Kautzky-Willer et al., 2016). Sociocultural factors, including disparities in healthcare access and physical activity, further shape these differences. Recognition of sex-specific risk profiles is essential for refining screening thresholds and tailoring prevention strategies across the life course (Table 1.4).

The incidence of T2DM is influenced by a combination of non-modifiable and modifiable risk factors. Age, ethnicity, family history, and genetic predisposition constitute key non-modifiable determinants. Genome-wide association studies have identified over 400 loci associated with glycemic traits, insulin secretion, and insulin sensitivity, confirming the strongly polygenic nature of T2DM (Mahajan et al., 2018). These variants individually confer modest risk but collectively shape susceptibility, particularly when interacting with adverse environmental exposures. Genetic insights have improved the understanding of disease heterogeneity but do not fully explain the rapid global rise in incidence.

Modifiable risk factors exert the greatest influence on T2DM incidence. Central obesity remains the strongest predictor, with individuals having a body mass index $\geq$30 kg/m^2 exhibiting more than a fivefold increased risk. Sedentary behavior, diets rich in refined carbohydrates and saturated fats, smoking, and psychosocial stress further exacerbate metabolic risk. Landmark prevention trials demonstrated that lifestyle interventions combining weight loss and physical activity can reduce T2DM incidence by up to 58% in high-risk individuals (Hu et al., 2011). These findings underscore prevention as a cornerstone of global diabetes control (Table 1.5).

Urbanization is a major driver of the contemporary T2DM epidemic. Rural-to-urban migration is consistently associated with reduced physical activity, increased

Table 1.4 Age- and sex-specific prevalence patterns of T2DM across selected global regions (Adults 20–79 years, 2024 estimates).

Region/Country	Age group (yrs)	Male prevalence (%)	Female prevalence (%)	References
United States	20–39	3.2	2.8	Mayer-Davis et al. (2017); IDF Atlas (2024)
	40–59	12.5	11.0	Gregg et al., 2018; IDF Atlas (2024)
	60–79	21.0	19.5	IDF Atlas (2024)
India	20–39	4.0	3.5	IDF Atlas (2024)
	40–59	11.8	10.2	IDF Atlas (2024)
	60–79	18.5	17.0	IDF Atlas (2024)
China	20–39	3.5	3.0	IDF Atlas (2024)
	40–59	12.0	10.5	IDF Atlas (2024)
	60–79	20.0	18.0	IDF Atlas (2024)
Europe (overall)	20–39	2.5	2.0	Kautzky-Willer et al. (2016); IDF Atlas (2024)
	40–59	9.5	8.5	IDF Atlas (2024)
	60–79	16.0	15.0	IDF Atlas (2024)
Middle East (Saudi Arabia, Egypt)	20–39	6.0	5.5	IDF Atlas (2024)
	40–59	17.5	16.0	IDF Atlas (2024)
	60–79	25.0	23.0	IDF Atlas (2024)

consumption of ultra-processed foods, and heightened psychosocial stress, accelerating insulin resistance in genetically susceptible individuals (Popkin, 2015). The nutrition transition accompanying economic development-characterized by high intake of refined carbohydrates, saturated fats, and sugar-sweetened beverages-has become a defining feature of diabetes epidemiology in rapidly developing regions. These shifts disproportionately affect LMICs, where public health responses often lag behind environmental change.

In many LMICs, urbanization intersects with early-life under nutrition, creating a "double burden" of malnutrition. Barker's developmental origins hypothesis posits that fetal and early childhood nutritional deprivation programs metabolic pathways toward energy conservation, increasing vulnerability to insulin resistance when exposed to caloric excess later in life (Barker et al., 2009). This dual exposure-early under nutrition followed by adult overnutrition-amplifies T2DM risk and represents a distinctive epidemiological challenge in transitioning economies, where economic growth coexists with persistent social inequities.

T2DM imposes a substantial and escalating economic burden globally. Direct medical costs include expenditures for outpatient care, hospitalizations, pharmacotherapy, glucose monitoring, and management of chronic complications such as cardiovascular disease and nephropathy. Indirect costs arising from lost productivity, disability, and premature mortality further magnify this burden. Global diabetes-related health

Table 1.5 Relative contribution of modifiable and non-modifiable risk factors to T2DM incidence (selected global studies).

Risk factor	Category	Relative risk	References
Age ≥60 years	Non-modifiable	2.5–3.0	IDF Atlas (2024); Gregg et al., 2018
Family history of diabetes	Non-modifiable	2.0–2.3	Mahajan et al. (2018)
South Asian ethnicity	Non-modifiable	1.8–2.2	Kautzky-Willer et al. (2016)
Obesity (BMI ≥30 kg/m^2)	Modifiable	5.0–6.0	Hu et al., 2011; IDF Atlas (2024)
Central adiposity (waist >102 cm men, >88 cm women)	Modifiable	4.5–5.5	Hu et al. (2011)
Sedentary lifestyle (<150 min/week activity)	Modifiable	2.0–2.5	Hu et al. (2011)
Unhealthy diet (high refined carbs, saturated fats)	Modifiable	1.8–2.2	Hu et al. (2011)
Tobacco use	Modifiable	1.3–1.5	WHO (2023)
Psychosocial stress	Modifiable	1.4–1.6	Gregg et al. (2018)

expenditure was estimated at approximately USD 850 billion annually, with continued growth projected alongside rising prevalence (Bommer et al., 2017). These costs disproportionately strain health systems in resource-limited settings (Table 1.6).

In low-resource settings, the financial burden of T2DM is frequently borne directly by patients and households. High out-of-pocket costs for medications, insulin, and glucose monitoring limit treatment adherence and contribute to poor glycemic control and higher complication rates. These economic barriers exacerbate health inequities, reinforcing cycles of poverty and disease. Disparities in access to essential diabetes care underscore the need for health financing reforms and universal coverage models that prioritize chronic disease management in LMICs.

Beyond economic consequences, T2DM profoundly affects quality of life and psychosocial well-being. Chronic disease management, dietary restrictions, and fear of complications contribute to emotional distress, while depression and anxiety are highly prevalent among individuals with T2DM. Diabetes-related distress is strongly associated with poor treatment adherence and suboptimal glycemic control, creating a bidirectional relationship between mental health and metabolic outcomes (Fisher et al., 2019). Addressing psychosocial dimensions is therefore integral to comprehensive diabetes care.

At the societal level, the rising prevalence of T2DM places sustained pressure on healthcare systems, social welfare structures, and workforce productivity. In many developing countries, T2DM disproportionately affects individuals in their most economically productive years, compounding national economic losses. The combined impact of healthcare expenditure, reduced labor participation, and long-term disability highlights T2DM as both a medical and socioeconomic challenge. Integrated policies addressing prevention, access to care, and social support are essential to mitigate its long-term societal impact.

Table 1.6 Estimated healthcare and societal costs attributable to T2DM globally (Adults 20–79 years, 2024 estimates).

Region/Country group	Direct costs (USD billions)	Indirect costs (USD billions)	Key drivers	References
North America & Caribbean	300–320	150–170	Hospitalization, pharmacotherapy, aging population	Bommer et al. (2017); IDF Atlas (2024)
Western Europe	150–160	80–90	Outpatient care, glucose monitoring, workforce loss	IDF Atlas (2024)
China	110–120	70–80	Urbanization, obesity, complication management	IDF Atlas (2024)
India	35–40	25–30	Out-of-pocket costs, limited preventive care	IDF Atlas (2024)
Middle East & North Africa	50–55	30–35	High prevalence, costly complication management	IDF Atlas (2024)
Latin America	40–45	25–30	Hospitalization, productivity loss	Bommer et al. (2017)
Sub-Saharan Africa	15–20	10–12	Out-of-pocket burden, limited access to insulin	WHO (2023)

3. Pathophysiology of type 2 diabetes mellitus

T2DM is a multifactorial metabolic disorder charaterized by progressive loss of glucose homeostasis due to insulin resistance and pancreatic β-cell dysfunction. Rather than a single lesion, T2DM represents a continuum of interrelated metabolic, cellular, and immunological disturbances shaped by genetic susceptibility, environmental exposures, and lifestyle factors. Central pathogenic processes include impaired insulin signaling, defective β-cell compensation, dysregulated lipid metabolism, and chronic low-grade inflammation, which together drive sustained hyperglycemia and downstream complications (DeFronzo et al., 2015; Prasad & Groop, 2015). This integrative framework underscores T2DM as a dynamic, systems-level disease rather than an isolated endocrine disorder (Fig. 1.1).

In healthy individuals, pancreatic β-cells maintain glucose homeostasis by coupling circulating glucose concentrations to insulin secretion. Glucose enters β-cells primarily through glucose transporter-2 (GLUT2), where its metabolism elevates intracellular ATP levels. The resulting ATP/ADP shift closes ATP-sensitive potassium (KATP) channels, leading to membrane depolarization, calcium influx, and insulin granule exocytosis (Ashcroft & Rorsman, 2012). Insulin secretion occurs in a biphasic pattern, with a rapid first phase followed by a sustained second phase, ensuring efficient postprandial glucose clearance and hepatic glucose suppression.

Following secretion, insulin binds to its transmembrane tyrosine kinase receptor on skeletal muscle, hepatic, and adipose tissues. Receptor activation initiates autophosphorylation and recruitment of insulin receptor substrates (IRS), triggering downstream

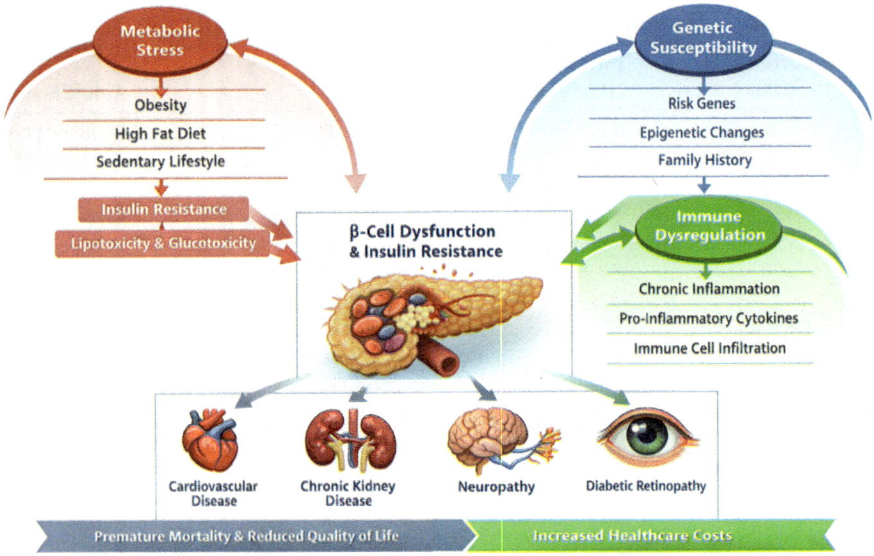

FIGURE 1.1 Conceptual model illustrating the interaction between metabolic dysfunction, genetic susceptibility, and immune pathways in T2DM.

Table 1.7 Major components of the insulin signaling pathway and their metabolic roles.

Component	Function in glucose homeostasis	References
Insulin receptor (IR)	Binds insulin, initiates autophosphorylation	Saltiel and Kahn (2001)
Insulin receptor substrates (IRS-1, IRS-2)	Docking proteins, activate PI3K	Saltiel and Kahn (2001)
PI3K (phosphatidylinositol 3-kinase)	Generates PIP3, activates Akt	Saltiel and Kahn (2001)
Akt (protein kinase B)	Stimulates GLUT4 translocation, glycogen synthesis	DeFronzo et al. (2015)
GLUT4 (skeletal muscle, adipose tissue)	Facilitates glucose uptake into cells	Ashcroft and Rorsman (2012)
GSK-3 (glycogen synthase kinase-3)	Regulates glycogen synthesis	Prasad and Groop (2015)
mTOR (mammalian target of rapamycin)	Controls protein synthesis and lipid metabolism	Saltiel and Kahn (2001)

signaling through the phosphatidylinositol-3-kinase (PI3K)-Akt pathway (Saltiel & Kahn, 2001). This cascade regulates glucose transport, glycogen synthesis, lipid metabolism, and protein synthesis, thereby coordinating systemic energy homeostasis. Disruption at any node of this pathway compromises insulin action and predisposes tissues to metabolic dysfunction, highlighting its central role in maintaining normoglycemia (Table 1.7).

Peripheral glucose uptake is mediated predominantly by GLUT4, an insulin-responsive transporter expressed in skeletal muscle and adipose tissue. Insulin signaling promotes GLUT4 translocation from intracellular vesicles to the plasma membrane, facilitating glucose entry into cells. In the liver, insulin suppresses gluconeogenesis while stimulating glycogen synthesis and lipogenesis, thereby limiting endogenous glucose production. These coordinated actions enable effective postprandial glucose disposal and prevent excessive glycemic excursions, maintaining metabolic equilibrium under physiological conditions.

Insulin resistance, a defining feature of T2DM, reflects a diminished biological response to normal or elevated insulin concentrations. In skeletal muscle, impaired GLUT4 translocation reduces postprandial glucose uptake. In adipose tissue, insulin resistance enhances lipolysis, increasing circulating free fatty acids that interfere with insulin signaling through lipotoxic mechanisms (Samuel & Shulman, 2016). Hepatic insulin resistance further disrupts glucose homeostasis by failing to suppress gluconeogenesis, resulting in excessive endogenous glucose production. Together, these tissue-specific defects substantially contribute to fasting and postprandial hyperglycemia.

Although insulin resistance often precedes T2DM, clinical disease emerges when pancreatic β-cells fail to meet increased insulin demand. Chronic hyperglycemia, elevated free fatty acids, oxidative stress, and endoplasmic reticulum stress progressively impair β-cell function and survival, a phenomenon termed glucolipotoxicity (Prentki & Nolan, 2006). Over time, β-cell mass declines through apoptosis and reduced regenerative capacity, leading to inadequate insulin secretion relative to metabolic needs. This progressive β-cell failure is central to disease progression and therapeutic failure in advanced T2DM.

In physiological states, insulin tightly regulates hepatic glucose production. In T2DM, hepatic insulin resistance disrupts this control, resulting in persistent gluconeogenesis and glycogenolysis even in the fed state. Elevated hepatic glucose output is a major driver of fasting hyperglycemia and contributes substantially to overall glycemic burden. This defect represents a critical therapeutic target, as suppressing hepatic glucose production can significantly improve fasting glucose levels and overall metabolic control in individuals with T2DM.

Adipose tissue functions as an active endocrine organ that secretes adipokines regulating metabolism and inflammation. Visceral adiposity is particularly pathogenic, releasing pro-inflammatory mediators such as tumor necrosis factor-α, interleukin-6, and resistin, while suppressing insulin-sensitizing adiponectin (Kershaw & Flier, 2004). This adipokine imbalance promotes systemic inflammation, disrupts insulin signaling, and exacerbates metabolic dysfunction. The close association between visceral fat accumulation and insulin resistance underscores the central role of adipose tissue biology in T2DM pathogenesis (Table 1.8).

T2DM commonly coexists with metabolic syndrome, a constellation of central obesity, hypertension, dyslipidemia, and impaired glucose regulation. Abdominal obesity is as a primary driver of insulin resistance and chronic inflammation, linking

Table 1.8 Major adipokines involved in insulin resistance and metabolic regulation.

Adipokine	Effect on metabolism	Role in T2DM pathogenesis	References
TNF-α	Promotes inflammation, inhibits insulin signaling	Elevated in obesity, impairs GLUT4 translocation	Kershaw and Flier (2004); Hotamisligil (2017)
IL-6	Stimulates hepatic gluconeogenesis, systemic inflammation	Elevated in visceral adiposity, predicts insulin resistance	Hotamisligil (2017)
Resistin	Increases hepatic glucose output	Associated with obesity-induced insulin resistance	Kershaw and Flier (2004)
Adiponectin	Enhances insulin sensitivity, anti-inflammatory	Reduced in obesity, protective against T2DM	Grundy (2016)
Leptin	Regulates appetite and energy balance	Leptin resistance contributes to obesity and metabolic syndrome	Kershaw and Flier (2004)

metabolic syndrome to the development of T2DM (Grundy, 2016). The interaction between obesity-related metabolic stress and inherited susceptibility accelerates disease progression and markedly increases cardiovascular risk. This clustering of risk factors explains the high burden of macrovascular complications observed in individuals with T2DM.

Chronic low-grade inflammation is a hallmark of T2DM pathophysiology. Expansion of adipose tissue promotes immune cell infiltration, particularly pro-inflammatory macrophages, which secrete cytokines that interfere with insulin signaling pathways (Hotamisligil, 2017). Circulating inflammatory markers, including C-reactive protein, interleukin-6, and tumor necrosis factor-α, are consistently elevated in individuals with T2DM and correlate with disease severity and risk of complications. These findings position inflammation as a mechanistic bridge between obesity and metabolic dysfunction.

Inflammatory processes in T2DM are increasingly recognized as genetically modulated. Variants in genes regulating innate immunity, cytokine signaling, and immune cell activation influence susceptibility to insulin resistance and β-cell dysfunction (Donath et al., 2019). This immunogenic framework highlights how genetic predisposition shapes inflammatory responses to metabolic stress, contributing to disease heterogeneity. Understanding these interactions provides a conceptual foundation for subsequent chapters exploring immune-metabolic pathways and personalized therapeutic strategies in T2DM.

4. Clinical features and diagnosis

T2DM is a clinically heterogeneous metabolic disorder, with manifestations ranging from asymptomatic hyperglycemia to overt metabolic decompensation. The disease develops insidiously through progressive insulin resistance and gradual pancreatic β-cell dysfunction, frequently delaying diagnosis for several years. During this prolonged subclinical phase, persistent hyperglycemia silently drives metabolic and vascular injury. Consequently, accurate recognition of clinical features and consistent application of standardized diagnostic criteria are essential for early intervention and prevention of long-term complications, including cardiovascular disease and microvascular damage (DeFronzo et al., 2015).

The classical triad of polyuria, polydipsia, and polyphagia reflects the physiological consequences of sustained hyperglycemia. When plasma glucose exceeds the renal threshold, glucosuria induces osmotic diuresis, leading to increased urinary volume and dehydration. The resulting fluid loss activates thirst centers, causing polydipsia, while impaired cellular glucose uptake creates an energy-deficient state that stimulates excessive hunger despite adequate caloric intake (Powers et al., 2022). These symptoms often indicate advanced metabolic dysregulation rather than early disease.

Despite its metabolic severity, T2DM frequently remains clinically silent in its early stages. Many individuals are diagnosed incidentally during routine health assessments or cardiovascular risk screening. Epidemiological data show that a significant proportion of patients already exhibit microvascular complications-retinopathy, nephropathy, or neuropathy-or macrovascular disease such as coronary artery disease or stroke at diagnosis, reflecting prolonged unrecognized hyperglycemia (Herman et al., 2015). This asymptomatic progression highlights the critical importance of targeted population-based screening among high-risk groups.

Diagnosis of T2DM is based on biochemical evidence of persistent hyperglycemia using internationally standardized thresholds (Table 1.9). Fasting plasma glucose levels ≥126 mg/dL (≥7.0 mmol/L) on two occasions confirm diabetes, while values between 100–125 mg/dL indicate impaired fasting glucose and increased future risk (ADA, 2024). A 2-hour plasma glucose ≥200 mg/dL following a 75-g oral glucose load reflects impaired postprandial regulation. Glycated hemoglobin ≥6.5% captures long-term glycemic exposure when standardized assays are used (WHO, 2011).

Accurate differential diagnosis is essential for optimal management (Table 1.10). Type 1 diabetes mellitus typically presents with abrupt onset, ketosis, and autoimmune β-cell

Table 1.9 Diagnostic criteria for diabetes mellitus and prediabetes according to international guidelines.

Test	Normal	Prediabetes	Diabetes	References
Fasting plasma glucose (FPG)	<100 mg/dL (<5.6 mmol/L)	100–125 mg/dL (5.6–6.9 mmol/L)	≥126 mg/dL (≥7.0 mmol/L)	ADA (2024)
2-h OGTT (75 g glucose)	<140 mg/dL (<7.8 mmol/L)	140–199 mg/dL (7.8–11.0 mmol/L)	≥200 mg/dL (≥11.1 mmol/L)	ADA (2024)
HbA1c	<5.7% (<39 mmol/mol)	5.7%–6.4% (39–47 mmol/mol)	≥6.5% (≥48 mmol/mol)	WHO (2011)

Table 1.10 Clinical and pathophysiological differences between Type 1 diabetes, Type 2 diabetes, and gestational diabetes.

Feature	Type 1 diabetes	Type 2 diabetes	Gestational diabetes	References
Onset	Acute, often childhood/adolescence	Gradual, adulthood	Pregnancy (2nd-3rd trimester)	Atkinson et al. (2014); ADA (2024)
Pathophysiology	Autoimmune β-cell destruction	Insulin resistance + β-cell dysfunction	Pregnancy-induced insulin resistance	Hattersley and Patel (2017)
Autoantibodies	Present (GAD, ICA, IA-2)	Absent	Absent	Atkinson et al. (2014)
Insulin requirement	Immediate, lifelong	Variable, progressive	Usually resolves postpartum	ADA (2024)
Risk factors	Genetic, autoimmune	Obesity, metabolic syndrome, family history	Pregnancy, obesity, family history	WHO (2011)

destruction, whereas T2DM shows gradual onset, insulin resistance, and relative insulin deficiency, commonly associated with obesity (Atkinson et al., 2014). Gestational diabetes mellitus develops during pregnancy and markedly the risk of future T2DM. Secondary hyperglycemia due to endocrine disorders, pancreatic disease, medications, or monogenic diabetes such as MODY should be considered in atypical presentations (Hattersley & Patel, 2017).

5. Molecular and genetic basis of type 2 diabetes mellitus

T2DM is a polygenic and multifactorial disorder in which inherited susceptibility converges with environmental exposures and lifestyle factors to shape disease onset and progression. Advances in genomics and immunology have reframed T2DM as more than a disorder of glucose metabolism, revealing intricate regulatory networks involving insulin signaling, pancreatic β-cell biology, inflammation, and immune modulation. Rather than acting in isolation, these pathways interact dynamically across tissues, producing marked interindividual variability in clinical presentation and progression. Understanding this genetic and immunological architecture is therefore essential for elucidating disease mechanisms and informing precision-based therapeutic strategies.

Strong familial aggregation of T2DM provides compelling evidence for a genetic contribution to disease susceptibility. Twin and family studies estimate heritability between 30%–70%, varying by population and study design (Lyssenko et al., 2005). Individuals with an affected first-degree relative have a substantially elevated lifetime risk, and concordance is consistently higher among monozygotic than dizygotic twins. Nonetheless, incomplete concordance in genetically identical twins highlights the critical role of environmental modifiers, indicating that genetic predisposition confers vulnerability rather than deterministic disease expression.

Genome-wide association studies have identified more than 400 loci associated with T2DM risk, most of which influence insulin secretion, β-cell development, and glucose homeostasis (Mahajan et al., 2018). Prominent susceptibility genes include *TCF7L2, PPARG, KCNJ11, SLC30A8,* and *FTO,* each with modest individual effects but substantial cumulative risk (Table 1.11). Many loci are expressed in pancreatic islets, liver, adipose tissue, and immune cells, underscoring the systemic nature of T2DM. These findings reinforce the concept that polygenic burden, rather than single-gene defects, underpins disease susceptibility.

Gene-environment interactions are central to translating genetic risk into clinical disease. Epigenetic mechanisms, including DNA methylation, histone modification, and non-coding RNA regulation-mediate environmentally responsive gene expression without altering the DNA sequence (Ling & Rönn, 2019). Nutritional status, physical activity, and metabolic stress shape these epigenetic marks, particularly during critical developmental windows. Early-life exposures, such as intrauterine undernutrition can induce persistent epigenetic changes that impair insulin sensitivity and β-cell function in adulthood, thereby contributing to long-term disease risk and phenotypic heterogeneity.

Lifestyle factors substantially modify the impact of inherited genetic risk. Large prospective cohort studies demonstrate that adherence to healthy dietary patterns, regular physical activity, and maintenance of normal body weight markedly attenuate T2DM risk, even among individuals with high polygenic risk scores (Hu et al., 2017). In contrast, obesogenic environments, sedentary behavior, and chronic psychosocial stress amplify genetic susceptibility, accelerating metabolic dysfunction. These observations highlight the plasticity of genetic risk and reinforce the public health value of lifestyle interventions across genetically diverse populations.

Although not classically autoimmune, T2DM is increasingly recognized as a disorder with significant immune involvement. Genetic variants affecting innate and adaptive immune pathways influence susceptibility to chronic low-grade inflammation, insulin resistance, and β-cell stress (Donath et al., 2019). Polymorphisms in genes encoding

Table 1.11 Key genetic variants associated with T2DM susceptibility and their functional implications.

Gene/Locus	Biological role	Functional implication	References
TCF7L2	Transcription factor in Wnt signaling	Strongest GWAS signal; regulates β-cell function and insulin secretion	Mahajan et al. (2018)
PPARG	Nuclear receptor regulating adipogenesis	Influences insulin sensitivity and lipid metabolism	Lyssenko et al. (2005)
KCNJ11	Potassium channel subunit in β-cells	Alters insulin secretion dynamics	Mahajan et al. (2018)
SLC30A8	Zinc transporter in β-cells	Modulates insulin granule formation	Mahajan et al. (2018)
FTO	Regulator of energy balance	Associated with obesity-related T2DM risk	Hu et al. (2017)

cytokines and immune regulators-including *IL6, TNFA, TLR4,* and HLA-associated loci-are linked to altered inflammatory tone and metabolic outcomes. These findings position immune dysregulation as a core contributor to disease pathogenesis rather than a secondary consequence.

Immune-metabolic crosstalk provides a unifying framework for T2DM pathophysiology. Metabolic tissues including adipose depots and pancreatic islets are infiltrated by immune cells that respond to nutrient excess and cellular stress. Activated macrophages and T cells release cytokines that disrupt insulin signaling and impair β-cell survival, while metabolic perturbations reciprocally alter immune cell function (Hotamisligil, 2017). This bidirectional interaction links genetic variation in immune regulation to metabolic dysfunction, forming the conceptual foundation for immunogenetic and precision-medicine approaches in diabetes care.

6. Metabolic and cellular mechanisms

The metabolic and cellular abnormalities underlying T2DM stem from chronic nutrient excess, which progressively disrupts insulin signaling, cellular energy balance, and organelle integrity. Sustained metabolic stress activates maladaptive intracellular pathways, linking over nutrition to insulin resistance, β-cell dysfunction, and systemic glucose dysregulation. These processes integrate defects in insulin signal transduction, lipid and glucose toxicity, oxidative stress, and inflammatory activation, establishing a self-reinforcing cycle of metabolic failure across multiple tissues (DeFronzo et al., 2015).

Insulin signaling disruption in T2DM primarily involves defects in the IRS-PI3K-AKT pathway. Under physiological conditions, insulin receptor activation phosphorylates IRS-1 and IRS-2, initiating downstream signaling. In T2DM, inflammatory cytokines, lipid intermediates, and stress-activated kinases promote serine phosphorylation of IRS proteins, reducing their signaling capacity (Saltiel & Kahn, 2001). Attenuated PI3K and AKT activation impairs glucose transport, glycogen synthesis, and lipid metabolism, while failure of AKT-mediated suppression of hepatic gluconeogenesis contributes to fasting hyperglycemia (Samuel & Shulman, 2016).

Defective glucose transporter dynamics further exacerbate insulin resistance. In healthy tissues, insulin stimulates the translocation of GLUT4 from intracellular vesicles to the plasma membrane, enabling efficient glucose uptake in skeletal muscle and adipose tissue. In T2DM, impaired upstream signaling disrupts this process, markedly reducing peripheral glucose disposal (Huang & Czech, 2007). Altered expression and function of GLUT2 in hepatocytes and pancreatic β-cells further impair glucose sensing and hepatic glucose regulation, amplifying postprandial and fasting hyperglycemia.

Lipotoxicity and glucotoxicity are central mechanisms linking nutrient excess to cellular dysfunction. Chronic elevation of free fatty acids promotes the accumulation of toxic lipid intermediates, including diacylglycerols and ceramides, which activate protein kinase C isoforms and inhibit insulin signaling cascades (Samuel & Shulman, 2016).

Concurrent hyperglycemia accelerates advanced glycation end-product formation and activates the polyol and hexosamine pathways, collectively disrupting redox balance and cellular integrity (Brownlee, 2005).

Pancreatic β-cells are uniquely vulnerable to nutrient-induced stress owning to limited antioxidant defenses. Prolonged exposure to elevated glucose and lipids induces endoplasmic reticulum stress, mitochondrial dysfunction, and activation of intrinsic apoptotic pathways. Although β-cells initially compensate by increased insulin synthesis, sustained metabolic pressure ultimately leads to secretory failure and cell loss, marking a critical transition from insulin resistance to overt diabetes (Prentki & Nolan, 2006).

Oxidative stress and mitochondrial dysfunction are key mediators of cellular injury in T2DM. Excess nutrient oxidation increases mitochondrial generation of reactive oxygen species, including superoxide and hydrogen peroxide, which interfere with insulin signaling and activate inflammatory pathways (Brownlee, 2005). β -cells are particularly susceptible due to low expression of antioxidant enzyme. Mitochondrial damage-characterized by impaired oxidative phosphorylation, reduced ATP production, and altered dynamics-further compromises cellular survival and metabolic flexibility (Lowell & Shulman, 2005).

7. Complications of type 2 diabetes mellitus

T2DM is accompanied by a broad spectrum of chronic complications that drive morbidity, premature mortality, and diminished quality of life. These complications develop through prolonged exposure to hyperglycemia, insulin resistance, dyslipidemia, and persistent low-grade inflammation, which collectively damage vascular, neural, and parenchymal tissues. On a clinical basis, complications are categorized into microvascular, macrovascular, and emerging non-classical manifestations, reflecting the systemic reach of metabolic dysregulation in T2DM (Forbes & Cooper, 2013).

Microvascular complications arise from injury to small blood vessels and correlate strongly with glycemic burden and disease duration. Chronic hyperglycemia induces endothelial dysfunction, basement membrane thickening, oxidative stress, and capillary occlusion, ultimately impairing tissue perfusion. These processes underlie diabetic retinopathy, nephropathy, and neuropathy, which collectively represent leading causes of blindness, renal failure, and disability among individuals with long-standing T2DM (Forbes & Cooper, 2013).

Diabetic retinopathy is the most common microvascular complication and a leading cause of preventable blindness in working-age adults worldwide. Sustained hyperglycemia damages retinal capillaries through endothelial dysfunction, pericyte loss, and microaneurysm formation (Cheung et al., 2010). Clinically, disease progression spans non-proliferative stages, marked by hemorrhages and exudates, to proliferative retinopathy characterized by pathological neovascularization and heightened risk of vitreous hemorrhage and retinal detachment.

Table 1.12 Stages of diabetic nephropathy and clinical characteristics.

Stage	Clinical features	Key pathophysiology	References
Early (microalbuminuria)	Albumin excretion 30–300 mg/day	Glomerular hyperfiltration, mesangial expansion	Tuttle et al. (2014)
Intermediate	Persistent proteinuria, declining GFR	Oxidative stress, fibrosis	Tuttle et al. (2014)
Advanced	ESRD, dialysis requirement	Progressive glomerulosclerosis	Tuttle et al. (2014)

Diabetic nephropathy is a principal cause of chronic kidney disease and end-stage renal failure worldwide. It presents clinically as persistent albuminuria, a declining glomerular filtration rate, and progressive renal fibrosis. Underlying mechanisms include glomerular hyperfiltration, mesangial expansion, oxidative stress, and activation of pro-fibrotic pathways (Tuttle et al., 2014). Early identification through microalbuminuria screening enables timely intervention and slows disease progression (Table 1.12).

Diabetic neuropathy comprises a heterogeneous group of disorders affecting sensory, motor, and autonomic nerves. Distal symmetric polyneuropathy is the most prevalent form, presenting with pain, paresthesia, numbness, and loss of protective sensation, particularly in the lower limbs (Callaghan et al., 2012). Autonomic involvement may disrupt cardiovascular, gastrointestinal, and genitourinary function, substantially increasing morbidity and mortality. Hyperglycemia-induced oxidative stress, ischemia, and inflammation are central pathogenic drivers.

Macrovascular complications reflect accelerated atherosclerosis in large and medium-sized arteries and are the leading cause of death in T2DM. Insulin resistance, dyslipidemia, endothelial dysfunction, and chronic inflammation synergistically promote plaque formation and instability, predisposing individuals to coronary artery disease, peripheral vascular disease, and stroke.

Coronary artery disease (CAD) is markedly overrepresented in T2DM, with a two-to fourfold higher risk of myocardial infarction than in non-diabetic populations (Haffner et al., 1998). Diabetes is often regarded as a coronary risk equivalent, emphasizing the need for aggressive cardiovascular risk reduction through glycemic control, lipid management, and blood pressure control.

Peripheral vascular disease (PVD) in T2DM results from progressive atherosclerotic occlusion of the lowerlimb arteries. Clinically, it presents with intermittent claudication, ischemic ulcers, impaired wound healing, and an increased risk of limb amputation. Coexisting neuropathy often masks symptoms, delaying diagnosis and worsening outcomes.

T2DM significantly increases the risk of both ischemic and hemorrhagic stroke. Hyperglycemia-driven endothelial dysfunction, hypertension, and pro-thrombotic states contribute to cerebrovascular injury and poorer neurological recovery (Emerging Risk Factors Collaboration, 2010). Stroke-related disability further amplifies healthcare burden and reduces long-term survival.

Table 1.13 Spectrum of microvascular, macrovascular, and emerging complications in T2DM.

Category	Complication	Mechanism	References
Microvascular	Retinopathy	Endothelial dysfunction, neovascularization	Cheung et al. (2010)
Microvascular	Nephropathy	Albuminuria, fibrosis, oxidative stress	Tuttle et al. (2014)
Microvascular	Neuropathy	Oxidative stress, ischemia, inflammation	Callaghan et al. (2012)
Macrovascular	CAD	Atherosclerosis, plaque instability	Haffner et al. (1998)
Macrovascular	PVD	Arterial occlusion, impaired healing	Emerging Risk Factors Collaboration (2010)
Macrovascular	Stroke	Endothelial dysfunction, pro-thrombotic state	Emerging Risk Factors Collaboration (2010)
Emerging	Cognitive impairment	Insulin resistance in brain, inflammation	Biessels and Despa (2018)
Emerging	NAFLD	Hepatic lipid accumulation, fibrosis	Younossi et al. (2019)

Beyond classical vascular disease, T2DM is increasingly associated with emerging complications that reflect its multisystem impact. Cognitive impairment is more prevalent among individuals with T2DM and includes mild cognitive decline, dementia, and Alzheimer's disease. Proposed mechanisms include cerebrovascular injury, brain insulin resistance, oxidative stress, and chronic inflammation (Biessels & Despa, 2018).

Non-alcoholic fatty liver disease (NAFLD) is highly prevalent in T2DM and is the hepatic manifestation of metabolic syndrome. Insulin resistance drives hepatic lipid accumulation, inflammation, and fibrosis, increasing the risk of non-alcoholic steatohepatitis, cirrhosis, and hepatocellular carcinoma (Younossi et al., 2019). NAFLD further exacerbates systemic insulin resistance, thereby reinforcing metabolic dysfunction (Table 1.13).

8. Summary and future directions

T2DM is a complex systemic disorder shaped by progressive metabolic dysfunction, genetic susceptibility, and immune-mediated mechanisms. Beyond chronic hyperglycemia, T2DM reflects dynamic interactions among defects in insulin signaling, adipose tissue biology, inflammatory pathways, and organ-specific damage. Insulin resistance and β-cell dysfunction evolve in parallel, reinforced by metabolic stress and immune activation, resulting in sustained dysglycemia and multisystem involvement. Integrating classical metabolic models with emerging immunogenetic insights provides a unifying framework for understanding disease heterogeneity, progression, and therapeutic failure (DeFronzo et al., 2015; Donath et al., 2019).

T2DM arises from the convergence of impaired insulin signaling, progressive β-cell failure, and chronic metabolic stress. Disruption of glucose transporter activity, glucotoxicity, lipotoxicity, and oxidative stress undermines glucose homeostasis and perpetuates hyperglycemia (Brownlee, 2005; Saltiel & Kahn, 2001). Visceral adiposity plays a central pathogenic role by promoting insulin resistance and inflammatory signaling through dysregulated adipokine secretion (Kershaw & Flier, 2004). Genetic susceptibility and epigenetic modification further shape individual variability in disease onset, progression, and complication risk (Ling & Rönn, 2019; Mahajan et al., 2018).

A defining feature of T2DM pathophysiology is chronic low-grade inflammation and immune-metabolic crosstalk. Metabolic tissues, including adipose tissue, liver, and pancreas function as immunologically active sites, where immune cell infiltration and cytokine release impair insulin action and β-cell integrity. Genetic variants influencing immune regulation and inflammatory signaling contribute to disease susceptibility and clinical heterogeneity, reinforcing the immunogenetic basis of T2DM (Donath et al., 2019; Hotamisligil, 2017). These interactions provide a conceptual foundation for understanding systemic complications and therapeutic resistance.

Despite substantial advances, critical gaps persist in T2DM research. The molecular triggers that initiate immune activation in metabolically stressed tissues are incompletely defined, and the temporal relationship among insulin resistance, inflammation, and β-cell failure remains unresolved (Prentki & Nolan, 2006). Population-specific genetic risk factors and their interactions with environmental exposures require deeper investigation, particularly in regions undergoing rapid epidemiological transitions (Hu et al., 2018). These gaps hinder precise risk prediction and limit the effectiveness of current interventions.

Identifying robust biomarkers for early detection, disease stratification, and treatment response is a major research priority. Promising candidates include inflammatory mediators, immune cell signatures, metabolomic and lipidomic profiles, epigenetic modifications, and genetic risk scores. Integrating multi-omics datasets offers a powerful strategy to capture disease heterogeneity and enable earlier, more personalized intervention (Fitipaldi et al., 2018) (Table 1.14).

Table 1.14 Emerging molecular, genetic, and immunological biomarkers in T2DM.

Category	Biomarker	Potential application	References
Inflammatory mediators	IL-6, TNF-α, CRP	Risk prediction, monitoring inflammation	Hotamisligil (2017)
Immune cell signatures	Macrophage/T-cell subsets	Disease stratification, immune profiling	Donath et al. (2019)
Metabolomics	Branched-chain amino acids, ceramides	Early detection, metabolic risk scoring	Hu et al. (2018)
Epigenetic markers	DNA methylation profiles	Predicting progression, therapeutic response	Ling and Rönn (2019)
Genetic risk scores	Polygenic risk scores (PRS)	Precision medicine, individualized risk	Mahajan et al. (2018)
Lipidomics	Altered lipid species	Stratification of cardiovascular risk	Franks & McCarthy (2016)

Recognition of T2DM as a heterogeneous disorder has accelerated interest in precision medicine. Stratifying patients using genetic, metabolic, and immune profiles may enable tailored prevention strategies and optimized therapeutic selection, moving beyond uniform treatment algorithms (Franks & McCarthy, 2016). Advances in genomics, bioinformatics, and systems biology are expected to translate mechanistic insights into clinically actionable tools, thereby improving long-term outcomes.

Integrating immunogenetic knowledge into routine clinical care creates new translational opportunities, including immune-modulatory therapies, targeted anti-inflammatory agents, and personalized lifestyle interventions informed by genetic risk (Donath et al., 2019). A deeper understanding of immune-metabolic interactions may also enable earlier identification of high-risk individuals and proactive prevention of complications. Achieving this integration will require interdisciplinary collaboration, standardized biomarkers, and rigorous clinical validation.

This chapter has provided a comprehensive overview of T2DM, covering its metabolic, genetic, immunological, and clinical dimensions. By framing the disease within an immunogenetic context, it lays the groundwork for further exploration of immune pathways and translational strategies. Continued research at the intersection of metabolism, genetics, and immunity remains essential to advance precision medicine and reducing the global burden of T2DM.

Acknowledgment

We sincerely thank Professor Neelavar Ananthram Aravind for his valuable insights, thoughtful comments and careful corrections, which greatly improved the clarity and presentation of this work.

References

Afrin, N. (2016). *Risk factors of diabetes mellitus; a review (Doctoral dissertation)*. East West University. Retrieved from http://dspace.ewubd.edu/handle/2525/1999.

Ahamd, A. (2022). Diabetes mellitus: Classification of diabetes. *Journal of Diabetes Medication & Care, 5* (6), 94–96. https://doi.org/10.37532/jdmc.2022

American Diabetes Association (ADA). (2024). Standards of medical care in diabetes—2024. *Diabetes Care, 47*(Suppl. 1), S1–S180. https://doi.org/10.2337/dc24-S001

Ashcroft, F. M., & Rorsman, P. (2012). Diabetes mellitus and the β cell: The last ten years. *Cell, 148*(6), 1160–1171. https://doi.org/10.1016/j.cell.2012.02.010

Athanasiadou, K. I., & Paschou, S. A. (2025). Gestational diabetes mellitus subtypes: From one-size-fits-all to precision medicine. *Hormones, 24,* 1153–1155. https://doi.org/10.1007/s42000-025-00700-z

Atkinson, M. A., Eisenbarth, G. S., & Michels, A. W. (2014). Type 1 diabetes. *The Lancet, 383*(9911), 69–82. https://doi.org/10.1016/S0140-6736(13)60591-7

Ayan, E., & DeMirci, H. (2023). A brief atlas of insulin. *Current Diabetes Reviews, 19*(6), 18–79. https://doi.org/10.2174/1573399819666220610150342

Barker, D. J., Osmond, C., Kajantie, E., & Eriksson, J. G. (2009). Growth and chronic disease: Findings in the Helsinki birth cohort. *Annals of Human Biology, 36*(5), 445–458. https://doi.org/10.1080/03014460902980295

Biessels, G. J., & Despa, F. (2018). Cognitive decline and dementia in diabetes mellitus: Mechanisms and clinical implications. *Nature Reviews Endocrinology, 14*, 591–604. https://doi.org/10.1038/s41574-018-0048-7

Bommer, C., Heesemann, E., Sagalova, V., Manne-Goehler, J., Atun, R., Bärnighausen, T., & Vollmer, S. (2017). The global economic burden of diabetes in adults aged 20–79 years: A cost-of-illness study. *The Lancet Diabetes & Endocrinology, 5*(6), 423–430. https://doi.org/10.1016/S2213-8587(17)30097-9

Brennan, C., Harkins, V., & Perry, I. J. (2008). Management of diabetes in primary care: A structured-care approach. *The European Journal of General Practice, 14*(4), 117–122. https://doi.org/10.1080/13814780802689154

Brigham, E. L. (2025). *Understanding barriers to addressing social determinants of health in diabetes: Perspectives of managed care administrators* (Doctoral dissertation). Franklin University.

Brownlee, M. (2005). The pathobiology of diabetic complications: A unifying mechanism. *Diabetes, 54*(6), 1615–1625. https://doi.org/10.2337/diabetes.54.6.1615

Callaghan, B. C., Cheng, H. T., Stables, C. L., Smith, A. L., & Feldman, E. L. (2012). Diabetic neuropathy: Clinical manifestations and current treatments. *The Lancet Neurology, 11*(6), 521–534. https://doi.org/10.1016/S1474-4422(12)70065-0

Carpenter, S., Rigaud, M., Barile, M., Priest, T. J., Perez, L., & Ferguson, J. B. (2006). The ebers papyrus. *Bard College Publications, 3*, 1–22.

Caruso, I., & Giorgino, F. (2022). SGLT-2 inhibitors as cardio-renal protective agents. *Metabolism, 127*, Article 154937. https://doi.org/10.1016/j.metabol.2021.154937

Cheung, N., Mitchell, P., & Wong, T. Y. (2010). Diabetic retinopathy. *The Lancet, 376*(9735), 124–136. https://doi.org/10.1016/S0140-6736(09)62124-3

Clarkson, A. K. (1926). *The discoveries associated with the name of Claude Bernard, and their results.* University of Edinburgh. Retrieved from http://hdl.handle.net/1842/29691.

Corremans, R. (2023). *Metformin: An old drug offering new opportunities in the battle against chronic kidney disease* (Doctoral dissertation). University of Antwerp.

DeFronzo, R. A., Ferrannini, E., Groop, L., et al. (2015). Type 2 diabetes mellitus. *Nature Reviews Disease Primers, 1*, Article 15019. https://doi.org/10.1038/nrdp.2015.19

Donath, M. Y., Dinarello, C. A., & Mandrup-Poulsen, T. (2019). Targeting innate immune mediators in type 1 and type 2 diabetes. *Nature Reviews Immunology, 19*, 734–746. https://doi.org/10.1038/s41577-019-0213-9

Dongiovanni, P., Paolini, E., Corsini, A., Sirtori, C. R., & Ruscica, M. (2021). Nonalcoholic fatty liver disease or metabolic dysfunction-associated fatty liver disease diagnoses and cardiovascular diseases: from epidemiology to drug approaches. *European Journal of Clinical Investigation, 51*(7), 98–121. https://doi.org/10.1111/eci.13519

Dushenkov, V. (2017). Can Avicenna help manage the diabetes epidemic in central Asia? *Central Asian Journal of Medical Sciences, 3*(3), 200–220. https://doi.org/10.24079/CAJMS.2017.11.002

Eknoyan, G. (2019). A historical overview of diabetic nephropathy. In J. Roelofs, & L. Vogt (Eds.), *Diabetic nephropathy*. Cham: Springer. https://doi.org/10.1007/978-3-319-93521-8_1

Emerging Risk Factors Collaboration. (2010). Diabetes mellitus, fasting glucose, and risk of cause-specific death. *New England Journal of Medicine, 364*(9), 829–841. https://doi.org/10.1056/NEJMoa1008862

Fisher, L., Mullan, J. T., Arean, P., Glasgow, R. E., Hessler, D., & Masharani, U. (2019). Diabetes distress but not depression is associated with glycemic control in both cross-sectional and longitudinal analyses. *Diabetes Care, 33*(1), 23–28. https://doi.org/10.2337/dc09-1238

Fitipaldi, H., McCarthy, M. I., Florez, J. C., & Franks, P. W. (2018). A global overview of precision medicine in type 2 diabetes. *Diabetes, 67*(10), 1911–1922. https://doi.org/10.2337/dbi17-0045

Forbes, J. M., & Cooper, M. E. (2013). Mechanisms of diabetic complications. *Physiological Reviews, 93* (1), 137–188. https://doi.org/10.1152/physrev.00045.2011

Franks, P. W., & McCarthy, M. I. (2016). Exposing the exposures responsible for type 2 diabetes and obesity. *Science, 354*(6308), 69–73. https://doi.org/10.1126/science.aaf5094

GBD 2021 Diabetes Collaborators. (2023). Global, regional, and national burden of diabetes from 1990 to 2021, with projections to 2050. *The Lancet, 402*(10397), 203–234. https://doi.org/10.1016/S0140-6736(23)01301-6

Grant, S. F. (2019). The TCF7L2 locus: A genetic window into the pathogenesis of type 1 and type 2 diabetes. *Diabetes Care, 42*(9), 1624–1629. https://doi.org/10.2337/dci19-0001

Gregg, E. W., Sattar, N., & Ali, M. K. (2018). The changing face of diabetes complications. *Lancet Diabetes & Endocrinology, 6*(6), 448–458. https://doi.org/10.1016/S2213-8587(17)30418-1

Grundy, S. M. (2016). Metabolic syndrome update. *Trends in Cardiovascular Medicine, 26*(4), 364–373. https://doi.org/10.1016/j.tcm.2015.10.004

Haffner, S. M., Lehto, S., Rönnemaa, T., Pyörälä, K., & Laakso, M. (1998). Mortality from coronary heart disease in subjects with type 2 diabetes and in nondiabetic subjects. *New England Journal of Medicine, 339*(4), 229–234. https://doi.org/10.1056/NEJM199807233390404

Hattersley, A. T., & Patel, K. A. (2017). Precision diabetes: Learning from monogenic diabetes. *Diabetologia, 60*(5), 769–777. https://doi.org/10.1007/s00125-017-4226-2

He, K. J., Wang, H., Xu, J., et al. (2024). Global burden of T2DMfrom 1990 to 2021, with projections to 2044: A systematic analysis across SDI levels. *Frontiers in Endocrinology, 15,* Article 1501690. https://doi.org/10.3389/fendo.2024.1501690

Herman, W. H., Ye, W., Griffin, S. J., et al. (2015). Early detection and treatment of type 2 diabetes reduce cardiovascular morbidity and mortality. *Diabetes Care, 38*(8), 1449–1455. https://doi.org/10.2337/dc14-2459

Hotamisligil, G. S. (2017). Inflammation, metaflammation and immunometabolic disorders. *Nature, 542* (7640), 177–185. https://doi.org/10.1038/nature21363

Hu, Y., Lu, Q., Powles, R., et al. (2017). Leveraging functional annotations in genetic risk prediction for human complex diseases. *PLoS Computational Biology, 13*(6), Article e1005589. https://doi.org/10.1371/journal.pcbi.1005589

Hu, F. B., Manson, J. E., Stampfer, M. J., et al. (2011). Diet, lifestyle, and the risk of T2DMin women. *New England Journal of Medicine, 345*(11), 790–797. https://doi.org/10.1056/NEJMoa010492

Hu, Y., Zong, G., Liu, G., Wang, M., Rosner, B., Pan, A., Willett, W. C., Manson, J. E., Hu, F. B., & Sun, Q. (2018). Smoking cessation, weight change, type 2 diabetes, and mortality. *New England Journal of Medicine, 379*(7), 623–632. https://doi.org/10.1056/NEJMoa1803626

Huang, S., & Czech, M. P. (2007). The GLUT4 glucose transporter. *Cell Metabolism, 5*(4), 237–252. https://doi.org/10.1016/j.cmet.2007.03.006

Huang, Q., Li, Y., Yu, M., et al. (2025). Global burden and risk factors of T2DMfrom 1990 to 2021, with forecasts to 2050. *Frontiers in Endocrinology, 16,* Article 1538143. https://doi.org/10.3389/fendo.2025.1538143

International Diabetes Federation. (2025). IDF diabetes atlas. In *Global, regional and national diabetes prevalence estimates for 2024 and projections for 2050* (11th ed.). The Lancet Diabetes & Endocrinology.

Jörgens, V. (2020). Oskar Minkowski and the discovery of pancreatic diabetes. *Unveiling Diabetes—Historical Milestones in Diabetology, 40,* 40–50. https://doi.org/10.1159/000506549

Jadon, A. S., Kaushik, M. P., Anitha, K., Bhatt, S., Bhadauriya, P., & Sharma, M. (2024). Types of diabetes mellitus, mechanism of insulin resistance and associated complications. In *Biochemical immunology of diabetes and associated complications* (pp. 1–18). Academic Press. https://doi.org/10.1016/B978-0-443-13195-0.00001-6

Jae, S. Y., Franklin, B. A., Choo, J., Yoon, E. S., Choi, Y. H., & Park, W. H. (2016). Fitness, body habitus, and the risk of incident T2DMin Korean men. *The American Journal of Cardiology, 117*(4), 585–589. https://doi.org/10.1016/j.amjcard.2015.11.046

Kautzky-Willer, A., Harreiter, J., & Pacini, G. (2016). Sex and gender differences in risk, pathophysiology and complications of type 2 diabetes mellitus. *Endocrine Reviews, 37*(3), 278–316. https://doi.org/10.1210/er.2015-1137

Kershaw, E. E., & Flier, J. S. (2004). Adipose tissue as an endocrine organ. *Journal of Clinical Endocrinology & Metabolism, 89*(6), 2548–2556. https://doi.org/10.1210/jc.2004-0395

Kim, S. H. (2011). Measurement of insulin action: A tribute to Sir Harold Himsworth. *Diabetic Medicine, 28*(12), 1487–1493. https://doi.org/10.1111/j.1464-5491.2011.03409.x

Laios, K., Karamanou, M., Saridaki, Z., et al. (2012). Aretaeus of Cappadocia and the first description of diabetes. *Hormones, 11*, 109–113. https://doi.org/10.1007/BF03401545

Lewis, G. F., & Brubaker, P. L. (2021). The discovery of insulin revisited: Lessons for the modern era. *Journal of Clinical Investigation, 131*(1), 1–9. https://doi.org/10.1172/JCI142239

Ling, C., & Rönn, T. (2019). Epigenetics in human obesity and type 2 diabetes. *Cell Metabolism, 29*(5), 1028–1044. https://doi.org/10.1016/j.cmet.2019.03.009

Liu, J., Ren, Z. H., Qiang, H., et al. (2020). Trends in the incidence of diabetes mellitus: Results from the global burden of disease study 2017 and implications for diabetes prevention. *BMC Public Health, 20*, 1415. https://doi.org/10.1186/s12889-020-09502-x

Lowell, B. B., & Shulman, G. I. (2005). Mitochondrial dysfunction and type 2 diabetes. *Science, 307*(5708), 384–387. https://doi.org/10.1126/science.1104343

Lyssenko, V., Almgren, P., Anevski, D., et al. (2005). Genetic prediction of future type 2 diabetes. *PLoS Medicine, 2*(12), Article e345. https://doi.org/10.1371/journal.pmed.0020345

Mahajan, A., Taliun, D., Thurner, M., et al. (2018). Fine-mapping type 2 diabetes loci to single-variant resolution using high-density imputation and islet-specific epigenome maps. *Nature Genetics, 50* (11), 1505–1513. https://doi.org/10.1038/s41588-018-0241-6

Mayer-Davis, E. J., Lawrence, J. M., Dabelea, D., et al. (2017). Incidence trends of type 1 and type 2 diabetes among youths, 2002–2012. *New England Journal of Medicine, 376*(15), 1419–1429. https://doi.org/10.1056/NEJMoa1610187

Mishra, L. C., & Adra, T. (2003). Diabetes mellitus (madhumeha). In *Scientific basis for ayurvedic therapies* (pp. 125–156). Routledge.

Narayan, A. J., Lieberman, A. F., & Masten, A. S. (2021). Intergenerational transmission and prevention of adverse childhood experiences (ACEs). *Clinical Psychology Review, 85*, Article 101997. https://doi.org/10.1016/j.cpr.2021.101997

Nauck, M. (2016). Incretin therapies: Highlighting common features and differences in the modes of action of GLP-1 receptor agonists and DPP-4 inhibitors. *Diabetes, Obesity and Metabolism, 18*(3), 203–216. https://doi.org/10.1111/dom.12591

Ornellas, F., Karise, I., Aguila, M. B., & Mandarim-de-Lacerda, C. A. (2020). Pancreatic islets of langerhans: Adapting cell and molecular biology to changes of metabolism. In J. Faintuch, & S. Faintuch (Eds.), *Obesity and diabetes*. Cham: Springer. https://doi.org/10.1007/978-3-030-53370-0_13

Pihoker, C., Gilliam, L. K., Hampe, C. S., & Lernmark, A. (2005). Autoantibodies in diabetes. *Diabetes, 54* (Suppl. 2), S52–S61. https://doi.org/10.2337/diabetes.54.suppl_2.S52

Popkin, B. M. (2015). Nutrition transition and the global diabetes epidemic. *Current Diabetes Reports, 15*, 64. https://doi.org/10.1007/s11892-015-0631-4

Powers, A. C., Niswender, K. D., & Evans-Molina, C. (2022). Diabetes mellitus: Diagnosis, classification, and pathophysiology. *Diabetes, 1000,* 415.

Pragati, G., & Paolo, P. (2025). Divergence in prediabetes guidelines—A global perspective. *Diabetes Research and Clinical Practice, 223,* Article 112142. https://doi.org/10.1016/j.diabres.2025.112142

Prasad, R. B., & Groop, L. (2015). Genetics of type 2 diabetes—Pitfalls and possibilities. *Genes, 6*(1), 87–123. https://doi.org/10.3390/genes6010087

Prentki, M., & Nolan, C. J. (2006). Islet β cell failure in type 2 diabetes. *Journal of Clinical Investigation, 116*(7), 1802–1812. https://doi.org/10.1172/JCI29103

Rodríguez-Gutiérrez, R., & Montori, V. M. (2016). Glycemic control for patients with type 2 diabetes mellitus. *Circulation: Cardiovascular Quality and Outcomes, 9*(5), 504–512. https://doi.org/10.1161/CIRCOUTCOMES.116.002901

Saini, V. (2010). Molecular mechanisms of insulin resistance in type 2 diabetes mellitus. *World Journal of Diabetes, 1*(3), 68–75. https://doi.org/10.4239/wjd.v1.i3.68

Saltiel, A. R., & Kahn, C. R. (2001). Insulin signalling and the regulation of glucose and lipid metabolism. *Nature, 414*(6865), 799–806. https://doi.org/10.1038/414799a

Samuel, V. T., & Shulman, G. I. (2016). The pathogenesis of insulin resistance. *Journal of Clinical Investigation, 126*(1), 12–22. https://doi.org/10.1172/JCI77812

Seshiah, V., Kalra, S., Gupte, S., et al. (2014). Classification of hyperglycemia in pregnancy. *Indian Journal of Endocrinology and Metabolism, 18*(4), 445–448. https://doi.org/10.4103/2230-8210.137484

Stranieri, A., Yatsko, A., Jelinek, H., & Venkatraman, S. (2015). Data-analytically derived flexible HbA1c thresholds for T2DMdiagnosis. *Artificial Intelligence Research, 5*(1), 111–134. https://doi.org/10.5430/air.v5n1p111

Tan, Q., Akindehin, S. E., Orsso, C. E., et al. (2022). Recent advances in incretin-based pharmacotherapies for the treatment of obesity and diabetes. *Frontiers in Endocrinology, 13,* Article 838410. https://doi.org/10.3389/fendo.2022.838410

Thomas, C. C., & Philipson, L. H. (2015). Update on diabetes classification. *Medical Clinics, 99*(1), 1–16. https://doi.org/10.1016/j.mcna.2014.08.015

Tomlinson, B., Patil, N. G., Fok, M., Chan, P., & Lam, C. W. K. (2022). The role of sulfonylureas in the treatment of type 2 diabetes. *Expert Opinion on Pharmacotherapy, 23*(3), 387–403. https://doi.org/10.1080/14656566.2021.1999413

Tuttle, K. R., Bakris, G. L., Bilous, R. W., et al. (2014). Diabetic kidney disease. *Diabetes Care, 37*(10), 2864–2883. https://doi.org/10.2337/dc14-1296

Von Mering, J., & Minkowski, O. (1889). Diabetes following pancreatectomy. *Centralblatt für Klinische Medizin, 23*(1), 394.

Weiskirchen, R., & Lonardo, A. (2025). Semaglutide from bench to bedside. *Medical Sciences, 13*(4), 1–26. Retrieved from https://www.mdpi.com/2076-3271/13/4/265.

World Health Organization. (2011). *Use of glycated haemoglobin (HbA1c) in diagnosis of diabetes mellitus (WHO/NMH/CHP/CPM/11.1).* Geneva: WHO. Retrieved from https://pesquisa.bvsalud.org/portal/resource/pt./who-70523.

World Health Organization. (2023). *Global report on diabetes.* Geneva: World Health Organization.

Younossi, Z., Tacke, F., Arrese, M., et al. (2019). Global perspectives on nonalcoholic fatty liver disease and nonalcoholic steatohepatitis. *Hepatology, 69*(6), 2672–2682.

Zimmet, P., Alberti, K. G., Magliano, D. J., & Bennett, P. H. (2016). Diabetes mellitus statistics on prevalence and mortality. *Nature Reviews Endocrinology, 12*(10), 616–622. https://doi.org/10.1038/nrendo.2016.105

2

Genetic and epigenetic landscape of type 2 diabetes mellitus

Pritee Chunarkar-Patil[1, a], Sahar Surve[1, a], Mohmmad Kaleem[2], Asaad Kayali[3] and Rishikesh Shankar Bachhav[2]

[1]DEPARTMENT OF BIOINFORMATICS, RAJIV GANDHI INSTITUTE OF IT AND BIOTECHNOLOGY, BHARATI VIDYAPEETH (DEEMED TO BE UNIVERSITY), PUNE, MAHARASHTRA, INDIA; [2]DEPARTMENT OF PHARMACOLOGY, R. G. SAPKAL COLLEGE OF PHARMACY, SAVITRIBAI PHULE PUNE UNIVERSITY, NASHIK, MAHARASHTRA, INDIA; [3]DEPARTMENT OF HEALTH SCIENCES, HIGHER COLLEGES OF TECHNOLOGY, ABU DHABI, UNITED ARAB EMIRATES

1. Introduction

Diabetes is one of the most significant global health issues of the 21st century, with an estimated 135.6 million individuals aged 65 to 99 having the disease worldwide in 2019. By 2030, that figure is predicted to rise to 195.2 million (Kaleem, Thool, et al., 2025). Type 2 diabetes mellitus (T2DM) is a widely researched metabolic disorder due to its increasing global prevalence, economic implications, and intricate biological origins. Recent data suggests that more than 530 million adults worldwide are currently living with T2DM, and this figure is projected to exceed 780 million by 2045 if current trends persist (International Diabetes Federation [IDF], 2023 (Rahu et al., 2025), are briefly explained in Fig. 2.1.

Diabetes has a major impact on macrovascular and microvascular consequences, including diabetic retinopathy, nephropathy, and neuropathy (microvascular disease) and ischemic heart disease, cerebral infarction, cardiac failure, and peripheral vascular disease (macrovascular) (Joseph et al., 2022; Ojha et al., 2016). Diabetic retinopathy is one of the main causes of blindness in working-age adults (Steinmetz et al., 2021), and type 2 diabetes is a major contributor to non-traumatic lower limb amputation and chronic kidney disease (CKD) (Koye et al., 2018). In comparison with the entire population, people with diabetes are two times more probable to lose their lives from cardiovascular (CV) disorders, and younger-onset type 2 diabetes is linked to a significantly greater prevalence and occurrence of CV vulnerability than persons detected subsequently (Anson et al., 2025).

[a]Both have equal contributions in writing the manuscript.

Type 2 Diabetes Mellitus. https://doi.org/10.1016/B978-0-443-33590-7.00012-5

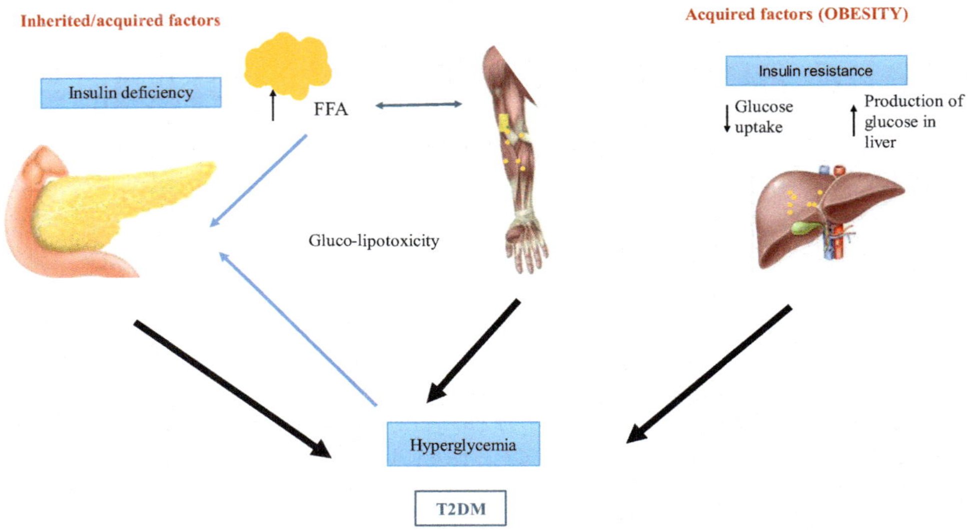

FIGURE 2.1 Factors leading to T2DM.

While factors related to lifestyle, such as dietary habits, physical inactivity, and obesity, are crucial in the onset of the disease, extensive research over the years has demonstrated that a significant genetic aspect also influences an individual's susceptibility to T2DM (Prasad & Groop, 2015). The interplay between genetic predisposition and environmental influences is now recognized as fundamental to the progression of the disease.

Extensive studies in the fields of epidemiology and molecular biology have convincingly demonstrated that genetic factors significantly influence an individual's susceptibility to type 2 diabetes mellitus (T2DM) (Prasad & Groop, 2015; Wheeler & Barroso, 2011). Understanding the interplay between genetic predisposition and environmental influences is now considered essential for comprehending the disease's progression.

Research involving families consistently indicates that individuals with a first-degree relative diagnosed with T2DM face an approximately threefold higher risk compared to those without such a family history (Lyssenko & Laakso, 2013). Evidence from twin studies further supports the notion of heritability, showing concordance rates for T2DM in identical twins to be between 60% and 70%, a figure significantly greater than that of fraternal twins, underscoring the importance of genetic factors (Hyttinen et al., 2003; Prasad & Groop, 2015). Notably, these studies also emphasize that genetic vulnerability does not operate in isolation, as environmental elements contribute significantly.

Variations among different ethnic groups highlight the interplay between genetics and environmental contexts. Populations undergoing rapid transitions in diet and lifestyle, such as South Asians, Pacific Islanders, and Indigenous communities, exhibit markedly elevated rates of type 2 diabetes mellitus (T2DM), even after accounting for factors like obesity and physical activity (Narayan et al., 2007). These observations suggest a genetic susceptibility that becomes more pronounced in modern environmental conditions.

In contrast to monogenic forms of diabetes, like maturity-onset diabetes of the young (MODY), T2DM does not adhere to simple Mendelian inheritance patterns. It arises from the collective impact of numerous common and rare genetic variants, each contributing modestly to the overall risk of the disease. These genetic variants interact with epigenetic factors, developmental processes, and environmental influences, culminating in a highly intricate genetic landscape (McCarthy, 2017).

Over the last 20 years, remarkable advancements in molecular genetics have taken place, including genome-wide association studies (GWAS), whole-exome sequencing, whole-genome sequencing, epigenomic profiling, single-cell transcriptomics, and integrative multi-omics strategies. These techniques have pinpointed hundreds of genetic loci associated with susceptibility to T2DM (Udler et al., 2018; Vujkovic et al., 2020). These discoveries have elucidated several critical biological pathways relevant to the progression of the disease, such as:

Differentiation, survival, and insulin secretion of β-cells (Ashcroft & Rorsman, 2012).

Biological processes of adipocytes and the distribution of visceral fat. Mechanisms of insulin signaling and glucose uptake. Mitochondrial functionality and metabolic activities (Khalilov & Abdullayeva, 2023). Circadian regulation of hormonal functions. Neuroendocrine regulation of appetite and energy homeostasis (Catalano et al., 2023; Chait & den Hartigh, 2020).

Despite these advancements, the genetic loci identified to date account for only about 10%–20% of the heritability estimated for T2DM, leaving a substantial proportion unexplained. This gap is often referred to as the "missing heritability" problem (Zuk et al., 2014).

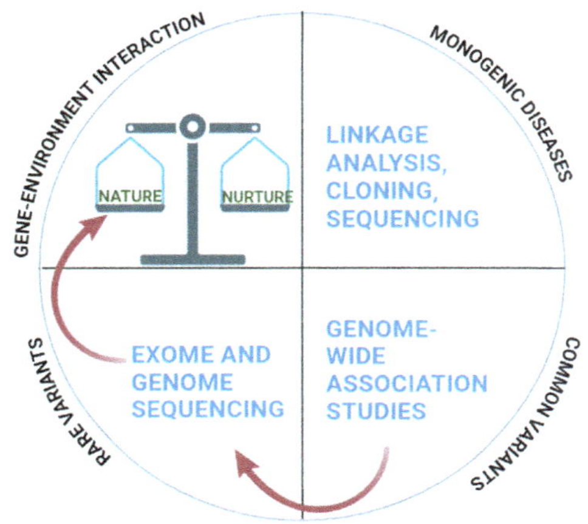

FIGURE 2.2 Techniques to study T2DM.

This chapter provides a comprehensive exploration of the genetic dimensions of T2DM, integrating traditional epidemiological perspectives with contemporary genomic discoveries, variations among distinct ethnic and population groups, molecular mechanisms, interactions between genes and the environment, and their practical implications in clinical settings, are briefly explained in Fig. 2.2.

2. Foundations and historical evolution of genetic research in T2DM

2.1 Early clinical insights and familial clustering

Long before molecular techniques emerged, healthcare providers noticed that type 2 diabetes mellitus (T2DM) often ran in families. Pedigree analyses done in the mid-20th century showed that siblings and children of affected individuals had a significantly higher risk (Kheriji et al., 2025). This finding helped establish the idea that T2DM has a genetic aspect, though its inheritance is too complicated for a simple Mendelian explanation.

2.1.1 Asymmetric risk

Diabetes in mothers carries a higher risk than in fathers, partly because of higher blood sugar levels during pregnancy (Dabelea, 2007).

2.1.2 High-risk populations

Certain groups, including Native Americans, South Asians, and communities from the Middle East, are more susceptible due to a mix of genetic and environmental factors (Mohan et al., 2012).

2.1.3 Phenotypic expression

The way the disease shows up varies due to environmental changes, socio-economic conditions, and dietary habits (Hu, 2011).

These early observations set the stage for understanding diabetes as a genetically complex but possibly changeable condition.

2.2 Twin studies and heritability estimates

Twin studies have been crucial in genetic epidemiology, especially in measuring the heritability of T2DM. Monozygotic twins have identical genetic makeups, while dizygotic twins share about half. The higher concordance rates in monozygotic twins compared to dizygotic twins highlight the genetic factors involved in T2DM (Lehtovirta et al., 2010; Willemsen et al., 2015). Monozygotic concordance: 60%–70%. Dizygotic concordance: 20%–30%. Heritability estimates: About 40%–70% across various populations (Kaprio et al., 1992). These results consistently show that T2DM has a strong genetic heritability, even though environmental factors also play a role.

2.3 Linkage studies: Limitations and learning

During the 1980s and 1990s, linkage analysis served as the main genetic approach for determining chromosomal areas connected to diseases within families. This technique was effective for disorders stemming from a single gene but faced difficulties with complex conditions such as type 2 diabetes mellitus (T2DM) due to several obstacles (Cole & Florez, 2020): Risk variants typically exert minor effects. The disease lacks distinct patterns of penetrance. Environmental factors can obscure genetic impacts. Establishing extensive, multigenerational family trees presents challenges. Although some potential regions were identified on chromosomes 2q, 10q, and 20q, the majority of findings were either inconsistent or weak (Kingdom & Wright, 2022).

2.4 Candidate-gene studies: Advantages and limitations

Candidate-gene studies, popular from the 1990s to the early 2000s, examined specific genes believed to affect glucose metabolism. Notable genes included: PPARG: Influences fat cell development (Altshuler et al., 2000). IRS1: Affects insulin signaling. KCNJ11: Involved in β-cell ion channels. HNF4A/HNF1A: Play a role in β-cell transcription (Muntean et al., 2022).

Although some associations were confirmed by genome-wide association studies (GWAS), many candidate-gene studies faced challenges like small sample sizes and inadequate replication.

2.5 The genomic revolution: From microarrays to sequencing

The completion of the Human Genome Project in 2003 and the advent of SNP microarray technology transformed genetic research. Scientists could now analyse hundreds of thousands, even millions, of genetic variants at once (Collins et al., 2003). Key developments during this period include should be replaced by key developments during this period has been covered in Table 2.1. These advances shifted diabetes genetics from a candidate-focused approach to data-driven exploration, revealing unexpected pathways and new biological mechanisms.

Table 2.1 Human genome project milestones.

Year/Period	Milestone	References
2007	First successful GWAS for T2DM	Sladek et al. (2007)
2010–15	Meta-analyses involving over 100,000 individuals	Mobasseri et al. (2020)
2015–Present	Whole-exome and whole-genome sequencing	Flannick et al. (2014)
2020s	Single-cell multi-omics and deep-learning genotypes	Bryois et al. (2020)

3. Genome-wide association studies (GWAS): Concepts, discoveries, and impact

3.1 GWAS methodology: A technical overview

A GWAS evaluates the frequency of genetic variants across a large number of single-nucleotide polymorphisms (SNPs) among individuals with type 2 diabetes mellitus (T2DM) compared to control groups. The statistical approach examines:

The strength of association (odds ratios), and levels of significance adjusted for multiple comparisons, Population stratification, and Verification in independent cohorts (Visscher et al., 2017). A typical Genome-Wide Association Study (GWAS) analyzes one to 10 million single-nucleotide polymorphisms (SNPs) using a stringent significance threshold of $P < 5 \times 10^{-8}$ to manage the high number of comparisons (Udayantha et al., 2025). Factors contributing to GWAS success include: High-density SNP arrays available. Global collaborations like DIAGRAM (Morris et al., 2012). Sample sizes of 50,000 to 500,000 participants. Access to biobanks like the UK Biobank and All of Us (Sudlow et al., 2015), are summarized in Fig. 2.3.

3.2 TCF7L2: A pioneering discovery

The identification of TCF7L2 in 2006 represented a significant advancement in the genetics of diabetes. This gene, which plays a role in Wnt signaling and β-cell functionality, exhibits the strongest known common-risk effect for T2DM (odds ratio ranging from approximately 1.4–1.9) (Lyssenko & Laakso, 2013). Its discovery was notable because:

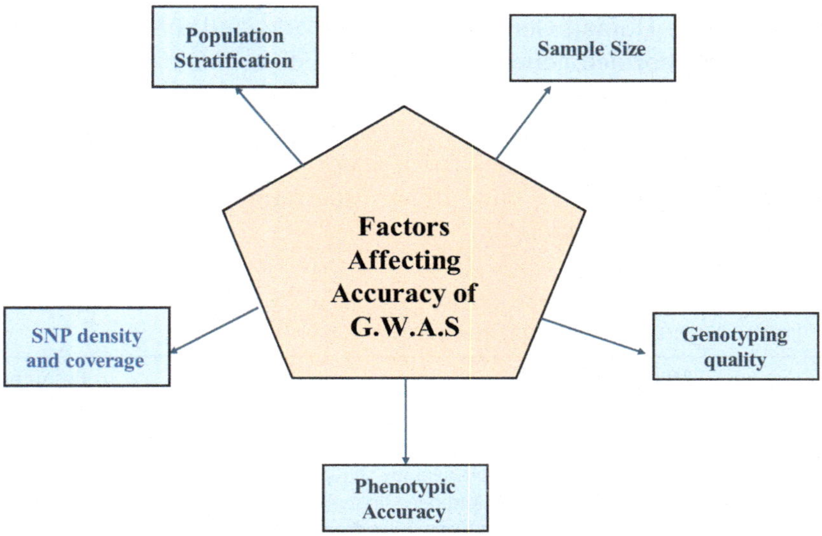

FIGURE 2.3 Factors affecting accuracy of GWAS.

It was not previously linked to type 2 diabetes mellitus (T2DM) and has a larger effect size than most common variants. This emphasizes the importance of incretin biology and pancreatic function. Risk alleles in TCF7L2 impair β-cells' insulin release in response to glucose, highlighting its clinical significance (Florez, 2008), are summarized in Fig. 2.4.

3.3 Expanded catalog of T2DM loci

Since the initial wave of genome-wide association studies (GWAS) in 2007, the identification of genetic regions associated with type 2 diabetes mellitus (T2DM) has dramatically accelerated. Extensive meta-analyses and research involving diverse ethnic populations have uncovered more than 400 regions linked to T2DM susceptibility in various groups (Mahajan et al., 2018; Vujkovic et al., 2020). These regions can be categorized based on their key biological roles.

3.3.1 Genes influencing β-cell function and insulin secretion

A considerable number of areas identified by GWAS have an impact on β-cell development and the capacity for insulin production and secretion. Notable examples include: SLC30A8 (ZnT8): Responsible for zinc transport into insulin granules, which is vital for the formation of insulin crystals. MTNR1B: Encodes a melatonin receptor, which connects circadian rhythms to insulin secretion (Suthon & Tangjittipokin, 2024). HHEX: Involved in the formation of the pancreas and liver. WFS1: Influences the stress response of the endoplasmic reticulum. GCK: Acts as the glucose sensor in pancreatic β-cells (Pasquali et al., 2014; Udler et al., 2018). Collectively, these genes underscore the significant importance of impaired insulin secretion as a key genetic contributor to type 2 diabetes mellitus (T2DM).

3.3.2 Genes related to insulin resistance and adiposity

While there are fewer in number, several GWAS-identified regions influence insulin sensitivity and the biology of fat tissue: for examples; IRS1, interferes with insulin

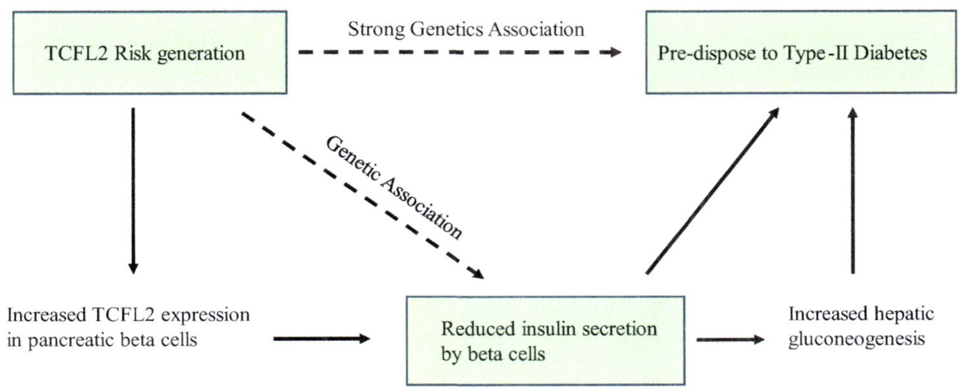

FIGURE 2.4 TCFL2 and its associations.

Table 2.2 Pathways revealed through GWAS.

Pathway	Key feature	References
β-Cell dysfunction	Main genetic risk: alleles impair β-cell development and insulin secretion.	Ashcroft and Rorsman (2012); McCarthy (2017)
Lipid metabolism & ectopic fat	Genes affect fat storage and metabolism; disruption causes insulin resistance.	Shulman (2014)
Neuroendocrine & circadian regulation	Variants in melatonin/circadian genes influence glucose homeostasis and T2DM risk.	Catalano et al. (2023)

signaling pathways, and PPARG, Regulates the development of fat cells and storage of fat while FTO Influences body mass index and energy consumption. Furthermore, KLF14: Governs gene expression in adipose tissue (Dimas et al., 2014).

Many loci associated with insulin resistance have indirect effects by increasing body fat, which exacerbates metabolic stress and glucose intolerance.

3.3.3 Genes for lipid and metabolic regulation

GWAS has revealed genes that play a role in glucose production in the liver, fat metabolism, and the accumulation of fat in inappropriate locations: GCKR: Modulates liver glucokinase activity. APOC3: Impacts the metabolism of triglycerides. PNPLA3: Strongly associated with liver fat and metabolic complications (Speliotes et al., 2011). These discoveries underscore the interconnectedness of lipid and glucose metabolism in T2DM, explained briefly in Table 2.2.

3.4 Pathways revealed through GWAS

3.4.1 β-Cell dysfunction as the primary genetic mechanism

One of the most reliable outcomes from GWAS is that β-cell dysfunction, rather than primary insulin resistance, accounts for the majority of genetic risk for T2DM (Ashcroft & Rorsman, 2012; McCarthy, 2017). The prevalent risk alleles impair β-cell development, insulin secretion, or the coupling of stimuli to secretion. This diminishes the capacity of β-cells to manage escalating metabolic demands. This shift in perspective has transformed our understanding of T2DM by placing β-cell failure at the center of genetic predisposition.

3.4.2 Lipid metabolism and ectopic fat accumulation

GWAS findings also underscore genes that regulate lipid metabolism, adipocyte growth, and the accumulation of fat in the liver and muscles. Deficiencies in these areas result in lipotoxicity, mitochondrial dysfunction, and subsequent insulin resistance (Shulman, 2014).

3.4.3 Neuroendocrine and circadian regulation

Genetic variants that affect melatonin signaling (MTNR1B) and circadian clock genes, such as CRY2, indicate that biological rhythms play a crucial role in regulating glucose homeostasis (Catalano et al., 2023; Marcheva et al., 2010). These findings help clarify the links between sleep disturbances, shift work, and an increased risk of T2DM.

3.5 Limitations of GWAS

Despite their notable contributions, GWAS have several acknowledged limitations:

The majority of identified variants exhibit small effect sizes (OR ~1.05–1.15).

A significant portion of heritability remains unexplained, often referred to as "missing heritability." (Zuk et al., 2014). Over 80% of GWAS participants are of European descent, restricting the global applicability (Sirugo et al., 2019). Many risk variants are found in non-coding regions, complicating functional interpretation. Establishing causality and identifying target genes continues to pose challenges (Gaulton, 2017).

These limitations have led researchers to integrate GWAS with rare-variant sequencing, epigenomics, single-cell transcriptomics, and functional genomics to enhance understanding of disease mechanisms.

4. Major genetic Loci associated with Type 2 diabetes mellitus (T2DM)

Over the last 2 decades, significant advancements in genome-wide association studies (GWAS), whole-exome sequencing, and functional genomics have resulted in the identification of numerous genetic loci associated with type 2 diabetes mellitus (T2DM). These loci are involved in a variety of biological functions, including pancreatic β-cell development and function, differentiation of fat cells, insulin signaling, lipid metabolism, mitochondrial energy production, and the effects of incretin hormones (Mccarthy, 2011; Udler et al., 2018). A principal observation across diverse populations is that the majority of common T2DM risk loci primarily influence β-cell function and insulin secretion rather than directly inducing insulin resistance. This indicates that challenges in insulin secretion are the main genetically influenced contributors to disease risk, while insulin resistance typically acts as an environmental or secondary element that exacerbates genetic susceptibility (Mahajan et al., 2018; McCarthy, 2017). The subsequent sections examine the main genetic loci associated with T2DM, classified according to their primary biological pathways.

4.1 Genes Affecting β-cell function and insulin secretion

Pancreatic β-cells are vital for regulating glucose levels. They secrete insulin in a well-coordinated manner in response to blood glucose levels. Genetic variations that impair β-cell development, survival, glucose detection, or the secretion of insulin

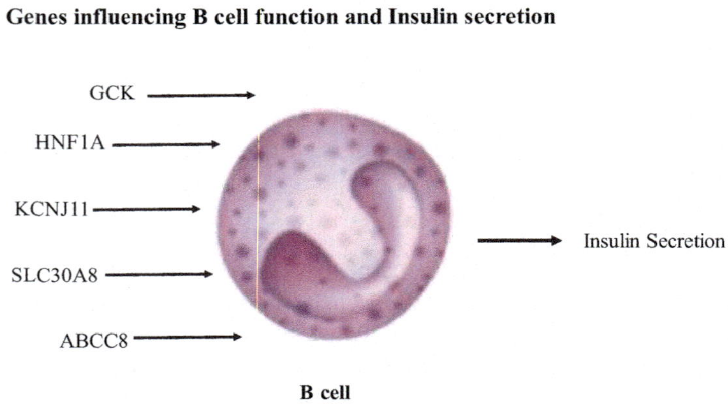

FIGURE 2.5 Genes affecting B-cell function & insulin secretion.

significantly increase the risk of T2DM. In fact, genes that affect β-cell biology represent the largest and most consistently replicated category of T2DM-related loci (Ashcroft & Rorsman, 2012; McCarthy, 2017), are summarized in Fig. 2.5.

4.1.1 *TCF7L2 (transcription factor 7-like 2)*

Recognized as the most significant common genetic risk factor for T2DM across various populations . It plays a vital role in Wnt signaling, incretin responsiveness, and the transcription of β-cell-associated genes. Risk alleles are associated with diminished insulin secretion, subpar proinsulin processing, and reduced GLP-1-triggered insulin release (Lyssenko et al., 2007).

4.1.2 *SLC30A8 (ZnT8; zinc transporter 8)*

This gene encodes a zinc transporter crucial for forming insulin crystals within secretory granules. Common risk variants diminish the effectiveness of zinc transport, leading to impaired insulin secretion (Sladek et al., 2007). Interestingly, rare loss-of-function variants confer protection against T2DM, suggesting the possibility of treating the condition through ZnT8 inhibition (Flannick et al., 2014).

4.1.3 *MTNR1B (melatonin receptor 1B)*

This gene links the regulation of circadian rhythms to glucose metabolism. Risk alleles are associated with elevated fasting glucose levels and decreased insulin release during the early phase (Prokopenko et al., 2009). This underscores the influence of sleep-wake cycles on β-cell functionality.

4.1.4 *HHEX, CDKAL1, and CDKN2A/B*

These genes are involved in pancreatic development, β-cell proliferation, and the regulation of the cell cycle. Variants are associated with lower insulin secretion and higher proinsulin levels, suggesting issues with β-cell maturation (Kommoju et al., 2016).

4.1.5 *KCNJ11 and ABCC8*

These genes encode components of the ATP-sensitive potassium (KATP) channel, which is essential for β-cell membrane depolarization. Common variants slightly elevate T2DM risk, while rare mutations can lead to neonatal diabetes or MODY (De Franco et al., 2020).

4.1.6 *PAX4, NKX6-1, and MAFA*

These transcription factors regulate β-cell identity, differentiation, and insulin gene expression. Variants exhibit significant effects in East Asian populations, revealing distinct genetic patterns across different groups (Aigha & Abdelalim, 2020).

4.1.7 *GLIS3*

This gene governs the survival of β-cells and the transcription of the insulin gene. Variants are associated with both type 1 and type 2 diabetes, indicating shared pathways that render β-cells susceptible (Nogueira et al., 2013). Genetic variations impacting β-cell pathways constitute the largest category of T2DM risk loci, underscoring insulin secretion difficulties as the principal genetically driven issue in the disease's development (Yau et al., 2025).

4.2 Genes related to insulin resistance and adiposity

Fewer genetic loci are mainly responsible for insulin resistance compared to those that affect β-cell function. However, several genes are consistently linked to adiposity, lipid metabolism, and insulin sensitivity. Understanding these genes helps to clarify the complex mechanisms behind type 2 diabetes mellitus (T2DM). Key Genes Implicated in Insulin Resistance and Adiposity (Brown & Walker, 2016).

4.2.1 *FTO (fat mass and obesity-associated gene)*

Recognized as one of the earliest and most significant loci linked to obesity. Contributes to a higher T2DM risk indirectly by raising body mass index (BMI). Plays a role in controlling energy intake, adipocyte differentiation, and hypothalamic signaling (Yang et al., 2017; da Fonseca et al., 2019).

4.2.2 *PPARG (Peroxisome Proliferator-activated receptor gamma)*

Acts as a master regulator of adipocyte differentiation. Serves as the main target for thiazolidinedione drugs used to manage diabetes. The Pro12Ala variant is linked to a lower risk of T2DM by improving insulin sensitivity (Jang et al., 2023).

4.2.3 *IRS1 (insulin receptor substrate 1)*

Helps with insulin signaling after the insulin receptor. Certain risk variants are associated with reduced adipose insulin signaling and higher ectopic fat deposition (Kilpeläinen et al., 2011).

4.2.4 LYPLAL1, GRB14, and ADIPOQ

These genes affect adipocyte metabolism and the production of adipokines. Variants can influence body fat distribution and contribute to insulin resistance (Enns et al., 2011; Sun et al., 2022).

4.2.5 LPL (lipoprotein lipase)

Regulates the removal of triglycerides from the bloodstream. Loss-of-function variants are linked to higher insulin resistance due to increased circulating triglycerides. Although these genes are well-linked to insulin resistance, it is important to note that their individual effects on T2DM risk are generally smaller than those of loci that impact β-cell function (Basu & Goldberg, 2020).

4.3 Genes involved in incretin signaling and metabolic regulation

Incretin hormones, like GLP-1 and GIP, are crucial for glucose-dependent insulin secretion. Several genetic loci have been found that influence this hormonal system, further affecting metabolic regulation and diabetes risk.

Notable Genes Affecting Incretin Signaling and Glucose Metabolism-

4.3.1 GIPR (GIP receptor)

Variants in this gene can reduce GIP-mediated insulin release, possibly leading to glucose intolerance (Lyssenko et al., 2011).

4.3.2 GLP1R (glucagon-like Peptide-1 receptor)

Affects the effectiveness of GLP-1–based diabetes therapies. Certain variants can change β-cell sensitivity to incretin hormones (Gaulton et al., 2015).

4.3.3 WFS1 (Wolframin ER Transmembrane protein)

Helps regulate endoplasmic reticulum (ER) stress. Variants are linked to impaired insulin secretion and shifts in incretin response (Sandhu et al., 2007).

4.3.4 G6PC2

Influences fasting glucose levels by affecting pancreatic glucose cycling (Pound et al., 2013).

4.3.5 GCK (glucokinase)

Acts as a glucose sensor within β-cells. Mildly harmful variants can raise fasting glucose and increase T2DM risk, while more severe mutations cause maturity-onset diabetes of the young type 2 (MODY2) (Stride et al., 2002).

Together, these genes illustrate the complex relationship between hormonal signaling and cellular glucose sensing in determining an individual's risk for type 2 diabetes, summarized in Fig. 2.6.

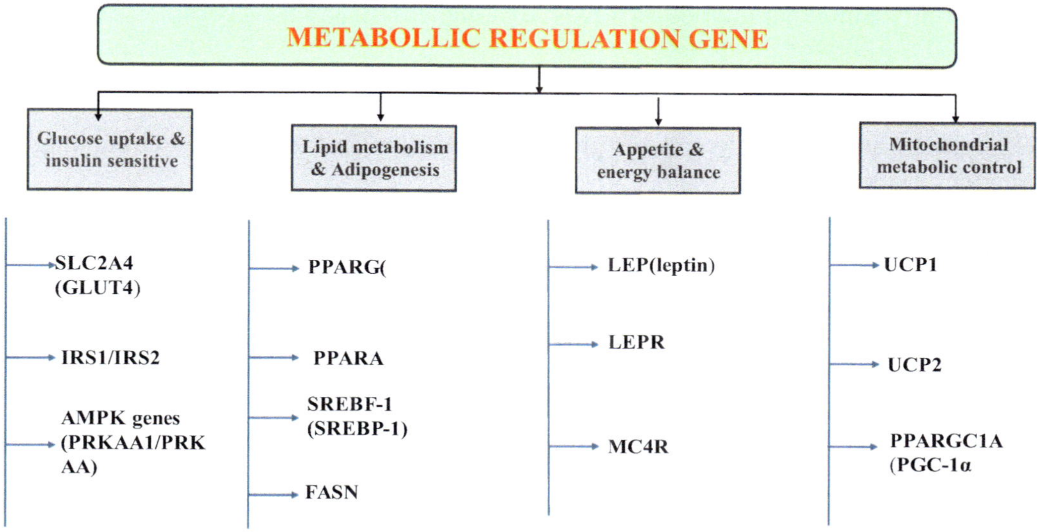

FIGURE 2.6 Genes involved in metabolic regulation.

4.4 Genes influencing lipid metabolism and mitochondrial function

Metabolic issues in the liver and muscle are closely related to lipid processing and mitochondrial function. Several genes are key in these processes and influence the risk and progression of metabolic diseases like type 2 diabetes mellitus (T2DM) (Mitrovic et al., 2023).

4.4.1 *SLC16A11*

Discovery: The SIGMA T2DM Consortium found SLC16A11 as a risk gene in Latino populations (Williams Amy et al., 2014).
Function: This gene encodes a transporter that helps with cellular metabolism.
Clinical Impact: People with the risk haplotype have lower mitochondrial fatty acid oxidation. This condition raises lipotoxicity and increases the chance of developing insulin resistance.

4.4.2 *CPT1A (Carnitine Palmitoyltransferase 1A)*

Role: CPT1A controls how fatty acids enter mitochondria, which is vital for energy production.
Variants: Rare genetic variants can disrupt β-oxidation and promote insulin resistance (Liang, 2023).

4.4.3 *Mitochondrial DNA variants*

Haplogroups: Changes in mitochondrial DNA (mtDNA) haplogroups affect the efficiency of oxidative phosphorylation.

Susceptibility: Some haplotypes are linked to a higher risk of T2DM complications (Fuku et al., 2007).

4.4.4 GCKR (glucokinase regulatory protein)

Metabolic Influence: GCKR impacts glucose production in the liver and circulating triglyceride levels.
Risk Variant: The common P446L variant is linked to a greater risk of T2DM by changing metabolic flow (Beer et al., 2009).

4.4.5 PNPLA3 and TM6SF2

Liver Health: Both genes are mainly related to liver fat and non-alcoholic fatty liver disease (NAFLD).
Indirect Effects: While their main influence is on liver fat, they also raise T2DM risk indirectly through ectopic lipid deposition. Together, these genetic loci highlight the complex relationships between lipid metabolism, mitochondrial function, and glucose balance (Oliveira et al., 2021), given in Table 2.3 and Fig. 2.7.

4.5 Protective genetic variants and loss-of-function

Protective genetic variants offer important insights into potential treatments. They reveal biological mechanisms that can reduce disease risk.

4.5.1 SLC30A8 loss-of-function variants

Unexpected Benefit: Some truncating variants in SLC30A8 lower the risk of T2DM by about 65% (Flannick & Florez, 2016). Therapeutic Implication: These findings indicate that blocking the ZnT8 protein may be a promising treatment strategy.

Table 2.3 Protective genetic variants and their respective functions.

Gene/Variant	Function/Role	Protective effect/Implication	References
SLC30A8 (LoF variants)	ZnT8 protein is involved in insulin secretion	Truncating variants reduce T2DM risk by ~65%; potential therapeutic target	Flannick et al. (2014)
PCSK9 (LoF variants)	Regulates LDL cholesterol	Lower LDL and reduced heart disease risk; improves overall metabolic health	Cohen et al. (2006)
CETP deficiency variants	Modulates HDL cholesterol	Higher HDL levels; may improve insulin sensitivity	Ølnes et al. (2023)
MTNR1B protective alleles	Melatonin receptor affects β-cell circadian response	Lowers fasting glucose; improves glucose regulation	Vella et al. (2024)
PAX4 protective alleles (east Asian)	β-cell survival under metabolic stress	Protects β-cells against T2DM	Lorenzo et al. (2015)

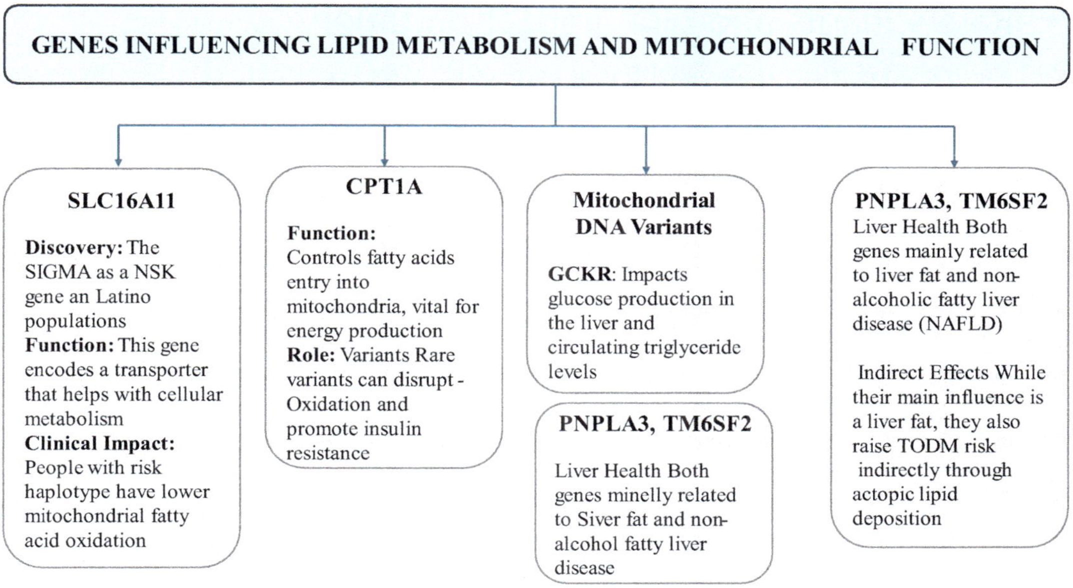

FIGURE 2.7 Genes influencing lipid metabolism and mitochondrial function.

4.5.2 PCSK9 loss-of-function variants

Cholesterol Management: People with these variants usually have lower LDL cholesterol and a decreased risk of heart disease. Broader Impact: While not specific to T2DM, these variants improve overall metabolic health and have helped develop new medications (Cohen et al., 2006).

4.5.3 CETP deficiency variants

HDL Levels: CETP deficiency is linked to higher HDL cholesterol. Insulin Sensitivity: In some groups, this may also improve insulin sensitivity (Ølnes et al., 2023).

4.5.4 MTNR1B Protective Allele

Glucose Regulation: Some MTNR1B variants help lower fasting glucose levels by improving the circadian response of pancreatic β-cells (Vella et al., 2024).

4.5.5 Transmission of Protective East Asian variants

PAX4 Alleles: Protective PAX4 variants help β-cells survive during metabolic stress, protecting against T2DM. These findings emphasize the important role that naturally occurring human genetic variants play in drug discovery and the development of future treatment strategies (Lorenzo et al., 2015).

5. Rare variants and high-impact mutations

While common genetic variants with moderate effect sizes contribute significantly to the population-level risk of type 2 diabetes mellitus (T2DM), there is growing awareness that rare and low-frequency variants also play an important role in disease susceptibility, particularly among those with early-onset or unusual phenotypes. These variants often have significant biological effects by altering protein-coding sequences, regulatory regions, or gene dosage, effectively linking monogenic and polygenic cases of diabetes (Bazzazzadehgan et al., 2025; Flannick & Florez, 2016).

The swift advancement of whole-exome sequencing (WES) and whole-genome sequencing (WGS) in large population studies has enabled the identification of many rare variants linked to T2DM risk. Although these variants usually account for a smaller share of the overall population risk in comparison to common variants, their considerable functional effects offer vital insights into disease mechanisms and potential therapeutic avenues (Zhou et al., 2021), summarized in Fig. 2.8.

5.1 Exome sequencing and rare-variant discovery

Whole-exome sequencing has changed how we identify rare coding variants linked to metabolic diseases. Unlike GWAS, which mainly investigates common single-nucleotide polymorphisms (SNPs) with minimal effects, WES targets protein-altering mutations that are more likely to have direct biological impacts (Flannick & Florez, 2016).

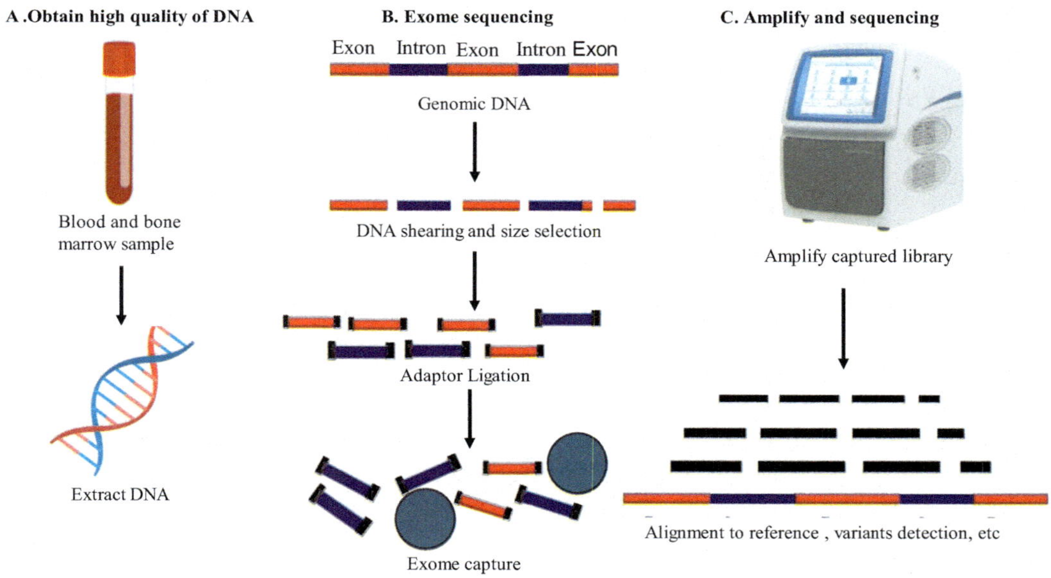

FIGURE 2.8 Exome sequencing.

5.1.1 Role of exome sequencing contributed to T2DM

Identification of high-impact mutations in established metabolic pathways:

Exome studies have found rare mutations in genes crucial for β-cell development, insulin processing, and mitochondrial function. Notably, these mutations can reflect the clinical features of monogenic diabetes, although their impact is not always complete (Flannick & Florez, 2016; Lv et al., 2022).

5.1.2 Discovery of unexpected gene targets

Large sequencing projects involving over 150,000 participants, like those by the UK Biobank and the AMP-T2D consortium, have identified novel rare variants in genes not previously linked to T2DM (Backman et al., 2021). For example, RFX6 truncating variants have been shown to lower insulin secretion, raising diabetes risk in certain individuals (Patel et al., 2017). PAM loss-of-function variants disrupt the amidation of GLP-1, linking rare genetic variation to incretin biology (Thomsen et al., 2018).

5.1.3 Clarification of previously unclear loci

Some genes that GWAS initially suggested were linked to T2DM have now been confirmed to carry rare variants with much stronger effects. This supports their role in developing the disease (Mahajan et al., 2018).

5.1.4 Identification of variants with protective effects

Rare variants in genes like SLC30A8, MC4R, and HSD17B13 have provided useful insights into natural defenses against metabolic disease (Abul-Husn et al., 2018; Flannick et al., 2014).

Overall, findings from whole-exome sequencing highlight an important point: even though rare variants may contribute only a small portion of the overall population risk, their significant biological effects are essential for understanding the complexities of T2DM. As research progresses, these discoveries are likely to reshape our understanding of disease mechanisms and create new options for targeted therapies.

5.2 Overlap with monogenic diabetes pathways

The genetic landscape of diabetes is more complex than just separating polygenic type 2 diabetes mellitus (T2DM) from monogenic forms like MODY or neonatal diabetes. Rare genetic variants often blur these lines. Many genes that cause monogenic diabetes when severely mutated also have milder variants that raise the risk of T2DM. This observation highlights a range of genetic effects, rather than a strict division between categories (Vaxillaire & Froguel, 2006).

5.2.1 Illustrative examples of monogenic-polygenic overlap

HNF1A: Severe mutations in this gene cause MODY3, a well-studied type of monogenic diabetes. However, even mild variants in HNF1A can increase the risk of T2DM in adults (Ellard & Colclough, 2006).

5.2.2 GCK (glucokinase)

Loss-of-function mutations in GCK lead to MODY2, which usually presents as stable, mild hyperglycemia. On the other hand, common variants in this gene have a small effect on fasting glucose levels and T2DM risk (Stride et al., 2002).

KCNJ11 and ABCC8: Severe mutations in these genes can result in neonatal diabetes. Yet, common variants are linked to a higher risk of T2DM, mainly through reduced insulin secretion (Gloyn et al., 2003).

PDX1 (Insulin Promoter Factor 1): Rare defects in PDX1 may lead to pancreatic agenesis or MODY4. At the same time, low-frequency variants can subtly impair β-cell function, contributing to the development of T2DM (Ebrahim et al., 2022).

WFS1: Homozygous mutations in WFS1 cause Wolfram syndrome, which includes early-onset diabetes. However, common variants are associated with T2DM and a reduced incretin effect (Sandhu et al., 2007). What does this continuum mean for understanding diabetes? It shows that genes essential for β-cell function often have effects that depend on their activity levels. Even slight decreases in gene function can make people more likely to develop T2DM, while larger disruptions may lead to monogenic forms of the disease. Recognizing this range is important for improving both research and clinical care in diabetes (Cernea & Dobreanu, 2013), summarized in Fig. 2.9.

5.3 Population-specific rare variants

Rare genetic variants often occur in specific geographic areas. This distribution is influenced by genetic drift, founder effects, and the unique histories of different populations. Discovering these variants requires including diverse groups in genomic research, which is a continual challenge due to the historical focus on European populations in many studies (Bentley et al., 2019). Why is this important? The effects of these rare variants can be significant, especially in populations where they are most common. Key Examples of Population-Specific Variants:

FIGURE 2.9 Monogenic polygenic overlap.

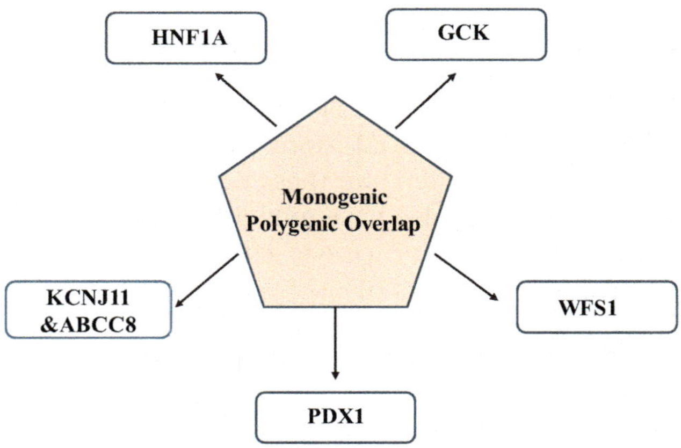

SLC16A11 (Latino Populations): First identified in a Mexican group and found to be rare among Europeans. This gene has a haplotype inherited from Neanderthals. It disrupts lipid metabolism, increasing the risk of type 2 diabetes mellitus (T2DM) by 20%–30% (Williams Amy et al., 2014).

PAX4 Variants (East Asians):

Missense mutations in PAX4 are common in East Asian populations but nearly absent in Europeans. These variants affect the survival of β-cells, raising the likelihood of T2DM (Kwak et al., 2018).

RREB1 Variants (South Asian Populations):

Rare coding variants in RREB1 are strongly linked to early-onset T2DM. They are crucial for regulating β-cell transcription networks (Mahajan et al., 2018).

TBC1D4 Variant (Inuit Populations):

A loss-of-function allele in this gene significantly increases postprandial insulin resistance (Moltke et al., 2014). These findings underscore an important point: rare variants can have a substantial impact within specific populations. To fully grasp and tackle the global diabetes burden, it is crucial to conduct equitable and inclusive genomic research.

5.4 Clinical significance of high-impact alleles

Rare genetic variants are not merely of academic interest; they have real clinical implications. Their importance is clear in diagnosing, selecting treatments, and advising families of individuals with unusual diabetes presentations. Let's look at how these high-impact alleles are influencing the future of precision medicine (Yvonnet et al., 2025).

5.5 Key Clinical Applications

5.5.1 Early and Atypical-onset T2DM

Individuals diagnosed with T2DM before age 30, or those with a normal body mass index, may carry rare variants that affect β-cell function (Ma, Lin, & Yu, 2025).

5.5.2 Pharmacogenomic implications

Certain mutations can predict how a patient will respond to specific treatments: KCNJ11 and ABCC8 variants can lead to significant improvement with sulfonylureas, often removing the need for insulin (Pearson et al., 2006). PPARG mutations may affect how well thiazolidinediones (TZDs) work.

5.5.3 Precision diagnostics

Identifying high-impact alleles can differentiate between maturity-onset diabetes of the young (MODY) and young-onset T2DM, resulting in more accurate treatment and prognosis (Tosur & Philipson, 2022).

5.5.4 Target discovery for drug development

Protective loss-of-function variants, like truncations in SLC30A8 or frameshifts in HSD17B13, provide natural models for developing new treatments (Abul-Husn et al., 2018).

5.5.5 Familial risk assessment

Because high-impact variants often show partial penetrance, genetic testing helps provide better counseling for family members at risk (Stein et al., 2014).

In summary, rare variants connect single-gene (monogenic) mechanisms to the complex features of polygenic diseases. Studying them not only enhances our understanding of diabetes but also creates new opportunities for personalized care and innovative treatments. Moving forward, we must commit to global inclusion, ensuring that the benefits of genomic medicine reach every community.

6. Ethnic and population-specific genetic architecture

The genetic landscape of type 2 diabetes mellitus (T2DM) varies greatly among different global populations. This diversity arises from evolutionary history, ancestry mixing, environmental exposures, and demographic changes. While many T2DM-related genetic markers appear worldwide, their impact, allele frequencies, and the existence of unique variants differ among ethnic groups (Mahajan et al., 2018). These genetic differences help explain variations in disease frequency, age at onset, and clinical symptoms across populations.

Historically, genomic research has focused mostly on individuals of European descent, leaving notable gaps in our understanding of other groups. Recently, global initiatives like DIAGRAM, SIGMA, AGEN, UK Biobank, and All of Us have started to fill this gap. Their work has highlighted the significant diversity in T2DM genetic risk (Rao et al., 2017).

In this section, we will systematically examine major ancestry groups, focusing on the most influential T2DM-related genetic markers within each group. We will also look at findings from trans-ethnic studies, which reveal both common and unique aspects of diabetes genetics.

6.1 South Asian genetic susceptibility

South Asians have some of the highest T2DM rates globally, often developing the disease at younger ages and lower body mass indices (BMI) compared to Europeans (Anjana et al., 2017). This pattern, sometimes called the "South Asian metabolic profile," appears to stem from genetic factors, prenatal influences, and environmental aspects.

6.1.1 Heightened genetic risk at lower adiposity

Genome-wide association studies (GWAS) in Indian, Pakistani, Bangladeshi, and Sri Lankan populations show that South Asians experience stronger effects at several β-cell-related genetic markers, indicating a primary issue with insulin secretion (Radha et al., 2011).

6.1.2 HNF4A and HNF1A variants

These variants are more strongly associated with South Asians than with Europeans and affect liver glucose production and β-cell gene expression (Im et al., 2024).

6.1.3 RREB1 (Ras-responsive element binding protein 1)

Rare coding variants found through exome sequencing significantly impact early-onset diabetes (Mahajan et al., 2018).

6.1.4 GRB14/COBLL1

This locus influences insulin signaling in fat tissue and shows a stronger effect size in South Asian and Middle Eastern populations (Kooner et al., 2011).

6.1.5 TMEM163 and ADCY5

These variants are more common and more closely linked to higher blood sugar levels in South Asians (Rees et al., 2011).

6.1.6 Distinct physiological patterns

Reduced β-cell capacity from early life. Increased abdominal fat, even at normal BMI. Higher levels of circulating non-esterified fatty acids (NEFAs). Greater vulnerability to glucotoxicity (Unnikrishnan et al., 2014).

Overall, these genetic and metabolic traits help explain why lifestyle changes often do not adequately reduce diabetes risk in this population.

6.2 East Asian genetic profiles

East Asian groups, including Chinese, Japanese, and Koreans, showcase a unique T2DM phenotype. This is marked by primary β-cell dysfunction, moderate obesity, and significant increases in blood sugar after meals (Yabe & Seino, 2016). T2DM tends to occur at lower BMI thresholds than in Europeans, indicating a greater genetic sensitivity to weight.

6.2.1 PAX4 variants

Missense variants like R192H and R192S are more frequent in East Asians and notably raise T2DM risk by affecting β-cell development (Kwak et al., 2018).

6.2.2 KCNQ1 locus

This is one of the most important East Asian-specific T2DM genetic markers, affecting insulin secretion and showing weaker effects in Europeans (Yasuda et al., 2008).

6.2.3 UBE2E2

This gene, found in Japanese studies, is linked to proinsulin processing and insulin release (Xu et al., 2016).

6.2.4 *GLIS3 and IDE-KIF11-HHEX regions*

These regions have higher allele frequencies or stronger connections in East Asians (Qian et al., 2012).

6.2.5 *ALDH2 variants (rs671)*

These are common in East Asians but nearly nonexistent in Europeans. They affect alcohol metabolism, weight, and T2DM risk. There is a rapid decline in β-cell function as individuals age, leading to high rates of isolated postprandial hyperglycemia. Additionally, there is an increased susceptibility to low-grade fat toxicity, even at lower BMI levels. These genetic and physiological traits help explain the effectiveness of incretin-based treatments in East Asian populations (Liu et al., 2024).

6.2.6 *Unique metabolic characteristics*

Rapid decline in β-cell function with age, with High rates of isolated postprandial high blood sugar, while increased susceptibility to low-grade fat toxicity, even at lower BMI.

These genetic and physiological traits help explain the effectiveness of incretin-based treatments in East Asian populations.

6.3 African and African-ancestry populations

African and African-ancestry groups, including African Americans and Afro-Caribbeans, have been historically underrepresented in genetic studies. However, available data show unique patterns reflecting both high genetic diversity and complex population histories (Atkinson et al., 2022).

6.3.1 *TCF7L2*

The rs7903146 variant shows some of the highest global effect sizes in African ancestry groups, significantly contributing to overall genetic risk (Helgason et al., 2007).

6.3.2 *APOL1 variants*

Though mainly tied to kidney disease, these variants also affect diabetes complications indirectly (Singhal & Skorecki, 2025).

6.3.3 *Insulin resistance physiology*

African ancestry groups generally have less visceral fat but greater insulin resistance at any BMI. Researchers are still exploring genetic factors, with INSR and IRS1 pathway variants receiving particular attention (Tan et al., 2015).

6.3.4 *Novel rare variants*

Advanced sequencing has revealed significant variants in genes like ZRANB3, a DNA repair gene associated with β-cell survival (Adeyemo et al., 2019).

6.3.5 Beta-cell secretion patterns

Compared to Europeans, individuals of African descent often show a stronger acute insulin response to glucose, possibly reflecting adaptations to ancestral diets (Keller et al., 2008).

Despite their limited representation in past studies, ongoing large-scale cohort research is set to uncover significant new findings in these groups.

7. Environmental and Lifestyle modifiers of genetic risk in Type 2 diabetes mellitus

7.1 Diet, obesity, and metabolic stress

For instance, certain anti-diabetic medications, like insulin, have been observed to enhance body weight, whereas anti-obesity medications may also have certain beneficial effects against diabetes. Surgery, particularly bariatric surgery, is more successful in treating obesity and type 2 diabetes. Further clinical and experimental research on the pathophysiology of these two diseases is necessary to enhance the effectiveness and safety of the current and novel therapies, in addition to ensuring that patients can take advantage of all current diagnostic and therapeutic approaches (Ruze et al., 2023).

7.1.1 Nutritional excess and insulin resistance

Genetic predisposition alone cannot account for the swift global rise in type 2 diabetes mellitus (T2DM). Environmental factors and lifestyle choices, instead, significantly influence whether genetic risks manifest clinically.

Increasing evidence highlights how diet, physical activity, obesity, socioeconomic factors, environmental pollutants, and psychological stress interact with genetic variants, affecting metabolic outcomes through both direct physiological effects and epigenetic modifications (Młynarska et al., 2025; Rönn & Ling, 2015).

Diet impacts T2DM risk not just by influencing energy balance but also by modifying the molecular pathways related to insulin signaling, fat metabolism, and β-cell function. Diets rich in saturated fats, refined carbohydrates, and sugary beverages contribute to insulin resistance through increased fat accumulation in undesired areas, oxidative stress, and low-grade inflammation. These effects are particularly pronounced in individuals with high-risk genetic variants such as PPARG Pro12Ala, FTO, and TCF7L2 (Hu, 2011; Omer et al., 2022; Petroni et al., 2021; Singh et al., 2024), which is summarized in Fig. 2.10.

For instance, individuals carrying the TCF7L2 rs7903146 risk variant experience reduced insulin secretion and diminished incretin responsiveness, especially when following a high-carbohydrate diet (Fry et al., 2022). This interaction of genetics and diet underscores the importance of moving away from universal dietary recommendations toward personalized nutrition approaches that account for individual genetic risks (Zeevi et al., 2015).

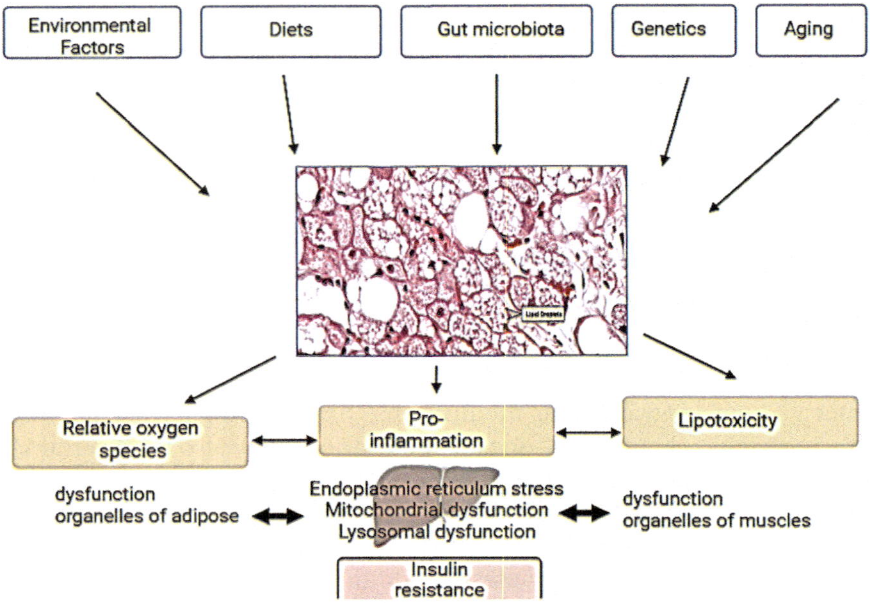

FIGURE 2.10 Role of various factors affecting T2DM.

7.1.2 Obesity as an Amplifier of genetic susceptibility

Obesity greatly enhances genetic risk rather than serving as a distinct factor. The expansion of fat tissue results in larger fat cells, immune cell infiltration, chronic inflammation, and toxic cellular stress, all of which exacerbate insulin resistance and β-cell dysfunction. These detrimental processes heighten the metabolic effects of risk variants located in genes such as IRS1, GCKR, SLC30A8, and FTO (Locke et al., 2015).

Importantly, for FTO, recognized as one of the most significant obesity-related genes, individuals with a body mass index (BMI) exceeding 30 kg/m^2 are at a significantly increased risk for developing T2DM compared to lean individuals with the same genotype (Khera et al., 2019). This relationship illustrates how obesity is a modifiable factor that can either exacerbate or mitigate inherited risk.

7.1.3 Dietary composition and gene-specific responses

The influence of diet on metabolism is heavily reliant on its composition and an individual's genetic profile. Diets abundant in fiber, whole grains, healthy fats, and plant-based foods—such as the Mediterranean diet—have been shown to lessen the detrimental effects of T2DM risk alleles (Ortega et al., 2017; Thomas et al., 2023).

For example, monounsaturated fatty acids improve insulin sensitivity and may help alleviate the negative metabolic consequences associated with the PPARG Pro12Ala variant. Similarly, individuals with risk variants in GIPR demonstrate increased insulin and incretin responses after consuming high-fat meals, indicating a need to adjust fat intake based on genetic backgrounds (He, 2009; Ortega et al., 2017). These findings reinforce the case for dietary interventions that consider genetic factors.

7.2 Physical activity and energy balance

7.2.1 Exercise as a buffer against genetic risk

Engaging in physical activity is one of the most effective non-pharmaceutical approaches to mitigate genetic susceptibilities related to type 2 diabetes mellitus (T2DM). Extensive research indicates that regular moderate-to-vigorous exercise can reduce the expression of T2DM risk alleles by approximately 40%–60% (Rung et al., 2009).

Genetic variants in FTO, IRS1, and TCF7L2 exhibit much weaker associations with insulin resistance, obesity, and elevated blood glucose levels among those who engage in physical activity. This implies that lifestyle decisions can have a greater impact than genetic predispositions (Loos & Yeo, 2014). Such findings reinforce public health initiatives that encourage physical activity, particularly for individuals predisposed to T2DM.

7.2.2 Mechanisms of gene-exercise interaction

Exercise enhances metabolic health through a range of biological mechanisms, many of which relate to genes implicated in T2DM. Physical activity increases mitochondrial generation, promotes glucose absorption via GLUT4 translocation, reduces fat accumulation in the liver, and activates AMP-activated protein kinase (AMPK) signaling (Richter & Hargreaves, 2013).

Individuals with risk alleles in PPARGC1A, a critical regulator of mitochondrial functionality, appear to experience significant metabolic benefits from aerobic exercise. This includes enhanced insulin sensitivity and improved oxidative capacity (Ling et al., 2007). These interactions between genes and exercise illustrate the potential advantages of tailored exercise regimens.

7.2.3 Sedentary behavior and risk enhancement

Conversely, prolonged sedentary behavior elevates post-meal glucose and insulin levels, even when accounting for overall physical activity levels. Extended periods of sitting exacerbate metabolic problems in those with gene variants that influence liver glucose production and circadian rhythms, such as GCKR and MTNR1B (Dong et al., 2024; Fritschi et al., 2016). These findings emphasize the importance of reducing sedentary time in addition to promoting physical activity.

7.3 Socioeconomic, cultural, and environmental modifiers

7.3.1 Socioeconomic status and metabolic gene expression

Socioeconomic status (SES) greatly impacts genetic risk, though its effects are often overlooked. Limited availability of nutritious foods, heightened stress levels, restricted access to healthcare, and lower levels of health literacy can all enhance the expression of genetic susceptibility (Stringhini et al., 2017).

Studies indicate that individuals with a high polygenic risk for T2DM face significantly higher rates of the disease in low SES environments compared to genetically similar individuals living in higher SES areas (Cromer et al., 2023). These findings underscore how social contexts can influence the manifestation of genetic risk within the body.

7.3.2 Urbanization and lifestyle changes

Rapid urban development has produced significant shifts in lifestyle, particularly in regions like South Asia, the Middle East, and sub-Saharan Africa. Decreased levels of physical activity, increased consumption of calorie-dense foods, and altered sleep patterns interact with obesity- and insulin resistance-related genes such as TMEM18, MC4R, and ADIPOQ. These elements accelerate the incidence of T2DM within these populations (Assah et al., 2011; Popkin, 2015).

7.3.3 Environmental exposures and endocrine disruptors

Environmental contaminants, including persistent organic pollutants (POPs), bisphenol A (BPA), and fine particulate matter, disrupt insulin signaling, mitochondrial performance, and inflammatory pathways. Genetic variations in detoxification and metabolism genes, including GSTM1 and CYP1A1, can alter individual responses to these exposures (Jaskulak et al., 2025; Manfredi et al., 2007).

Furthermore, air pollution has been associated with exacerbating the diabetogenic impacts of inflammatory gene variants, particularly those in IL6 and TNF, linking environmental exposures to gene-driven metabolic inflammation (Panasevich et al., 2013).

7.3.4 Psychosocial stress and neuroendocrine interactions

Chronic psychosocial stress stimulates the hypothalamic–pituitary–adrenal (HPA) axis, resulting in sustained increases in cortisol and catecholamines. These hormonal fluctuations contribute to abdominal fat accumulation, enhanced glucose production in the liver, and insulin resistance. Individuals carrying variants in NR3C1 and other stress-response genes may be particularly vulnerable to these effects (McEwen, 2007).

7.4 Epigenetic consequences of environmental exposures

Epigenetics is the scientific investigation in which the environment affects the genome functions instead of altering its sequence (Kaleem, Perwaiz, et al., 2021, 2022). Although they are functionally significant, epigenetic modifications are (often reversible) alterations of the genome (chromatin) that have no influence on the DNA's nucleotide sequence. These include DNA methylation, and Histone alterations along with micro-RNA and post-Translation modification (Chunarkar-patil et al., 2024; Mijač et al., 2024).

7.4.1 DNA methylation links between lifestyle and metabolic disease

Our environment leaves lasting molecular marks that can influence disease risk long-term. Lifestyle factors can change DNA methylation at key T2DM-related sites, including PPARGC1A, KCNQ1, and H19 (Dayeh et al., 2014). Obesity, in particular, causes methylation changes in fat tissue that impede insulin signaling and β-cell function, creating a direct link between lifestyle and gene activity (Parrillo et al., 2019).

7.4.2 Nutritional modulation of epigenetic signatures

The foods we eat can either support or harm our metabolic health at the epigenetic level. Dietary fiber, polyphenols, and omega-3 fatty acids have been shown to positively affect methylation and histone acetylation in genes linked to inflammation and glucose metabolism (Milagro et al., 2013). In contrast, high-fat diets can cause chromatin changes that promote fat production and liver fat buildup.

7.4.3 Early-life Programming and fetal exposure

The roots of T2DM risk can begin before birth. Maternal obesity, gestational diabetes, and undernutrition during pregnancy can cause lasting epigenetic changes that affect a person's risk for metabolic disease throughout their life. Historical events, like the Dutch Hunger Winter, show this clearly: individuals exposed to famine in the womb have lower methylation at IGF2 and are more likely to have metabolic disorders as adults (Laker et al., 2013).

7.4.4 Intergenerational transmission of metabolic risk

Remarkably, epigenetic changes caused by parental high blood sugar and obesity can pass down to future generations without changing the DNA sequence (Lillycrop & Burdge, 2012). Animal studies have confirmed that changes in sperm methylation patterns related to metabolic genes can increase risk, highlighting the lasting impact of environmental exposures.

In summary, genetic predisposition alone cannot explain the global trends in type 2 diabetes mellitus. The interplay between risk alleles and environmental factors—ranging from diet and obesity to inactivity, pollutants, and stress—determines whether genetic susceptibility leads to disease. Epigenetic mechanisms play a crucial role in translating environmental influences into long-term metabolic consequences. Understanding these interactions not only enhances our grasp of T2DM's complexity but also provides the tools to intervene more powerfully, allowing for prevention efforts even among those at the highest genetic risk.

8. Epigenetic regulation in Type 2 diabetes mellitus (T2DM)

Epigenetic regulation plays a key role in our understanding of Type 2 Diabetes Mellitus (T2DM). It helps explain how environmental and lifestyle factors can affect disease risk, even among people with similar genetic backgrounds. These heritable but reversible changes to chromatin structure do not alter the DNA sequence, yet they significantly influence which genes are active and when. Research indicates that interactions among our environment, aging, diet, and developmental exposures can leave unique epigenetic marks. These marks can lead to very different metabolic outcomes (Khalaf et al., 2021).

Epigenetic dysregulation has become a crucial factor linking environmental stressors to problems like impaired pancreatic β-cell function, insulin resistance, and overall metabolic dysfunction. The changing nature of these modifications connects our genetic traits to the actual development and progression of T2DM (Dayeh & Ling, 2015), given in Fig. 2.11.

8.1 DNA methylation patterns

8.1.1 Principles of methylation and metabolic Relevance

DNA methylation predominantly occurs at cytosine residues within CpG dinucleotides and plays a crucial role in regulating gene expression (Kaleem, Perwaiz, et al., 2021; Kaleem, Azmi, et al., 2025). In metabolic tissues such as pancreatic islets, liver, adipose tissue, and skeletal muscle, particular methylation patterns are essential for sustaining glucose regulation, fat metabolism, and mitochondrial function (Volkmar et al., 2012).

Abnormalities in methylation can inappropriately inhibit or activate genes, leading to decreased insulin secretion, impaired mitochondrial function, disrupted fat cell formation, and increased glucose output from the liver. Collectively, these molecular alterations contribute to insulin resistance and β-cell dysfunction, which are significant characteristics of type 2 diabetes (T2DM) (Xiao Liang, 2024), summarized in Fig. 2.12.

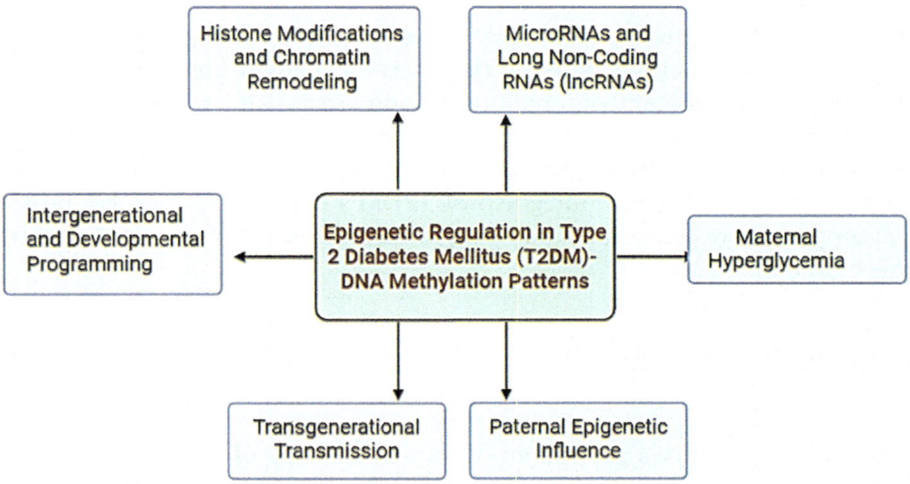

FIGURE 2.11 Role of epigenetic regulation in T2DM.

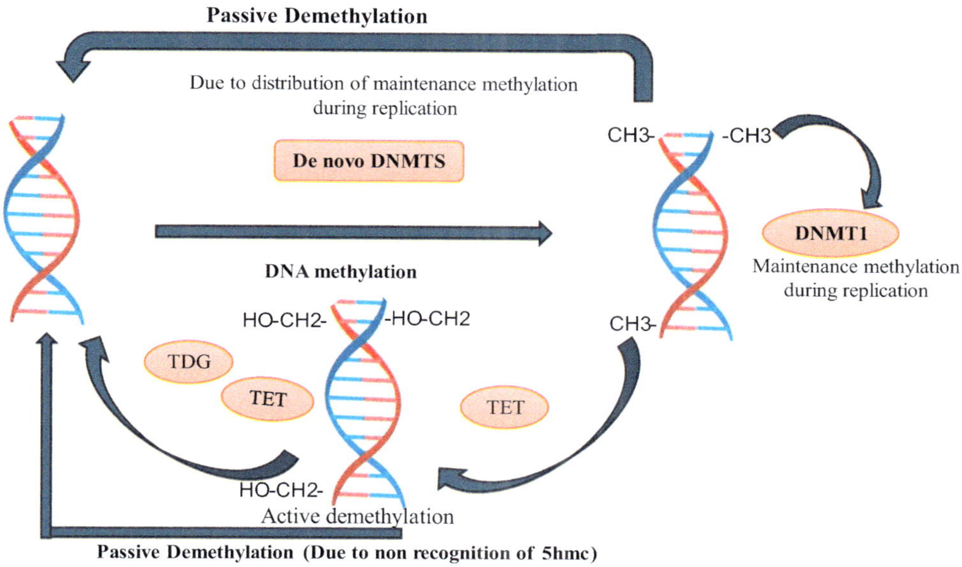

FIGURE 2.12 Role of DNA methylation in T2DM.

8.1.2 Methylation changes in pancreatic β-cells

Research on human pancreatic islets has revealed notable differences in methylation between individuals with type 2 diabetes mellitus (T2DM) and those with normal glucose levels. Vital genes related to β-cell identity and insulin synthesis, including PDX1, NKX6-1, MAFA, and INS, exhibit modified methylation in islets from diabetic patients (Volkmar et al., 2012).

Increased methylation of the PDX1 promoter reduces its transcriptional activity, leading to compromised β-cell development and lower insulin production (Dayeh et al., 2014). Moreover, prolonged elevated blood sugar levels trigger additional methylation alterations in enhancer regions that regulate insulin secretion. This results in a cycle where metabolic stress exacerbates the epigenetic decline in β-cell functionality (El-Osta et al., 2008).

8.1.3 Methylation and insulin resistance

Skeletal muscle, the primary site for insulin-stimulated glucose uptake, exhibits changes in the methylation of genes that govern mitochondrial development and energy metabolism, such as PPARGC1A, MEF2A, and NDUFB6 (Ling et al., 2007). Reduced expression of these genes leads to insufficient fat oxidation and insulin resistance.

In adipose tissue, the methylation alterations associated with obesity affect inflammatory genes like TNF and IL6, in addition to genes related to adipokines such as ADIPOQ and LEP. These alterations contribute to a pro-inflammatory milieu that exacerbates overall insulin resistance (Kirchner et al., 2013).

8.1.4 Blood-based methylation biomarkers

Recent extensive studies have identified consistent methylation markers in peripheral blood that can indicate the risk of developing T2DM. Changes in methylation at CpG sites within genes such as ABCG1, PHOSPHO1, SREBF1, and TXNIP are linked to new diabetes cases, independent of traditional risk factors (Nadiger et al., 2024).

Although blood-based markers may not fully reflect tissue-specific epigenetic changes, they provide a convenient and less invasive method for early risk assessment and population screening Fig. 2.13.

8.2 Histone Modifications and Chromatin Remodeling

8.2.1 Histone acetylation and gene activation

Histone acetylation loosens the structure of chromatin by neutralizing the positive charges present on histone tails, facilitating the access of transcription factors to the DNA (Kaleem, Alhosin, et al., 2021). In pancreatic β-cells, a proper balance between histone acetyltransferases (HATs) and histone deacetylases (HDACs) is essential for the expression of genes that regulate insulin production, vesicle trafficking, and glucose sensing (van Arensbergen et al., 2013). Metabolic stressors such as prolonged high blood sugar levels and elevated free fatty acids disrupt histone acetylation in the enhancer regions of β-cell-specific genes. This disturbance negatively impacts the transcriptional networks critical for insulin secretion and the survival of β-cells (Ahmed et al., 2017).

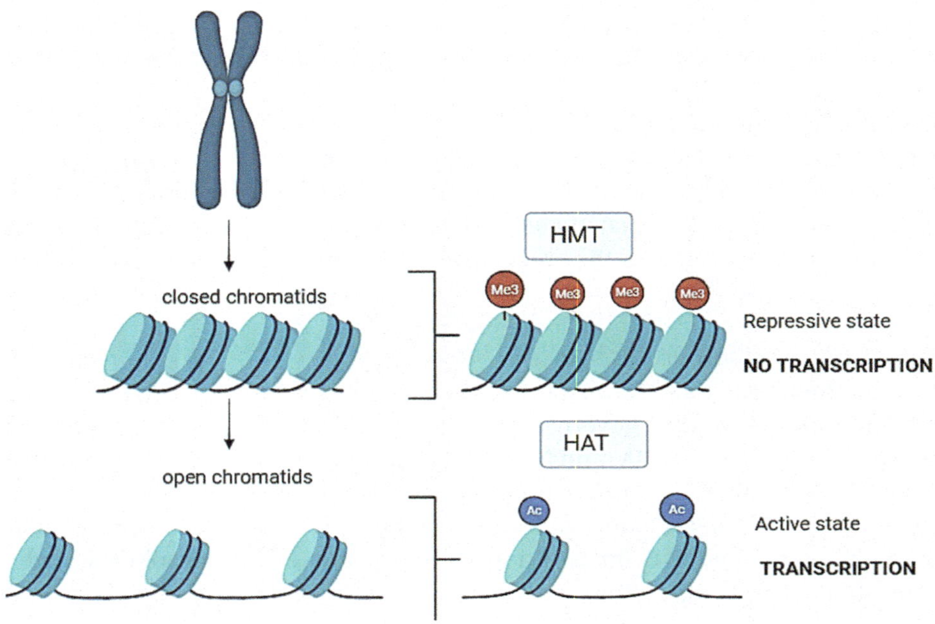

FIGURE 2.13 Histone modifications and chromatin remodeling in T2DM.

8.2.2 Histone methylation and metabolic repression

Histone methylation has the potential to either promote or inhibit transcription, influenced by the specific residue modified and the extent of methylation. Repressive modifications such as H3K9me2 and H3K27me3 silence genes that are important for mitochondrial functions, energy production, and insulin signaling (Ravassard et al., 2011). In adipose tissue, obesity induces histone alterations that increase the expression of pro-inflammatory genes while suppressing pathways associated with insulin sensitivity. This phenomenon contributes to overarching metabolic disorders (Steger et al., 2010).

8.2.3 Chromatin remodeling complexes

ATP-dependent chromatin remodeling complexes, including the SWI/SNF family, reposition nucleosomes to manage gene accessibility. Key components like BRG1 play a crucial role in β-cell growth, responsiveness to glucose, and defense against oxidative stress (McDonnell et al., 2016). Interfering with these remodeling mechanisms diminishes the adaptability of β-cells to metabolic stress, rendering them more susceptible to damage resulting from high glucose and fatty acids, summarized in Fig. 2.12.

8.3 MicroRNAs and long non-coding RNAs (lncRNAs)

8.3.1 MicroRNAs in β-cell differentiation and function

MicroRNAs (miRNAs) are brief non-coding RNAs that control gene expression post-transcriptionally (Kaleem et al., 2024). They target mRNA molecules for degradation or inhibit their translation. Within pancreatic β-cells, miRNAs play a vital role in differentiation, insulin synthesis, and insulin secretion capabilities. For example, miR-375 is one of the most prevalent miRNAs observed in islets. It regulates β-cell mass and the release of insulin.

Disruption of this miRNA leads to elevated blood glucose levels and a reduction in β-cell numbers (Poy et al., 2004). In islets affected by diabetes, excessive levels of miR-29 and miR-34a impair insulin secretion and promote cell death when exposed to detrimental glucose and fatty acid conditions.

8.3.2 miRNAs and insulin resistance

In the context of obesity and Type 2 diabetes, alterations in miRNA expression within adipose tissue and the liver contribute to insulin resistance. miR-27a, miR-103/107, and miR-143 play significant roles in the development of adipocytes, lipid metabolism, and insulin responsiveness (Jordan et al., 2011). In detail, miR-103/107 specifically targets caveolin-1, an essential component of insulin receptor signaling, which diminishes insulin sensitivity in the liver and adipose tissues (Trajkovski et al., 2011).

8.3.3 Long non-coding RNAs in metabolic regulation

Long non-coding RNAs (lncRNAs) influence chromatin architecture, transcriptional activity, and RNA stability. In Type 2 diabetes, lncRNAs such as H19 and MEG3 affect pancreatic development, β-cell proliferation, and insulin secretion (López–Noriega & Rutter, 2021).

For instance, MEG3 decreases insulin production by activating p53-dependent apoptotic pathways. Conversely, H19 is associated with β-cell proliferation and glucose regulation (Zhu et al., 2016). Additionally, outside of the pancreatic environment, lncRNAs also affect inflammatory responses and lipid regulation in the liver and adipose tissue, summarized in Fig. 2.14.

8.4 Intergenerational and developmental programming

8.4.1 The fetal origins of adult disease hypothesis

The "fetal origins of adult disease," suggests that negative conditions in the womb can lead to chronic diseases like T2DM later in life. Low birth weight—a common sign of poor nutrition in the womb—has been linked to smaller β-cell mass and a greater risk of developing T2DM as an adult (Guo et al., 2022).

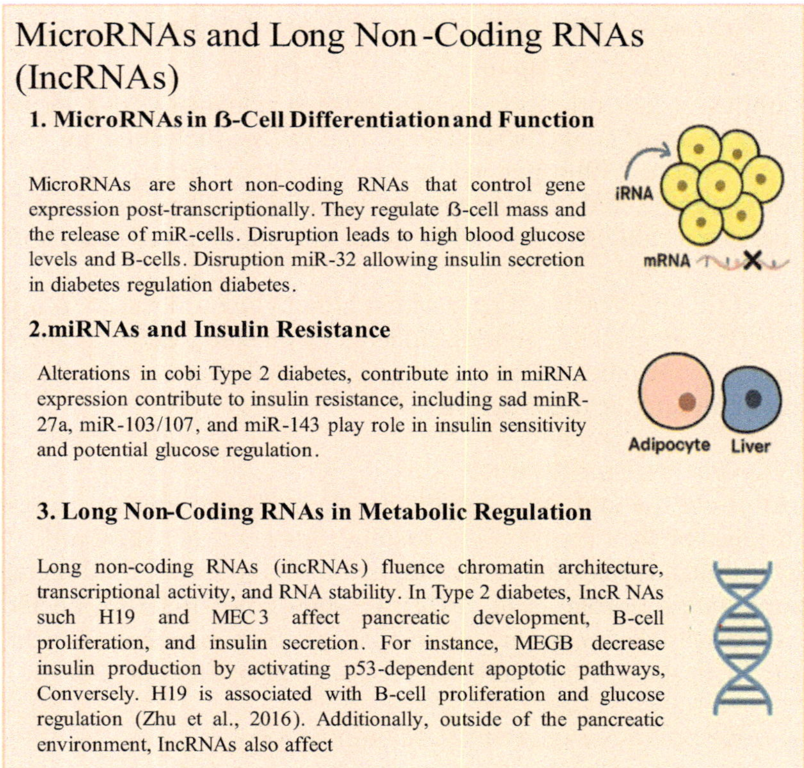

FIGURE 2.14 MicroRNAs and long non-coding RNAs (lncRNAs) functions (Zhu et al., 2016).

8.4.2 Maternal hyperglycemia and epigenetic inheritance

A mother's health during pregnancy creates lasting effects. Maternal obesity and gestational diabetes expose the growing fetus to high levels of glucose and fats, changing the methylation of key genes such as LEP, ABCG1, and MEG3 (Li, 2022). These epigenetic changes may last into adulthood, increasing the offspring's risk of metabolic disease for their lifetime.

8.4.3 Paternal epigenetic influence

Fathers also play a role in shaping their children's metabolic future. Animal studies show that a father's high-fat diet can change sperm methylation patterns in genes related to metabolism, leading to impaired glucose tolerance in the next generation (Ng et al., 2009).

8.4.4 Transgenerational transmission

Interestingly, some epigenetic marks seem to be passed down beyond the directly exposed generation, suggesting the possibility of inheriting metabolic traits across generations. While evidence in humans is still developing, studies of cohorts affected by historical famines indicate that grandchildren of individuals facing severe nutritional deprivation may face higher metabolic risks (Painter et al., 2008).

Epigenetic regulation links our environment to our genes, shaping the risk and progression of T2DM. Through processes like DNA methylation, histone modifications, and actions of non-coding RNAs, these mechanisms control insulin secretion, sensitivity, fat cell growth, and inflammation. Remarkably, epigenetic changes can begin in fetal development and may even pass through generations. This highlights the urgent need for interventions throughout life, including preconception care, to break the cycle of metabolic disease and encourage healthier futures (Stančáková & Laakso, 2016).

9. Polygenic risk scores (PRS): A new frontier in understanding Type 2 diabetes risk

Imagine looking at your genetic makeup to see your personal risk for developing type 2 diabetes mellitus (T2DM). This is what polygenic risk scores (PRS) aim to do. By combining the small effects of many common genetic variants, PRS gives an individual's inherited risk for T2DM a single, useful number. Unlike monogenic diabetes, where one gene can greatly change disease risk, T2DM results from the combined influence of hundreds of genetic locations. Each contributes a small effect (Vujkovic et al., 2020). PRS captures this overall genetic impact. It allows clinicians and researchers to categorize individuals by lifetime risk, chances of early onset, and metabolic changes (Khera et al., 2018). As genome-wide association studies (GWAS) and multi-ancestry sequencing continue to identify new risk factors, PRS is quickly becoming essential for precision prevention. However, challenges remain, especially in ensuring fair and meaningful use across different populations which is summarized in Table 2.4.

Table 2.4 Construction methods and advantages.

Step/Method	Description	Key notes/Advantages	References
SNP selection & weighting	Choose tens to hundreds of thousands of SNPs; assign weights based on GWAS β-coefficients	Newer models include lower-impact variants to capture more heritability	Chatterjee et al. (2016)
Clumping & thresholding (C + T)	Removes related SNPs and applies *P*-value cut-offs	Selects most informative variants; simple and widely used	Venkat et al. (2025)
Bayesian models (LDpred, PRS-CS)	Accounts for linkage disequilibrium (LD) to estimate SNP effects	More precise SNP effect sizes; improves prediction	Vilhjálmsson et al. (2015)
Machine learning frameworks	Elastic net regression, gradient boosting, mixed models	Captures nonlinear interactions; enhances predictive accuracy	Mak et al. (2017)
Multi-ancestry reference panels	Incorporates diverse population data for LD estimation	Improves PRS applicability across populations	Martin et al. (2019)

9.1 Construction and statistical foundations

9.2 Clinical utility and predictive performance

9.2.1 Risk stratification

The strength of PRS is its ability to categorize individuals by their risk. Those with high PRS can have a two-to fourfold increase in lifetime risk of developing T2DM compared to those with the lowest scores (Khera et al., 2018). This categorization is particularly useful for identifying young adults at higher risk—individuals who might not yet show obesity or high blood sugar but would benefit from early intervention.

9.2.2 Prediction of early-onset diabetes

Early-onset T2DM is usually more influenced by genetics and has a worse cardiometabolic outlook. High PRS not only predicts an earlier onset but also indicates a quicker decline in β-cell function (Suzuki et al., 2024). In some studies, PRS has done better than traditional measurements in predicting early-onset disease.

9.2.3 Integration with family history and clinical markers

Interestingly, PRS offers risk information that stands apart from family history, capturing inherited factors that traditional family analysis might miss (Do et al., 2013). When PRS is paired with clinical markers like BMI, fasting glucose, HbA1c, and lifestyle factors, predictive models become significantly stronger (Meigs et al., 2000).

9.2.4 Use in gestational diabetes prediction

PRS is also useful in predicting gestational diabetes mellitus (GDM). Women with high T2DM PRS are more likely to develop GDM, showing a shared metabolic background (Kwak et al., 2012). These women often show impaired β-cell function during pregnancy, highlighting the connections between genetic risk across diabetes types.

9.3 Limitations in diverse populations

9.3.1 Reduced accuracy outside european ancestry

One major drawback of current PRS models is their lack of accuracy in non-European populations. Since most GWAS data come from European groups, PRS often performs poorly for African, South Asian, and Latino individuals (Martin et al., 2019). Differences in LD structure, allele frequencies, and environmental factors limit the general applicability of these scores.

9.3.2 Gene–environment heterogeneity

PRS based on European data often do not account for the complex gene–environment interactions found in other populations. For instance, South Asians have stronger gene–adiposity interactions that can greatly change PRS risk estimates compared to Europeans (Geng & Huang, 2020).

9.3.3 Socioeconomic and environmental Confounding

Environmental factors—like food availability, chronic stress, pollution, and cultural norms—can either conceal or exaggerate genetic risk. In areas where environmental conditions vary widely, the predictive power of PRS may be weakened (Hindorff et al., 2018).

9.3.4 The imperative for multi-ethnic reference Panels

To promote fairness in PRS application, the research must include multi-ancestry meta-analyses, diverse LD reference sets, and cross-ethnic mapping. Without broad representation, the understanding of global T2DM risk will remain incomplete (Fatumo et al., 2022a).

9.4 Integration with traditional risk factors

9.4.1 PRS combined with lifestyle factors

The connection between genetics and lifestyle is clear. When PRS is combined with diet, exercise, obesity metrics, and socioeconomic status, risk prediction becomes much more accurate (Hüls et al., 2021; Meigs et al., 2000). Notably, people with high genetic risk gain the most significant benefit from lifestyle changes.

9.4.2 PRS and metabolic biomarkers

Adding metabolic biomarkers—such as fasting insulin, triglycerides, HDL cholesterol, and C-reactive protein—further enhances prediction models and may help identify distinct pathways related to T2DM (Mukherjee & Im, 2025).

9.4.3 Integration with imaging and Anthropometry

Advanced imaging techniques, including liver fat measurement, visceral fat assessment, and pancreatic volume assessment, can improve risk prediction when combined with PRS. This is particularly valuable for detecting early-onset or lean T2DM when traditional risk factors may not be as useful (Lim et al., 2011).

9.4.4 Clinical feasibility

Even with its potential, the broad use of PRS in clinical settings depends on several factors: standardized analysis methods, validated risk thresholds, affordable genetic testing, and clear guidelines for patient communication (Liao et al., 2025). Ethical questions and challenges in interpretation also need careful consideration before PRS can become part of routine care.

Polygenic risk scoring is leading a shift in diabetes risk assessment. By bringing together information from hundreds of common—and increasingly rare—genetic variants, PRS presents unmatched opportunities for risk categorization, early detection, and a better understanding of the complex nature of T2DM development. However, to realize its full potential, the field must address ongoing challenges in diverse populations and work for global representation in genomics. Ultimately, combining PRS with lifestyle, biomarkers, imaging, and clinical data will be key to translating this powerful tool into precision medicine (Ashenhurst et al., 2022).

10. Translational and clinical implications

Recent advances in genomics, including genome-wide association studies (GWAS), sequencing, multi-omics approaches, and large-scale biobank analyses, are changing how we manage type 2 diabetes mellitus (T2DM). Though T2DM is complex and affected by lifestyle factors, using genetic data is starting to improve risk predictions, personalize treatment choices, inform prevention strategies, and open new pathways for drug development (Tian et al., 2025). Despite the challenges of translating genomic insights into practical clinical tools, ongoing technological and methodological advancements are helping connect genetic research with everyday medical practice.

10.1 Pharmacogenomics in T2DM therapy

Pharmacogenomics looks at how genetic differences affect a person's response to medications, including how drugs are processed and the risk of side effects. Because T2DM shows a wide range of symptoms, using genetic markers could help optimize and tailor treatment plans (Pollastro et al., 2015).

10.1.1 Metformin transport and response

Metformin is the primary treatment for T2DM worldwide. Yet, about 30% of patients do not achieve good glycemic control. Variants in genes for organic cation transporters, especially SLC22A1 (OCT1), SLC22A2 (OCT2), and SLC47A1 (MATE1), significantly affect metformin's availability and uptake by the liver (Mato et al., 2018; Zhou et al., 2011). People with less active OCT1 variants usually have lower liver levels of metformin and a weaker glycemic response (Dujic et al., 2015). These insights highlight the potential for future personalized metformin dosing plans.

10.1.2 Sulfonylureas and β-cell gene variants

Sulfonylureas promote insulin release from pancreatic β-cells through KATP channels. Genetic variants in KCNJ11 and ABCC8, which code for these channel subunits, can change how individuals respond to the drug. Loss-of-function variants are often linked to increased sensitivity to sulfonylureas, suggesting a future for genotype-guided therapy with this medication type (Song et al., 2017).

10.1.3 Thiazolidinediones (TZDs) and PPARG

The PPARG Pro12Ala variant influences how patients respond to TZDs, with carriers of Ala12 showing stronger insulin-sensitizing effects. Considering the known side effects of TZDs, predictive biomarkers could help identify which patients are most likely to benefit from these drugs (Jang et al., 2023).

10.1.4 DPP-4 inhibitors and incretin genes

Variants in genes related to incretins, such as TCF7L2 and WFS1, can affect how β-cells respond and may change the effectiveness of DPP-4 inhibitors (Bhargave et al., 2022). Although these findings are still in early stages for clinical use, they hint at better-targeted incretin therapies (Zimdahl et al., 2014).

10.1.5 SGLT2 inhibitors and Renal glucose handling

Polymorphisms in SLC5A2, which encodes SGLT2, might affect how individuals respond to SGLT2 inhibitors, though clear clinical links are still being researched (Xu et al., 2023). As this research grows, pharmacogenomic approaches could help refine treatment, especially in varied patient populations, summarized in Table 2.5.

10.2 Personalized prevention strategies

10.2.1 Risk stratification using genetic information

Polygenic risk scores (PRS) combine the effects of many genetic variants to predict a person's risk of developing T2DM. Individuals with a high PRS are more likely to benefit

Table 2.5 Role of anti-diabetic drugs in targeting gene and their responses.

Drug class	Gene/Variant	Effect on drug response	References
Metformin	SLC22A1 (OCT1), SLC22A2 (OCT2), SLC47A1 (MATE1)	Variants reduce hepatic uptake of metformin → weaker glycemic response	Al-Eitan et al. (2019); Dujic et al. (2015)
Sulfonylureas	KCNJ11, ABCC8	Loss-of-function variants → increased drug sensitivity; affects insulin release from β-cells	Vedovato et al. (2024)
Thiazolidinediones (TZDs)	PPARG Pro12Ala	Ala12 carriers → stronger insulin-sensitizing response	Jang et al. (2023)
DPP-4 inhibitors	TCF7L2, WFS1	Variants affect β-cell response → may alter drug effectiveness	Bhargave et al. (2022)
SGLT2 inhibitors	SLC5A2	Polymorphisms may influence renal glucose excretion and response to therapy	Xu et al. (2023)

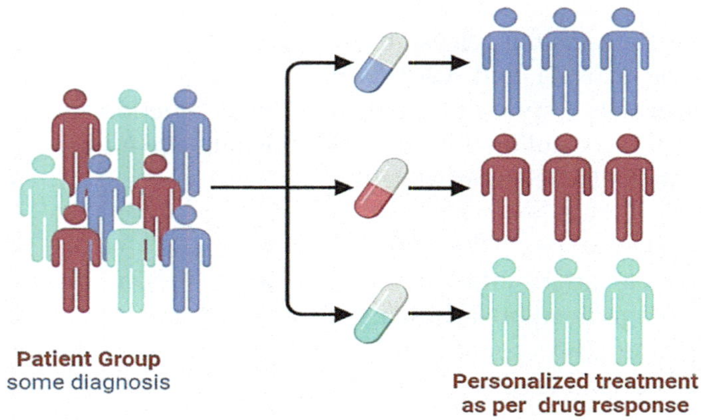

FIGURE 2.15 Personalized treatment in T2DM.

from early lifestyle changes like weight management, exercise, and dietary improvements (Liu et al., 2023). This approach encourages proactive screening and tailored prevention advice as indicated in Fig. 2.15.

10.2.2 Lifestyle modification tailored to genotype

New evidence indicates that some genetic profiles can affect how people react to dietary changes. For example, PPARG variants might influence responses to monounsaturated fats, while TCF7L2 variants interact with carbohydrate intake to impact blood sugar levels (Qi & Liang, 2010). Similarly, genetic variations, especially in genes like PPARGC1A, may determine how effective exercise interventions.

10.2.3 Population-specific prevention

Ethnic differences in insulin secretion and resistance require prevention strategies that respect cultural backgrounds. For instance, South Asian populations, who often face greater β-cell vulnerability and higher genetic risks, may need earlier and more aggressive interventions (Chambers et al., 2015).

10.3 Genetic counseling and ethical considerations

10.3.1 Communicating complex risk

Genetic counseling is vital for helping patients understand risk information and how it relates to lifestyle, environment, and social factors (Garg et al., 2025). Clear communication must explain the polygenic nature of T2DM and protect against misunderstanding risk scores.

10.3.2 Avoiding genetic determinism

An ongoing ethical issue is the false belief that genetic risk leads to certain disease. Counselors should stress that genetic predispositions can change—lifestyle interventions can significantly lower or even negate genetic risk for most people (Khera et al., 2018).

10.3.3 Equity and global genomic disparities

The dominance of European populations in genetic research risks widening gaps in prediction accuracy and clinical benefits. Ethical practices require more inclusive datasets, community involvement, and equal access to genetic testing (Hindorff et al., 2018).

10.3.4 Data privacy and genomic security

As genetic testing becomes more common, protecting genomic data is crucial. Data breaches can lead to discrimination or loss of personal freedom. Strong governance and strict adherence to data protection standards are necessary (Tavani & Moor, 2001), given in figure.

10.4 Emerging therapeutic targets from genetic discovery

10.4.1 β-cell transcriptional regulators

GWAS and sequencing have identified key transcription factors, like NKX6-1, HNF1A, HNF4A, and MAFA, as essential for β-cell identity and function (Morris et al., 2012). Aiming at these pathways through gene editing or small-molecule treatments could help preserve or restore β-cell health.

10.4.2 Incretin biology and intestinal gene networks

Variants in genes like GIPR and GLP1R have provided new chances for manipulating the incretin pathway. These findings have already spurred the development of new incretin-based treatments, including GLP-1 receptor agonists and dual agonists (Nauck & Meier, 2018).

10.4.3 Lipid metabolism and hepatic fat regulation

Genes linked to lipid metabolism, such as GCKR, PNPLA3, and TM6SF2, have shed light on the mechanisms behind liver fat accumulation and insulin resistance (Davis et al., 2010). Targeting these pathways could offer benefits beyond just controlling blood sugar.

10.4.4 Mitochondrial function and oxidative stress

Both rare and common genetic variants involve genes that manage mitochondrial functions, energy production, and defense against harmful molecules. New treatments aimed at improving mitochondrial quality control are currently in development (Hebert & Myatt, 2021).

10.4.5 Immune and inflammatory pathways

Studies on genes related to obesity and inflammation, such as IL6 and TNF, support exploring anti-inflammatory treatments. These could include macrophage modulators and cytokine inhibitors, which may provide new options for addressing T2DM (Donath, 2013).

The rapid growth in genetic discovery is reshaping the prevention and treatment of T2DM. Pharmacogenomics is creating new opportunities for personalized medication approaches, while polygenic risk scores and genetic markers are improving risk assessment and enabling earlier detection. However, successfully integrating these advances into clinical practice requires careful attention to ethical issues, including equity, effective communication, and strong data governance. Meanwhile, ongoing discovery of new genes continues to uncover targets for precision interventions that tackle the challenges of β-cell dysfunction and insulin resistance (Venkatachalapathy et al., 2021).

11. Future prospective

The ongoing merging of genomics, multi-omics, and data-driven technologies is changing how we understand Type 2 Diabetes Mellitus (T2DM). While the field has seen significant progress, many key questions remain unanswered. In the future, research must explore the biological mechanisms behind T2DM more deeply, improve predictive models, expand the diversity of genomic resources, and ensure clinical applications are guided by strong ethical principles. Progress in these areas will ultimately shape the success of precision medicine in diabetes care (Singh et al., 2024; Tian et al., 2025) Table 2.6.

11.1 Integrating multi-omics for systems-level understanding

11.1.1 Harmonizing genomics with other omics layers

A major challenge in T2DM research is combining different omics datasets, such as genomics, transcriptomics, epigenomics, proteomics, and metabolomics, into cohesive and meaningful models of disease biology. T2DM arises from complex interactions among β-cell dysfunction, insulin resistance, changes in fat tissue, inflammation, and environmental factors. Using just one omics approach gives a limited view of this complexity. Future studies should create advanced computational frameworks that can align these varied data streams into clear, causal networks, leading to a more complete understanding of disease mechanisms (Nafie et al., 2025).

Table 2.6 Role of multi-omics integration in T2DM.

Aspect	Key feature	References
Multi-omics integration	Combine genomics, transcriptomics, epigenomics, proteomics, and metabolomics for a systems-level view of T2DM	Li et al. (2025)
Temporal & spatial profiling	Longitudinal and single-cell/spatial analyses to track disease progression and cell interactions	Olaniru et al. (2023); Segerstolpe et al. (2016)
Functional validation	Use CRISPR, β-cell organoids, and iPSC-derived tissues to confirm gene/pathway roles	Dutta et al. (2017)

11.1.2 Temporal and spatial multi-omics

Most current omics datasets are cross-sectional, capturing only a moment in time. We need longitudinal multi-omics profiling to track molecular changes as individuals move from prediabetes to full diabetes. Such studies could clarify the sequence of harmful events and find early markers of disease onset. Additionally, techniques like single-cell and spatial transcriptomics can enhance our understanding of pancreatic islet structure and the complex interactions among different cell types (Song et al., 2025).

11.2 Expanding diversity in genomic research

11.2.1 Addressing eurocentric bias

A major limitation of current genomic research is the heavy focus on individuals of European ancestry, as over 80% of participants in genome-wide association studies (GWAS) belong to this group. This imbalance restricts the discovery of population-specific genetic variations and affects the accuracy of polygenic risk scores for non-European groups. It's urgent to include African, South Asian, Indigenous, Middle Eastern, and Latin American populations to ensure equitable scientific insights (Fatumo et al., 2022b).

11.3 Artificial intelligence and machine learning in T2DM genomics

11.3.1 AI-assisted variant interpretation

Deep learning models are increasingly capable of identifying important genetic variants based on their predicted regulatory functions, chromatin accessibility, and transcription factor binding. These tools will speed up the identification of causal genes and pathways in T2DM (Wesolowska-Andersen et al., 2020).

11.3.2 AI-driven precision therapeutics

Artificial intelligence (AI) systems that blend multi-omics data, electronic health records, and real-time glucose monitoring could suggest personalized treatment plans. In the future, these systems may even adjust medication doses on the fly based on a patient's metabolic profile. AI offers significant potential to improve diabetes care and save healthcare costs, but its effective application necessitates overcoming a number of obstacles, such as legal restrictions and guaranteeing fair access to technology. Therefore, it is especially important for physicians to use AI to simplify data management, accurately evaluate data, enhance clinical decision-making, and aid in therapy. In the coming years, we believe AI can anticipate a significant role in the medical field of diabetes, with prospective for the future (Ma, Zhang, et al., 2025).

11.3.3 Automated drug discovery

AI-driven protein modeling platforms, such as AlphaFold, along with ligand-receptor prediction tools, are set to speed up the discovery of new treatments targeting genetically validated pathways in T2DM (Jarallah et al., 2025).

11.4 Ethical and societal considerations

11.4.1 Fairness and accessibility

As genomics becomes more embedded in clinical practice, ensuring fair access to these advancements is critical. Without appropriate policy measures, there is a risk that precision medicine could worsen existing health inequities worldwide. Precision medicine for diabetes has gained attention due to the increasing diversity of genetic and electronic medical information among huge populations, which is an effective research tool (Floyd & Psaty, 2016).

11.4.2 Addressing genetic discrimination

Robust legal and ethical protections are needed to prevent the misuse of genetic risk information by insurers, employers, or other organizations. Openness in governance and building public trust will be vital for responsibly adopting genomic medicine (Hazin et al., 2013).

11.4.3 Cultural sensitivity and community engagement

Future research must emphasize culturally sensitive approaches, especially in low- and middle-income countries where diabetes rates are rapidly increasing. Involving communities in the research process will be crucial for making sure scientific advancements lead to real health benefits (Zehra et al., 2025).

Looking ahead, research in T2DM should focus on integrating multi-omics data, including diverse populations, improving predictive models, advancing gene-editing techniques, and applying artificial intelligence to personalized therapeutics. Achieving these goals will require strong ethical frameworks, international teamwork, and a commitment to fair clinical translation. Together, these efforts could change diabetes care, moving from reactive disease management to proactive, tailored prevention and treatment (Herder et al., 2025), summarized Table 2.5.

12. Conclusions

Over the past 20 years, advances in genetic and genomic research have transformed how we understand Type 2 Diabetes Mellitus (T2DM). This condition was once seen mainly as a metabolic disorder influenced by lifestyle choices. It is now recognized as a complex polygenic disease. This change reflects a deeper understanding of how genetic predisposition, environmental factors, and epigenetic modifications interact.

Achieving this vision will require ongoing interdisciplinary collaboration, a commitment to diversity in populations, and a focus on turning scientific breakthroughs into real health improvements. As the field progresses, genetic research in T2DM is positioned at the forefront of precision medicine, promising more effective, personalized, and fair solutions for one of the world's most common chronic diseases.

Abbreviations

AMPK AMP-activated Protein Kinase
CpG Cytosine-phosphate-Guanine
CPT1A Carnitine Palmitoyltransferase 1A
CV Cardiovascular
DPP-4 inhibitors Dipeptidyl Peptidase-4 Inhibitors
FTO Fat Mass and Obesity-Associated Gene
G6PC2 Glucose-6-Phosphatase Catalytic Subunit 2
GCK Glucokinase
GCKR Glucokinase Regulatory Protein
GDM Gestational Diabetes Mellitus
GIPR GIP Receptor
GLP1R Glucagon-Like Peptide-1 Receptor
GLUT4 Glucose Transporter Type 4
GWAS Genome-wide Association Studies
HATs Histone Acetyltransferases
HDACs Histone Deacetylases
HPA Hypothalamic–Pituitary–Adrenal
IRS1 Insulin Receptor Substrate 1
LD Linkage Disequilibrium
lncRNAs Long Non-coding RNAs
LPL Lipoprotein Lipase
miRNAs MicroRNAs
MODY Maturity-onset Diabetes of the Young
MTNR1B Melatonin Receptor 1B
NAFLD Non-alcoholic Fatty Liver Disease
NEFAs Non-esterified Fatty Acids
PDX1 Insulin Promoter Factor 1
PPARG Peroxisome Proliferator-Activated Receptor Gamma
PRS Polygenic Risk Scores
SES Socioeconomic Status
SGLT2 Sodium-Glucose Cotransporter 2
SLC5A2 Solute Carrier Family 5 Member 2
SNPs Single-nucleotide Polymorphisms
T2DM Type 2 Diabetes Mellitus
TZDs Thiazolidinediones
WFS1 Wolframin ER Transmembrane Protein

Acknowledgments

The authors extended their gratitude to for having an opportunity to work at Ravindra Gambhirrao Sapkal College of Pharmacy, Department of Pharmacology in Nashik (India).

Conflict of interest

The Authors declare no conflict of interest.

References

Abul-Husn, N. S., Cheng, X., Li, A. H., Xin, Y., Schurmann, C., Stevis, P., et al. (2018). A protein-truncating HSD17B13 variant and protection from chronic liver disease. *New England Journal of Medicine, 378.* https://doi.org/10.1056/nejmoa1712191

Adeyemo, A. A., Zaghloul, N. A., Chen, G., Doumatey, A. P., Leitch, C. C., Hostelley, T. L., et al. (2019). ZRANB3 is an african-specific type 2 diabetes locus associated with beta-cell mass and insulin response. *Nature Communications, 10.* https://doi.org/10.1038/s41467-019-10967-7

Ahmed, M., de Winther, M. P. J., & Van den Bossche, J. (2017). Epigenetic mechanisms of macrophage activation in type 2 diabetes. *Immunobiology, 222.* https://doi.org/10.1016/j.imbio.2016.08.011

Aigha, I. I., & Abdelalim, E. M. (2020). NKX6.1 transcription factor: A crucial regulator of pancreatic β cell development, identity, and proliferation. *Stem Cell Research & Therapy, 11.* https://doi.org/10.1186/s13287-020-01977-0

Al-Eitan, L. N., Almomani, B. A., Nassar, A. M., Elsaqa, B. Z., & Saadeh, N. A. (2019). Metformin pharmacogenetics: Effects of SLC22A1, SLC22A2, and SLC22A3 polymorphisms on glycemic control and HBA1c levels. *Journal of Personalized Medicine, 9.* https://doi.org/10.3390/jpm9010017

Altshuler, D., Hirschhorn, J. N., Klannemark, M., Lindgren, C. M., Vohl, M. C., Nemesh, J., et al. (2000). The common PPARγ Pro12Ala polymorphism is associated with decreased risk of type 2 diabetes. *Nature Genetics, 26.* https://doi.org/10.1038/79216

Anjana, R. M., Deepa, M., Pradeepa, R., Mahanta, J., Narain, K., Das, H. K., et al. (2017). Prevalence of diabetes and prediabetes in 15 states of India: Results from the ICMR–INDIAB population-based cross-sectional study. *Lancet Diabetes & Endocrinology, 5.* https://doi.org/10.1016/S2213-8587(17)30174-2

Anson, M., Henney, A. E., Edwards, H., Ibarburu, G. H., Mordi, I., Jaffar, S., et al. (2025). The rapidly increasing incidence of type 2 diabetes and macrovascular and microvascular complications disproportionately affects younger age groups: A decade of evidence from an international federated database. *Diabetes Research and Clinical Practice, 228.* https://doi.org/10.1016/j.diabres.2025.112431

Ashcroft, F. M., & Rorsman, P. (2012). Diabetes mellitus and the β cell: The last ten years. *Cell, 148.* https://doi.org/10.1016/j.cell.2012.02.010

Ashenhurst, J. R., Sazonova, O. V., Svrchek, O., Detweiler, S., Kita, R., Babalola, L., et al. (2022). A polygenic score for type 2 diabetes improves risk stratification beyond current clinical screening factors in an ancestrally diverse sample. *Frontiers in Genetics, 13.* https://doi.org/10.3389/fgene.2022.871260

Assah, F. K., Ekelund, U., Brage, S., Mbanya, J. C., & Wareham, N. J. (2011). Urbanization, physical activity, and metabolic health in Sub-Saharan Africa. *Diabetes Care, 34.* https://doi.org/10.2337/dc10-0990

Atkinson, E. G., Dalvie, S., Pichkar, Y., Kalungi, A., Majara, L., Stevenson, A., et al. (2022). Genetic structure correlates with ethnolinguistic diversity in eastern and Southern Africa. *The American Journal of Human Genetics, 109.* https://doi.org/10.1016/j.ajhg.2022.07.013

Backman, J. D., Li, A. H., Marcketta, A., Sun, D., Mbatchou, J., Kessler, M. D., et al. (2021). Exome sequencing and analysis of 454,787 UK biobank participants. *Nature, 599.* https://doi.org/10.1038/s41586-021-04103-z

Basu, D., & Goldberg, I. J. (2020). Regulation of lipoprotein lipase-mediated lipolysis of triglycerides. *Current Opinion in Lipidology, 31.* https://doi.org/10.1097/MOL.0000000000000676

Bazzazzadehgan, S., Shariat-Madar, Z., & Mahdi, F. (2025). Distinct roles of common genetic variants and their contributions to diabetes: MODY and uncontrolled T2DM. *Biomolecules, 15.* https://doi.org/10.3390/biom15030414

Beer, N. L., Tribble, N. D., McCulloch, L. J., Roos, C., Johnson, P. R. V., Orho-Melander, M., et al. (2009). The P446L variant in GCKR associated with fasting plasma glucose and triglyceride levels exerts its effect through increased glucokinase activity in liver. *Human Molecular Genetics, 18.* https://doi.org/10.1093/hmg/ddp357

Bentley, A. R., Sung, Y. J., Brown, M. R., Winkler, T. W., Kraja, A. T., Ntalla, I., et al. (2019). Multi-ancestry genome-wide gene–smoking interaction study of 387,272 individuals identifies new loci associated with serum lipids. *Nature Genetics, 51.* https://doi.org/10.1038/s41588-019-0378-y

Bhargave, A., Devi, K., Ahmad, I., Yadav, A., & Gupta, R. (2022). Genetic variation in DPP-IV gene linked to predisposition of T2DM: A case control study. *Journal of Diabetes and Metabolic Disorders, 21.* https://doi.org/10.1007/s40200-022-01131-y

Brown, A. E., & Walker, M. (2016). Genetics of insulin resistance and the metabolic syndrome. *Current Cardiology Reports, 18.* https://doi.org/10.1007/s11886-016-0755-4

Bryois, J., Skene, N. G., Hansen, T. F., Kogelman, L. J. A., Watson, H. J., Liu, Z., et al. (2020). Genetic identification of cell types underlying brain complex traits yields insights into the etiology of Parkinson's disease. *Nature Genetics, 52.* https://doi.org/10.1038/s41588-020-0610-9

Catalano, F., De Vito, F., Cassano, V., Fiorentino, T. V., Sciacqua, A., & Hribal, M. L. (2023). Circadian clock desynchronization and insulin resistance. *International Journal of Environmental Research and Public Health, 20.* https://doi.org/10.3390/ijerph20010029

Cernea, S., & Dobreanu, M. (2013). Diabetes and beta cell function: From mechanisms to evaluation and clinical implications. *Biochemia Medica, 23.* https://doi.org/10.11613/BM.2013.033

Chait, A., & den Hartigh, L. J. (2020). Adipose tissue distribution, inflammation and its metabolic consequences, including diabetes and cardiovascular disease. *Frontiers in Cardiovascular Medicine, 7.* https://doi.org/10.3389/fcvm.2020.00022

Chambers, J. C., Loh, M., Lehne, B., Drong, A., Kriebel, J., Motta, V., et al. (2015). Epigenome-wide association of DNA methylation markers in peripheral blood from Indian Asians and Europeans with incident type 2 diabetes: A nested case-control study. *Lancet Diabetes & Endocrinology, 3.* https://doi.org/10.1016/S2213-8587(15)00127-8

Chatterjee, N., Shi, J., & García-Closas, M. (2016). Developing and evaluating polygenic risk prediction models for stratified disease prevention. *Nature Reviews Genetics, 17.* https://doi.org/10.1038/nrg.2016.27

Chunarkar-patil, P., Kaleem, M., Mishra, R., Ray, S., Ahmad, A., Verma, D., et al. (2024). *Anticancer drug discovery based on natural products: From computational approaches to clinical studies, 1–35.*

Cohen, J. C., Boerwinkle, E., Mosley, T. H., & Hobbs, H. H. (2006). Sequence variations in PCSK9, low LDL, and protection against coronary heart disease. *New England Journal of Medicine, 354.* https://doi.org/10.1056/nejmoa054013

Cole, J. B., & Florez, J. C. (2020). Genetics of diabetes mellitus and diabetes complications. *Nature Reviews Nephrology, 16.* https://doi.org/10.1038/s41581-020-0278-5

Collins, F. S., Morgan, M., & Patrinos, A. (2003). The human genome project: Lessons from large-scale biology. *Science,* (80-), 300. https://doi.org/10.1126/science.1084564

Cromer, S. J., Lakhani, C. M., Mercader, J. M., Majarian, T. D., Schroeder, P., Cole, J. B., et al. (2023). Association and interaction of genetics and area-level socioeconomic factors on the prevalence of type 2 diabetes and obesity. *Diabetes Care, 46.* https://doi.org/10.2337/dc22-1954

da Fonseca, A. C. P., Abreu, G. M., Zembrzuski, V. M., Campos Junior, M., Carneiro, J. R. I., Neto, J. F. N., et al. (2019). The association of the fat mass and obesity-associated gene (FTO) rs9939609 polymorphism and the severe obesity in a Brazilian population. *Diabetes, Metabolic Syndrome and Obesity, 12.* https://doi.org/10.2147/DMSO.S199542

Dabelea, D. (2007). The predisposition to obesity and diabetes in offspring of diabetic mothers. *Diabetes Care, 30.* https://doi.org/10.2337/dc07-s211

Davis, J. N., Le, K. A., Walker, R. W., Vikman, S., Spruijt-Metz, D., Weigensberg, M. J., et al. (2010). Increased hepatic fat in overweight Hispanic youth influenced by interaction between genetic variation in PNPLA3 and high dietary carbohydrate and sugar consumption. *American Journal of Clinical Nutrition, 92.* https://doi.org/10.3945/ajcn.2010.30185

Dayeh, T., & Ling, C. (2015). Does epigenetic dysregulation of pancreatic islets contribute to impaired insulin secretion and type 2 diabetes?1. *Biochemistry and Cell Biology, 93*. https://doi.org/10.1139/bcb-2015-0057

Dayeh, T., Volkov, P., Salö, S., Hall, E., Nilsson, E., Olsson, A. H., et al. (2014). Genome-wide DNA methylation analysis of human pancreatic islets from type 2 diabetic and non-diabetic donors identifies candidate genes that influence insulin secretion. *PLoS Genetics, 10*. https://doi.org/10.1371/journal.pgen.1004160

De Franco, E., Saint-Martin, C., Brusgaard, K., Knight Johnson, A. E., Aguilar-Bryan, L., Bowman, P., et al. (2020). Update of variants identified in the pancreatic β-cell KATP channel genes KCNJ11 and ABCC8 in individuals with congenital hyperinsulinism and diabetes. *Human Mutation, 41*. https://doi.org/10.1002/humu.23995

Dimas, A. S., Lagou, V., Barker, A., Knowles, J. W., Mägi, R., Hivert, M. F., et al. (2014). Impact of type 2 diabetes susceptibility variants on quantitative glycemic traits reveals mechanistic heterogeneity. *Diabetes, 63*. https://doi.org/10.2337/db13-0949

Do, R., Willer, C. J., Schmidt, E. M., Sengupta, S., Gao, C., Peloso, G. M., et al. (2013). Common variants associated with plasma triglycerides and risk for coronary artery disease. *Nature Genetics, 45*. https://doi.org/10.1038/ng.2795

Donath, M. Y. (2013). Targeting inflammation in the treatment of type 2 diabetes. *Diabetes, Obesity and Metabolism, 15*. https://doi.org/10.1111/dom.12172

Dong, Y., Pan, Y., Zhang, X., He, Q., Chen, S., Du, L., et al. (2024). Impact of prolonged sitting interruption on blood glucose, insulin and triacylglycerol in adults: A systematic review and meta-analysis. *Applied Sciences, 14*. https://doi.org/10.3390/app14083201

Dujic, T., Zhou, K., Donnelly, L. A., Tavendale, R., Palmer, C. N. A., & Pearson, E. R. (2015). Association of organic cation transporter 1 with intolerance to metformin in type 2 diabetes: A GoDARTS study. *Diabetes, 64*. https://doi.org/10.2337/db14-1388

Dutta, D., Heo, I., & Clevers, H. (2017). Disease modeling in stem cell-derived 3D organoid systems. *Trends in Molecular Medicine, 23*. https://doi.org/10.1016/j.molmed.2017.02.007

Ebrahim, N., Shakirova, K., & Dashinimaev, E. (2022). PDX1 is the cornerstone of pancreatic β-cell functions and identity. *Frontiers in Molecular Biosciences, 9*. https://doi.org/10.3389/fmolb.2022.1091757

Ellard, S., & Colclough, K. (2006). Mutations in the genes encoding the transcription factors hepatocyte nuclear factor 1 alpha (HNF1A) and 4 alpha (HNF4A) in maturity-onset diabetes of the young. *Human Mutation, 27*. https://doi.org/10.1002/humu.20357

El-Osta, A., Brasacchio, D., Yao, D., Pocai, A., Jones, P. L., Roeder, R. G., et al. (2008). Transient high glucose causes persistent epigenetic changes and altered gene expression during subsequent normoglycemia. *Journal of Experimental Medicine, 205*. https://doi.org/10.1084/jem.20081188

Enns, J. E., Taylor, C. G., & Zahradka, P. (2011). Variations in adipokine genes AdipoQ, lep, and LepR are associated with risk for obesity-related metabolic disease: The modulatory role of gene-nutrient interactions. *Journal of Obesity.* , Article 2011. https://doi.org/10.1155/2011/168659

Fatumo, S., Chikowore, T., Choudhury, A., Ayub, M., Martin, A. R., & Kuchenbaecker, K. (2022a). A roadmap to increase diversity in genomic studies. *Nature Medicine, 28*. https://doi.org/10.1038/s41591-021-01672-4

Fatumo, S., Chikowore, T., Choudhury, A., Ayub, M., Martin, A. R., & Kuchenbaecker, K. (2022b). Diversity in genomic studies: A roadmap to address the imbalance. *Nature Medicine, 28*.

Flannick, J., & Florez, J. C. (2016). Type 2 diabetes: Genetic data sharing to advance complex disease research. *Nature Reviews Genetics, 17*. https://doi.org/10.1038/nrg.2016.56

Flannick, J., Thorleifsson, G., Beer, N. L., Jacobs, S. B. R., Grarup, N., Burtt, N. P., et al. (2014). Loss-of-function mutations in SLC30A8 protect against type 2 diabetes. *Nature Genetics, 46*. https://doi.org/10.1038/ng.2915

Florez, J. C. (2008). Newly identified loci highlight beta cell dysfunction as a key cause of type 2 diabetes: Where are the insulin resistance genes? *Diabetologia, 51*. https://doi.org/10.1007/s00125-008-1025-9

Floyd, J. S., & Psaty, B. M. (2016). The application of genomics in diabetes: Barriers to discovery and implementation. *Diabetes Care, 39*. https://doi.org/10.2337/dc16-0738

Fritschi, C., Park, H., Richardson, A., Park, C., Collins, E. G., Mermelstein, R., et al. (2016). Association between daily time spent in sedentary behavior and duration of hyperglycemia in type 2 diabetes. *Biological Research For Nursing, 18*. https://doi.org/10.1177/1099800415600065

Fry, J. L., Munson, B. D., Thompson, K. L., Fry, C. S., Paddon-Jones, D., & Arentson-Lantz, E. J. (2022). The T allele of TCF7L2 rs7903146 is associated with decreased glucose tolerance after bed rest in healthy older adults. *Scientific Reports, 12*. https://doi.org/10.1038/s41598-022-10683-1

Fuku, N., Park, K. S., Yamada, Y., Nishigaki, Y., Cho, Y. M., Matsuo, H., et al. (2007). Mitochondrial haplogroup N9a confers resistance against type 2 diabetes in Asians. *The American Journal of Human Genetics, 80*. https://doi.org/10.1086/512202

Garg, A., Pandey, P., Singh, V., & Ashique, S. (2025). Ethical considerations of cancer immunotherapy and patient perspectives on the benefits and risks of treatment. In *Nanotechnology based strategies for cancer immunotherapy: Concepts, design, and clinical applications*. https://doi.org/10.1007/978-981-97-7022-9_16

Gaulton, K. J., Ferreira, T., Lee, Y., Raimondo, A., Mägi, R., Reschen, M. E., et al. (2015). Genetic fine mapping and genomic annotation defines causal mechanisms at type 2 diabetes susceptibility loci. *Nature Genetics, 47*. https://doi.org/10.1038/ng.3437

Gaulton, K. J. (2017). Mechanisms of type 2 diabetes risk loci. *Current Diabetes Reports, 17*. https://doi.org/10.1007/s11892-017-0908-x

Geng, T., & Huang, T. (2020). Gene-environment interactions and type 2 diabetes. *Asia Pacific Journal of Clinical Nutrition, 29*. https://doi.org/10.6133/apjcn.202007_29(2).0002

Gloyn, A. L., Weedon, M. N., Owen, K. R., Turner, M. J., Knight, B. A., Hitman, G., et al. (2003). Large-scale association studies of variants in genes encoding the pancreatic β-cell KATP channel subunits Kir6.2 (KCNJ11) and SUR1 (ABCC8) confirm that the KCNJ11 E23K variant is associated with type 2 diabetes. *Diabetes, 52*. https://doi.org/10.2337/diabetes.52.2.568

Guo, J., Wu, J., He, Q., Zhang, M., Li, H., & Liu, Y. (2022). The potential role of PPARs in the fetal origins of adult disease. *Cells, 11*. https://doi.org/10.3390/cells11213474

Hazin, R., Brothers, K. B., Malin, B. A., Koenig, B. A., Sanderson, S. C., Rothstein, M. A., et al. (2013). Ethical, legal, and social implications of incorporating genomic information into electronic health records. *Genetics in Medicine, 15*. https://doi.org/10.1038/gim.2013.117

He, W. (2009). PPARγ2Pro12Ala polymorphism and human health. *PPAR Research*. . https://doi.org/10.1155/2009/849538

Hebert, J. F., & Myatt, L. (2021). Placental mitochondrial dysfunction with metabolic diseases: Therapeutic approaches. *Biochimica et Biophysica Acta, Molecular Basis of Disease, 1867*. https://doi.org/10.1016/j.bbadis.2020.165967

Helgason, A., Pálsson, S., Thorleifsson, G., Grant, S. F. A., Emilsson, V., Gunnarsdottir, S., et al. (2007). Refining the impact of TCF7L2 gene variants on type 2 diabetes and adaptive evolution. *Nature Genetics, 39*. https://doi.org/10.1038/ng1960

Herder, C., Pritlove, C., Chaturvedi, N., & Mulder, H. (2025). Diabetes prevention and treatment: A global perspective. *Diabetologia, 68*. https://doi.org/10.1007/s00125-025-06511-6

Hindorff, L. A., Bonham, V. L., Brody, L. C., Ginoza, M. E. C., Hutter, C. M., Manolio, T. A., et al. (2018). Prioritizing diversity in human genomics research. *Nature Reviews Genetics, 19.* https://doi.org/10.1038/nrg.2017.89

Hu, F. B. (2011). Globalization of diabetes: The role of diet, lifestyle, and genes. *Diabetes Care.* . https://doi.org/10.2337/dc11-0442

Hüls, A., Wright, M. N., Bogl, L. H., Kaprio, J., Lissner, L., Molnár, D., et al. (2021). Polygenic risk for obesity and its interaction with lifestyle and sociodemographic factors in European children and adolescents. *International Journal of Obesity, 45.* https://doi.org/10.1038/s41366-021-00795-5

Hyttinen, V., Kaprio, J., Kinnunen, L., Koskenvuo, M., & Tuomilehto, J. (2003). Genetic liability of type 1 diabetes and the onset age among 22, 650 young Finnish twin pairs: A nationwide follow-up study. *Diabetes, 52.* https://doi.org/10.2337/diabetes.52.4.1052

Im, C., Neupane, A., Baedke, J. L., Lenny, B., Delaney, A., Dixon, S. B., et al. (2024). Trans-ancestral genetic risk factors for treatment-related type 2 diabetes mellitus in survivors of childhood cancer. *Journal of Clinical Oncology, 42.* https://doi.org/10.1200/JCO.23.02281

Jang, E. J., Lee, D. H., Im, S. S., Yee, J., & Gwak, H. S. (2023). Correlation between PPARG Pro12Ala polymorphism and therapeutic responses to thiazolidinediones in patients with type 2 diabetes: A meta-analysis. *Pharmaceutics, 15.* https://doi.org/10.3390/pharmaceutics15061778

Jarallah, S. J., Almughem, F. A., Alhumaid, N. K., Fayez, N. A. L., Alradwan, I., Alsulami, K. A., et al. (2025). Artificial intelligence revolution in drug discovery: A paradigm shift in pharmaceutical innovation. *International Journal of Pharmacy, 680.* https://doi.org/10.1016/j.ijpharm.2025.125789

Jaskulak, M., Zimowska, M., Rolbiecka, M., & Zorena, K. (2025). Understanding the role of endocrine disrupting chemicals as environmental obesogens in the obesity epidemic: A comprehensive overview of epidemiological studies between 2014 and 2024. *Ecotoxicology and Environmental Safety, 299.* https://doi.org/10.1016/j.ecoenv.2025.118401

Jordan, S. D., Krüger, M., Willmes, D. M., Redemann, N., Wunderlich, F. T., Brönneke, H. S., et al. (2011). Obesity-induced overexpression of miRNA-143 inhibits insulin-stimulated AKT activation and impairs glucose metabolism. *Nature Cell Biology, 13.* https://doi.org/10.1038/ncb2211

Joseph, J. J., Deedwania, P., Acharya, T., Aguilar, D., Bhatt, D. L., Chyun, D. A., et al. (2022). Comprehensive management of cardiovascular risk factors for adults with type 2 diabetes: A scientific statement from the American heart Association. *Circulation, 145.* https://doi.org/10.1161/CIR.0000000000001040

Kaleem, M., Alhosin, M., Khan, K., Ahmad, W., Hosawi, S., Nur, S. M., et al. (2021). *Epigenetic basis of polyphenols in cancer prevention and therapy.* https://doi.org/10.1007/978-981-16-4935-6_6

Kaleem, M., Perwaiz, M., Nur, S. M., Abdulrahman, A. O., Ahmad, W., Al-Abbasi, F. A., et al. (2021). Epigenetics of triple-negative breast cancer via natural compounds. *Current Medicinal Chemistry, 29,* 1436–1458. https://doi.org/10.2174/0929867328666210707165530

Kaleem, M., Dalhat, M. H., Azmi, L., Asar, T. O., Ahmad, W., Alghanmi, M., et al. (2022). An insight into molecular targets of breast cancer brain metastasis. *International Journal of Molecular Sciences, 23.* https://doi.org/10.3390/ijms231911687

Kaleem, M., Thool, M., Dumore, N. G., Abdulrahman, A. O., Ahmad, W., Almostadi, A., et al. (2024). Management of triple-negative breast cancer by natural compounds through different mechanistic pathways. *Frontiers in Genetics, 15,* 1–18. https://doi.org/10.3389/fgene.2024.1440430

Kaleem, M., Azmi, L., Shahzad, N., Taha, M., Kumar, S., Mujtaba, M. A., et al. (2025). Epigenetic dynamics and molecular mechanisms in oncogenesis, tumor progression, and therapy resistance. *Naunyn-Schmiedeberg's Archives of Pharmacology.* . https://doi.org/10.1007/s00210-025-04217-5

Kaleem, M., Thool, M., Shahzad, N., Mujtaba, M. A., Almutairy, A. F., Kayali, A., et al. (2025). Revolutionizing diabetic foot ulcer management: Exploring the therapeutic potential of natural products. *Current Pharmaceutical Design.* . https://doi.org/10.2174/0113816128398467250922104224

Kaprio, J., Tuomilehto, J., Koskenvuo, M., Romanov, K., Reunanen, A., Eriksson, J., et al. (1992). Concordance for type 1 (insulin-dependent) and Type 2 (non-insulin-dependent) diabetes mellitus in a population-based cohort of twins in Finland. *Diabetologia, 35.* https://doi.org/10.1007/BF02221682

Keller, M. P., Choi, Y. J., Wang, P., Davis, D. B., Rabaglia, M. E., Oler, A. T., et al. (2008). A gene expression network model of type 2 diabetes links cell cycle regulation in islets with diabetes susceptibility. *Genome Research, 18.* https://doi.org/10.1101/gr.074914.107

Khalaf, A., Khalaf, A., Abdulrahman, A. O., Kaleem, M., Nur, S. M., Asseri, A. H., et al. (2021). Comparative analysis of the impact of urolithins on the composition of the gut microbiota in normal-diet Fed rats. *Nutrients, 13.* https://doi.org/10.3390/NU13113885

Khalilov, R., & Abdullayeva, S. (2023). Mechanisms of insulin action and insulin resistance. *Advances in Biolgy and Earth Science, 8.*

Khera, A. V., Chaffin, M., Aragam, K. G., Haas, M. E., Roselli, C., Choi, S. H., et al. (2018). Genome-wide polygenic scores for common diseases identify individuals with risk equivalent to monogenic mutations. *Nature Genetics, 50.* https://doi.org/10.1038/s41588-018-0183-z

Khera, A. V., Chaffin, M., Wade, K. H., Zahid, S., Brancale, J., Xia, R., et al. (2019). Polygenic prediction of weight and obesity trajectories from birth to adulthood. *Cell, 177.* https://doi.org/10.1016/j.cell.2019.03.028

Kheriji, N., Dallali, H., Gharbi, M., Krir, A., Bahlous, A., Ben Ahmed, M., et al. (2025). Genomic insights into unspecified monogenic forms of diabetes and their associated comorbidities: Implication for treatment. *Current Issues in Molecular Biology, 47.* https://doi.org/10.3390/cimb47121055

Kilpeläinen, T. O., Zillikens, M. C., Stančákova, A., Finucane, F. M., Ried, J. S., Langenberg, C., et al. (2011). Genetic variation near IRS1 associates with reduced adiposity and an impaired metabolic profile. *Nature Genetics, 43.* https://doi.org/10.1038/ng.866

Kingdom, R., & Wright, C. F. (2022). Incomplete penetrance and variable expressivity: From clinical studies to population cohorts. *Frontiers in Genetics, 13.* https://doi.org/10.3389/fgene.2022.920390

Kirchner, H., Osler, M. E., Krook, A., & Zierath, J. R. (2013). Epigenetic flexibility in metabolic regulation: Disease cause and prevention? *Trends in Cell Biology, 23.* https://doi.org/10.1016/j.tcb.2012.11.008

Kommoju, U. J., Samy, S. K., Maruda, J., Irgam, K., Kotla, J. P., Velaga, L., et al. (2016). Association of CDKAL1, CDKN2A/B & HHEX gene olymorphisms with type 2 diabetes mellitus in the population of Hyderabad, India. *Indian Journal of Medical Research, 143.* https://doi.org/10.4103/0971-5916.184303

Kooner, J. S., Saleheen, D., Sim, X., Sehmi, J., Zhang, W., Frossard, P., et al. (2011). Genome-wide association study in individuals of South Asian ancestry identifies six new type 2 diabetes susceptibility loci. *Nature Genetics, 43.* https://doi.org/10.1038/ng.921

Koye, D. N., Magliano, D. J., Nelson, R. G., & Pavkov, M. E. (2018). The global epidemiology of diabetes and kidney disease. *Advances in Chronic Kidney Disease, 25.* https://doi.org/10.1053/j.ackd.2017.10.011

Kwak, S. H., Jang, H. C., & Park, K. S. (2012). Finding genetic risk factors of gestational diabetes. *Genomics Inform, 10.* https://doi.org/10.5808/gi.2012.10.4.239

Kwak, S. H., Chae, J., Lee, S., Choi, S., Koo, B. K., Yoon, J. W., et al. (2018). Nonsynonymous variants in PAX4 and GLP1R are associated with type 2 diabetes in an East Asian population. *Diabetes.* . https://doi.org/10.2337/db18-0361

Laker, R. C., Wlodek, M. E., Connelly, J., & Yan, Z. (2013). Epigenetic origins of metabolic disease: The impact of the maternal condition to the offspring epigenome and later health consequences. *Food Science and Human Wellness, 2.* https://doi.org/10.1016/j.fshw.2013.03.002

Lehtovirta, M., Pietiläinen, K. H., Levälahti, E., Heikkilä, K., Groop, L., Silventoinen, K., et al. (2010). Evidence that BMI and type 2 diabetes share only a minor fraction of genetic variance: A follow-up study of 23,585 monozygotic and dizygotic twins from the Finnish twin cohort study. *Diabetologia, 53.* https://doi.org/10.1007/s00125-010-1746-4

Li, W., Cheng, Y., Cui, A., Huang, M., Huang, Q., Wang, Q., et al. (2025). Multiomics integration of epigenetics, proteomics, and metabolomics identifies putative drug targets and improves early prediction for diabetes. *Diabetes, 74.* https://doi.org/10.2337/db25-0354

Li, Y. (2022). Epigenetic modifications in obesity and type 2 diabetes. *The Open Biochemistry Journal, 16.* https://doi.org/10.2174/1874091x-v16-e2206271

Liang, K. (2023). Mitochondrial CPT1A: Insights into structure, function, and basis for drug development. *Frontiers in Pharmacology, 14.* https://doi.org/10.3389/fphar.2023.1160440

Liao, W. L., Yang, J. S., Liu, T. Y., Lu, H. F., Chang, Y. W., & Tsai, F. J. (2025). Pathway insights and predictive modeling for type 2 diabetes using polygenic risk scores. *Scientific Reports, 15.* https://doi.org/10.1038/s41598-025-13391-8

Lillycrop, K. A., & Burdge, G. C. (2012). Epigenetic mechanisms linking early nutrition to long term health. *Best Practice & Research Clinical Endocrinology & Metabolism, 26.* https://doi.org/10.1016/j.beem.2012.03.009

Lim, E. L., Hollingsworth, K. G., Aribisala, B. S., Chen, M. J., Mathers, J. C., & Taylor, R. (2011). Reversal of type 2 diabetes: Normalisation of beta cell function in association with decreased pancreas and liver triacylglycerol. *Diabetologia, 54.* https://doi.org/10.1007/s00125-011-2204-7

Ling, C., Poulsen, P., Simonsson, S., Rönn, T., Holmkvist, J., Almgren, P., et al. (2007). Genetic and epigenetic factors are associated with expression of respiratory chain component NDUFB6 in human skeletal muscle. *Journal of Clinical Investigation, 117.* https://doi.org/10.1172/JCI30938

Liu, J., Wang, L., Cui, X., Shen, Q., Wu, D., Yang, M., et al. (2023). Polygenic risk score, lifestyles, and type 2 diabetes risk: A prospective Chinese cohort study. *Nutrients, 15.* https://doi.org/10.3390/nu15092144

Liu, R., Peng, M., Zhang, J., Qiu, K., Zeng, T., & Chen, L. (2024). The ALDH2 gene rs671 polymorphism is associated with cardiometabolic risk factors in East Asian population: An updated meta-analysis. *Frontiers in Endocrinology, 15.* https://doi.org/10.3389/fendo.2024.1333595

Locke, A. E., Kahali, B., Berndt, S. I., Justice, A. E., Pers, T. H., Day, F. R., et al. (2015). Genetic studies of body mass index yield new insights for obesity biology. *Nature, 518.* https://doi.org/10.1038/nature14177

Loos, R. J. F., & Yeo, G. S. H. (2014). The bigger picture of FTO - The first GWAS-identified obesity gene. *Nature Reviews Endocrinology, 10.* https://doi.org/10.1038/nrendo.2013.227

López–Noriega, L., & Rutter, G. A. (2021). Long non-coding RNAs as key modulators of pancreatic β-Cell mass and function. *Frontiers in Endocrinology, 11.* https://doi.org/10.3389/fendo.2020.610213

Lorenzo, P. I., Fuente-Martín, E., Brun, T., Cobo-Vuilleumier, N., Jimenez-Moreno, C. M., Herrera Gomez, G., et al. (2015). PAX4 defines an expandable β-cell subpopulation in the adult pancreatic islet. *Scientific Reports, 5.* https://doi.org/10.1038/srep15672

Lv, B., Yang, X., An, T., Wu, Y., He, Z., Li, B., et al. (2022). Combined analysis of whole-exome sequencing and RNA sequencing in type 2 diabetes mellitus patients with thirst and fatigue. *Diabetology & Metabolic Syndrome, 14.* https://doi.org/10.1186/s13098-022-00884-z

Lyssenko, V., & Laakso, M. (2013). Genetic screening for the risk of type 2 diabetes: Worthless or valuable? *Diabetes Care, 36*(Suppl. 2), S120–S126. https://doi.org/10.2337/dcS13-2009

Lyssenko, V., Lupi, R., Marchetti, P., Del Guerra, S., Orho-Melander, M., Almgren, P., et al. (2007). Mechanisms by which common variants in the TCF7L2 gene increase risk of type 2 diabetes. *Journal of Clinical Investigation, 117.* https://doi.org/10.1172/JCI30706

Lyssenko, V., et al. (2011). Pleiotropic effects of a variant in the GIPR gene on islet function and risk of type 2 diabetes. *Diabetes, 60.*

Ma, R. C. W., Lin, H., & Yu, G. (2025). Unravelling diabetes endotypes and associated pathophysiology for precision medicine in diabetes: Ready for prime time? *Diabetes Care, 48.* https://doi.org/10.2337/dci25-0067

Ma, S., Zhang, M., Sun, W., Gao, Y., Jing, M., Gao, L., et al. (2025). Artificial intelligence and medical-engineering integration in diabetes management: Advances, opportunities, and challenges. *Healthcare and Rehabilitation, 1.* https://doi.org/10.1016/j.hcr.2024.100006

Mahajan, A., Taliun, D., Thurner, M., Robertson, N. R., Torres, J. M., Rayner, N. W., et al. (2018). Fine-mapping type 2 diabetes loci to single-variant resolution using high-density imputation and islet-specific epigenome maps. *Nature Genetics, 50.* https://doi.org/10.1038/s41588-018-0241-6

Mak, T. S. H., Porsch, R. M., Choi, S. W., Zhou, X., & Sham, P. C. (2017). Polygenic scores via penalized regression on summary statistics. *Genetic Epidemiology, 41.* https://doi.org/10.1002/gepi.22050

Manfredi, S., Federici, C., Picano, E., Botto, N., Rizza, A., & Andreassi, M. G. (2007). GSTM1, GSTT1 and CYP1A1 detoxification gene polymorphisms and susceptibility to smoking-related coronary artery disease: A case-only study. *Mutation Research, Fundamental and Molecular Mechanisms of Mutagenesis*, 621. https://doi.org/10.1016/j.mrfmmm.2007.02.014

Marcheva, B., Ramsey, K. M., Buhr, E. D., Kobayashi, Y., Su, H., Ko, C. H., et al. (2010). Disruption of the clock components CLOCK and BMAL1 leads to hypoinsulinaemia and diabetes. *Nature, 466.* https://doi.org/10.1038/nature09253

Martin, A. R., Kanai, M., Kamatani, Y., Okada, Y., Neale, B. M., & Daly, M. J. (2019). Clinical use of current polygenic risk scores may exacerbate health disparities. *Nature Genetics, 51.* https://doi.org/10.1038/s41588-019-0379-x

Mato, E. P. M., Guewo-Fokeng, M., Essop, M. F., & Owira, P. M. O. (2018). Genetic polymorphisms of organic cation transporter 1 (OCT1) and responses to metformin therapy in individuals with type 2 diabetes. *Médica Sur, 97.* https://doi.org/10.1097/MD.0000000000011349

Mccarthy, M. I. (2011). From hype to hope? A journey through the genetics of Type 2 diabetes. *Diabetic Medicine, 28,* 132–140. https://doi.org/10.1111/j.1464-5491.2010.03194.x

McCarthy, M. I. (2017). Painting a new picture of personalised medicine for diabetes. *Diabetologia, 60.* https://doi.org/10.1007/s00125-017-4210-x

McDonnell, E., Crown, S. B., Fox, D. B., Kitir, B., Ilkayeva, O. R., Olsen, C. A., et al. (2016). Lipids reprogram metabolism to become a major carbon source for histone acetylation. *Cell Reports, 17.* https://doi.org/10.1016/j.celrep.2016.10.012

McEwen, B. S. (2007). Physiology and neurobiology of stress and adaptation: Central role of the brain. *Physiological Reviews, 87.* https://doi.org/10.1152/physrev.00041.2006

Meigs, J. B., Cupples, L. A., & Wilson, P. W. F. (2000). Parental transmission of type 2 diabetes: The Framingham offspring study. *Diabetes, 49.* https://doi.org/10.2337/diabetes.49.12.2201

Mijač, S., Banić, I., Genc, A. M., Lipej, M., & Turkalj, M. (2024). The effects of environmental exposure on epigenetic modifications in allergic diseases. *Med, 60.* https://doi.org/10.3390/medicina60010110

Milagro, F. I., Mansego, M. L., De Miguel, C., & Martínez, J. A. (2013). Dietary factors, epigenetic modifications and obesity outcomes: Progresses and perspectives. *Molecular Aspects of Medicine, 34.* https://doi.org/10.1016/j.mam.2012.06.010

Mitrovic, B., Gluvic, Z. M., Obradovic, M., Radunovic, M., Rizzo, M., Banach, M., et al. (2023). Non-alcoholic fatty liver disease, metabolic syndrome, and type 2 diabetes mellitus: Where do we stand today? *Archives of Medical Science, 19.* https://doi.org/10.5114/aoms/150639

Młynarska, E., Czarnik, W., Dzieża, N., Jędraszak, W., Majchrowicz, G., Prusinowski, F., et al. (2025). Type 2 diabetes mellitus: New pathogenetic mechanisms, treatment and the Most important complications. *International Journal of Molecular Sciences, 26.* https://doi.org/10.3390/ijms26031094

Mobasseri, M., Shirmohammadi, M., Amiri, T., Vahed, N., Fard, H. H., & Ghojazadeh, M. (2020). Prevalence and incidence of type 1 diabetes in the world: A systematic review and meta-analysis. *Health Promotion Perspectives, 10.* https://doi.org/10.34172/hpp.2020.18

Mohan, V., Sandeep, S., Deepa, R., Shah, B., & Varghese, C. (2012). Epidemiology of type 2 diabetes: Indian scenario. *Indian Journal of Medical Research, 136.*

Moltke, I., Grarup, N., Jørgensen, M. E., Bjerregaard, P., Treebak, J. T., Fumagalli, M., et al. (2014). A common Greenlandic TBC1D4 variant confers muscle insulin resistance and type 2 diabetes. *Nature, 512.* https://doi.org/10.1038/nature13425

Morris, A. P., Voight, B. F., Teslovich, T. M., Ferreira, T., Segrè, A. V., Steinthorsdottir, V., et al. (2012). Large-scale association analysis provides insights into the genetic architecture and pathophysiology of type 2 diabetes. *Nature Genetics, 44.* https://doi.org/10.1038/ng.2383

Mukherjee, S., & Im, S. S. (2025). Decoding health: Exploring essential biomarkers linked to metabolic dysfunction-associated steatohepatitis and type 2 diabetes mellitus. *Biomedicines, 13.* https://doi.org/10.3390/biomedicines13020359

Muntean, C., Sasaran, M. O., Crisan, A., & Banescu, C. (2022). Effects of PPARG and PPARGC1A gene polymorphisms on obesity markers. *Frontiers in Public Health, 10.* https://doi.org/10.3389/fpubh.2022.962852

Nadiger, N., Veed, J. K., Chinya Nataraj, P., & Mukhopadhyay, A. (2024). DNA methylation and type 2 diabetes: A systematic review. *Clinical Epigenetics, 16.* https://doi.org/10.1186/s13148-024-01670-6

Nafie, M. S., Abu-Elsaoud, A. M., & Diab, M. K. (2025). A comprehensive review on computational metabolomics: Advancing multiscale analysis through in-silico approaches. *Computational and Structural Biotechnology Journal, 27.* https://doi.org/10.1016/j.csbj.2025.07.016

Narayan, K. M. V., Boyle, J. P., Thompson, T. J., Gregg, E. W., & Williamson, D. F. (2007). Effect of BMI on lifetime risk for diabetes in the U.S. *Diabetes Care, 30.* https://doi.org/10.2337/dc06-2544

Nauck, M. A., & Meier, J. J. (2018). Incretin hormones: Their role in health and disease. *Diabetes, Obesity and Metabolism, 20.* https://doi.org/10.1111/dom.13129

Ng, S. B., Turner, E. H., Robertson, P. D., Flygare, S. D., Bigham, A. W., Lee, C., et al. (2009). Targeted capture and massively parallel sequencing of 12 human exomes. *Nature, 461.* https://doi.org/10.1038/nature08250

Nogueira, T. C., Paula, F. M., Villate, O., Colli, M. L., Moura, R. F., Cunha, D. A., et al. (2013). GLIS3, a susceptibility gene for type 1 and type 2 diabetes, modulates pancreatic beta cell apoptosis via regulation of a splice variant of the BH3-Only protein bim. *PLoS Genetics, 9.* https://doi.org/10.1371/journal.pgen.1003532

Ojha, S., Kurdi, A., Sadek, B., Kaleem, M., Cai, L., A. Kamal, M., et al. (2016). Phytochemicals as prototypes for pharmaceutical leads towards drug development against diabetic cardiomyopathy. *Current Pharmaceutical Design, 22,* 3058–3070. https://doi.org/10.2174/1381612822666160322145255

Olaniru, O. E., Kadolsky, U., Kannambath, S., Vaikkinen, H., Fung, K., Dhami, P., et al. (2023). Single-cell transcriptomic and spatial landscapes of the developing human pancreas. *Cell Metabolism, 35.* https://doi.org/10.1016/j.cmet.2022.11.009

Oliveira, A. I. N., Malta, F. M., Zitelli, P. M. Y., Salles, A. P. M., Gomes-Gouvea, M. S., Nastri, A. C. S., et al. (2021). The role of PNPLA3 and TM6SF2 polymorphisms on liver fibrosis and metabolic abnormalities in Brazilian patients with chronic hepatitis C. *BMC Gastroenterology, 21.* https://doi.org/10.1186/s12876-021-01654-3

Ølnes, Å. S., Teigen, M., Laerdahl, J. K., Leren, T. P., Strøm, T. B., & Bjune, K. (2023). Variants in the CETP gene affect levels of HDL cholesterol by reducing the amount, and not the specific lipid transfer activity, of secreted CETP. *PLoS One, 18.* https://doi.org/10.1371/journal.pone.0294764

Omer, A. B., Dalhat, M. H., Khan, M. K., Afzal, O., Altamimi, A. S. A., Alzarea, S. I., et al. (2022). Butin mitigates memory impairment in Streptozotocin-induced diabetic rats by inhibiting oxidative stress and inflammatory responses. *Metabolites, 12*. https://doi.org/10.3390/metabo12111050

Ortega, Á., Berná, G., Rojas, A., Martín, F., & Soria, B. (2017). Gene-diet interactions in type 2 diabetes: The chicken and egg debate. *International Journal of Molecular Sciences, 18*. https://doi.org/10.3390/ijms18061188

Painter, R. C., Osmond, C., Gluckman, P., Hanson, M., Phillips, D. I. W., & Roseboom, T. J. (2008). Transgenerational effects of prenatal exposure to the Dutch famine on neonatal adiposity and health in later life. *BJOG: An International Journal of Obstetrics and Gynaecology, 115*. https://doi.org/10.1111/j.1471-0528.2008.01822.x

Panasevich, S., Leander, K., Ljungman, P., Bellander, T., De Faire, U., Pershagen, G., et al. (2013). Interaction between air pollution exposure and genes in relation to levels of inflammatory markers and risk of myocardial infarction. *BMJ Open, 3*. https://doi.org/10.1136/bmjopen-2013-003058

Parrillo, L., Spinelli, R., Nicolò, A., Longo, M., Mirra, P., Raciti, G. A., et al. (2019). Nutritional factors, dna methylation, and risk of type 2 diabetes and obesity: Perspectives and challenges. *International Journal of Molecular Sciences, 20*. https://doi.org/10.3390/ijms20122983

Pasquali, L., Gaulton, K. J., Rodríguez-Seguí, S. A., Mularoni, L., Miguel-Escalada, I., Akerman, I., et al. (2014). Pancreatic islet enhancer clusters enriched in type 2 diabetes risk-associated variants. *Nature Genetics, 46*. https://doi.org/10.1038/ng.2870

Patel, K. A., Kettunen, J., Laakso, M., Stančáková, A., Laver, T. W., Colclough, K., et al. (2017). Heterozygous RFX6 protein truncating variants are associated with MODY with reduced penetrance. *Nature Communications, 8*. https://doi.org/10.1038/s41467-017-00895-9

Pearson, E. R., Flechtner, I., Njølstad, P. R., Malecki, M. T., Flanagan, S. E., Larkin, B., et al. (2006). Switching from insulin to oral sulfonylureas in patients with diabetes due to Kir6.2 mutations. *New England Journal of Medicine, 355*. https://doi.org/10.1056/nejmoa061759

Petroni, M. L., Brodosi, L., Marchignoli, F., Sasdelli, A. S., Caraceni, P., Marchesini, G., et al. (2021). Nutrition in patients with type 2 diabetes: Present knowledge and remaining challenges. *Nutrients, 13*. https://doi.org/10.3390/nu13082748

Pollastro, C., Ziviello, C., Costa, V., & Ciccodicola, A. (2015). Pharmacogenomics of drug response in type 2 diabetes: Toward the definition of tailored therapies? *PPAR Research, 2015*. https://doi.org/10.1155/2015/415149

Popkin, B. M. (2015). Nutrition transition and the global diabetes epidemic. *Current Diabetes Reports, 15*. https://doi.org/10.1007/s11892-015-0631-4

Pound, L. D., Oeser, J. K., O'Brien, T. P., Wang, Y., Faulman, C. J., Dadi, P. K., et al. (2013). G6PC2: A negative regulator of basal glucose-stimulated insulin secretion. *Diabetes, 62*. https://doi.org/10.2337/db12-1067

Poy, M. N., Eliasson, L., Krutzfeldt, J., Kuwajima, S., Ma, X., MacDonald, P. E., et al. (2004). A pancreatic islet-specific microRNA regulates insulin secretion. *Nature, 432*. https://doi.org/10.1038/nature03076

Prasad, R. B., & Groop, L. (2015). Genetics of type 2 diabetes—pitfalls and possibilities. *Genes, 6*. https://doi.org/10.3390/genes6010087

Prokopenko, I., Langenberg, C., Florez, J. C., Saxena, R., Soranzo, N., Thorleifsson, G., et al. (2009). Variants in MTNR1B influence fasting glucose levels. *Nature Genetics, 41*. https://doi.org/10.1038/ng.290

Qi, L., & Liang, J. (2010). Interactions between genetic factors that predict diabetes and dietary factors that ultimately impact on risk of diabetes. *Current Opinion in Lipidology, 21*. https://doi.org/10.1097/MOL.0b013e3283346cb6

Qian, Y., Lu, F., Dong, M., Lin, Y., Li, H., Chen, J., et al. (2012). Genetic variants of IDE-KIF11-HHEX at 10q23.33 associated with type 2 diabetes risk: A fine-mapping study in chinese population. *PLoS One, 7*. https://doi.org/10.1371/journal.pone.0035060

Radha, V., Kanthimathi, S., & Mohan, V. (2011). Genetics of Type 2 diabetes in Asian Indians. *Diabetes Management, 1*. https://doi.org/10.2217/dmt.11.14

Rahu, M. A., Shaikh, Q., Jabeen, M., & Perveen, S. (2025). Regulation of hyperglycemia in type 2 diabetes mellitus: Insights into current therapeutic pathways. *Letters in Drug Design and Discovery*. . https://doi.org/10.1016/j.lddd.2025.100204

Rao, D. C., Sung, Y. J., Winkler, T. W., Schwander, K., Borecki, I., Adrienne Cupples, L., et al. (2017). Multiancestry study of gene-lifestyle interactions for cardiovascular traits in 610 475 individuals from 124 cohorts: Design and rationale. *Circulation: Cardiovascular Genetics, 10*. https://doi.org/10.1161/CIRCGENETICS.116.001649

Ravassard, P., Hazhouz, Y., Pechberty, S., Bricout-Neveu, E., Armanet, M., Czernichow, P., et al. (2011). A genetically engineered human pancreatic β cell line exhibiting glucose-inducible insulin secretion. *Journal of Clinical Investigation, 121*. https://doi.org/10.1172/JCI58447

Rees, S. D., Hydrie, M. Z. I., O'Hare, J. P., Kumar, S., Shera, A. S., Basit, A., et al. (2011). Effects of 16 genetic variants on fasting glucose and type 2 diabetes in South Asians: ADCY5 and GLIS3 variants may predispose to type 2 diabetes. *PLoS One, 6*. https://doi.org/10.1371/journal.pone.0024710

Richter, E. A., & Hargreaves, M. (2013). Exercise, GLUT4, and skeletal muscle glucose uptake. *Physiological Reviews, 93*. https://doi.org/10.1152/physrev.00038.2012

Rönn, T., & Ling, C. (2015). DNA methylation as a diagnostic and therapeutic target in the battle against Type 2 diabetes. *Epigenomics, 7*. https://doi.org/10.2217/epi.15.7

Rung, J., Cauchi, S., Albrechtsen, A., Shen, L., Rocheleau, G., Cavalcanti-Proença, C., et al. (2009). Genetic variant near IRS1 is associated with type 2 diabetes, insulin resistance and hyperinsulinemia. *Nature Genetics, 41*. https://doi.org/10.1038/ng.443

Ruze, R., Liu, T., Zou, X., Song, J., Chen, Y., Xu, R., et al. (2023). Obesity and type 2 diabetes mellitus: Connections in epidemiology, pathogenesis, and treatments. *Frontiers in Endocrinology, 14*. https://doi.org/10.3389/fendo.2023.1161521

Sandhu, M. S., Weedon, M. N., Fawcett, K. A., Wasson, J., Debenham, S. L., Daly, A., et al. (2007). Common variants in WFS1 confer risk of type 2 diabetes. *Nature Genetics, 39*. https://doi.org/10.1038/ng2067

Segerstolpe, Å., Palasantza, A., Eliasson, P., Andersson, E. M., Andréasson, A. C., Sun, X., et al. (2016). Single-cell transcriptome profiling of human pancreatic islets in health and type 2 diabetes. *Cell Metabolism, 24*. https://doi.org/10.1016/j.cmet.2016.08.020

Shulman, G. I. (2014). Ectopic fat in insulin resistance, dyslipidemia, and cardiometabolic disease. *New England Journal of Medicine, 371*. https://doi.org/10.1056/nejmra1011035

Singh, S., Kriti, M.,K. S.,A., Sarma, D. K., Verma, V., Nagpal, R., et al. (2024). Deciphering the complex interplay of risk factors in type 2 diabetes mellitus: A comprehensive review. *Metabolism Open, 22*. https://doi.org/10.1016/j.metop.2024.100287

Singhal, P. C., & Skorecki, K. (2025). APOL1 dynamics in diabetic kidney disease and hypertension. *Biomolecules, 15*. https://doi.org/10.3390/biom15020205

Sirugo, G., Williams, S. M., & Tishkoff, S. A. (2019). The missing diversity in human genetic studies. *Cell, 177*. https://doi.org/10.1016/j.cell.2019.02.048

Sladek, R., Rocheleau, G., Rung, J., Dina, C., Shen, L., Serre, D., et al. (2007). A genome-wide association study identifies novel risk loci for type 2 diabetes. *Nature, 445*. https://doi.org/10.1038/nature05616

Song, J., Yang, Y., Mauvais-Jarvis, F., Wang, Y. P., & Niu, T. (2017). KCNJ11, ABCC8 and TCF7L2 polymorphisms and the response to sulfonylurea treatment in patients with type 2 diabetes: A bioinformatics assessment. *BMC Medical Genetics, 18.* https://doi.org/10.1186/s12881-017-0422-7

Song, J., Wang, C., Zhao, T., Zhang, Y., Xing, J., Zhao, X., et al. (2025). Multi-omics approaches for biomarker discovery and precision diagnosis of prediabetes. *Frontiers in Endocrinology, 16.* https://doi.org/10.3389/fendo.2025.1520436

Speliotes, E. K., Yerges-Armstrong, L. M., Wu, J., Hernaez, R., Kim, L. J., Palmer, C. D., et al. (2011). Genome-wide association analysis identifies variants associated with nonalcoholic fatty liver disease that have distinct effects on metabolic traits. *PLoS Genetics, 7.* https://doi.org/10.1371/journal.pgen.1001324

Stančáková, A., & Laakso, M. (2016). Genetics of type 2 diabetes. *Endocrine Development, 31.* https://doi.org/10.1159/000439418

Steger, D. J., Grant, G. R., Schupp, M., Tomaru, T., Lefterova, M. I., Schug, J., et al. (2010). Propagation of adipogenic signals through an epigenomic transition state. *Genes & Development, 24.* https://doi.org/10.1101/gad.1907110

Stein, S. A., Maloney, K. A., & Pollin, T. I. (2014). Genetic counseling for diabetes mellitus. *Current Genetic Medicine Reports, 2.* https://doi.org/10.1007/s40142-014-0039-5

Steinmetz, J. D., Bourne, R. R. A., Briant, P. S., Flaxman, S., Taylor, H. R., Jonas, J. B., et al. (2021). Causes of blindness and vision impairment in 2020 and trends over 30 years, and prevalence of avoidable blindness in relation to VISION 2020: The right to sight: An analysis for the global burden of disease study. *Lancet Global Health, 9.* https://doi.org/10.1016/S2214-109X(20)30489-7

Stride, A., Vaxillaire, M., Tuomi, T., Barbetti, F., Njølstad, P. R., Hansen, T., et al. (2002). The genetic abnormality in the beta cell determines the response to an oral glucose load. *Diabetologia, 45.* https://doi.org/10.1007/s00125-001-0770-9

Stringhini, S., Carmeli, C., Jokela, M., Avendaño, M., Muennig, P., Guida, F., et al. (2017). Socioeconomic status and the 25 × 25 risk factors as determinants of premature mortality: A multicohort study and meta-analysis of 1·7 million men and women. *Lancet, 389.* https://doi.org/10.1016/S0140-6736(16)32380-7

Sudlow, C., Gallacher, J., Allen, N., Beral, V., Burton, P., Danesh, J., et al. (2015). UK biobank: An open access resource for identifying the causes of a wide range of complex diseases of middle and old age. *PLoS Medicine, 12.* https://doi.org/10.1371/journal.pmed.1001779

Sun, C., Förster, F., Gutsmann, B., Moulla, Y., Stroh, C., Dietrich, A., et al. (2022). Metabolic effects of the waist-to-hip ratio associated locus GRB14/COBLL1 are related to GRB14 expression in adipose tissue. *International Journal of Molecular Sciences, 23.* https://doi.org/10.3390/ijms23158558

Suthon, S., & Tangjittipokin, W. (2024). Mechanisms and physiological roles of polymorphisms in gestational diabetes mellitus. *International Journal of Molecular Sciences, 25.* https://doi.org/10.3390/ijms25042039

Suzuki, K., Hatzikotoulas, K., Southam, L., Taylor, H. J., Yin, X., Lorenz, K. M., et al. (2024). Genetic drivers of heterogeneity in type 2 diabetes pathophysiology. *Nature, 627.* https://doi.org/10.1038/s41586-024-07019-6

Tan, V. M. H., Lee, Y. S., Venkataraman, K., Khoo, E. Y. H., Tai, E. S., Chong, Y. S., et al. (2015). Ethnic differences in insulin sensitivity and beta-cell function among Asian men. *Nutrition & Diabetes, 5.* https://doi.org/10.1038/nutd.2015.24

Tavani, H. T., & Moor, J. H. (2001). Privacy protection, control of information, and privacy-enhancing technologies. *ACM SIGCAS Computers and Society, 31.* https://doi.org/10.1145/572277.572278

Thomas, M. S., Calle, M., & Fernandez, M. L. (2023). Healthy plant-based diets improve dyslipidemias, insulin resistance, and inflammation in metabolic syndrome. A narrative review. *Advances in Nutrition, 14.* https://doi.org/10.1016/j.advnut.2022.10.002

Thomsen, S. K., Raimondo, A., Hastoy, B., Sengupta, S., Dai, X. Q., Bautista, A., et al. (2018). Type 2 diabetes risk alleles in PAM impact insulin release from human pancreatic β-cells. *Nature Genetics, 50.* https://doi.org/10.1038/s41588-018-0173-1

Tian, X., Wang, L., Zhong, L., Zhang, K., Ge, X., Luo, Z., et al. (2025). The research progress and future directions in the pathophysiological mechanisms of type 2 diabetes mellitus from the perspective of precision medicine. *Frontiers of Medicine, 12.* https://doi.org/10.3389/fmed.2025.1555077

Tosur, M., & Philipson, L. H. (2022). Precision diabetes: Lessons learned from maturity-onset diabetes of the young (MODY). *Journal of Diabetes Investigation, 13.* https://doi.org/10.1111/jdi.13860

Trajkovski, M., Hausser, J., Soutschek, J., Bhat, B., Akin, A., Zavolan, M., et al. (2011). MicroRNAs 103 and 107 regulate insulin sensitivity. *Nature, 474.* https://doi.org/10.1038/nature10112

Udayantha, H. M. V., Kim, J., Kim, G., Lee, J., Lee, S., Park, C. U., et al. (2025). Genome-wide association and genomic prediction of thermal tolerance in olive flounders (Paralichthys olivaceus): A validation study. *Aquaculture Reports, 45.* https://doi.org/10.1016/j.aqrep.2025.103205

Udler, M. S., Kim, J., von Grotthuss, M., Bonàs-Guarch, S., Cole, J. B., Chiou, J., et al. (2018). Type 2 diabetes genetic loci informed by multi-trait associations point to disease mechanisms and subtypes: A soft clustering analysis. *PLoS Medicine, 15.* https://doi.org/10.1371/journal.pmed.1002654

Unnikrishnan, R., Anjana, R. M., & Mohan, V. (2014). Diabetes in South Asians: Is the phenotype different? *Diabetes, 63.* https://doi.org/10.2337/db13-1592

van Arensbergen, J., García-Hurtado, J., Maestro, M. A., Correa-Tapia, M., Rutter, G. A., Vidal, M., et al. (2013). Ring1b bookmarks genes in pancreatic embryonic progenitors for repression in adult β cells. *Genes & Development, 27.* https://doi.org/10.1101/gad.206094.112

Vaxillaire, M., & Froguel, P. (2006). Genetic basis of maturity-onset diabetes of the young. *Endocrinology and Metabolism Clinics of North America, 35.* https://doi.org/10.1016/j.ecl.2006.02.009

Vedovato, N., Salguero, M. V., Greeley, S. A. W., Yu, C. H., Philipson, L. H., & Ashcroft, F. M. (2024). A loss-of-function mutation in KCNJ11 causing sulfonylurea-sensitive diabetes in early adult life. *Diabetologia, 67.* https://doi.org/10.1007/s00125-024-06103-w

Vella, M., Mohan, S., Christie, H., Bailey, K. R., Cobelli, C., Man, C. D., et al. (2024). Diabetes-associated genetic variation in MTNR1B and its effect on islet function. *Journal of Endocrine Society, 8.* https://doi.org/10.1210/jendso/bvae130

Venkat, V., Clark, K., Jeng, X. J., Yao, T. C., Tsai, H. J., Lu, T. P., et al. (2025). Exploring random forest in genetic risk score construction. *Genetic Epidemiology, 49.* https://doi.org/10.1002/gepi.70022

Venkatachalapathy, P., Padhilahouse, S., Sellappan, M., Subramanian, T., Kurian, S. J., Miraj, S. S., et al. (2021). Pharmacogenomics and personalized medicine in type 2 diabetes mellitus: Potential implications for clinical practice. *Pharmgenomics and Personalized Medicine, 14.* https://doi.org/10.2147/PGPM.S329787

Vilhjálmsson, B. J., Yang, J., Finucane, H. K., Gusev, A., Lindström, S., Ripke, S., et al. (2015). Modeling linkage disequilibrium increases accuracy of polygenic risk scores. *The American Journal of Human Genetics, 97.* https://doi.org/10.1016/j.ajhg.2015.09.001

Visscher, P. M., Wray, N. R., Zhang, Q., Sklar, P., McCarthy, M. I., Brown, M. A., et al. (2017). 10 years of GWAS discovery: Biology, function, and translation. *The American Journal of Human Genetics, 101.* https://doi.org/10.1016/j.ajhg.2017.06.005

Volkmar, M., Dedeurwaerder, S., Cunha, D. A., Ndlovu, M. N., Defrance, M., Deplus, R., et al. (2012). DNA methylation profiling identifies epigenetic dysregulation in pancreatic islets from type 2 diabetic patients. *The EMBO Journal, 31.* https://doi.org/10.1038/emboj.2011.503

Vujkovic, M., Keaton, J. M., Lynch, J. A., Miller, D. R., Zhou, J., Tcheandjieu, C., et al. (2020). Discovery of 318 new risk loci for type 2 diabetes and related vascular outcomes among 1.4 million participants in a multi-ancestry meta-analysis. *Nature Genetics, 52.* https://doi.org/10.1038/s41588-020-0637-y

Wesolowska-Andersen, A., Yu, G. Z., Nylander, V., Abaitua, F., Thurner, M., Torres, J. M., et al. (2020). Deep learning models predict regulatory variants in pancreatic islets and refine type 2 diabetes association signals. *eLife, 9*. https://doi.org/10.7554/eLife.51503

Wheeler, E., & Barroso, I. (2011). Genome-wide association studies and type 2 diabetes. *Briefings in Functional Genomics, 10*. https://doi.org/10.1093/bfgp/elr008

Willemsen, G., Ward, K. J., Bell, C. G., Christensen, K., Bowden, J., Dalgård, C., et al. (2015). The concordance and heritability of type 2 diabetes in 34,166 twin pairs from international twin registers: The discordant twin (DISCOTWIN) consortium. *Twin Research and Human Genetics, 18*. https://doi.org/10.1017/thg.2015.83

Williams Amy, A. L., Jacobs Suzanne, S. B. R., Moreno-Macías, H., Huerta-Chagoya, A., Churchhouse, C., Márquez-Luna, C., et al. (2014). Sequence variants in SLC16A11 are a common risk factor for type 2 diabetes in Mexico. *Nature, 506*. https://doi.org/10.1038/nature12828

Xiao Liang, K. (2024). Interplay of mitochondria and diabetes: Unveiling novel therapeutic strategies. *Mitochondrion, 75*. https://doi.org/10.1016/j.mito.2024.101850

Xu, K., Jiang, L., Zhang, M., Zheng, X., Gu, Y., Wang, Z., et al. (2016). Type 2 diabetes risk allele UBE2E2 is associated with decreased glucose-stimulated insulin release in elderly Chinese Han individuals. *Médica Sur, 95*. https://doi.org/10.1097/MD.0000000000003604

Xu, B., Li, S., Kang, B., Fan, S., Chen, C., Li, W., et al. (2023). Role of SLC5A2 polymorphisms and effects of genetic polymorphism on sodium glucose cotransporter 2 inhibitorsinhibitor response. *Molecular Biology Reports, 50*. https://doi.org/10.1007/s11033-023-08836-0

Yabe, D., & Seino, Y. (2016). Type 2 diabetes via β-cell dysfunction in East Asian people. *Lancet Diabetes & Endocrinology, 4*. https://doi.org/10.1016/S2213-8587(15)00389-7

Yang, Q., Xiao, T., Guo, J., & Su, Z. (2017). Complex relationship between obesity and the fat mass and obesity locus. *International Journal of Biological Sciences, 13*. https://doi.org/10.7150/ijbs.17051

Yasuda, K., Miyake, K., Horikawa, Y., Hara, K., Osawa, H., Furuta, H., et al. (2008). Variants in KCNQ1 are associated with susceptibility to type 2 diabetes mellitus. *Nature Genetics, 40*. https://doi.org/10.1038/ng.207

Yau, B., Ghislain, J., Kebede, M. A., Hughes, J., & Poitout, V. (2025). The role of the beta cell in type 2 diabetes: New findings from the last 5 years. *Diabetologia, 68*. https://doi.org/10.1007/s00125-025-06499-z

Yvonnet, S., Reim, P. K., & Thuesen, A. C. B. (2025). Actionability of genetic variants in diabetes: Core aspects and applied examples. *Diabetes Spectrum, 38*. https://doi.org/10.2337/ds24-0081

Zeevi, D., Korem, T., Zmora, N., Israeli, D., Rothschild, D., Weinberger, A., et al. (2015). Personalized nutrition by prediction of glycemic responses. *Cell, 163*. https://doi.org/10.1016/j.cell.2015.11.001

Zehra, A., Gerstle, D., Ali, F. M., Ali, M., Mejia-Lancheros, C., & Fazli, G. S. (2025). A scoping review on community-based diabetes screening interventions: Paving the pathway to early care and prevention of diabetes. *Current Diabetes Reports, 25*. https://doi.org/10.1007/s11892-025-01605-2

Zhou, K., Bellenguez, C., Spencer, C. C. A., Bennett, A. J., Coleman, R. L., Tavendale, R., et al. (2011). Common variants near ATM are associated with glycemic response to metformin in type 2 diabetes. *Nature Genetics, 43*. https://doi.org/10.1038/ng.735

Zhou, X., Guo, W., Yin, H., Chen, J., Ma, L., Yang, Q., et al. (2021). Whole exome sequencing study in a family with type 2 diabetes mellitus. *International Journal of General Medicine, 14*. https://doi.org/10.2147/IJGM.S335090

Zhu, X., Wu, Y. B., Zhou, J., & Kang, D. M. (2016). Upregulation of lncRNA MEG3 promotes hepatic insulin resistance via increasing FoxO1 expression. *Biochemical and Biophysical Research Communications, 469*. https://doi.org/10.1016/j.bbrc.2015.11.048

Zimdahl, H., Ittrich, C., Graefe-Mody, U., Boehm, B. O., Mark, M., Woerle, H. J., et al. (2014). Influence of TCF7L2 gene variants on the therapeutic response to the dipeptidylpeptidase-4 inhibitor linagliptin. *Diabetologia, 57*. https://doi.org/10.1007/s00125-014-3276-y

Zuk, O., Schaffner, S. F., Samocha, K., Do, R., Hechter, E., Kathiresan, S., et al. (2014). Searching for missing heritability: Designing rare variant association studies. *Proceedings of the National Academy of Sciences of the United States of America, 111*. https://doi.org/10.1073/pnas.1322563111

3

The immune system and type 2 diabetes mellitus (T2DM)

Abhishek Sharma, Shivanshi Madeshiya, Neha Raj and Waseem Ahmad Siddiqui

INTERDISCIPLINARY BIOTECHNOLOGY UNIT, FACULTY OF LIFE SCIENCES, ALIGARH MUSLIM UNIVERSITY, ALIGARH, UTTAR PRADESH, INDIA

1. Introduction

The hallmark of diabetes mellitus, a major global health concern, is persistent hyperglycemia caused by insulin resistance, decreased insulin production, or pancreatic β-cell dysfunction. Type 1 diabetes mellitus (T1DM), which occurs due to autoimmune destruction of pancreatic β-cells, and type 2 diabetes mellitus (T2DM), which is primarily caused by peripheral insulin resistance and progressive β-cell dysfunction, are the two main forms of the disease that are clinically categorized as diabetes mellitus. Chronic hyperglycemia causes macrovascular issues, such as atherosclerotic cardiovascular disease, and microvascular sequelae, such as retinopathy, nephropathy, and neuropathy, which harm organs such as the brain, kidneys, heart, and eyes (Sharma et al., 2026).

1.1 Overview of type 2 diabetes mellitus

Over half a billion people worldwide suffer from diabetes mellitus (DM), a serious global health issue.It is among the main reasons why people die young and a major contributor to the burden of chronic illnesses worldwide. It is anticipated that The quantity of individuals with diabetes will increase steadily over the next several decades, reaching an estimated 783 million by 2045. Around USD 966 billion was spent globally in 2021 on healthcare related to diabetes, a 316% increase over the preceding 15 years. Effective preventative techniques, early diagnosis, and better diabetes care are critically needed, as evidenced by the growing economic and health costs (https://www.idf.org/). There is mounting evidence that the pathophysiology of type 2 diabetes mellitus (T2DM) involves both the innate and adaptive immune systems. Attenuated insulin action, a major risk

Type 2 Diabetes Mellitus. https://doi.org/10.1016/B978-0-443-33590-7.00010-1

factor for type 2 diabetes, has been demonstrated to be significantly influenced by immune-mediated mechanisms. Specifically, persistent inflammation in adipose tissue encourages aberrant immune cell activation and recruitment from both arms of the immune system. This immunological dysregulation exacerbates insulin resistance and accelerates the development of type 2 diabetes (Michailidou et al., 2022).

1.2 The immune system: innate and adaptive immunity

Comprising various immune cells, specialized organs, and signaling molecules, the immune system represents an elaborate and adaptable biological network that responds continuously to changing conditions that works together to protect the host from harmful assaults and preserve tissue homeostasis. Innate and adaptive immunity are the two main interrelated branches (Mokhtar & Abdelhafez, 2021). The first line of defense is innate immunity, which is defined by quick, non-specific reactions mediated by pattern recognition receptors (PRRs) expressed on cells such as natural killer (NK) cells, dendritic cells (DCs), and macrophages. In contrast, antigen-specific T and B cells, which produce highly specialized immune responses and create long-term immunological memory, mediate adaptive immunity. There is mounting evidence that the pathophysiology of metabolic illnesses, especially type 2 diabetes mellitus (T2DM), is significantly influenced by the dysregulation of these immunological pathways. Tissue remodeling and metabolic inflammation complexly regulate the immune system, both innate and adaptive. The pancreas, liver, and adipose tissue are metabolically active organs, and obesity and chronic malnutrition promote the infiltration and initiation of immune cell responses. Insulin resistance and β-cell impairment emerge as a result of immune cell invasion, which triggers a low-grade, protracted inflammatory response that interferes with insulin signaling. Immune function and metabolic processes interact in both directions, according to recent developments in immunometabolism (Sun et al., 2020). Innate immune responses can be triggered by metabolic stress, such as lipotoxicity, hyperglycemia, and hyperlipidemia, which can result in persistent systemic inflammation. For example, adipose tissue macrophages polarize toward a pro-inflammatory M1 phenotype due to metabolic disruptions, which are linked to the release of cytokines such as interleukin-6 (IL-6), interleukin-1β (IL-1β), and tumor necrosis factor-alpha (TNF-α). By disrupting insulin receptor signaling in peripheral organs, these cytokines worsen insulin resistance and prolong metabolic dysfunction. Finding new treatment approaches for type 2 diabetes that emphasize enhancing insulin sensitivity and reducing inflammation (requires knowledge of the intricate interactions between metabolic pathways and immunological responses) (Dahik et al., 2020) (Tables 3.1–3.6).

1.3 Connecting immunity and metabolism

Immune cells depend on specific metabolic pathways for their activation, differentiation, and effector functions, highlighting the close physiological relationship between immunity and metabolism. Conversely, metabolic tissues, including adipose tissue, liver,

Table 3.1 The effects of high blood sugar levels on several immune cell types.

The impact of glucose on cell type	Type of immune cell	References
Research has demonstrated that pro-inflammatory mediators, such as tumor necrosis factor-alpha (TNF-α) and interleukin-6 (IL-6), are expressed at higher levels in isolated human monocytes. Superoxide anions, which are reactive oxygen species (ROS) that intensify oxidative stress and stimulate inflammatory reactions, are also produced in greater quantities by these cells.	Monocytes	Esser et al. (2014)
It lowers the generation of superoxide anions, inhibits immune cell motility and phagocytosis, and reduces the capacity of immune cells to eradicate microorganisms. furthermore, it causes apoptosis, resulting in the death of these immune cells dying on their own.	Neutrophils	Deleo and Allen (2020)
The addition of sugar molecules to proteins, known as glycosylation, prevents the activation of the complement system. Consequently, it hinders opsonization, making it challenging for immune proteins, such as immunoglobulins, to bind to the surfaces of pathogens or target cells.	Lymphocytes (B cells)	Xiao et al. (2016)
T Cells exhibit reduced activation and responsiveness when signaling through CD28 and CD3 molecules is weakened. Furthermore, regulatory T cells (Tregs), which are essential for regulating immunological responses, become less numerous and less active with age.	Lymphocytes (T cells)	Simone et al. (2008)
Superoxide anions, a type of reactive oxygen species, are produced at an increased rate. These substances may make the body more prone to inflammation and oxidative stress.	Macrophages	Newsholme et al. (2016)
A diminished immune response results from a reduction in the quantity and function of these lymphocytes.	Natural Killer Cells	Cheent and Khakoo (2009)

and skeletal muscle, play crucial roles in immune modulation and support both systemic and local immune responses (Hotamisligil, 2017a, 2017b). This reciprocal relationship has given rise to the emerging field of immunometabolism, which investigates how metabolic changes influence immune cell function and how immune responses impact metabolic homeostasis (O'Neill et al., 2016). Among the many cellular disruptions brought on by cellular metabolic burden in the context of obesity are oxidative stress, endoplasmic reticulum (ER) stress, and the production of damage-associated molecular patterns (DAMPs). These factors promote the activation of innate immune cells, especially macrophages and dendritic cells,Tumor necrosis factor-alpha (TNF-α), interleukin-6 (IL-6), and interleukin-1 beta (IL-1β) are pro-inflammatory cytokines that are made when these immune cells are activated. These cytokines exacerbate insulin resistance, which is essential for disrupting insulin receptor signalingpathways (Donath & Shoelson, 2011). Significant new information about the functions of various immune cell subsets and signaling cascades in the pathophysiology of type 2 diabetes mellitus (T2DM) has been made possible by developments in immunological techniques and single-cell analyses (Tang et al., 2019). Chronic, low-grade inflammation is caused by

Table 3.2 Adaptive immune components in T2DM: Roles, recent discoveries & therapeutic implications.

Immune component	Role in T2DM pathogenesis	Therapeutic implications	References
Th1 cells	In visceral adipose tissue, Th1 cells are important mediators of persistent low-grade inflammation. They influence insulin signaling, cause adipocyte dysfunction, and increase M1 macrophage polarization by secreting pro-inflammatory cytokines such as IFN-γ and TNF-α. In T2DM, a lingering Th1 bias has been found. According to recent research, Th1 cells play an early role in metabolic disturbance by being linked to greater HbA1c and fasting glucose levels when they are activated	It may be possible to reduce inflammation-induced insulin resistance by modifying Th1 differentiation or focusing on IFN-γ pathways. Monoclonal antibodies against IFN-γ are undergoing preclinical testing.	Donath and Shoelson (2011); Nishimura et al. (2009); Mahlangu et al. (2020)
Th17 cells	Th17 cells cause oxidative stress, poor insulin signaling, and endothelial dysfunction in metabolic organs by secreting IL-17A and IL-21. They are prevalent in the adipose tissue of diabetics and work in concert with TNF-α to exacerbate inflammation.In new research revealed that Trefoil Factor 3 (TFF3) promotes Th17 development in diabetic settings, adding to our knowledge of Th17-driven tissue inflammation.	Inhibitors of the IL-17 pathway, such as Secukinumab, are being considered for repurposing in metabolic disorders such as NAFLD and type 2 diabetes.	Ahmed and Gaffen (2010); Lin et al. (2024)
Treg cells	Tregs lower inflammation and maintain immune tolerance. In type 2 diabetes, insulin resistance and unchecked inflammation are associated with decreased FOXP3 Tregs. The hepatic and adipose tissues are especially susceptible to the Th17/Treg imbalance. Current research (2023–24) indicates that there is a negative relationship between HbA1c levels and Treg counts, as well as a decrease in PD-1^{+}. Problems like retinopathy are associated with retinocytes in the diabetic retina.	Adoptive Treg transfer and low-dose IL-2 therapy are being investigated to preserve β-cell function and restore immunological balance in T2DM.	Feuerer et al. (2009); Llorián-Salvador et al. (2024)

Table 3.2 Adaptive immune components in T2DM: Roles, recent discoveries & therapeutic implications.—cont'd

Immune component	Role in T2DM pathogenesis	Therapeutic implications	References
$CD8^+$ Cytotoxic T Lymphocytes (CTLs)	CD8 T cells promote adipose inflammation by mediating adipocyte death and facilitating macrophage recruitment via granzyme B and perforin. Additionally, they might be involved in the destruction of β-cells in the pancreatic islets.In single-cell transcriptomics show that diabetic adipose and islet tissues have enriched activated $CD8^+$ T cells with gene signatures that overlap β-cell exhaustion markers.	In T2DM, β-cell function may be preserved by blocking granzyme B or by activating checkpoint molecules (like PD-1).	Nishimura et al. (2009); Zhao and Fang (2025)
B Cells	Apart from producing antibodies, B cells in type 2 diabetes also release IL-6 and TNF-α and expose T cells to antigens, which perpetuates inflammation. They also exacerbate β-cell stress by encouraging the development of autoreactive T cells. According to recent animal research elevated IgG2a and IgG1 subclasses exacerbate adipose inflammation by activating macrophage FcRnreceptors.	Rituximab and other anti-CD20 treatments are being researched to lessen B cell-mediated inflammation in insulin-resistant conditions.	DeFuria et al. (2013); Winer et al. (2011); Yu et al. (2024); Sharma et al. (2024a)
Autoantibodies (in LADA)	Antibodies (such as GAD65 and IA-2) that target pancreatic β-cells are seen in LADA, a slow-onset autoimmune type of diabetes. Progressive insulin dependence is the outcome of this Studies conducted in show that people with multiple autoantibodies lose β-cells more quickly, highlighting the importance of early intervention.	In order to preserve residual β-cell mass in LADA patients, autoantibody screening allows for an earlier diagnosis and prompt insulin therapy.	Naik et al. (2009)

macrophages in the adipose tissue of obese people changing phenotypically from the anti-inflammatory M2 state to the pro-inflammatory M1 state. Furthermore, T-helper 1 (Th1) and T-helper 17 (Th17) cells contribute to this inflammatory environment by secreting cytokines like interleukin-17 (IL-17) and interferon-gamma (IFN-γ) (Winer et al., 2009). On the other hand, anti-inflammatory mediators such as interleukin-10 (IL-

Table 3.3 Immune components & their effects.

Immune factor	Effect on insulin sensitivity	Effect on insulin secretion	References
Macrophages M1	Impair sensitivity via TNF-α, IL-6	Promote β-cell stress and dysfunction	Chen et al. (2008)
Macrophages M2	Support sensitivity via IL-10	Help preserve β-cell function	Acosta et al. (2019)
T Cells that regulate (Tregs)	Improve sensitivity through anti-inflammatory pathways	Ensure that β-cells receive protective measures.	Varanasi et al. (2012)
IL-1β, TNF-α, IFN-γ	Disrupt insulin signaling pathways	Contribute to cell death and the dysfunction of β-cells.	Xie et al. (2018)

Table 3.4 Immunometabolism in type 2 diabetes.

Immune cell type	Metabolic pathways involved	Activation state	Key cytokines/ Markers	Role in T2DM	References
M1 macrophages (pro-inflammatory)	Glycolysis ↑ OXPHOS ↓	Activated by LPS, IFN-γ	TNF-α, IL-6, IL-1β	Promote inflammation, insulin resistance in adipose tissue	Gindri Dos Santos and Goedeke (2023); Pinheiro-Machado (2020)
M2 macrophages (anti-inflammatory)	OXPHOS ↑ FAO ↑	Activated by IL-4, IL-13	IL-10, Arg1, MRC1	Anti-inflammatory, improve insulin sensitivity	Gindri Dos Santos and Goedeke (2023); Li et al. (2025)
$CD8^+$ T cells	Glycolysis ↑	Effector T cells	IFN-γ, Granzyme B	Infiltrate adipose tissue, promote inflammation	Daryabor et al. (2020); Hu et al. (2024)
$CD4^+$ Th1 cells	Glycolysis ↑	Differentiated from naïve $CD4^+$	IFN-γ, TNF-α	Support M1 macrophage activation, exacerbate inflammation	Pinheiro-Machado et al. (2020), Lee and Wolfrum (2018)
$CD4^+$ Th2 cells	FAO ↑ OXPHOS ↑	Differentiated from naïve $CD4^+$	IL-4, IL-10, IL-13	Counterbalance inflammation, favor M2 polarization	Lee and Wolfrum (2018); Li et al. (2025)
Regulatory T cells (Tregs)	FAO ↑ OXPHOS ↑	Foxp3+ cells	IL-10, TGF-β	Suppress inflammation, maintain insulin sensitivity	Daryabor et al. (2020); Li et al. (2025)
B cells	Glycolysis (in plasma cells)	Activated in obesity	IL-6, IgG	Pro-inflammatory B cells contribute to insulin resistance	Pinheiro-Machado et al. (2020); Hu et al., 2024
Dendritic cells (DCs)	Glycolysis ↑ (in pro-inflammatory state)	Activated by DAMPs/ PAMPs	IL-12, TNF-α	Activate T cells, promote Th1 responses	Daryabor et al. (2020); Hu et al. (2024)
Neutrophils	Glycolysis ↑	Activated in obesity	ROS, MPO, NETs	Contribute to inflammation and β-cell damage	Lee and Wolfrum (2018); Pinheiro-Machado (2020)
NKT cells	FAO and glycolysis	Activated by lipid antigens	IFN-γ, IL-4	Can modulate inflammation; role context-dependent	Li et al. (2025); Daryabor et al. (2020)

Table 3.5 Targeting immune checkpoints in type 2 diabetes (T2DM).

Immune checkpoint	Ligand(s)	Expressed on	Function in immune regulation	Role in T2DM	Therapeutic potential	References
PD-1 (programmed Death-1) is a protein that plays a crucial role in regulating the immune system's response to cells.	PD-L1, PD-L2	T cells, B cells	It postpones the activation of T cells and promotes tolerance.	Elevated PD-1 expression linked to T cell exhaustion and chronic inflammation in T2DM	Targeting PD-1/PD-L1 axis may restore immune balance and reduce chronic inflammation	Pauken and Wherry (2015)
Cytotoxic T lymphocyte antigen 4, commonly referred to as CTLA-4, is a protein important in regulating immune responses.	CD80, CD86	Tregs, Activated T cells	Competes with CD28 for co-stimulatory ligands to downregulate immune responses	May contribute to impaired immune regulation and low-grade inflammation	Enhancing CTLA-4 signaling could suppress inflammation and autoimmunity in metabolic disorders	Rowshanravan et al. (2018); Eizirik et al. (2020)
Lymphocyte activation gene 3, commonly known as LAG-3.	MHC class II	Activated T cells, Tregs	Negatively regulates T cell expansion and cytokine production	Associated with altered T cell regulation and insulin resistance	Modulation may improve T cell homeostasis and metabolic outcomes	Andrews et al. (2017)
TIM-3, which includes the T-cell immunoglobulin and mucin domain, plays a significant role in immune regulation.	Galectin-9, phosphatidylserine	Th1 cells, DCs, macrophages	Inhibits Th1 responses and maintains tolerance	TIM-3 dysfunction may lead to pro-inflammatory responses in obesity and T2DM	Targeting TIM-3 could modulate macrophage and T cell responses in adipose tissue	Anderson et al. (2016); Das et al. (2017)
TIGIT (T cell immunoreceptor with Ig and ITIM domains)	CD155, CD112	Tregs, memory T cells	Suppresses NK and T cell activity, enhances regulatory responses	Emerging evidence suggests role in maintaining T cell tolerance in metabolic tissues	Agonists may enhance Treg-mediated suppression of inflammation	Chauvin and Zarour (2020); Hoseini-Aghdam et al. (2020)
V-domain immunoglobulin suppressor of T cell activation, commonly known as VISTA.	VSIG-3, unknown	Myeloid cells, T cells	Dampens T cell activation and supports immune quiescence	May influence inflammation in adipose and liver tissue	Targeting VISTA could offer novel anti-inflammatory strategies in T2DM	Wang et al. (2019)

Table 3.6 Personalized medicine approaches in type 2 diabetes.

Approach	Description	Immune-related target	Clinical application	References
Genetic profiling	Identification of polymorphisms in genes involved in insulin signaling, beta-cell function, or inflammation.	HLA haplotypes, IL-6, TNF-α, TCF7L2 genes	Risk stratification, early diagnosis, and preventive interventions	Kim et al. (2021)
Epigenetic markers	DNA methylation, histone modification, and miRNA expression patterns associated with T2DM and immune response.	miR-146a, miR-21, and histone deacetylases (HDACs)	Predictive biomarkers and development of HDAC inhibitors for immune modulation	Ling and Rönn (2019)
Transcriptomic profiling	Analysis of changes in gene expression in immune cells, including T cells, macrophages, and adipose tissue, in patients with type 2 diabetes.	Toll-like receptors (TLRs), NOD-like receptor pyrin domain-containing 3 (NLRP3), and pro-inflammatory cytokines such as tumor necrosis factor-alpha (TNF-α) and interleukin-1 beta (IL-1β).	Stratification of patients by inflammatory status for targeted anti-inflammatory therapy	Li et al. (2025); Dongre (2025); Sharma et al. (2025a)
Proteomic biomarkers	Study of circulating proteins, cytokines, and chemokines associated with T2DM pathology and immune activation.	CRP, IL-6, MCP-1	Patient monitoring and personalized anti-inflammatory interventions	Kurgan et al. (2024); Sharma et al. (2024b), (2025b)
mRNA-based therapeutics	Targeting immune-modulatory molecules involved in T2DM using mRNA or RNAi-based therapies.	TLRs, NLRP3, IL-1β	Personalized immune suppression or activation strategies	Vu et al. (2024)
Metabolomic profiling	Identification of metabolic intermediates that link immune activation with insulin resistance.	Branched-chain amino acids, ceramides, and lipopolysaccharides	Identifying metabolic signatures for customized lifestyle and dietary interventions	Guo, Callaway et al. (2015); Guo, Milburn, et al. (2015)
Gut microbiome analysis	Characterization of gut microbial communities influencing systemic inflammation and glucose metabolism.	LPS-producing bacteria, SCFA-producing microbiota	Use of probiotics/ prebiotics or fecal microbiota transplant (FMT) in selected patients	Gurung et al. (2020).
Immune cell phenotyping	Analysis of immune cell subsets in peripheral and adipose tissues, including regulatory T cells and M1/ M2 macrophages.	$CD4^+$ T cells, $CD8^+$ T cells, macrophage polarization markers	Selection of immunomodulatory therapies like IL-1 antagonists or TNF-α blockers	Li et al. (2023)

Table 3.6 Personalized medicine approaches in type 2 diabetes.—cont'd

Approach	Description	Immune-related target	Clinical application	References
Pharmacogenomics	Assessment of how genetic variations affect individual responses to anti-diabetic and anti-inflammatory drugs	Variants affecting response to metformin, thiazolidinediones	Drug selection and dosing tailored to genetic profile	Shukla et al. (2025a), Shukla et al. (2025b); Zeng et al. (2020)
Digital health & wearable devices	Continuous monitoring of glucose, insulin, and inflammatory biomarkers using wearable sensors and AI algorithms.	Dynamic changes in glucose and inflammatory markers	Real-time feedback for medication adjustments and lifestyle modifications	Guan et al. (2023)

10) and regulatory T cells (Tregs) work to combat inflammation; however, obesity frequently reduces their activity and numbers, making them insufficient to restore immunological homeostasis (Feuerer et al., 2009).

2. Pathophysiology of type 2 diabetes

Chronic hyperglycemia brought on by a combination of insulin resistance and impaired pancreatic beta cell function is a hallmark of type 2 diabetes mellitus (T2DM), a complex, multifactorial disease. Obesity and metabolic syndrome, which lead to insulin resistance and an increased workload for beta-cells, significantly worsen the disease's progression (Defronzo, 2009; Kahn et al., 2014) (Fig. 3.1).

An intricate network of genetic and environmental components contributes to the onset and progression of type 2 diabetes (T2D) and obesity. There is a hereditary

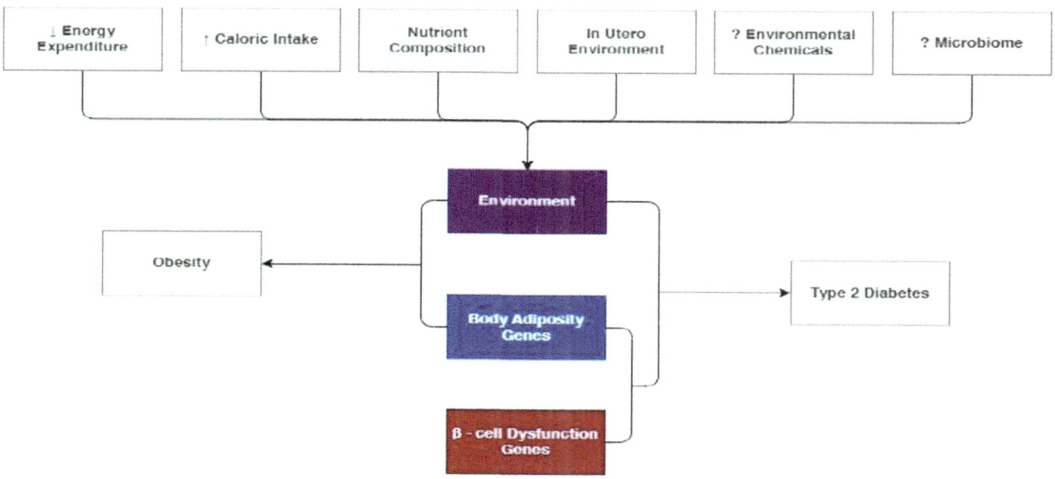

FIGURE 3.1 Type 2 diabetes and obesity are influenced by both genetic and environmental factors.

component to obesity, or excess body fat. Insulin resistance combined with obesity can result from the interaction of these genetic predispositions with environmental variables, including sedentary lifestyles, high-calorie diets, and physical inactivity. However, an additional genetic susceptibility—specifically, It typically takes mutations that affect pancreatic β-cell function to advance from obesity and insulin resistance to type 2 diabetes. In other words, during adverse environmental conditions, type 2 diabetes must fully develop due to both hereditary variables that encourage excessive fat formation and those that impair β-cells' ability to secrete insulin.

2.1 Insulin resistance

The reduced ability of peripheral tissues, primarily skeletal muscle, adipose tissue, and the liver, to respond effectively to insulin is known as insulin resistance. This condition is one of the primary anomalies linked to type 2 diabetes (T2DM) (Samuel & Shulman, 2012). Insulin is essential for preventing the liver from producing glucose and encouraging the skeletal muscles to absorb it.However, these processes are compromised by insulin resistance, which raises blood glucose levels. Basal inflammatory activity and intracellular lipid accumulation are closely linked to insulin resistance (Hotamisligil, 2006). Several serine/threonine kinases, including c-Jun N-terminal kinase (JNK), protein kinase C (PKC), and IκB kinase β (IKKβ), are activated by elevated levels of lipid intermediates, including ceramides, diacylglycerol (DAG), and free fatty acids (FFAs). By phosphorylating insulin receptor substrate (IRS) proteins at serine residues, these kinases disrupt insulin signaling (Samuel & Shulman, 2012). Additionally, macrophages in adipose tissue release pro-inflammatory cytokines like interleukin-6 (IL-6) and tumor necrosis factor alpha (TNF-α), which worsen insulin resistance by interfering with insulin signaling pathways (Hotamisligil, 2006) (Fig. 3.2).

When the insulin binds to the cell surface receptor, an enzyme called insulin receptor tyrosine kinase is activated. This enzyme gives the protein IRS1 phosphate groups. This activates Akt2, another crucial protein, through a series of processes. GLUT4, a unique glucose transporter protein, is transported to the cell surface with the aid of Akt2. Glucose can enter cells thanks to these transporters. Akt2 also promotes the storage of glucose as glycogen for later use (Fig. 3.3).

When insulin attaches to its cell surface receptor, an enzyme known as insulin receptor tyrosine kinase is activated. This enzyme adds phosphate groups to two important proteins, IRS1 and IRS2. This action triggers a signaling cascade that activates the Akt2 protein. Once activated, Akt2 helps the cell store glucose as glycogen, inhibits gluconeogenesis (the liver's synthesis of glucose) and encourages de novo lipogenesis (DNL), which is the process of fat production.

- **Case Study of insulin resistance—**

A Case of Insulin Resistance in an Underweight Woman with Polycystic Ovary Syndrome (PCOS).

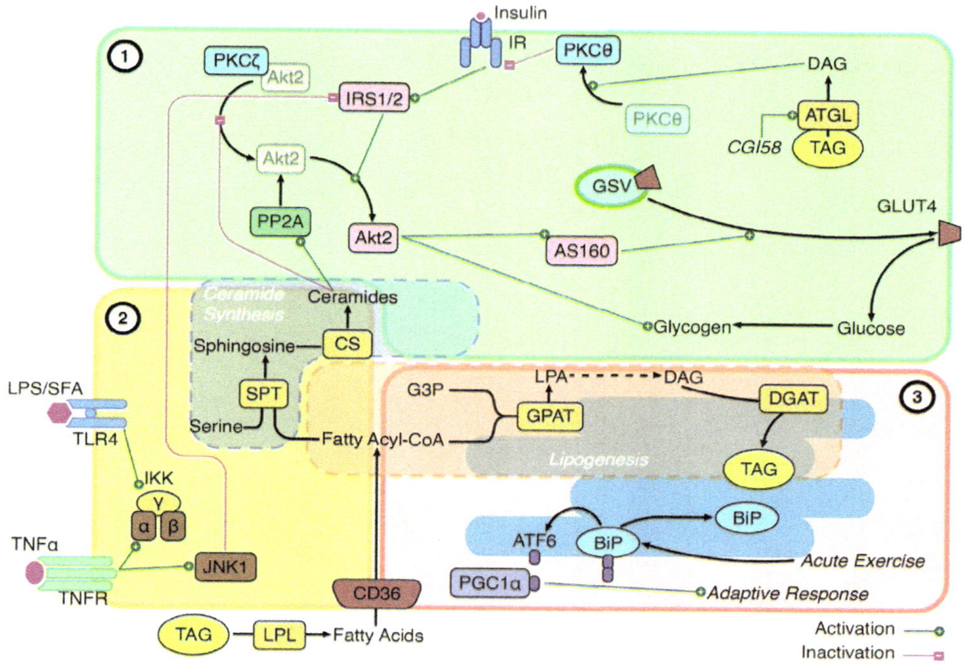

FIGURE 3.2 Diagrammatic representation of the processes underlying muscular insulin resistance.

A 24-year-old woman with a low body mass index (BMI: 15.9 kg/m2) showed signs of irregular menstrual periods, acne, and hirsutism. Her insulin resistance and PCOS diagnosis were confirmed by an oral glucose tolerance test (OGTT), even though she was underweight. Her menstrual cycle, acne, and hirsutism were significantly improved after 6 months of metformin and dexamethasone medication. This instance emphasizes the significance of a thorough diagnostic approach by showing that insulin resistance can develop in PCOS patients independent of their body weight (GacaferriLumezi et al., 2025) (Fig. 3.4).

2.2 Beta-cell dysfunction

The initiation of type 2 diabetes is significantly impacted by beta-cell dysfunction in the pancreas, which leads to insulin resistance and overt hyperglycemia (Kahn, 2003). Beta cells first produce more insulin to make up for insulin resistance. Nonetheless, chronic exposure to elevated FFAs (lipotoxicity) and hyperglycemia (glucotoxicity) results in beta cell stress, which reduces insulin synthesis and ultimately leads to beta cell death. Beta-cell failure is linked to mitochondrial dysfunction, endoplasmic reticulum (ER) stress, and oxidative stress (Prentki & Nolan, 2006). The production of reactive oxygen species (ROS), which oxidatively harm cellular components, is increased by chronic hyperglycemia. Additionally, the unfolded protein response (UPR), which can be lethal if

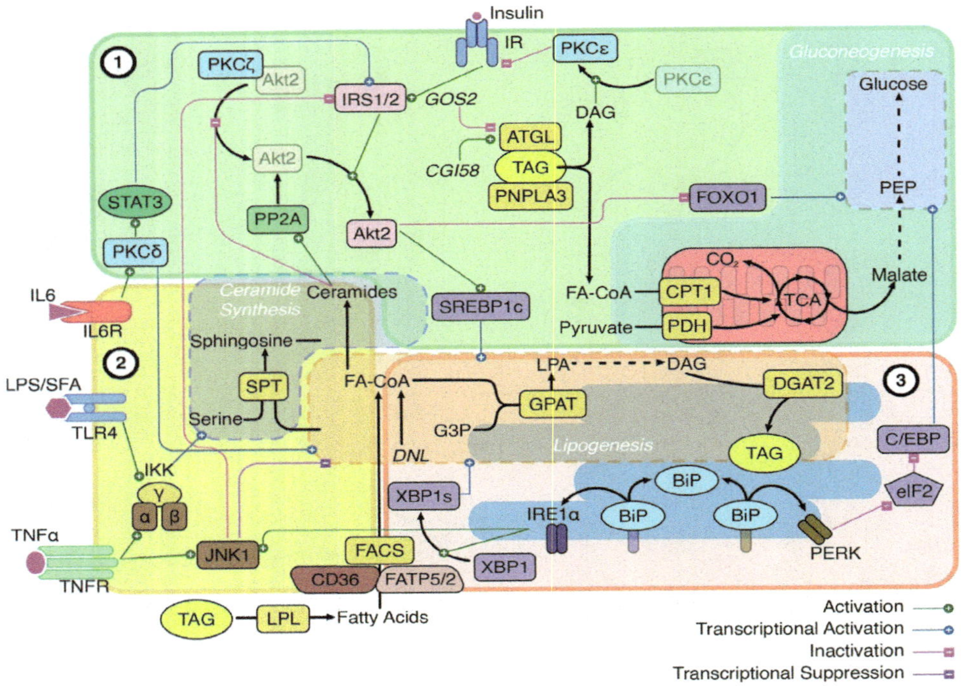

FIGURE 3.3 Diagrammatic illustration of the mechanisms underlying hepatic insulin resistance.

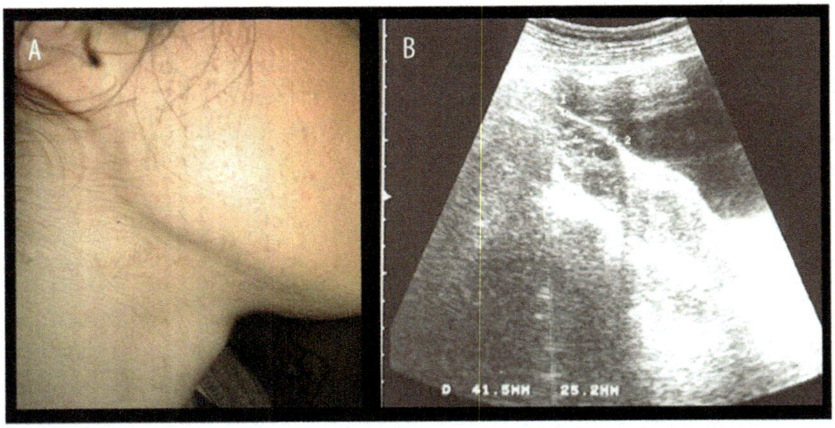

FIGURE 3.4 Insulin resistance and polycystic ovarian syndrome (PCOS) are identified in a female patient aged 24. She exhibits profuse facial hair growth, especially around her sideburns (A). Her right ovary's ultrasound shows that it has grown in size, measuring 41.5 × 25.2 mm. Numerous follicles of various sizes are also seen on the ultrasound, the largest of which is 10 mm (B).

untreated, is brought on by the buildup of misfolded proteins in the ER (Poitout & Robertson, 2008). In type 2 diabetes, another harmful feature that results in beta-cell death is pancreatic aggregation of islet amyloid polypeptide (IAPP) (Hull et al., 2004).

- **Beta cell failure mechanisms in type 2 diabetes-**

Long-term maintenance of normal glucose tolerance (NGT) depends on the ability of islet β cells to address insulin resistance, as long as they are healthy. However, if acquired or inherited factors render β cells vulnerable, this compensatory mechanism can fail (Hu et al., 2011). When the compensatory mechanism is compromised, β cells malfunction, leading to conditions like impaired glucose tolerance (IGT) and early type 2 diabetes (T2D). Once hyperglycemia is established, it activates several additional mechanisms collectively referred to as glucotoxicity, resulting in severe β cell failure and progression to overt and late-stage type 2 diabetes. This process involves the signaling networks associated with AMPK/malonyl-CoA (Prentki & Nolan, 2006) (Fig. 3.5).

- **Case Study of Beta-cell dysfunction-**

People with initial phase oftype2diabetes experience rapid beta-cell loss at diagnosis.

Following an urgent presentation of severe hyperglycemic hyperosmolar state (HHS, Type 2 diabetes has been identified in a 45-year-old male. Interestingly, a test of oral glucose tolerance (OGTT) conducted only 4 months earlier revealed decreased first-phase insulin secretion without obvious diabetes symptoms. The patient had severe beta-cell failure despite early treatment, requiring long-term exogenous insulin administration. This instance highlights how T2DM can develop abnormally quickly from poor glucose metabolism to severe beta-cell failure.

2.3 Metabolic Syndrome and Obesity

The onset of type 2 diabetes is closely linked to metabolic syndrome, a group of metabolic disorders that includes central obesity, dyslipidemia, hypertension, and impaired glucose (Alberti et al., 2009). Particularly significant is central obesity because visceral adipose tissue acts as an endocrine organ that secretes a range of adipokines and pro-inflammatory cytokines that exacerbate insulin resistance and systemic inflammation (Wajchenberg, 2000). Insulin resistance is further aggravated by dysregulation of adipokines, which is typified by elevated levels of leptin and resistin and decreased levels of adiponectin (Kershaw & Flier, 2004). A common problem for people with type 2 diabetes and metabolic syndrome, this combination of factors not only increases insulin resistance but also cardiovascular risk.

- **Case study of Metabolic Syndrome and Obesity-**

The link between Metabolic Syndrome and Obesity in Rishikesh, Uttarakhand's Urban Dwellers: In Rishikesh, Uttarakhand, a cross-sectional survey of 478 urban adults found that the prevalence of MetS was 38.2%, with a greater prevalence among females

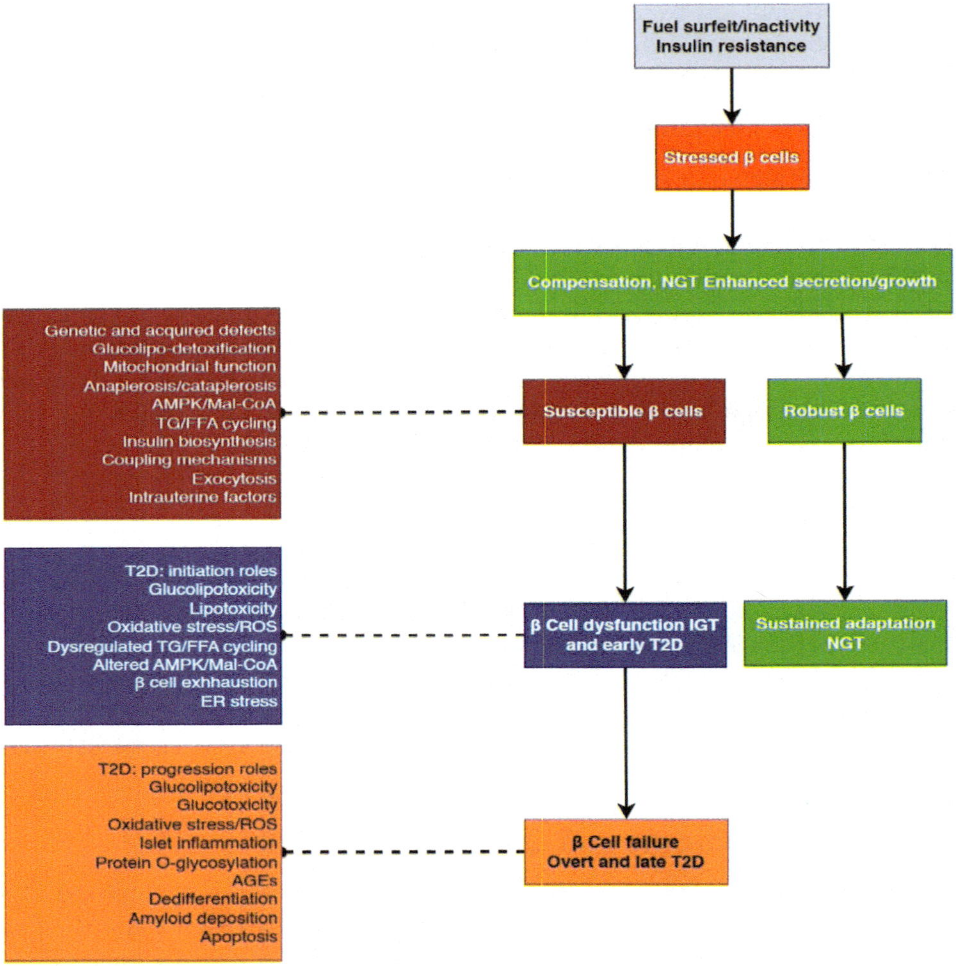

FIGURE 3.5 Mechanisms of beta cell failure in type 2 diabetes.

(40.5%) than among males (33.9%). Overall, 61.9% of participants were overweight or obese, and 64.2% of participants had central obesity. Increased body mass index (BMI) was found to be significantly associated with the likelihood of developing MetS, highlighting the urgent need for focused interventions in urban populations (Dakshinamurthy et al., 2020) (Fig. 3.6).

3. Innate immunity and inflammation in T2DM

Type 2 diabetes mellitus (T2DM) is increasingly recognized as a metabolic disease characterized by chronic low-grade inflammation.Components of the innate immune

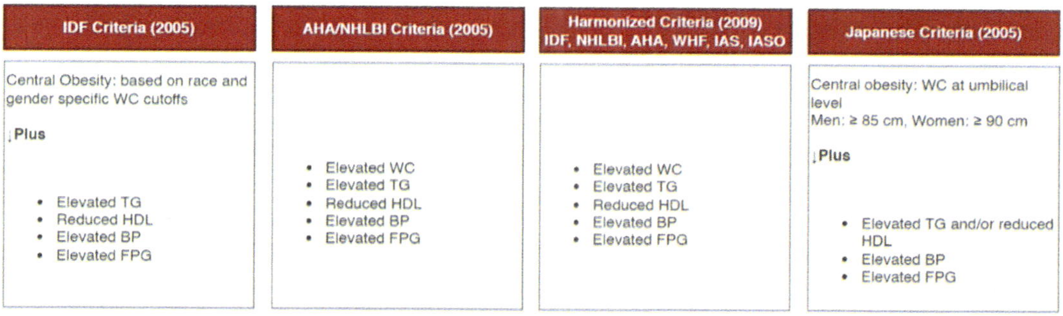

FIGURE 3.6 Criteria of metabolic syndrome.

system, such as dendritic cells (DCs), Toll-like receptors (TLRs), macrophages, and inflammasomes like NLRP3, have a important role in initiating and maintaining an inflammatory state. Systemic metabolic dysregulation, beta-cell dysfunction, and insulin signaling pathways are all disrupted by the inflammatory environment (Gora et al., 2021; Hameed et al., 2015; Wang et al., 2020).

3.1 Macrophages and adipose tissue inflammation

Adipose tissue is a dynamic organ that plays active roles in both the immune system and endocrine functions. One of the biggest threat for type 2 diabetes mellitus (T2DM) is being obese. In lean individuals, adipose tissue macrophages (ATMs) generally exhibit an anti-inflammatory M2 phenotype, which aids in tissue repair, insulin sensitivity, and overall homeostasis. However, in cases of obesity and malnutrition, adipocytes can expand and, in some instances, undergo necrosis. This process attracts circulating monocytes to the tissue (Cai et al., 2022; Dahdah et al., 2024; Li et al., 2020). As these monocytes differentiate into pro-inflammatory M1 macrophages, the immune environment of adipose tissue changes. M1 macrophages release moreproinflammatorycytokines, including intraleukin-6 (IL-6), tumor necrosis factor-alpha (TNF-α), andmonocyte chemoattractant protein-1 (MCP-1). By triggering stress kinases such as c-Jun N-terminal kinase (JNK) and IκB kinase β (IKKβ), these cytokines encourage the serine phosphorylation of insulin receptor substrate (IRS) proteins (Lee et al., 2003; Engin, 2017a, 2017b). The disruption of insulin signaling is the mechanismthatpromotesinsulinresistance.Adipose tissue's chronic inflammatory response makes insulin resistance and glucose intolerance worse, which eventually damages the liver and skeletal muscles, two peripheral metabolic organs. The chronic inflammatory environment is perpetuated and exacerbated by the ongoing recruitment and activation of monocytes and macrophages. This creates a self-reinforcing feedback loop linking adipose tissue inflammation to metabolic abnormalities in type 2 diabetes (Banu & Sur, 2023; Odegaard et al., 2007; Szukiewicz, 2023) (Fig. 3.7).

Excessive dietary intake and obesity lead to lipid buildup in adipocytes, which activates stress-responsivesignaling pathways, including NF-κB and JNK, that cause cellular

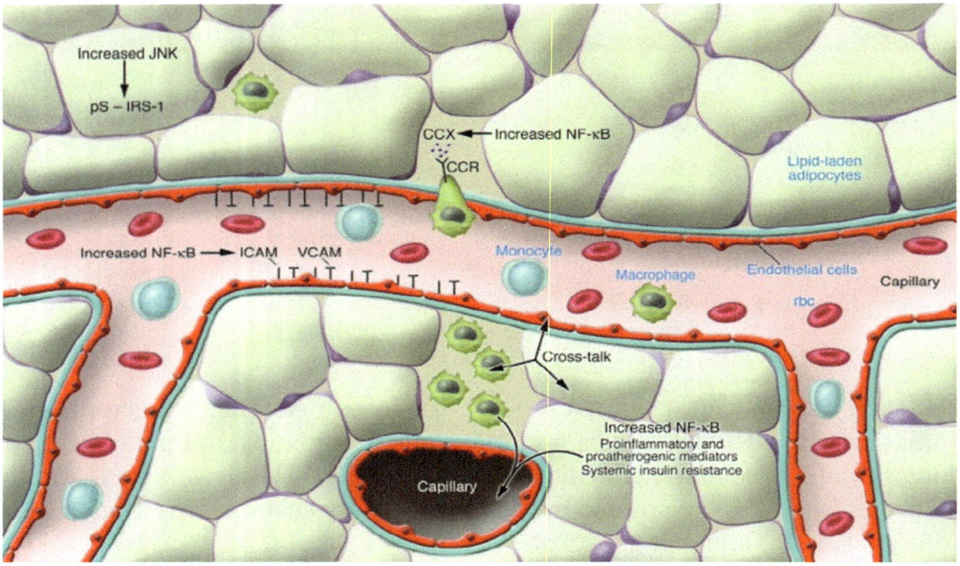

FIGURE 3.7 Possible pathways by which inflammation in adipose tissue is triggered.

stress. The initiation of these inflammatory pathways regulates protein phosphorylation and transcriptional programs,resulting in a rise in the release of pro-inflammatory cytokines like TNF-α, IL-6, leptin, and resistin, as well as pro-atherogenic mediators like PAI-1 and chemokines like MCP-1. At the same time, molecules that adhere to endothelium (e.g., A. Chemoattractant molecules and integrins and chemokine receptors (CCR) on monocytes interact with ICAM-1 and VCAM-1, facilitating their recruitment to adipose tissue. Once recruited, monocytes differentiate into macrophages, they produce a variety of cytokines and chemokines, including thosereleasedby adipocytes, which further intensify the inflammatory response. This process promotes local inflammation and contributes to systemic inflammatory responses. Additionally, the phosphorylation of serine residues (pS) plays aimportant role in modulating these signaling networks and metabolic dysfunction (Engin, 2017a, 2017b, 2024).

3.2 Role of toll-like receptors (TLRs)

Both endogenous danger signals released during metabolic stress and conserved microbial motifs can be recognized by the class of pattern recognition receptors called toll-like receptors. Among these, TLR2 and TLR4 are particularly relevant to metabolic inflammation. Saturated fatty acids such as palmitate and lipopolysaccharide (LPS) activate TLR4,which in turn activates the MAPK and NF-κBsignaling cascades (Kim & Sears, 2010). This signaling cascade results in the transcription of inflammatory genes, which leads to insulin resistance and metabolic dysfunction. Experimental models indicate that mice lacking the TLR4 gene experience reduced inflammation in their adipose (fat) tissue and are protected against insulin resistance caused by a high-fat diet (Tsukumo et al., 2007). Additionally, the improved insulin sensitivity and glucose tolerance observed in TLR2 mutant animals highlight the role of TLR2 receptors in linking innate immune signaling to metabolic regulation (Himes & Smith, 2010) (Fig. 3.8).

3.3 Inflammasomes (NLRP3)

The innate immune system greatly depends on cytosolic multiprotein complexes known as inflammasomes, which play an important role in identifying pathogenic microorganisms and various endogenous danger-associated molecular patterns (DAMPs). These complexes help caspase-1 in its autocatalytic activation, leading to the cleavage of pro-inflammatory cytokines pro-IL-1β and pro-IL-18 into their mature and bioactive forms. The most extensively studied inflammasome in relation to metabolic diseases, particularly type 2 diabetes and inflammation associated with obesity, is the NLRP3 inflammasome (NOD-like receptor family pyrin domain-containing 3) (Broz & Dixit, 2016;

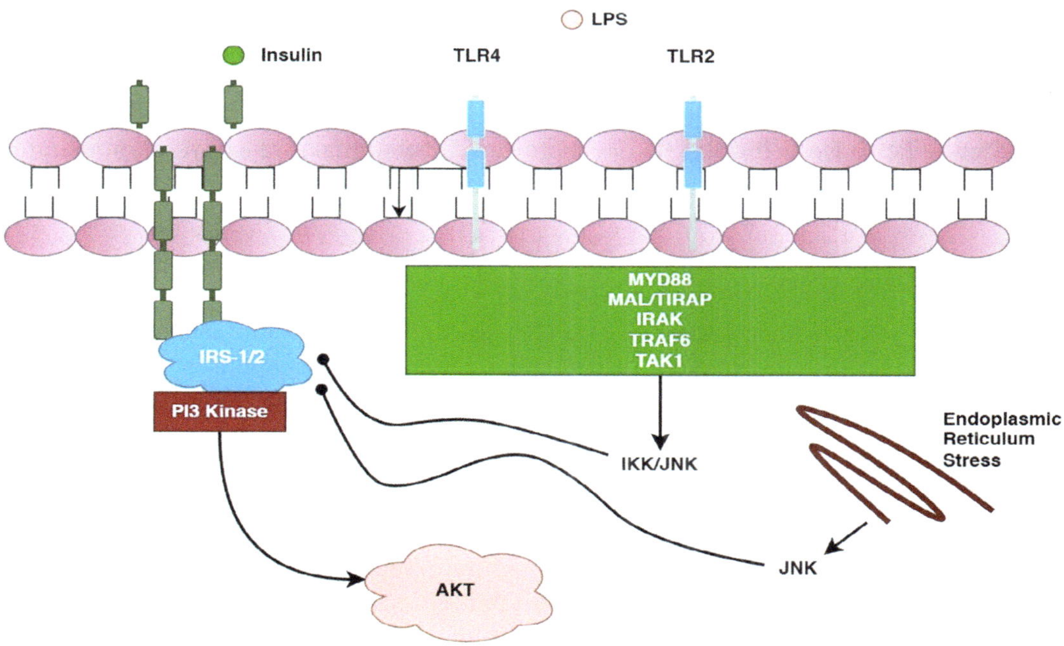

FIGURE 3.8 The toll-like receptor (TLR) two and TLR4 mechanism play a crucial role in regulating insulin signaling by interacting with various intracellular mediators. Key signaling components involved in this process include phosphoinositide 3-kinase (PI3K), protein kinase B (AKT), IκB kinase (IKK), and c-Jun N-terminal kinase (JNK). The inflammatory signaling cascade that intersects with insulin action is coordinated by adapter molecules such as myeloid differentiation primary response protein 88 (MyD88) and MyD88-adapter-like (MAL/TIRAP). Additionally, downstream effectors like TNFR-associated factor 6 (TRAF6) and transforming growth factor β-activated kinase 1 (TAK1) contribute to this regulatory network.

Stienstra et al., 2010). As a molecular sensor, NLRP3 incorporates a variety of environmental and metabolic stresses. Reactive oxygen species (ROS) buildup, mitochondrial dysfunction, high glucose levels, excess saturated fatty acids, and islet amyloid polypeptide (IAPP) are some of the factors that cause its activation in the context of type 2 diabetes (T2DM) (Masters et al., 2010; Wen et al., 2011).

These stimuli start a two-step activation process: a priming signal (Signal 1), usually through Toll-like receptors (TLRs) or cytokines like TNF-α, which causes transcriptional upregulation of NLRP3 and pro-IL-1β through NF-κB activation; and an activation signal (Signal 2), like potassium efflux, lysosomal rupture, or ROS production, which causes NLRP3 to oligomerize with pro-caspase-1 and ASC (apoptosis-associated speck-like protein containing a CARD) to form the active inflammasome complex (Guo, Callaway et al., 2015; Guo, Milburn, et al., 2015).

Pro-IL-1β and pro-IL-18, two crucial mediators of sterile inflammation, are cleaved into their active forms by activated caspase-1. In type 2 diabetes, IL-1β particularly has two detrimental effects. It first disrupts insulin signaling in peripheral organs by serine phosphorylating IRS-1 and preventing the formation of insulin receptors. Furthermore, by increasing oxidative stress and promoting endoplasmic reticulum stress within the islets, it directly leads to pancreatic β-cell dysfunction and death (Dinarello, 2011; Donath & Shoelson, 2011). The NLRP3 inflammasome has been linked with the development of type 2 diabetes, as indicated by both preclinical and clinical studies (Stienstra et al., 2010; Vandanmagsar et al., 2011). Additionally, treatment trials targeting IL-1 signaling—like those using the IL-1 receptor antagonist anakinra—have demonstrated that patients with type 2 diabetes experience improved glucose control and decreased inflammatory markers (Larsen et al., 2007) (Fig. 3.9).

3.4 Dendritic cells

Professional antigen-presenting cells (APCs), particularly dendritic cells (DCs), play a crucial role in initiating and regulating adaptive immune responses. Beyond their traditional function in adaptive immunity, DCs are increasingly recognized for their involvement in innate immune responses and chronic inflammation, particularly in metabolic disorders such as Type 2 Diabetes Mellitus (T2DM) (Soedono & Cho, 2021; Osborn & Olefsky, 2012). One of the primary risk factors for type 2 diabetes (T2D) is obesity, which leads to the infiltration of dendritic cells (DCs) into visceral adipose tissue, where they develop a pro-inflammatory phenotype. During this transition, co-stimulatory molecules such as CD80 and CD86 are upregulated, while pro-inflammatory cytokines like interleukin-6 (IL-6), interleukin-12 (IL-12), and tumor necrosis factor-α (TNF-α) are released more frequently (Soedono & Cho , 2021). This inflammatory microenvironment exacerbates both local and systemic inflammation, as T helper (Th) cells become more polarized toward Th1 and Th17 lineages, which produce cytokines like IL-17 and interferon-γ (IFN-γ) (Reynolds et al., 2012). These immunological changes disrupt insulin receptor signaling in key metabolic tissues,

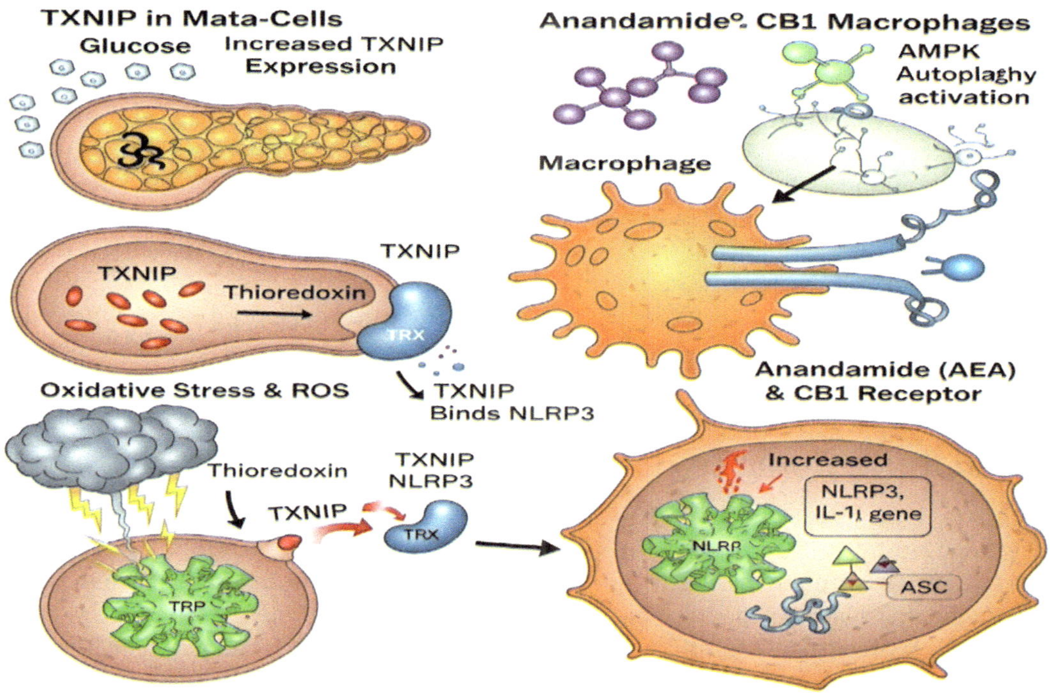

FIGURE 3.9 In type 2 diabetes (T2D), both macrophages and pancreatic islet β-cells play a role in initiating the NLRP3 inflammasome. Under hyperglycemic conditions, the expression of thioredoxin-interacting protein (TXNIP) is increased in β-cells. Reactive oxygen species (ROS) produced during oxidative stress cause TXNIP to dissociate from its binding partner, thioredoxin (TRX). This allows TXNIP to interact with NLRP3, initiating the assembly of the inflammasome. Meanwhile, the endocannabinoid anandamide binds to cannabinoid receptor 1 (CB1) on macrophages and other myeloid cells, which enhances the expression of NLRP3, the interleukin-1 beta (IL-1β) gene, and the adapter protein ASC. All of these elements are essential for activating the inflammasome. Saturated fatty acids (SFAs) further worsen this process by inhibiting AMP-activated protein kinase (AMPK), an enzyme that senses energy and regulates autophagy. Impaired AMPK signaling reduces autophagic clearance, leading to mitochondrial dysfunction and an accumulation of mitochondrial ROS (mtROS), which further activates the NLRP3 inflammasome. Additionally, macrophages take up soluble islet amyloid polypeptide (IAPP) through the scavenger receptor CD36. Inside the cells, IAPP aggregates into amyloid fibrils that destabilize lysosomes, releasing cathepsin proteases that serve as additional triggers for NLRP3 activation. In T2D patients, the progressive deposition of IAPP within pancreatic islets and its uptake by immune cells amplify inflammasome activity, worsening β-cell dysfunction and systemic inflammation (Masters et al., 2010; Zhou et al., 2010; Wen et al., 2011).

including the liver, adipose tissue, and skeletal muscle, ultimately leading to insulin resistance. In addition to their role in adipose tissue inflammation, DCs also have pathogenic effects in pancreatic islets, further worsening β-cell dysfunction and contributing to disease progression. Their capacity to internalize and transfer autoantigens produced by β-cells to T cells may cause or exacerbate autoreactive immune responses that result in apoptosis and β-cell dysfunction. This interaction might be especially significant as T2DM worsens because β-cell failure is a major determinant of the disease's severity (Ferris et al., 2014). The inflammatory loop in adipose tissue is exacerbated by the interaction between dendritic cells (DCs) and adipocytes, driven by the release of various cytokines and chemokines. Adipocytes secrete substances such as resistin, leptin, and free fatty acids (FFAs) that can activate DCs. In turn, the cytokines released by DCs, including TNF-α and IL-6, promote insulin resistance in adipocytes (McNelis & Olefsky, 2014; Osborn & Olefsky, 2012). This creates a cycle that amplifies metabolic inflammation in a bidirectional manner. An illustration of the interaction between immunological and metabolic pathways that results in type 2 diabetes is this reciprocal relationship. Recent findings indicate that dendritic cells in metabolic organs play a crucial role in both innate and adaptive immune responses, fulfilling various functions. These dendritic cells could be a promising intervention point for type 2 diabetes management because of their involvement in chronic low-grade inflammation, which contributes to insulin resistance and may directly impact β-cell function.

4. Adaptive immune responses in T2DM

Cytotoxic T lymphocytes, also known as $CD8^+$ T cells, are associated with insulin resistance and β-cell dysfunction in type 2 diabetes mellitus (T2DM). Within adipose tissue, $CD8^+$ T lymphocytes contribute to increased inflammation and decreased insulin sensitivity by triggering macrophage activation and adipocyte death (Nishimura et al., 2009; Park & Shastri, 2022). Additionally, they directly encourage the death of β-cells in the pancreatic islets, which lowers the amount of insulin secreted (Walter & Santamaria, 2005). According to Velikova et al. (2021), B cells and autoantibodies also aid in the advancement of the disease by releasing pro-inflammatory cytokines such TNF-α and IL-6, which worsen insulin resistance.Furthermore, B cells have the ability to deliver antigens, which can activate T cells and prolong chronic inflammation (DeFuria et al., 2013).Autoantibodies like GAD65 and IA-2 speed up β-cell death in Latent Autoimmune Diabetes in Adults (LADA), resulting in early insulin dependence (Grasso et al., 2001; Joneset al., 2021) (Fig. 3.10).

The relationships between various immune cells and signaling pathways in diabetes are shown in Fig. 4.2. The process starts with hypertrophic adipocytes, which trigger antigen-presenting cells like dendritic cells and macrophages by releasing stress signals and danger-associated molecular patterns (DAMPs). These activated cells promote the onset of naïve T cells in local lymphoid tissues into more pro-inflammatory subsets, such as Th1 and Th17 cells. Interferon-gamma (IFN-γ) and tumor necrosis factor-alpha (TNF-α), which are produced by Th1 cells, encourage M1 macrophage polarization and local tissue inflammation. Insulin signaling in peripheral organs like the liver and muscles is further disrupted by Th17 cells' production of interleukin-17 (IL-17) and interleukin-21 (IL-21), which causes oxidative stress and endothelial dysfunction.

At the same time, regulatory T cells (Tregs), which typically regulate immune activation and preserve tolerance, are noticeably declining. This regulatory axis is weakened by a decreased presence of FOXP3 Tregs, which permits inflammation to continue. In patients with type 2 diabetes, metabolic dysregulation and elevated insulin resistance

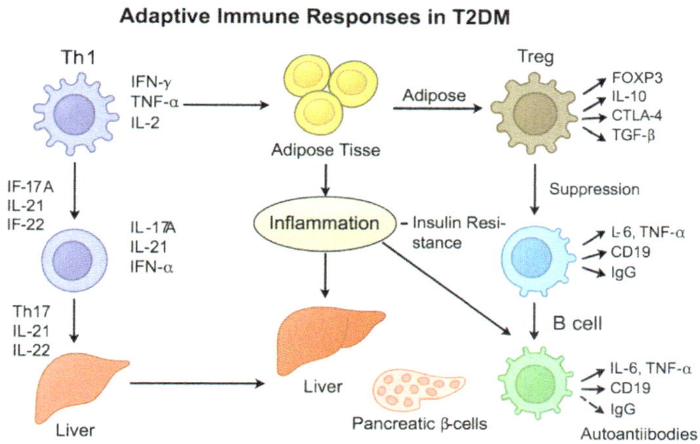

FIGURE 3.10 Gives a visual depiction of how various immune cells and signaling pathways interact in diabetic disorders.

have been associated with Treg cell depletion (Yang et al., 2018). Upon entering adipose tissue and pancreatic islets, $CD8^+$ cytotoxic T lymphocytes release perforin and Granzyme B, resulting in β-cell dysfunction and adipocyte death. The cytotoxic effects that have been observed are one of the main reasons for immune-mediated β-cell death in type 2 diabetes (Wang et al., 2018).

In autoimmune diseases like Latent Autoimmune Diabetes in Adults (LADA), B cells have two functions. They not only secrete proinflammatory cytokines but also produce autoantibodies that contribute to β-cell loss. These autoantibodies impair insulin production and exacerbate immunological dysfunction associated with diabetes (Fousteri et al., 2017). The diabetic condition is exacerbated by these adaptive immune changes that impair insulin responsiveness and secretion. The pathways depicted are currently being actively studied for therapeutic intervention; targets include immune checkpoints, cytokines, and cell-specific inhibitors with the goal of re-establishing metabolic health and immune balance. Recent advances in immune modulation therapies have shown potential in addressing the immune component of insulin resistance (Hotamisligil, 2017a, 2017b).

5. Role of gut microbiota and the immune system in T2DM

The gut microbiota plays more widely recognized for a critical role in the etiology of type 2 diabetes mellitus (T2DM) through several complex processes. An imbalance in the gut microbiota composition and function is known as dysbiosis, which significantly impacts immunological dysregulation, chronic inflammation, and metabolic disorders. The development of type 2 diabetes may be facilitated by this change in microbial communities, which may result in a situation in which harmful microorganisms multiply and beneficial microorganisms are reduced (Zhang et al., 2021; Zhou et al., 2022). Type 2 diabetes mellitus (T2DM) is associated with two significant microbial metabolites produced by the gut microbiota: short-chain fatty acids (SCFAs) and lipopolysaccharides (LPS). Research has shown that SCFAs, which are generated when beneficial bacteria ferment dietary fibers, have strong anti-inflammatory effects, help regulate glucose levels, and enhance insulin sensitivity. Conversely, LPS can trigger inflammation and immune responses when they translocate into the bloodstream, exacerbating the metabolic dysfunctions associated with T2DM (Zhang et al., 2021).

Furthermore, it is becoming more well acknowledged that gut microbiota influence host epigenetics, which is defined as stable, heritable gene expression changes independent of DNA sequence alteration. These microbiological effects have the ability to modify metabolic signaling pathways and inflammatory responses, which in turn helps to activate the NLRP3 inflammasome, a vital part of the innate immune system. This inflammasome's activation intensifies inflammatory cascades, which worsen metabolic abnormalities and hasten the development of type 2 diabetes (Sharma et al., 2022).

The intestinal barrier, a vital defensive system that prevents potentially dangerous bacteria and metabolites from entering the bloodstream, may be weakened in people with type 2 diabetes. This disruption allows harmful entities to infiltrate the circulatory system, which can result in systemic inflammation and multi-organ damage, contributing to the complications frequently observed in diabetes, such as cardiovascular diseases and neuropathy (Chong et al. ,2025). Therapeutic approaches that target the alteration of gut microbiota have garnered significant attention for the prevention and treatment of type 2 diabetes mellitus (T2DM) due to continuous research developments. Among these, probiotics—live microorganisms that aid in the restoration of a healthy microbial balance—and prebiotics—non-digestible dietary components that specifically promote the growth and activity of beneficial microbes—have demonstrated encouraging promise. Another potential strategy for restoring microbial balance and opening up new treatment options for type 2 diabetes is fecal microbiota transplantation (FMT), a process that involves transferring intestinal microbial populations from healthy donors to recipients. Additionally, dietary interventions that emphasize the consumption of fiber-rich and nutrient-dense foods support the growth of beneficial gut bacteria, which can lead to improved metabolic outcomes. When combined, these strategies seek to enhance the health and lifestyle of patients with type 2 diabetes by improving its outcomes and reducing associated problems (Riedel et al., 2022).

The significance of gut health in preventing and treating type 2 diabetes is highlighted by the intricate relationship between metabolic health and the gut bacteria (Fig. 3.11).

5.1 Dysbiosis and increased gut permeability

Maintaining metabolic health and regulating immunological responses throughout the body heavily depend on gut bacteria. The emergence of type 2 Diabetes Mellitus (T2DM)

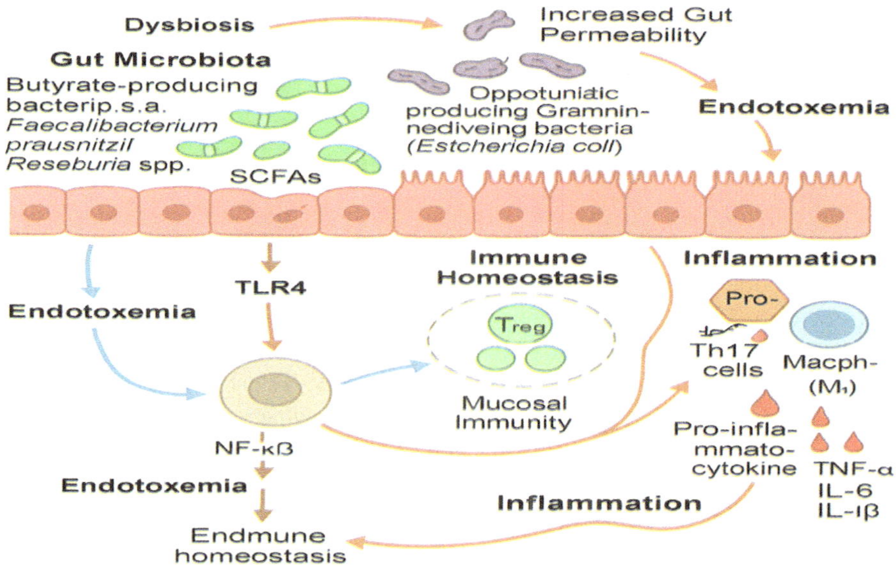

FIGURE 3.11 The connection between inflammation, the immune system, and gut microbiota in type 2 diabetes mellitus (T2DM) is crucial. A decrease in bacteria that produce short-chain fatty acids (SCFAs) and an excess of Gram-negative bacteria that are rich in lipopolysaccharides (LPS) are signs of gut microbiota dysbiosis, which affects the integrity of the intestinal barrier and encourages endotoxemia in people with type 2 diabetes mellitus (T2DM). Pro-inflammatory cytokines like interleukin-6 (IL-6), interleukin-1 beta (IL-1β), and tumor necrosis factor-alpha (TNF-α) are released continuously when circulating LPS levels are elevated. Thus, systemic inflammation and metabolic dysfunction are sustained by activating nuclear factor kappa-light-chain-enhancer of activated B cells (NF-κB) and stimulating toll-like receptor 4 (TLR4) signaling within immune cells.This persistent inflammation disrupts insulin signaling and alters the mucosal immune environment, leading to an increase in Th17 cells and M1 macrophages, while decreasing regulatory T cells (Tregs). Ultimately, these changes contribute to insulin resistance, which is characteristic of type 2 diabetes.

has been closely linked to dysbiosis, a state of microbial imbalance, according to a recent study. Increased intestinal permeability can result from the breakdown of tight connections between the epithelial cells lining the gut, caused by a disturbance in the delicate balance of gut bacteria (Chong et al., 2025).

This increased permeability becomes a gateway for various bacterial components, particularly lipopolysaccharides (LPS), to enter the bloodstream. The translocation of LPS is known to provoke significant systemic inflammation, an issue that is exacerbated by the impaired barrier function of the gut (Burcelin, 2016). When gut defenses deteriorate, the equilibrium between gut bacteria and host immunological responses is upset.

Thus, a series of negative consequences, such as the development of chronic inflammation, increased oxidative stress, and disturbances in insulin signaling pathways, are hallmarks of the pathophysiology of type 2 diabetes.The intricate relationships between different elements highlight the critical role that gut bacteria play in both preserving metabolic health and causing metabolic disorders like type 2 diabetes. Gaining a better understanding of these interactions may lead to new therapeutic approaches aimed at restoring gut health, which could help reduce the incidence of diabetes (Yoo et al., 2020).

5.2 Endotoxemia and metabolic inflammation

Metabolic endotoxemia occurs when bacterial products, particularly lipopolysaccharides (LPS), enter the bloodstream due to a compromised intestinal barrier. After activation, macrophages and antigen-presenting cells release pro-inflammatory cytokines, including tumor necrosis factor-alpha (TNF-α), interleukin-1 beta (IL-1β), and interleukin-6 (IL-6). Additionally, immunological receptors, such as Toll-like receptor 4 (TLR4), are activated as a result of this activation. These inflammatory mediators significantly disrupt insulin receptor signaling, affecting metabolic control in peripheral tissues such as skeletal muscle, liver, and adipose tissue. This disruption leads to insulin resistance, impairing the cells' ability to absorb glucose and resulting in glucose dysregulation, which is a hallmark of metabolic diseases such as type 2 Diabetes Mellitus (Berbudi et al., 2025; Fuke et al., 2019).

A chronic pro-inflammatory environment linked to microbial dysbiosis—an imbalance in the gut microbiota—exacerbates insulin resistance in both type 1 and type 2 diabetes. This ongoing inflammation reduces immunological tolerance and increases the risk of autoimmune reactions in the body. Additionally, it adversely affects pancreatic β-cell function, leading to impaired insulin production and worsening insulin deficiency (Bielka et al., 2022).

In summary, the relationship between endotoxemia and metabolic inflammation is crucial for understanding diabetes pathology. Addressing these factors provides a pathway for innovative therapeutic strategies aimed at improving insulin sensitivity and overall metabolic health.

5.3 Gut immune homeostasis

Under normal physiological conditions, the gut microbiota is crucial for maintaining immune balance in the gastrointestinal tract by regulating pro-inflammatory and anti-inflammatory responses. Short-chain fatty acids (SCFAs), particularly butyrate, propionate, and acetate, are produced when beneficial bacteria ferment dietary fibers and play a significant role in regulating this process. In addition to their well-known roles in metabolic processes, SCFAs have powerful immunomodulatory effects that support the integrity of the epithelial barrier and help maintain the overall health of the immune system.One of the primary functions of SCFAs is to strengthen the intestinal barrier, which is crucial for preventing harmful infections and toxins from leaking through the gut lining into the bloodstream of the host. By promoting this barrier function, SCFAs act as guardians of the gut. Additionally, FOXP3-regulatory T cells (Tregs), a specialized subset of immune cells essential for modulating and attenuating immune responses, are stimulated to proliferate and differentiate, which is essential for maintaining tolerance to the divese array of microorganisms in the gut and preventing excessive inflammatory reactions. In the stomach, short-chain fatty acids (SCFAs) stimulate the synthesis of anti-inflammatory cytokines, such as interleukin-10 (IL-10), to further reduce inflammation and preserve a balanced immunological milieu (Ali et al., 2022; Ratajczak et al., 2019; Yap & Mariño, 2020).

However, when dysbiosis occurs—characterized by a disruption in the microbial community and a subsequent decline in SCFA production—the equilibrium that was so carefully maintained begins to falter. This shift often leads to a predominance of pro-inflammatory responses, effectively weakening mucosal immunity and setting the stage for a host of complications, particularly in the context of Type 2 diabetes. The decreased production of SCFAs removes essential protective effects, paving the way for heightened oxidative stress and promoting systemic inflammation. This discord not only hampers local immune responses but also disrupts essential metabolic functions, including glucose homeostasis and the proper functioning of pancreatic β-cells (Roelofsen et al., 2010; Yoo et al., 2020).

Understanding the crucial interactions between the immune system and gut microbiota reveals exciting opportunities for developing therapeutic approaches to manage diabetes. By recognizing the gut-immune axis, researchers can develop innovative methods to enhance immune regulation and restore microbial balance. Interventions aimed at promoting a healthy gut microbiota composition, including dietary changes and the use of probiotics, synbiotics, and prebiotics, are currently being actively explored. These strategies aim to elevate SCFA production, reduce inflammation, and bolster overall metabolic health. By fostering a healthier gut environment, these approaches not only hold promise for managing diabetes but also for achieving long-term health and vitality (Baghel et al., 2024; Chu et al., 2025) (Fig. 3.12).

6. Autoimmunity and type 2 diabetes

Autoimmunity has been strongly linked to the onset and progression of type 2 diabetes (T2D), according to recent scientific investigations. Researchers have found that islet autoantibodies and self-reactive T cells are present in the blood of individuals with type 2 diabetes.This complex interaction highlights the significant autoimmune response that contributes to the pathophysiology of this disease (de Candia et al., 2019; Itariu & Stulnig, 2014).

The detection of autoimmune indicators is essential because they are associated with a significantly faster decline in β cell function. β-cells, located in the pancreatic islets, produce and release insulin, which is crucial for regulating blood glucose levels. Researchers assess β-cell function using fasting C-peptide levels and responses to

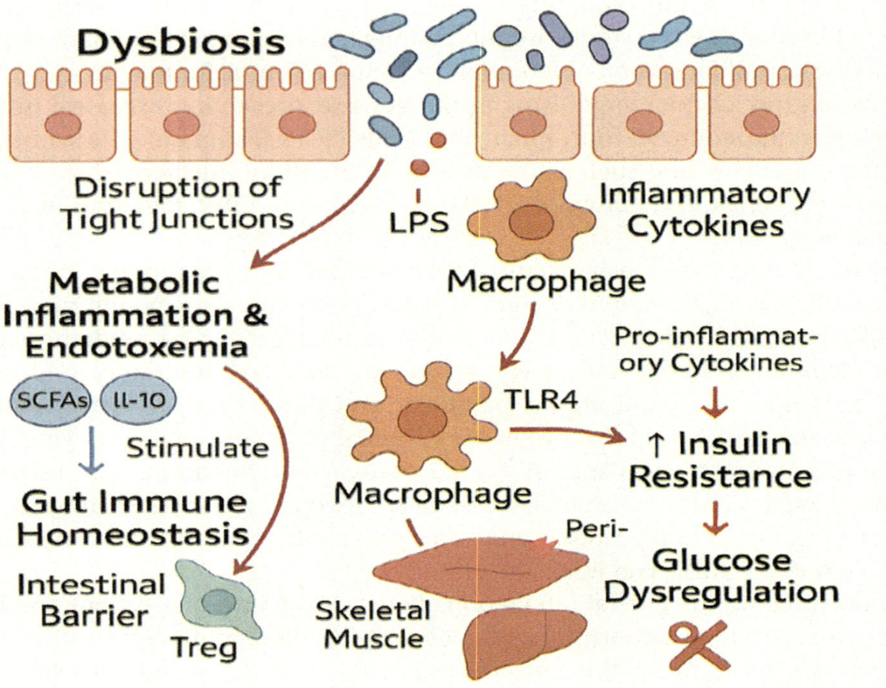

FIGURE 3.12 Gut dysbiosis and immune imbalance: A pathway to metabolic inflammation in type 2 diabetes.

glucagon stimulation—two critical measures that illuminate how effectively these cells continue to perform their vital roles as T2D progresses (Brooks-Worrell et al., 2014).

Adding another layer of complexity to this picture is the chronic low-grade inflammation that typifies T2D. This persistent inflammatory state may trigger autoimmune activation by exposing previously masked "self" antigens to the immune system. Autoreactive cells become active when the immune system targets these antigens, which are normally protected by immune defenses. Additionally, the involvement of innate immune systems, particularly macrophages, along with T cells, significantly compounds the inflammatory processes that occur in T2D (de Candia et al., 2019).

The emergence of islet autoimmunity in patients with T2D has been shown to dramatically accelerate the functional decline of β-cells. As these immune processes impair the ability of β-cells to produce sufficient insulin, patients experience increasing levels of hyperglycemia, further complicating the already challenging nature of the disease.

These findings have significant implications, highlighting the importance of considering autoimmunity as a crucial factor in the pathophysiology of type 2 diabetes. This perspective ought to coexist alongside other pivotal mechanisms, such as autophagy—the cellular process responsible for degrading and recycling damaged cellular components—and β-cell dedifferentiation, which refers to the loss of the specialized characteristics and functions of mature β-cells (Zhang, 2023). Exploring the complex relationships among these variables may lead to new treatment strategies that address more than just T2D symptoms, but also addressing the underlying autoimmune processes to enhance patient outcomes significantly (Fig. 3.13).

6.1 Islet autoimmunity in T2DM

Type 2 diabetes (T2D), traditionally defined by insulin resistance and metabolic dysfunction, has a complex and intriguing relationship with islet autoimmunity, as highlighted in recent studies. Once primarily associated with type 1 diabetes, islet autoimmunity is now recognized to play aimportant role in type 2 diabetes. Current research indicates that 41.3% of people with type 2 diabetes exhibit cellular islet autoimmunity, whereas 13.5% show signs of humoral islet autoimmunity. Moreover, approximately 5.3% of these patients demonstrate both humoral and cellular immune responses against pancreatic islet cells, further underscoring the importance of islet autoimmunity in T2D (Brooks-Worrell et al., 2022).

The implications of these findings are profound, particularly regarding the progression and management of T2D. A quicker decline in the function of β-cells, which are insulin-producing cells in the pancreas, has been linked to islet autoimmunity. This functional decline can lead to significantly poorer glycemic control, making it

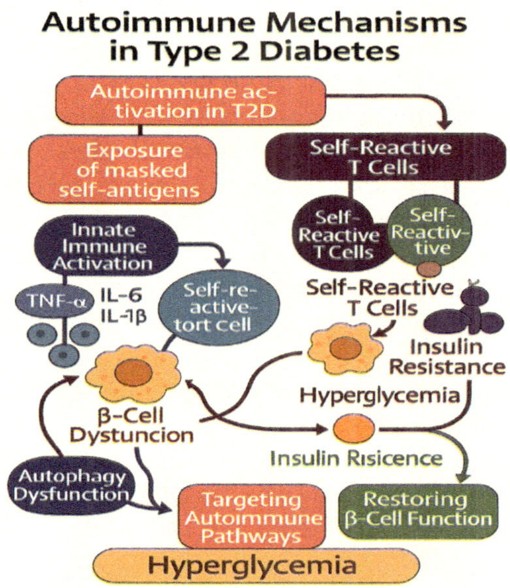

FIGURE 3.13 Autoimmune mechanisms in type 2 diabetes: From inflammation to β-cell dysfunction.

increasingly challenging for patients to regulate their blood sugar levels (Brooks-Worrell et al., 2014, 2022). As β-cells deteriorate, patients may find themselves requiring more aggressive treatment strategies to manage their diabetes effectively. Several underlying mechanisms may contribute to the onset of islet autoimmunity in T2D, with chronic systemic inflammation being a notable suspect. This type of inflammation is often observed in individuals with obesity and can serve as a catalyst for an autoimmune response targeting the pancreatic islets. Such inflammatory processes can trigger heightened endoplasmic reticulum stress within β-cells, thereby compromising their health and functionality (Brooks-Worrell & Palmer, 2019). Furthermore, research has demonstrated a clear connection between the progressive decline in β-cell function and the autoimmune response affecting islet cells, highlighting the significant role that these autoimmune reactions may play in the onset of type 2 diabetes (Brooks-Worrell et al., 2013). The recognition of islet autoimmunity as a vital component of T2D holds substantial promise for the future of diabetes research and treatment. By acknowledging the autoimmune underpinnings of T2D, researchers and clinicians can pave the way for transformative changes in the classification and management of the disease. This fresh viewpoint could result in the creation of novel treatment strategies that explicitly target autoimmune pathways, which would ultimately improve outcomes for a sizable portion of T2D patients.The medical community can improve patient management techniques and tailor therapeutic treatments more successfully by gaining a better understanding of these intricate underlying systems (Brooks-Worrell et al., 2020; Pilla et al., 2024) (Fig. 3.14).

6.2 Overlap with latent autoimmune diabetes in adults (LADA)

A distinct kind of diabetes that combines elements of type 1 and type 2 diabetes mellitus is called latent autoimmune diabetes in adults (LADA). This condition is typically diagnosed in adults who exhibit symptoms of type 2 diabetes while also having characteristics of type 1 diabetes-associated autoantibodies (Naik et al., 2009). This distinction is crucial as it affects the approach to treatment and management. Genetically, LADA shows significant overlap with type 1 diabetes, particularly in associations with certain HLA region variants. However, the effect sizes in LADA tend to be smaller compared to classic type 1 diabetes (Andersen & Hansen, 2010). This relationship suggests a nuanced genetic background that may influence disease onset and progression.

The development of latent autoimmune diabetes in adults (LADA) is significantly influenced by environmental variables. Insulin resistance may be involved in LADA since risk factors such being overweight and living a sedentary lifestyle closely mimic those linked to type 2 diabetes. This overlap in risk profiles complicates the clinical classification of diabetes subtypes and offers critical understanding of disease mechanisms.

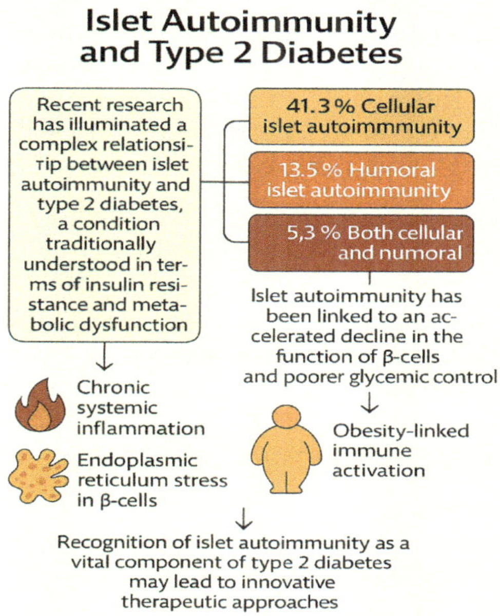

FIGURE 3.14 Islet autoimmunity in type 2 diabetes: Mechanisms and clinical implications.

Disease advancement in LADA is typically more aggressive than in type 2 diabetes; many patients often progress to requiring insulin therapy shortly after their diagnosis (Carlsson, 2019). Some studies suggest that glitazones may be beneficial in the early stages of LADA, although insulin remains the primary treatment for individuals with this condition. Effective management and therapy necessitate a comprehensive understanding of LADA, as misclassification can lead to inappropriate therapy strategies (Pollak & Vásquez, 2012).

7. The immune system's impact on insulin sensitivity and secretion

The immune system plays a crucial role in managing metabolic health, especially concerning insulin activity. This regulation becomes particularly significant in conditions like obesity and type 2 diabetes (T2D), where inflammatory processes interfere with insulin's ability to function effectively (Hotamisligil, 2017a, 2017b).

In a healthy state, the immune system supports insulin activity. However, chronic low-grade inflammation significantly impairs insulin signaling, particularly in cases of obesity. Increased levels of pro-inflammatory cytokines, including interleukin-6 (IL-6), interleukin-1 beta (IL-1β), and tumor necrosis factor-alpha (TNF-α), are frequently seen in the circulation and adipose (fat) tissue during obesity (Zatterale et al., 2020).

These cytokines lead to abnormal phosphorylation of insulin receptor substrates (IRS-1 and IRS-2) by activating intracellular stress pathways such as JNK1 and IKKβ. This change impacts insulin signaling in tissues like muscle and liver, resulting in insulin resistance (McArdle et al., 2013).

7.1 Immune cell shifts and metabolic inflammation

- In lean individuals, immune cells with anti-inflammatory roles—such as M2 macrophages, regulatory T cells (Tregs), and eosinophils—are more active. These cells help maintain insulin sensitivity through cytokines like TGF-β and IL-10.
- Obesity leads to an increase in Th1 cells, $CD8^+$ T cells, and M1 macrophages in adipose tissue. The inflammatory cytokines released by these cells directly impair insulin signaling (Chawla et al., 2011)

7.2 Mechanisms of impaired insulin sensitivity

- Activation of stress kinases like JNK and IKKβ
- IRS proteins are typically phosphorylated on serine residues instead of tyrosine, which is more common in other proteins.
- Inhibition of the PI3K/AKT signaling **pathway**
- Decreased glucose uptake due to disrupted GLUT4 translocation (Acosta-Martinez & Cabail, 2022)

  ➢**Immune Influence on Insulin Secretion**

The immune system affects how pancreatic β-cells secrete insulin. These β-cells, found in the islets of Langerhans, are extremely sensitive to inflammatory situations (Dludla et al., 2023).

➢ **Cytokine Effects on β-Cells**

Interferon-gamma (IFN-γ), tumor necrosis factor-alpha (TNF-α), and interleukin-1 beta (IL-1β) are examples of cytokines that can:

- Cause endoplasmic reticulum (ER) stress and oxidative stress.
- Induce cell death (apoptosis) or disrupt β-cell function.
- Decreased secretion and expression of the insulin gene (Lambelet et al., 2018; Eizirik et al., 2009)

➢ **Chronic Inflammation and Autoimmunity**

- In type 1 diabetes, the immune system mistakenly targets the β-cells, which are important for producing insulin.
- In type 2 diabetes, prolonged inflammation contributes to gradual β-cell dysfunction, often leading to dedifferentiation—a process where β-cells lose their insulin-producing identity (Atkinson et al., 2014; Donath, 2014).

➢ **Immune-β-Cell Cross-talk**

Long-term inflammation can alter the cellular environment of pancreatic islets, disrupting communication and structure, and further impairing insulin production (Eguchi & Nagai, 2017).

7.3 Immune mediators affecting insulin receptor signaling

1. TNF-α, which stands for tumor necrosis factor-alpha, is a cytokine involved in systemic inflammation.
   - Produced by adipocytes and M1 macrophages**.**
   - Action: Activates JNK and IKKβ, causing abnormal phosphorylation of IRS proteins. It also upregulates SOCS3, which promotes IRS degradation.
   - Result: Marked decrease in insulin responsiveness in muscle, liver, and fat tissues (Xu et al., 2002).

2. **Interleukin-6 (IL-6)**
   - Produced by immune cells located in adipose tissue.
   - **Action:** Engages the JAK/STAT pathway, leading to increased SOCS3 expression. SOCS3 blocks IRS-1 and flags it for degradation.
   - **Result:** Reduced insulin sensitivity, especially in the liver (Fasshauer et al., 2004).

3. **Interleukin-1β (IL-1β)**
   - Produced by: Macrophages and pancreatic immune cells
   - Action: Induces oxidative and ER stress in both β-cells and peripheral tissue. Suppresses IRS expression.
   - Result: Disrupts both insulin action and insulin production (Burke et al., 2015).

4. **Interferon-gamma (IFN-γ)**
   - Produced by natural killer (NK) cells and T helper 1 (Th1) cells.
   - Action: Amplifies inflammation by activating STAT1 and SOCS pathways, which interfere with insulin signaling.
   - **Result:** Worsens insulin resistance through inflammatory reinforcement (Wada et al., 2011).

5. **C-reactive Protein (CRP)**
   - Produced in response to systemic inflammation
   - Action: While not directly involved in signaling, elevated CRP levels are associated with impaired **endothelial insulin response.**
   - Result: Marker of metabolic stress and insulin resistance in clinical settings (Bahceci et al., 2004).

7.4 Cytokine-induced beta-cell dysfunction

Cytokine	Source	Effects on β-Cells
IL-1β	Macrophages, β-cells	ER stress, oxidative damage, insulin gene suppression, apoptosis
TNF-α	Macrophages	JNK activation, apoptosis, insulin signaling inhibition
IFN-γ	Th1 cells, NK cells	STAT1 activation, immune targeting, synergistic toxicity

➢ **Clinical Relevance & Therapeutic Insight**
- Blocking IL-1β (e.g., with Anakinra) has shown promise in improving β-cell function in T2D.
- Anti-TNF therapies, commonly used in autoimmune diseases, are being explored for metabolic benefits.
- Understanding the inflammatory landscape in adipose tissue and pancreatic islets is key to identifying new diabetes treatments.

Both type 1 and type 2 diabetes involve interactions between the immune system and insulin function.Understanding the signaling mechanisms and immune mediators involved opens the door for targeted therapies—such as anti-inflammatory drugs, cytokine inhibitors, and immunomodulators—to improve metabolic outcomes in affected individuals (Larsen et al., 2007; Gonzalez-Gay et al., 2006; Hotamisligil, 2017a, 2017b; Gupta et al., 2025).

8. Therapeutic modulation of the immune system in T2DM

Research on the regulation of the immune system for therapeutic purposes in type 2 Diabetes Mellitus (T2DM) is advancing swiftly. While T2DM has traditionally been regarded as a metabolic disorder, it is now understood that insulin resistance and β-cell dysfunction primarily result from dysregulation of the immune system and chronic low-grade inflammation (Hameed et al., 2015). The immune system in people with type 2 diabetes (T2DM) tends to remain moderately active at all times, leading to a persistently low-grade inflammatory state. This is often caused by excess fat, particularly in the abdomen. Fat cells release inflammatory substances known as cytokines, such as TNF-α, IL-6, and IL-1β, which interfere with insulin action. This makes it harder for the body to manage blood sugar levels properly. To counter this, researchers are exploring anti-inflammatory treatments. IL-1 blockers like canakinumab and anakinra are being used to reduce inflammation in the pancreas, which may help improve insulin production. TNF-α blockers, typically used in conditions like rheumatoid arthritis, have also been tested for diabetes, though results have been mixed. IL-6 blockers like tocilizumab are still being studied to see if they might increases the body's ability to respond to insulin (Al-Hilu, 2025; Macedo, 2019, pp. 145–167; Porto et al., 2006). Interestingly, some common diabetes medications also have anti-inflammatory effects. Metformin, for example, not only lowers blood sugar but also reduces inflammation by calming certain immune system pathways. Thiazolidinediones (TZDs), such as pioglitazone, enhance the function of fat cells and reduce the inflammatory response of immune cells. Likewise, SGLT2 inhibitors may decrease oxidative stress and inflammation in the body by promoting the excretion of excess sugar through urine (Weinberg Sibony et al., 2024; Kim et al., 2013).

An immunological cell imbalance is associated with type 2 diabetes mellitus (T2DM). There are frequently too many "aggressive" immune cells, like M1 macrophages and pro-inflammatory T-cells like Th1 and Th17, and too few "peacekeeping" cells, called regulatory T-cells (Tregs). Researchers are working on ways to fix this imbalance. One approach involves boosting Tregs using low doses of IL-2. Another strategy is to help macrophages switch from their aggressive M1 form to the more calming M2 type. Researchers are also investigating the potential benefits of enhancing gut health through fecal transplants, probiotics, or prebiotics on inflammation and immunological response (Juan et al., 2015; Kartika & Wibowo, 2020; Zeng et al., 2011).

Lifestyle modifications can significantly influence immune system function. Chronic inflammation can be reduced through practices such as intermittent fasting and following anti-inflammatory diets like the Mediterranean diet. Certain natural substances have shown promise in promoting immune balance, including vitamin D, resveratrol (found in red wine and grapes), omega-3 fatty acids, and curcumin (found in turmeric). Additionally, regular exercise is an effective strategy as it helps lower inflammation throughout the body and supports the regulation of immune cells (Dragičević Tomičić et al., 2025; Razavi et al., 2017).

Looking ahead, there are several promising and experimental treatments in development. These include vaccines designed to target specific inflammatory pathways, monoclonal antibodies that block immune system triggers, and stem cell therapy aimed at regenerating insulin-producing cells in the pancreas. Researchers are also exploring immune "checkpoint" therapies—similar to those used in cancer treatment—as a way to reset the actions of the immune system in people with type 2 diabetes (Wehbe, 2024).

8.1 Anti-inflammatory treatments for type 2 diabetes (T2DM)

In Type 2 Diabetes, the body doesn't just struggle with sugar—it's also dealing with chronic, low-level inflammation.This ongoing inflammation can damage the pancreatic cells responsible for producing insulin and hinder insulin's ability to function properly. That's why scientists and doctors are looking at anti-inflammatory treatments as a way to help manage and possibly improve diabetes.

8.1.1 Targeting inflammatory signals (cytokine inhibitors)

Certain immune chemicals, called cytokines, are elevated in people with T2DM and contribute to the problem. New medications are trying to block these troublemakers.

- IL-1β Inhibitors (like *Anakinra* and *Canakinumab*) These help calm inflammation in the pancreas and may improve how well it produces insulin. Some studies show they can lower blood sugar and inflammation.
- TNF-α Inhibitors (like *Etanercept* and *Infliximab*) These block TNF-α, another inflammatory signal. While they've been helpful in autoimmune diseases, results in diabetes are mixed—some people benefit, others not as much.
- IL-6 Inhibitors (like *Tocilizumab*) Still being studied, but early signs suggest they might help the body respond better to insulin (Bashir et al., 2022; Peiró et al., 2017)

8.1.2 Diabetes medications that also fight inflammation

Some commonly used diabetes drugs don't just control blood sugar—they also help reduce inflammation:

- MetforminA first-line diabetes drug that also calms the immune system by turning off certain inflammatory signals in the body (Natali & Ferrannini, 2006).
- TZDs (Thiazolidinediones) like *Pioglitazone*These help cells become more sensitive to insulin and shift immune cells into a more anti-inflammatory mode (Lee et al., 2021).
- SGLT2 Inhibitors (like *Dapagliflozin* and *Empagliflozin*) These lower blood sugar by making the kidneys flush out excess glucose—and they also help reduce inflammation and stress in the body (Vivian, 2014).

8.1.3 Natural & lifestyle-based anti-inflammatory options

Sometimes, simple lifestyle changes can make a big difference:

- Anti-inflammatory diets, like the Mediterranean diet, focus on healthy fats, fish, whole grains, and plenty of fruits and vegetables. These foods help lower inflammation naturally (Grosso et al., 2022).
- Consuming fewer calories or practicing intermittent fasting can increase the body's capability to manage sugar and offer a break for the immune system.
- Supplements like:
  - Fish oil is rich in omega-3 fatty acids, which help to reduce inflammation.
  - *Vitamin D*—supports immune balance.
  - Key plant compounds with anti-inflammatory properties include curcumin, found in turmeric, and resveratrol, found in grapes and red wine.
- One of the most effective ways to reduce inflammation is through exercise. It reduces the body's chronic inflammation and helps balance immunological responses (Poles et al., 2021)

8.1.4 New and experimental treatments

Exciting new approaches are being explored in research labs and clinical trials:

- Low-dose IL-2 therapy—This boosts "peacekeeper" immune cells (Tregs) to bring inflammation under control (Dong et al., 2021).

- Monoclonal antibodies—These are lab-made proteins designed to block specific inflammation triggers in the body.
- Vaccines targeting inflammatory molecules—Still in early stages, but they aim to train the immune system to calm down.
- Gut microbiome therapy—The bacteria in our gut strongly influence inflammation. Treatments like probiotics, prebiotics, or even fecal transplants are being studied to reset the gut and improve immune (Sankararaman et al., 2023).

8.2 Immunomodulators

Immunomodulators are substances—such as drugs, biologics, or even nutrients—that help regulate the immune system. They can either calm it down when it's too active or give it a boost when it's too weak. The majority of immunomodulators are used to treat Type 2 Diabetes (T2DM), a condition significantly influenced by harmful inflammation. It is commonly known that long-term low-grade inflammation harms the beta cells in the pancreas that produce insulin. Additionally, this inflammation raises the release of inflammatory cytokines and upsets the equilibrium of immune cells, including macrophages and T-cells, which hinders the body's reaction to insulin (Sharma, Arora, et al., 2024).

The purpose of immunomodulators in type 2 diabetes is to reduce insulin resistance, protect or preserve the beta cells responsible for insulin production, and improve overall blood sugar regulation. Currently, the potential of various types of immunomodulators in diabetes treatment is being explored.

One major group is cytokine inhibitors, which are biological drugs that block inflammatory molecules. For example, Anakinra and canakinumab, both IL-1β inhibitors, are used to reduce pancreatic inflammation and may improve insulin secretion. TNF-α inhibitors such as *Etanercept* and *Infliximab* are also being tested, although results in diabetes have been mixed. Another cytokine, IL-6, is being targeted by *Tocilizumab*, which is currently under study for its possible effects on insulin sensitivity (Larsen et al., 2007; Van Poppel et al., 2014).

Another promising approach is boosting the body's natural "peacekeeping" immune cells—regulatory T-cells (Tregs)—which help keep inflammation in check. Low-dose IL-2 therapy is one way to increase Treg levels and reduce the kind of autoimmune-like inflammation often seen in T2DM (Tahvildari & Dana, 2019).

Interestingly, some well-known diabetes medications also have immunomodulatory effects. While not traditional immune drugs, medications like Metformin help reduce inflammation by calming down certain immune signaling pathways like NF-κB. Pioglitazone, a drug in the TZD class, helps switch immune cells into a more anti-inflammatory mode, and SGLT2 inhibitors like *Dapagliflozin* or *Empagliflozin* may lower oxidative stress and inflammation while also improving glucose control.

Researchers are examining the alteration of gut microbiota due to its strong connection to the immune system. To lessen systemic inflammation and reestablish a healthy balance in the gut, treatments like fecal microbiota transplantation (FMT), probiotics, and prebiotics are being investigated.

Several natural substances, known as nutraceuticals, have shown promise as mild immune modulators. These include vitamin D, omega-3 fatty acids from fish oil, resveratrol found in grapes and berries, and curcumin derived from turmeric. These substances may help reduce inflammatory cytokine levels and promote a balanced immune system.

In summary, immunomodulators offer a fresh and promising way to approach Type 2 Diabetes—not just by lowering blood sugar, but by tackling the underlying inflammation and immune system imbalance. Although research on these treatments is still in progress, people with type 2 diabetes may benefit from combining them with traditional medication to improve long-term outcomes and quality of life (Mwaura, 2025; Xia et al., 2024; Zhou et al., 2022).

8.3 Vaccines and immune tolerance strategies

Researchers are currently exploring vaccine-like strategies to manage chronic diseases, particularly type 2 diabetes (T2DM). Despite the fact that vaccination is usually linked to avoiding diseases, their focus is on the immune system's function in terms of inflammation and insulin resistance. Chronic, low-grade inflammation is a major factor in type 2 diabetes because it harms beta cells that produce insulin and exacerbates insulin resistance. The aim of immunology-based approaches, including immune tolerance techniques and therapeutic vaccinations, is to diminish the overactive immune response that contributes to the disease development (Mathur et al., 2023; Sharma et al., 2025c; Singh et al., 2025).

One strategy currently being researched involves the use of vaccinations aimed at specific inflammatory molecules, such as pro-inflammatory cytokines, including TNF-α and IL-1β. The goal of these vaccinations is to "train" the immune system to neutralize or block these cytokines to reduce inflammation in the pancreas and insulin-sensitive organs. For instance, early research is testing whether vaccines that generate antibodies against IL-1β can improve glucose control and protect beta cell function.

Another exciting area is immunotolerance therapy. Tolerance techniques aim to retrain the immune system to stop attacking or overreacting to the body's tissues. This differs from traditional vaccinations, which stimulate the immune system. The aim of these treatments is to enhance the activity of regulatory T-cells (Tregs), which are essential for preserving immunological balance and reducing harmful inflammation. Low-dose IL-2 therapy is one way to increase Treg activity, and it has demonstrated promise in establishing a less inflammatory and more tolerant immune environment. Other tolerance strategies include exposing the immune system to small doses of antigens (such as insulin or specific peptides) to gradually "desensitize" it, preventing harmful immune attacks that may contribute to beta-cell decline (Moorman et al., 2021; Prame Kumar et al., 2023).

In addition, scientists are looking into nanoparticle-based vaccines that can deliver diabetes-related antigens directly to immune cells in a way that promotes tolerance instead of triggering inflammation. These are still experimental, but they represent a promising new generation of precision immunotherapies (Feng et al., 2020; Shruti et al., 2026).

Overall, both vaccine approaches and immune tolerance therapies represent a forward-thinking way to manage T2DM—not just by treating symptoms like high blood sugar, but by addressing the root cause: an imbalanced, overactive immune system. While most of these strategies are still in the research phase, they offer hope for long-term disease modification and improved outcomes in the future.

9. Emerging research and future directions

The complex relationship between immune dysfunction and metabolic disorders is increasingly acknowledged as the underlying mechanism of Type 2 Diabetes Mellitus (T2DM). In the present scenario, advances in systems biology, genomics, and immunology have thrown up several new areas of research that hold tremendous promise in exploring effective ways for treating T2DM. Among these, the immunometabolic aspect, personalized medicine, and modulation of immune checkpoints have drawn considerable attention. A reality although Journal of Experimental Medicine is something more convoluted (Chen & Gerszten, 2020; Raut, 2026).

9.1 Immunometabolism

Immunometabolism refers to the influence of metabolism on immune cell function. The pathophysiology of type 2 diabetes primarily results from immune cell dysregulation and persistent low-grade inflammation. Using single-cell RNA-sequencing, an independent study identified substantial differences in immune-cell subpopulations between T2DM patients with a predominance of monocytes and decrease in $CD4^+$ T cells (Chang et al., 2022). These alterations indicate an affected immune regulation which may be involved in insulin resistance and β-cell failure. Further research highlights tissue-specific immune responses that impair metabolic processes, particularly in adipose tissue, gut, muscle, liver, and pancreas.These interactions between immune cells and metabolic tissues underscore the complexity of T2DM pathogenesis (Lackey & Olefsky, 2016).

9.2 Targeting immune checkpoints

Immune checkpoints are proteins that regulate T cell activation, ensuring that the immune system remains balanced and preventing autoimmunity. The most recognized immune checkpoint proteins are CTLA-4 (cytotoxic T-lymphocyte-associated protein 4), PD-1 (programmed death-1), and PD-L1. Inputs from these systems can contribute to the chronic inflammation to which T2DM contributes. Accumulating evidence has suggested that immune checkpoints are involved in the pathophysiology of metabolic derangements, including their implication in cancer and autoimmune diseases. PD-1 expression within T cells is upregulated in obesity, and blockade in mice has improved T cell capacity and adipose tissue inflammation. This implies that immune checkpoint pathways would thus contribute to inflammation and insulin resistance secondary to obesity (Palmer et al., 2019).Interestingly, new-onset diabetes resembling type 1 diabetes has been associated to the use of immune checkpoint inhibitors (ICIs) in cancer patients suggesting that these pathways are also critical for maintaining β-cell integrity. It indicates the twin-natured action requiring caution in tampering with immune checkpoints in metabolic disorders.Therapeutic modulation of checkpoint pathways might facilitate fine-tuning of immune activation for diabetes. Such a possibility would include enhancing PD-1 signaling, which could alleviate adipose tissue inflammation while maintaining the β-cell life, and particular CTLA-4 modulation which could possibly moderate autoaggressive immune responses while sparing defense against exogenous sources.

9.3 Personalized medicine approaches

Personalized medicine for diabetes (PMFD) represents a transformative approach in the management and treatment of diabetes, leveraging an individual's unique genetic and molecular profile to optimize healthcare outcomes. PMFD aims to tailor diabetes prevention, early diagnosis, treatment, and monitoring plans for every patient's unique genetic, biochemical, and environmental factors (Sugandh et al., 2023).

10. Conclusion

Key features of type 2 diabetes include immunological dysfunction and chronic inflammation, which lead to insulin resistance and metabolic abnormalities. The strong correlation between type 2 diabetes mellitus (T2DM) and immunology opens the door to novel treatment strategies. Immune-based therapies offer promise in reducing inflammation, improving insulin sensitivity, and potentially altering the disease course, paving the way for innovative strategies for diabetes management.

References

Acosta, J. R., Arner, P., Kulyté, A., Tavira, B., Laurencikiene, J., Douagi, I., & Rydén, M. (2019). Human-specific function of IL-10 in adipose tissue linked to insulin resistance. *The Journal of Clinical Endocrinology & Metabolism, 104*(10), 4552–4562. https://doi.org/10.1210/jc.2019-00341

Acosta-Martinez, M., & Cabail, M. Z. (2022). The PI3K/Akt pathway in meta-inflammation. *International Journal of Molecular Sciences, 23*(23), 15330. https://doi.org/10.3390/ijms232315330

Ahmed, M., & Gaffen, S. L. (2010). IL-17 in obesity and adipogenesis. *Cytokine & Growth Factor Reviews, 21*(6), 449–453. https://doi.org/10.1016/j.cytogfr.2010.10.005

Al-Hilu, M. (2025). The role of inflammation IL-6, TNF-α in type -2 diabetes mellitus. *Al-Kufa University Journal for Biology, 17*(2), 89–97. https://doi.org/10.36320/ajb/v17.i2.19615

Alberti, K. G., Eckel, R. H., Grundy, S. M., Zimmet, P. Z., Cleeman, J. I., Donato, K. A., Fruchart, J. C., James, W. P., Loria, C. M., Smith, S. C., Jr., & International Diabetes Federation Task Force on Epidemiology and Prevention, Hational Heart, Lung, and Blood Institute, American Heart Association, World Heart Federation, International Atherosclerosis Society, & International Association for the Study of Obesity. (2009). Harmonizing the metabolic syndrome: A joint interim statement of the international diabetes Federation task force on epidemiology and prevention; national heart, lung, and blood institute; American heart association; world heart Federation; international atherosclerosis society; and international association for the study of obesity. *Circulation, 120*(16), 1640–1645. https://doi.org/10.1161/CIRCULATIONAHA.109.192644

Ali, Q., Gao, Z., Cui, Y., Guo, Z., Li, D., La, S., Zhu, X., Ma, S., Wang, Z., Farooq, U., Liu, B., & Shi, Y. (2022). Microbial short-chain fatty acids: A bridge between dietary fibers and poultry gut health — A review. *Animal Bioscience, 35*(10), 1461–1478. https://doi.org/10.5713/ab.21.0562

Andersen, M. K., Lundgren, V., Turunen, J. A., Forsblom, C., Isomaa, B., Groop, P. H., Groop, L., & Tuomi, T. (2010). Latent autoimmune diabetes in adults differs genetically from classical type 1 diabetes diagnosed after the age of 35 years. *Diabetes Care, 33*(9), 2062–2064. https://doi.org/10.2337/dc09-2188

Anderson, A. C., Joller, N., & Kuchroo, V. K. (2016). Lag-3, Tim-3, and TIGIT: Co-inhibitory receptors with specialized functions in immune regulation. *Immunity, 44*(5), 989–1004. https://doi.org/10.1016/j.immuni.2016.05.001

Andrews, L. P., Marciscano, A. E., Drake, C. G., & Vignali, D. A. A. (2017). LAG3 (CD223) as a cancer immunotherapy target. *Immunological Reviews, 276*(1), 80–96. https://doi.org/10.1111/imr.12519

Atkinson, M. A., Eisenbarth, G. S., & Michels, A. W. (2014). Type 1 diabetes. *Lancet (London, England), 383*(9911), 69–82. https://doi.org/10.1016/S0140-6736(13)60591-7

Baghel, K., Khan, A., & Kango, N. (2024). Role of synbiotics (Prebiotics and probiotics) as dietary supplements in type 2 diabetes mellitus induced health complications. *Journal of Dietary Supplements, 21*(5), 677–708. https://doi.org/10.1080/19390211.2024.2340509

Bahceci, M., Tuzcu, A., Canoruc, N., Tuzun, Y., Kidir, V., & Aslan, C. (2004). Serum C-Reactive protein (CRP) levels and insulin resistance in non-obese women with polycystic ovarian syndrome, and effect of bicalutamide on hirsutism, CRP levels and insulin resistance. *Hormone Research in Paediatrícs, 62*(6), 283–287. https://doi.org/10.1159/000081973

Banu, S., & Sur, D. (2023). Role of macrophage in type 2 diabetes mellitus: Macrophage polarization a new paradigm for treatment of type 2 diabetes mellitus. *Endocrine, Metabolic & Immune Disorders - Drug Targets, 23*(1), 2–11. https://doi.org/10.2174/1871530322666220630093359

Bashir, H., Hayat Bhat, M., & Majid, S. (2022). Molecular pathogenesis of inflammatory cytokines in insulin resistance diabetes mellitus. *Intechopen.* . https://doi.org/10.5772/intechopen.100971

Berbudi, A., Khairani, S., & Tjahjadi, A. I. (2025). Interplay between insulin resistance and immune dysregulation in type 2 diabetes mellitus: Implications for therapeutic interventions. *ImmunoTargets and Therapy, 14*, 359–382. https://doi.org/10.2147/ITT.S499605

Bielka, W., Przezak, A., & Pawlik, A. (2022). The role of the gut microbiota in the pathogenesis of diabetes. *International Journal of Molecular Sciences, 23*(1), 480. https://doi.org/10.3390/ijms23010480

Brooks-Worrell, B., Shojaie, A., Cohen, R. M., Balasubramanyam, A., Palmer, J. P., Rasouli, N., Hampe, C. S., Desouza, C., Younes, N., Valencia, W. M., Kahn, S. E., Mather, K., Johnson, M., Utzschneider, K., Gonzalez, E., Park, J., Larkin, M., Flórez, H., Palomino, B., & Zangeneh, S. (2020). 254-OR: Islet autoimmunity is highly prevalent and associated with diminished beta-cell function in patients with type 2 diabetes (T2D) in the GRADE study. *Diabetes, 69*(Suppl. 1). https://doi.org/10.2337/db20-254-or

Brooks-Worrell, B. M., Boyko, E. J., & Palmer, J. P. (2014). Impact of islet autoimmunity on the progressive β-cell functional decline in type 2 diabetes. *Diabetes Care, 37*(12), 3286–3293. https://doi.org/10.2337/dc14-0961

Brooks-Worrell, B., Hampe, C. S., Hattery, E. G., Palomino, B., Zangeneh, S. Z., Utzschneider, K., Kahn, S. E., Larkin, M. E., Johnson, M. L., Mather, K. J., Younes, N., Rasouli, N., Desouza, C., Cohen, R. M., Park, J. Y., Florez, H. J., Valencia, W. M., GRADE Beta-cell Ancillary Study Network, Shojaie, A., Palmer, J. P., … Balasubramanyam, A. (2022). Islet autoimmunity is highly prevalent and associated with diminished β-Cell function in patients with type 2 diabetes in the grade study. *Diabetes, 71*(6), 1261–1271. https://doi.org/10.2337/db21-0590. Advance online publication.

Brooks-Worrell, B., Narla, R., & Palmer, J. P. (2013). Islet autoimmunity in phenotypic type 2 diabetes patients. *Diabetes, Obesity and Metabolism, 15*(Suppl. 3), 137–140. https://doi.org/10.1111/dom.12167 (0 3).

Brooks-Worrell, B. M., & Palmer, J. P. (2019). Setting the stage for islet autoimmunity in type 2 diabetes: Obesity-associated chronic systemic inflammation and endoplasmic reticulum (ER) stress. *Diabetes Care, 42*(12), 2338–2346. https://doi.org/10.2337/dc19-0475

Broz, P., & Dixit, V. M. (2016). Inflammasomes: Mechanism of assembly, regulation and signalling. *Nature Reviews Immunology, 16*(7), 407–420. https://doi.org/10.1038/nri.2016.58

Burcelin, R. (2016). Gut microbiota and immune crosstalk in metabolic disease. *Molecular Metabolism, 5* (9), 771–781. https://doi.org/10.1016/j.molmet.2016.05.016

Burke, S. J., Stadler, K., Lu, D., Karlstad, M. D., Collier, J. J., Donohoe, D. R., Gleason, E., Rogers, R. C., Hermann, G. E., & Han, A. (2015). IL-1β reciprocally regulates chemokine and insulin secretion in pancreatic β-cells via NF-κB. *American Journal of Physiology-Endocrinology and Metabolism, 309*(8), E715–E726. https://doi.org/10.1152/ajpendo.00153.2015

Cai, Z., Huang, Y., & He, B. (2022). New insights into adipose tissue macrophages in obesity and insulin resistance. *Cells, 11*(9), 1424. https://doi.org/10.3390/cells11091424

Carlsson, S. (2019). Etiology and pathogenesis of latent autoimmune diabetes in adults (LADA) compared to type 2 diabetes. *Frontiers in Physiology, 10,* 320. https://doi.org/10.3389/fphys.2019.00320

Chang, J. G., Tu, S. J., Huang, C. M., Chen, Y. C., Chiang, H. S., Lee, Y. T., Yen, J. C., Lin, C. L., Chung, C. C., Liu, T. C., & Chang, Y. S. (2022). Single-cell RNA sequencing of immune cells in patients with acute gout. *Scientific Reports, 12*(1), 22130. https://doi.org/10.1038/s41598-022-25871-2

Chauvin, J. M., & Zarour, H. M. (2020). TIGIT in cancer immunotherapy. *Journal for Immunotherapy of Cancer, 8*(2), e000957. https://doi.org/10.1136/jitc-2020-000957

Chawla, A., Nguyen, K. D., & Goh, Y. P. (2011). Macrophage-mediated inflammation in metabolic disease. *Nature Reviews Immunology, 11*(11), 738–749. https://doi.org/10.1038/nri3071

Cheent, K., & Khakoo, S. I. (2009). Natural killer cells: Integrating diversity with function. *Immunology, 126*(4), 449–457. https://doi.org/10.1111/j.1365-2567.2009.03045.x

Chen, X., Andresen 1, B. T., Hill, M., Zhang, J., Booth, F., & Zhang, C. (2008). Role of reactive oxygen species in tumor necrosis factor-alpha induced endothelial dysfunction. *Current Hypertension Reviews, 4*(4), 245–255. https://doi.org/10.2174/157340208786241336

Chen, Z. Z., & Gerszten, R. E. (2020). Metabolomics and proteomics in type 2 diabetes. *Circulation Research, 126*(11), 1613–1627. https://doi.org/10.1161/CIRCRESAHA.120.315898

Chong, S., Lin, M., Chong, D., Jensen, S., & Lau, N. S. (2025). A systematic review on gut microbiota in type 2 diabetes mellitus. *Frontiers in Endocrinology, 15,* 1486793. https://doi.org/10.3389/fendo.2024.1486793

Chu, X., Xing, H., Chao, M., Xie, P., & Jiang, L. (2025). Gut microbiota modulation in osteoporosis: Probiotics, prebiotics, and natural compounds. *Metabolites, 15*(5), 301. https://doi.org/10.3390/metabo15050301

Dahdah, N., Tercero-Alcázar, C., Malagón, M. M., Garcia-Roves, P. M., & Guzmán-Ruiz, R. (2024). Interrelation of adipose tissue macrophages and fibrosis in obesity. *Biochemical Pharmacology, 225*, 116324. https://doi.org/10.1016/j.bcp.2024.116324

Dahik, V. D., Frisdal, E., & Le Goff, W. (2020). Rewiring of lipid metabolism in adipose tissue macrophages in obesity: Impact on insulin resistance and type 2 diabetes. *International Journal of Molecular Sciences, 21*(15), 5505. https://doi.org/10.3390/ijms21155505

Dakshinamurthy, S., Saxena, V., Kumari, R., Mirza, A. A., & Dhar, M. (2020). Association of obesity and metabolic syndrome among urban dwellers of rishikesh, Uttarakhand. *Indian Journal of Community Medicine: Official Publication of Indian Association of Preventive & Social Medicine, 45*(4), 516–521. https://doi.org/10.4103/ijcm.IJCM_24_20

Daryabor, G., Atashzar, M. R., Kabelitz, D., Meri, S., & Kalantar, K. (2020). The effects of type 2 diabetes mellitus on organ metabolism and the immune system. *Frontiers in Immunology, 11*, 1582. https://doi.org/10.3389/fimmu.2020.01582

Das, M., Zhu, C., & Kuchroo, V. K. (2017). Tim-3 and its role in regulating anti-tumor immunity. *Immunological Reviews, 276*(1), 97–111. https://doi.org/10.1111/imr.12520

de Candia, P., Prattichizzo, F., Garavelli, S., De Rosa, V., Galgani, M., Di Rella, F., Spagnuolo, M. I., Colamatteo, A., Fusco, C., Micillo, T., Bruzzaniti, S., Ceriello, A., Puca, A. A., & Matarese, G. (2019). Type 2 diabetes: How much of an autoimmune disease? *Frontiers in Endocrinology, 10*, 451. https://doi.org/10.3389/fendo.2019.00451

Defronzo, R. A. (2009). Banting lecture. From the triumvirate to the ominous octet: A new paradigm for the treatment of type 2 diabetes mellitus. *Diabetes, 58*(4), 773–795. https://doi.org/10.2337/db09-9028

DeFuria, J., Belkina, A. C., Jagannathan-Bogdan, M., Snyder-Cappione, J., Carr, J. D., Nersesova, Y. R., Markham, D., Strissel, K. J., Watkins, A. A., Zhu, M., Allen, J., Bouchard, J., Toraldo, G., Jasuja, R., Obin, M. S., McDonnell, M. E., Apovian, C., Denis, G. V., & Nikolajczyk, B. S. (2013). B cells promote inflammation in obesity and type 2 diabetes through regulation of T-cell function and an inflammatory cytokine profile. *Proceedings of the National Academy of Sciences of the United States of America, 110*(13), 5133–5138. https://doi.org/10.1073/pnas.1215840110

DeLeo, F. R., & Allen, L. H. (2020). Phagocytosis and neutrophil extracellular traps. *Faculty reviews, 9*, 25. https://doi.org/10.12703/r/9-25

Dinarello, C. A. (2011). Interleukin-1 in the pathogenesis and treatment of inflammatory diseases. *Blood, 117*(14), 3720–3732. https://doi.org/10.1182/blood-2010-07-273417

Dludla, P. V., Mabhida, S. E., Ziqubu, K., Nkambule, B. B., Mazibuko-Mbeje, S. E., Hanser, S., Basson, A. K., Pheiffer, C., & Kengne, A. P. (2023). Pancreatic β-cell dysfunction in type 2 diabetes: Implications of inflammation and oxidative stress. *World Journal of Diabetes, 14*(3), 130–146. https://doi.org/10.4239/wjd.v14.i3.130

Donath, M. Y. (2014). Targeting inflammation in the treatment of type 2 diabetes: Time to start. *Nature Reviews Drug Discovery, 13*(6), 465–476. https://doi.org/10.1038/nrd4275

Donath, M. Y., & Shoelson, S. E. (2011). Type 2 diabetes as an inflammatory disease. *Nature Reviews Immunology, 11*(2), 98–107. https://doi.org/10.1038/nri2925

Dong, G., Sun, J., Yang, M., Wang, Y., Sun, B., Hu, Q., Gao, F., Li, C., & Mao, L. (2021). Low-dose IL-2 treatment affords protection against subarachnoid hemorrhage injury by expanding peripheral regulatory T cells. *ACS Chemical Neuroscience, 12*(3), 430–440. https://doi.org/10.1021/acschemneuro.0c00611

Dongre, S. (2025). Enigma of AMP-activated protein kinase subunit expression in glioma. *Academia Oncology*. https://doi.org/10.20935/AcadOnco7881

Dragičević Tomičić, D., Lešić, N., Škrlec, I., Steigmann, L., Tseneva, K., ČalušićŠarac, M., Crnić, T., Tomičić, I., PerićKačarević, Ž., & Čandrlić, M. (2025). Effects of vitamin D, melatonin, and Omega-3 fatty acids on periodontal health: A narrative review. *Dentistry Journal, 13*(4), 178. https://doi.org/10.3390/dj13040178

Eguchi, K., & Nagai, R. (2017). Islet inflammation in type 2 diabetes and physiology. *Journal of Clinical Investigation, 127*(1), 14–23. https://doi.org/10.1172/JCI88877

Eizirik, D. L., Colli, M. L., & Ortis, F. (2009). The role of inflammation in insulitis and beta-cell loss in type 1 diabetes. *Nature Reviews Endocrinology, 5*(4), 219–226. https://doi.org/10.1038/nrendo.2009.21

Eizirik, D. L., Pasquali, L., & Cnop, M. (2020). Pancreatic β-cells in type 1 and type 2 diabetes mellitus: Different pathways to failure. *Nature Reviews Endocrinology, 16*(7), 349–362. https://doi.org/10.1038/s41574-020-0355-7

Engin, A. (2017a). The pathogenesis of obesity-associated adipose tissue inflammation. *Advances in Experimental Medicine & Biology, 960*, 221–245. https://doi.org/10.1007/978-3-319-48382-5_9

Engin, A. B. (2017b). Adipocyte-macrophage cross-talk in obesity. *Advances in Experimental Medicine & Biology, 960*, 327–343. https://doi.org/10.1007/978-3-319-48382-5_14

Engin, A. (2024). Reappraisal of adipose tissue inflammation in obesity. *Advances in Experimental Medicine & Biology, 1460*, 297–327. https://doi.org/10.1007/978-3-031-63657-8_10

Esser, N., Legrand-Poels, S., Piette, J., Scheen, A. J., & Paquot, N. (2014). Inflammation as a link between obesity, metabolic syndrome and type 2 diabetes. *Diabetes Research and Clinical Practice, 105*(2), 141–150. https://doi.org/10.1016/j.diabres.2014.04.006

Fasshauer, M., Bluher, M., Klein, J., Klier, M., Paschke, R., Lossner, U., & Kralisch, S. (2004). Insulin resistance-inducing cytokines differentially regulate SOCS mRNA expression via growth factor- and Jak/Stat-signaling pathways in 3T3-L1 adipocytes. *Journal of Endocrinology, 181*(1), 129–138. https://doi.org/10.1677/joe.0.1810129

Feng, X., Xu, W., Liu, J., Li, G., & Ding, J. (2020). Tackling autoimmunity with nanomedicines. *Nanomedicine, 15*(16), 1585–1597. https://doi.org/10.2217/nnm-2020-0102

Ferris, S. T., Carrero, J. A., Mohan, J. F., Calderon, B., Murphy, K. M., & Unanue, E. R. (2014). A minor subset of Batf3-dependent antigen-presenting cells in islets of Langerhans is essential for the development of autoimmune diabetes. *Immunity, 41*(4), 657–669. https://doi.org/10.1016/j.immuni.2014.09.012

Feuerer, M., Herrero, L., Cipolletta, D., Naaz, A., Wong, J., Nayer, A., Lee, J., Goldfine, A. B., Benoist, C., Shoelson, S., & Mathis, D. (2009). Lean, but not obese, fat is enriched for a unique population of regulatory T cells that affect metabolic parameters. *Nature Medicine, 15*(8), 930–939. https://doi.org/10.1038/nm.2002

Fousteri, G., Ippolito, E., Ahmed, R., & Hamad, A. R. A. (2017). Beta-cell specific autoantibodies: Are they just an indicator of type 1 diabetes? *Current Diabetes Reviews, 13*(3), 322–329. https://doi.org/10.2174/1573399812666160427104157

Fuke, N., Nagata, N., Suganuma, H., & Ota, T. (2019). Regulation of gut microbiota and metabolic endotoxemia with dietary factors. *Nutrients, 11*(10), 2277. https://doi.org/10.3390/nu11102277

GacaferriLumezi, B., & Lokaj-Berisha, V. (2025). Insulin resistance in an underweight woman with polycystic ovary syndrome: A case study. *The American journal of case reports, 26*, e945814. https://doi.org/10.12659/AJCR.945814

Gonzalez-Gay, M. A., De Matias, J. M., Gonzalez-Juanatey, C., Garcia-Porrua, C., Sanchez-Andrade, A., Martin, J., & Llorca, J. (2006). Anti-tumor necrosis factor-alpha blockade improves insulin resistance in patients with rheumatoid arthritis. *Clinical & Experimental Rheumatology, 24*(1), 83–86.

Gora, I. M., Ciechanowska, A., & Ladyzynski, P. (2021). NLRP3 inflammasome at the interface of inflammation, endothelial dysfunction, and type 2 diabetes. *Cells, 10*(2), 314. https://doi.org/10.3390/cells10020314

Grasso, Y. Z., Reddy, S. K., Rosenfeld, C. R., Hussein, W. I., Hoogwerf, B. J., Faiman, C., & Gupta, M. K. (2001). Autoantibodies to IA-2 and GAD65 in patients with type 2 diabetes mellitus of varied duration: Prevalence and correlation with clinical features. *Endocrine Practice: Official Journal of the American College of Endocrinology and the American Association of Clinical Endocrinologists, 7*(5), 339–345. https://doi.org/10.4158/EP.7.5.339

Grosso, G., Laudisio, D., Frías-Toral, E., Barrea, L., Muscogiuri, G., Savastano, S., & Colao, A. (2022). Anti-inflammatory nutrients and obesity-associated metabolic-inflammation: State of the art and future direction. *Nutrients, 14.*

Guan, Z., Li, H., Liu, R., Cai, C., Liu, Y., Li, J., Wang, X., Huang, S., Wu, L., Liu, D., Yu, S., Wang, Z., Shu, J., Hou, X., Yang, X., Jia, W., & Sheng, B. (2023). Artificial intelligence in diabetes management: Advancements, opportunities, and challenges. *Cell Reports Medicine, 4*(10), 101213. https://doi.org/10.1016/j.xcrm.2023.101213

Guo, H., Callaway, J. B., & Ting, J. P. Y. (2015). Inflammasomes: Mechanism of action, role in disease, and therapeutics. *Nature Medicine, 21*(7), 677–687. https://doi.org/10.1038/nm.3893

Guo, L., Milburn, M. V., Ryals, J. A., Lonergan, S. C., Mitchell, M. W., Wulff, J. E., Alexander, D. C., Evans, A. M., Bridgewater, B., Miller, L., Gonzalez-Garay, M. L., & Caskey, C. T. (2015). Plasma metabolomic profiles enhance precision medicine for volunteers of normal health. *Proceedings of the National Academy of Sciences of the United States of America, 112*(35), E4901–E4910. https://doi.org/10.1073/pnas.1508425112

Gupta, S., et al. (2025). From development to clinical success: The journey of established and next-generation BTK inhibitors. *Investigational New Drugs.* https://doi.org/10.1007/s10637-025-01513-y

Gurung, M., et al. (2020). Role of gut microbiota in type 2 diabetes pathophysiology. *EBioMedicine, 51*, 102590. https://doi.org/10.1016/j.ebiom.2019.11.051

Hameed, I., Masoodi, S. R., Mir, S. A., Nabi, M., Ghazanfar, K., & Ganai, B. A. (2015). Type 2 diabetes mellitus: From a metabolic disorder to an inflammatory condition. *World Journal of Diabetes, 6*(4), 598–612. https://doi.org/10.4239/wjd.v6.i4.598

Himes, R. W., & Smith, C. W. (2010). Tlr2 is critical for diet-induced metabolic syndrome in a murine model. *The FASEB Journal: Official Publication of the Federation of American Societies for Experimental Biology, 24*(3), 731–739. https://doi.org/10.1096/fj.09-141929

Hoseini-Aghdam, M., Sheikh, V., Eftekharian, M. M., Rezaeepoor, M., & Behzad, M. (2020). Enhanced expression of TIGIT but not neuropilin-1 in patients with type 2 diabetes mellitus. *Immunology Letters, 225*, 1–8. https://doi.org/10.1016/j.imlet.2020.06.003

Hotamisligil, G. S. (2006). Inflammation and metabolic disorders. *Nature, 444*(7121), 860–867. https://doi.org/10.1038/nature05485

Hotamisligil, G. S. (2017a). Foundations of immunometabolism and implications for metabolic health and disease. *Immunity, 47*(3), 406–420. https://doi.org/10.1016/j.immuni.2017.08.009

Hotamisligil, G. S. (2017b). Inflammation, metaflammation and immunometabolic disorders. *Nature, 542*(7640), 177–185. https://doi.org/10.1038/nature21363

Hu, T., et al. (2024). Metabolic regulation of the immune system in health and disease. *Signal Transduction and Targeted Therapy, 9*, 113. https://doi.org/10.1038/s41392-024-01954-6

Hu, Y., Li, L., Xu, Y., Yu, T., Tong, G., Huang, H., Bi, Y., Weng, J., & Zhu, D. (2011). Short-term intensive therapy in newly diagnosed type 2 diabetes partially restores both insulin sensitivity and β-cell function in subjects with long-term remission. *Diabetes Care, 34*(8), 1848–1853. https://doi.org/10.2337/dc10-2105

Hull, R. L., Westermark, G. T., Westermark, P., & Kahn, S. E. (2004). Islet amyloid: A critical entity in the pathogenesis of type 2 diabetes. *Journal of Clinical Endocrinology & Metabolism, 89*(8), 3629–3643. https://doi.org/10.1210/jc.2004-0405

Itariu, B. K., & Stulnig, T. M. (2014). Autoimmune aspects of type 2 diabetes mellitus - A mini-review. *Gerontology, 60*(3), 189–196. https://doi.org/10.1159/000356747

Jones, A. G., McDonald, T. J., Shields, B. M., Hagopian, W., & Hattersley, A. T. (2021). Latent autoimmune diabetes of adults (LADA) is likely to represent a mixed population of autoimmune (type 1) and nonautoimmune (type 2) diabetes. *Diabetes Care, 44*(6), 1243–1251. https://doi.org/10.2337/dc20-2834

Juan, G.-F., Edgar, L.-P., Saúl, R.-D. L. S., Sergio, L.-B., & Victoriano, P.-V. (2015). Relationship between Th17 and regulatory T cells in patients with type 2 diabetes mellitus. *Frontiers in Immunology, 6*. https://doi.org/10.3389/conf.fimmu.2015.05.00042

Kahn, S. E. (2003). The relative contributions of insulin resistance and beta-cell dysfunction to the pathophysiology of type 2 diabetes. *Diabetologia, 46*(1), 3–19. https://doi.org/10.1007/s00125-002-1009-0

Kahn, S. E., Cooper, M. E., & Del Prato, S. (2014). Pathophysiology and treatment of type 2 diabetes: Perspectives on the past, present, and future. *Lancet (London, England), 383*(9922), 1068–1083. https://doi.org/10.1016/S0140-6736(13)62154-6

Kartika, R., & Wibowo, H. (2020). Impaired function of regulatory T cells in type 2 diabetes mellitus. *Molecular and Cellular Biomedical Sciences, 4*(1), 1. https://doi.org/10.21705/mcbs.v4i1.64

Kershaw, E. E., & Flier, J. S. (2004). Adipose tissue as an endocrine organ. *Journal of Clinical Endocrinology & Metabolism, 89*(6), 2548–2556. https://doi.org/10.1210/jc.2004-0395

Kim, D. S., Gloyn, A. L., & Knowles, J. W. (2021). Genetics of type 2 diabetes: Opportunities for precision medicine: JACC focus seminar. *Journal of the American College of Cardiology, 78*(5), 496–512. https://doi.org/10.1016/j.jacc.2021.03.346

Kim, J. J., & Sears, D. D. (2010). TLR4 and insulin resistance. *Gastroenterology Research and Practice, 2010*, 212563. https://doi.org/10.1155/2010/212563

Kim, M.-S., Woo, J. R., Yamamoto, Y., Shoelson, S. E., Lee, J., Kim, K., Moore, K., Shimada, T., Liu, L., & Kamei, N. (2013). Regulation of diet-induced adipose tissue and systemic inflammation by salicylates and pioglitazone. *PLoS One, 8*(12), e82847. https://doi.org/10.1371/journal.pone.0082847

Kurgan, N., Kjærgaard Larsen, J., & Deshmukh, A. S. (2024). Harnessing the power of proteomics in precision diabetes medicine. *Diabetologia, 67*(5), 783–797. https://doi.org/10.1007/s00125-024-06097-5

Lackey, D. E., & Olefsky, J. M. (2016). Regulation of metabolism by the innate immune system. *Nature Reviews Endocrinology, 12*(1), 15–28. https://doi.org/10.1038/nrendo.2015.189

Lambelet, M., Terra, L. F., Fukaya, M., Meyerovich, K., Labriola, L., Cardozo, A. K., & Allagnat, F. (2018). Dysfunctional autophagy following exposure to pro-inflammatory cytokines contributes to pancreatic β-cell apoptosis. *Cell Death & Disease, 9*(2), 96. https://doi.org/10.1038/s41419-017-0121-5

Larsen, C. M., Faulenbach, M., Vaag, A., Vølund, A., Ehses, J. A., Seifert, B., Mandrup-Poulsen, T., & Donath, M. Y. (2007). Interleukin-1-receptor antagonist in type 2 diabetes mellitus. *New England Journal of Medicine, 356*(15), 1517–1526. https://doi.org/10.1056/NEJMoa065213

Lee, Y. H., Giraud, J., Davis, R. J., & White, M. F. (2003). c-Jun N-terminal kinase (JNK) mediates feedback inhibition of the insulin signaling cascade. *Journal of Biological Chemistry, 278*(5), 2896–2902. https://doi.org/10.1074/jbc.M208359200

Lee, J., Noh, S., Lim, S., & Kim, B. (2021). Plant extracts for type 2 diabetes: From traditional medicine to modern drug discovery. *Antioxidants, 10*(1), 81. https://doi.org/10.3390/antiox10010081

Lee, Y. S., & Wolfrum, C. (2018). An integrated view of immunometabolism. *Cell, 172*(1–2), 22–40. https://doi.org/10.1016/j.cell.2017.12.025

Li, J., Niu, Q., Wu, A., Zhang, Y., Hong, L., & Wang, H. (2023). Causal relationship between circulating immune cells and the risk of type 2 diabetes: A Mendelian randomization study. *Frontiers in Endocrinology, 14*, 1210415. https://doi.org/10.3389/fendo.2023.1210415

Li, Y., Yun, K., & Mu, R. (2020). A review on the biology and properties of adipose tissue macrophages involved in adipose tissue physiological and pathophysiological processes. *Lipids in Health and Disease, 19*(1), 164. https://doi.org/10.1186/s12944-020-01342-3

Li, H., Zou, L., Long, Z., & Zhan, J. (2025). Immunometabolic alterations in type 2 diabetes mellitus revealed by single-cell RNA sequencing: Insights into subtypes and therapeutic targets. *Frontiers in Immunology, 15*, 1537909. https://doi.org/10.3389/fimmu.2024.1537909

Lin, Z., Zhang, J., Duan, T., Yang, J., & Yang, Y. (2024). Trefoil factor 3 can stimulate Th17 cell response in the development of type 2 diabetes mellitus. *Scientific Reports, 14*. https://doi.org/10.1038/s41598-024-60426-7. Article 10340.

Ling, C., & Rönn, T. (2019). Epigenetics in human obesity and type 2 diabetes. *Cell Metabolism, 29*(5), 1028–1044. https://doi.org/10.1016/j.cmet.2019.03.009

Llorián-Salvador, M., Pérez-Martínez, D., Tang, M., Duarri, A., García-Ramirez, M., Deàs-Just, A., Álvarez-Guaita, A., Ramos-Pérez, L., Bogdanov, P., Gomez-Sanchez, J. A., Stitt, A. W., Hernández, C., de la Fuente, A. G., & Simó, R. (2024). Regulatory T cell expansion prevents retinal degeneration in type 2 diabetes. *Journal of Neuroinflammation, 21*(1), 328. https://doi.org/10.1186/s12974-024-03323-0

Macedo, R. G. (2019). *The immune system and inflammation in type 2 diabetes*. Springer. https://doi.org/10.1007/978-3-030-11815-0_11

Mahlangu, T., Dludla, P. V., Nyambuya, T. M., Mxinwa, V., Mazibuko-Mbeje, S. E., Cirilli, I., Marcheggiani, F., Tiano, L., Louw, J., & Nkambule, B. B. (2020). A systematic review on the functional role of Th1/Th2 cytokines in type 2 diabetes and related metabolic complications. *Cytokine, 126*, 154892. https://doi.org/10.1016/j.cyto.2019.154892

Masters, S. L., Dunne, A., Subramanian, S. L., Hull, R. L., Tannahill, G. M., Sharp, F. A., Becker, C., Franchi, L., Yoshihara, E., Chen, Z., Mullooly, N., Mielke, L. A., Harris, J., Coll, R. C., Mills, K. H. G., Mok, K. H., Newsholme, P., Nuñez, G., & O'Neill, L. A. J. (2010). Activation of the NLRP3 inflammasome by islet amyloid polypeptide provides a mechanism for enhanced IL-1β in type 2 diabetes. *Nature Immunology, 11*(10), 897–904. https://doi.org/10.1038/ni.1935

Mathur, A., Patra, S., Asthana, S., & Jana, P. (2023). A review on current Type-2 diabetes mellitus treatment by selected phytoconstituents. *Research Journal of Pharmacology and Pharmacodynamics*, 205–211. https://doi.org/10.52711/2321-5836.2023.00036

McArdle, M. A., Finucane, O. M., Connaughton, R. M., McMorrow, A. M., & Roche, H. M. (2013). Mechanisms of obesity-induced inflammation and insulin resistance: Insights into the emerging role of nutritional strategies. *Frontiers in Endocrinology, 4*, 52. https://doi.org/10.3389/fendo.2013.00052

McNelis, J. C., & Olefsky, J. M. (2014). Macrophages, immunity, and metabolic disease. *Immunity, 41*(1), 36–48. https://doi.org/10.1016/j.immuni.2014.05.010

Michailidou, Z., Gomez-Salazar, M., & Alexaki, V. I. (2022). Innate immune cells in the adipose tissue in health and metabolic disease. *Journal of Innate Immunity, 14*(1), 4–30. https://doi.org/10.1159/000515117

Mokhtar, D. M., & Abdelhafez, E. A. (2021). An overview of the structural and functional aspects of immune cells in teleosts. *Histology & Histopathology, 36*(4), 399–414. https://doi.org/10.14670/HH-18-302

Moorman, C. D., Phee, H., & Sohn, S. J. (2021). Emerging therapeutics for immune tolerance: Tolerogenic vaccines, T cell therapy, and IL-2 therapy. *Frontiers in Immunology, 12*(Suppl. 2 2). https://doi.org/10.3389/fimmu.2021.657768

Mwaura, J.,N. (2025). The role of gut microbiota modulation through fecal microbiota transplantation (FMT) in managing type 1 diabetes: A scoping review. *Research Invention Journal of Scientific and Experimental Sciences, 5*(2), 97–100. https://doi.org/10.59298/rijses/2025/5297100

Naik, R. G., Brooks-Worrell, B. M., & Palmer, J. P. (2009). Latent autoimmune diabetes in adults. *Journal of Clinical Endocrinology & Metabolism, 94*(12), 4635–4644. https://doi.org/10.1210/jc.2009-1120

Natali, A., & Ferrannini, E. (2006). Effects of metformin and thiazolidinediones on suppression of hepatic glucose production and stimulation of glucose uptake in type 2 diabetes: A systematic review. *Diabetologia, 49*(3), 434–441. https://doi.org/10.1007/s00125-006-0141-7

Newsholme, P., Cruzat, V. F., Keane, K. N., Carlessi, R., & de Bittencourt, P. I., Jr. (2016). Molecular mechanisms of ROS production and oxidative stress in diabetes. *Biochemical Journal, 473*(24), 4527–4550. https://doi.org/10.1042/BCJ20160503C

Nishimura, S., Manabe, I., Nagasaki, M., Eto, K., Yamashita, H., Ohsugi, M., Otsu, M., Hara, K., Ueki, K., Sugiura, S., Yoshimura, K., Kadowaki, T., & Nagai, R. (2009). CD8+ effector T cells contribute to macrophage recruitment and adipose tissue inflammation in obesity. *Nature Medicine, 15*(8), 914–920. https://doi.org/10.1038/nm.1964

O'Neill, L. A., Kishton, R. J., & Rathmell, J. (2016). A guide to immunometabolism for immunologists. *Nature Reviews Immunology, 16*(9), 553–565. https://doi.org/10.1038/nri.2016.70

Odegaard, J. I., Ricardo-Gonzalez, R. R., Goforth, M. H., Morel, C. R., Subramanian, V., Mukundan, L., Red Eagle, A., Vats, D., Brombacher, F., Ferrante, A. W., & Chawla, A. (2007). Macrophage-specific PPARgamma controls alternative activation and improves insulin resistance. *Nature, 447*(7148), 1116–1120. https://doi.org/10.1038/nature05894

Osborn, O., & Olefsky, J. M. (2012). The cellular and signaling networks linking the immune system and metabolism in disease. *Nature Medicine, 18*(3), 363–374. https://doi.org/10.1038/nm.2627

Palmer, A. K., Xu, M., Zhu, Y., Pirtskhalava, T., Weivoda, M. M., Hachfeld, C. M., Prata, L. G., van Dijk, T. H., Verkade, E., Casaclang-Verzosa, G., Johnson, K. O., Cubro, H., Doornebal, E. J., Ogrodnik, M., Jurk, D., Jensen, M. D., Chini, E. N., Miller, J. D., Matveyenko, A., Stout, M. B., … Kirkland, J. L. (2019). Targeting senescent cells alleviates obesity-induced metabolic dysfunction. *Aging Cell, 18*(3), e12950. https://doi.org/10.1111/acel.12950

Park, C. S., & Shastri, N. (2022). The role of T cells in obesity-associated inflammation and metabolic disease. *Immune Network, 22*(1), e13. https://doi.org/10.4110/in.2022.22.e13

Pauken, K. E., & Wherry, E. J. (2015). Overcoming T cell exhaustion in infection and cancer. *Trends in Immunology, 36*(4), 265–276. https://doi.org/10.1016/j.it.2015.02.008

Peiró, C., Lorenzo, Ó., Carraro, R., & Sánchez-Ferrer, C. F. (2017). IL-1β inhibition in cardiovascular complications associated to diabetes mellitus. *Frontiers in Pharmacology, 8*(e10091). https://doi.org/10.3389/fphar.2017.00363

Pilla, S. J., Mathioudakis, N. N., Zhao, N., Knowler, W. C., Lin, D., Balasubramanyam, A., Clark, J., Maruthur, N. M., Anderson, A. M., Lernmark, Å., Hampe, C. S., Bancks, M., & Pietropaolo, S. (2024). 1993-LB: Subgroups of type 2 diabetes (T2D) by clinical features and islet autoimmunity. *Diabetes, 73* (Suppl. 1). https://doi.org/10.2337/db24-1993-lb

Pinheiro-Machado, E., Gurgul-Convey, E., & Marzec, M. T. (2020). Immunometabolism in type 2 diabetes mellitus: Tissue-specific interactions. *Archives of Medical Science: AMS, 19*(4), 895–911. https://doi.org/10.5114/aoms.2020.92674

Poitout, V., & Robertson, R. P. (2008). Glucolipotoxicity: Fuel excess and beta-cell dysfunction. *Endocrine Reviews, 29*(3), 351–366. https://doi.org/10.1210/er.2007-0023

Poles, J., Karhu, E., McGill, M., McDaniel, H. R., & Lewis, J. E. (2021). The effects of twenty-four nutrients and phytonutrients on immune system function and inflammation: A narrative review. *Journal of clinical and translational research, 7*(3), 333–376.

Pollak, F., & Vásquez, T. (2012). Diabetes autoinmune (latente) del adulto [Latent autoimmune diabetes in adults]. *Revista Medica de Chile, 140*(11), 1476–1481. https://doi.org/10.4067/S0034-98872012001100015

Porto, F. D., Triaca, V., Laganà, B., Aloe, L., D'Amelio, R., & Nofroni, I. (2006). Nerve growth factor and brain-derived neurotrophic factor levels in patients with rheumatoid arthritis treated with TNF-α blockers. *Annals of the New York Academy of Sciences, 1069*(1), 438–443. https://doi.org/10.1196/annals.1351.042

Prame Kumar, K., Ooi, J. D., & Goldberg, R. (2023). The interplay between the microbiota, diet and T regulatory cells in the preservation of the gut barrier in inflammatory bowel disease. *Frontiers in Microbiology, 14*. https://doi.org/10.3389/fmicb.2023.1291724

Prentki, M., & Nolan, C. J. (2006). Islet beta cell failure in type 2 diabetes. *Journal of Clinical Investigation, 116*(7), 1802–1812. https://doi.org/10.1172/JCI29103

Ratajczak, W., Rył, A., Mizerski, A., Walczakiewicz, K., Sipak, O., & Laszczyńska, M. (2019). Immunomodulatory potential of gut microbiome-derived short-chain fatty acids (SCFAs). *Acta Biochimica Polonica, 66*(1). https://doi.org/10.18388/abp.2018_26483

Raut, S. S. (2026). A decade of bibliometric and biotechnological advances in microbial polyhydroxyalkanoate (PHA) for biomedical applications: Developments in economical production, biosynthetic pathways, physicochemical properties, and therapeutic potential: A review. *International Journal of Biological Macromolecules*. https://doi.org/10.1016/j.ijbiomac.2025.149477

Razavi, M., Jamilian, M., Samimi, M., Afshar Ebrahimi, F., Taghizadeh, M., Bekhradi, R., Seyed Hosseini, E., Haddad Kashani, H., Karamali, M., & Asemi, Z. (2017). The effects of vitamin D and omega-3 fatty acids co-supplementation on biomarkers of inflammation, oxidative stress and pregnancy outcomes in patients with gestational diabetes. *Nutrition & Metabolism, 14*(1). https://doi.org/10.1186/s12986-017-0236-9

Reynolds, C. M., McGillicuddy, F. C., Harford, K. A., Finucane, O. M., Mills, K. H., & Roche, H. M. (2012). Dietary saturated fatty acids prime the NLRP3 inflammasome via TLR4 in dendritic cells-implications for diet-induced insulin resistance. *Molecular Nutrition & Food Research, 56*(8), 1212–1222. https://doi.org/10.1002/mnfr.201200058

Riedel, S., Pheiffer, C., Johnson, R., Louw, J., & Muller, C. J. F. (2022). Intestinal barrier function and immune homeostasis are missing links in obesity and type 2 diabetes development. *Frontiers in Endocrinology, 12*, 833544. https://doi.org/10.3389/fendo.2021.833544

Roelofsen, H., Priebe, M. G., & Vonk, R. J. (2010). The interaction of short-chain fatty acids with adipose tissue: Relevance for prevention of type 2 diabetes. *Beneficial Microbes, 1*(4), 433–437. https://doi.org/10.3920/BM2010.0028

Rowshanravan, B., Halliday, N., & Sansom, D. M. (2018). CTLA-4: A moving target in immunotherapy. *Blood, 131*(1), 58–67. https://doi.org/10.1182/blood-2017-06-741033

Samuel, V. T., & Shulman, G. I. (2012). Mechanisms for insulin resistance: Common threads and missing links. *Cell, 148*(5), 852–871. https://doi.org/10.1016/j.cell.2012.02.017

Sankararaman, S., Noriega, K., Velayuthan, S., et al. (2023). Gut microbiome and its impact on obesity and obesity-related disorders. *Current Gastroenterology Reports, 25*(1), 31–44. https://doi.org/10.1007/s11894-022-00859-0

Sharma, Y., Arora, M., & Bala, K. (2024). The potential of immunomodulators in shaping the future of healthcare. *Discovery Medicine, 1*, 37. https://doi.org/10.1007/s44337-024-00029-3

Sharma, A., et al. (2024a). Navigating the landscape of cancer-induced thrombocytopenia: Current challenges and emerging advances. *Industrial Microbiology and Biotechnology*. https://doi.org/10.1007/978-981-97-6270-5_14

Sharma, A., et al. (2024). *DDX3X* dynamics, glioblastoma's genetic landscape, therapeutic advances, and autophagic interplay. *Medical Oncology*. https://doi.org/10.1007/s12032-024-02525-z

Sharma, A., et al. (2025a). From tissue architecture to clinical insights: Spatial transcriptomics in solid tumor studies. *Seminars in Oncology*. https://doi.org/10.1016/j.seminoncol.2025.152389

Sharma, A., et al. (2025b). Deciphering the relevance of dead box RNA helicases in gliomagenesis and autophagy. *Human Cell*. https://doi.org/10.1007/s13577-025-01329-1

Sharma, A., et al. (2025c). Phytochemical triad in lung cancer: Synergistic mechanisms and clinical translation of genistein, piperine, and resveratrol. *Molecular Nutrition & Food Research*. https://doi.org/10.1002/mnfr.70348

Sharma, A., et al. (2026). Therapeutic targeting of the mitochondrial dysfunction-PANoptosis axis: Mechanistic insights and emerging strategies. *Translational Research*. https://doi.org/10.1016/j.trsl.2026.03.004

Sharma, B., Kumar, A., Sharma, U., Pal, D., & Prashar, S. (2022). The potential role of gut microbiota in the pathogenesis of type 2 diabetes mellitus *via* epigenetics and inflammasome. *Endocrine, Metabolic & Immune Disorders - Drug Targets, 22*(14), 1331–1343. https://doi.org/10.2174/1871530322666220331152809

Shruti, R., et al. (2026). Biological green synthesis of nanoparticles: A sustainable platform for agricultural, environmental, food, and cosmetic applications. *Journal of Environmental Chemical Engineering*. . https://doi.org/10.1016/j.jece.2026.121102

Shukla, A., et al. (2025a). Antitumor potential of ivermectin against T-cell lymphoma-bearing hosts. *Medical Oncology*. https://doi.org/10.1007/s12032-025-02726-0

Shukla, A. (2025b). Structure-guided discovery of a novel BTK inhibitor inducing apoptosis and G1 phase arrest in tumor cells. *Molecular Diversity*. https://doi.org/10.1007/s11030-025-11334-z

Simone, R., Zicca, A., & Saverino, D. (2008). The frequency of regulatory $CD3^{+}CD8^{+}CD28^{-}CD25^{+}$ T lymphocytes in human peripheral blood increases with age. *Journal of Leukocyte Biology, 84*(6), 1454–1461. https://doi.org/10.1189/jlb.0907627

Singh, S., et al. (2025). Silibinin: A natural flavonoid with multifaceted anticancer potential and therapeutic challenges. *Medicinal Chemistry Research*. . https://doi.org/10.1007/s00044-025-03466-6

Soedono, S., & Cho, K. W. (2021). Adipose tissue dendritic cells: Critical regulators of obesity-induced inflammation and insulin resistance. *International Journal of Molecular Sciences, 22*(16), 8666. https://doi.org/10.3390/ijms22168666

Stienstra, R., Joosten, L. A. B., Koenen, T., van Tits, L. J. H., van Diepen, J. A., van den Berg, S. A. A., Rensen, P. C. N., Voshol, P. J., Fantuzzi, G., Hijmans, A., Kersten, S., Müller, M., van den Berg, W. B., van Rooijen, N., Wabitsch, M., Kanneganti, T. D., Tack, C. J., de Winther, M. P. J., & Netea, M. G. (2010). The inflammasome-mediated caspase-1 activation controls adipocyte differentiation and insulin sensitivity. *Cell Metabolism, 12*(6), 593–605. https://doi.org/10.1016/j.cmet.2010.11.011

Sugandh, F., Chandio, M., Raveena, F., Kumar, L., Karishma, F., Khuwaja, S., Memon, U. A., Bai, K., Kashif, M., Varrassi, G., Khatri, M., & Kumar, S. (2023). Advances in the management of diabetes mellitus: A focus on personalized medicine. *Cureus, 15*(8), e43697. https://doi.org/10.7759/cureus.43697

Sun, L., Xi, S., He, G., Li, Z., Gang, X., Sun, C., Guo, W., & Wang, G. (2020). Two to Tango: Dialogue between adaptive and innate immunity in type 1 diabetes. *Journal of Diabetes Research, 2020*, 4106518. https://doi.org/10.1155/2020/4106518

Szukiewicz, D. (2023). Molecular mechanisms for the vicious cycle between insulin resistance and the inflammatory response in obesity. *International Journal of Molecular Sciences, 24*(12), 9818. https://doi.org/10.3390/ijms24129818

Tahvildari, M., & Dana, R. (2019). Low-dose IL-2 therapy in transplantation, autoimmunity, and inflammatory diseases. *The Journal of Immunology, 203*(11), 2749–2755. https://doi.org/10.4049/jimmunol.1900733

Tang, H. Y., Jiang, A. J., Ma, J. L., Wang, F. J., & Shen, G. M. (2019). Understanding the signaling pathways related to the mechanism and treatment of diabetic peripheral neuropathy. *Endocrinology, 160*(9), 2119–2127. https://doi.org/10.1210/en.2019-00311

Tsukumo, D. M., Carvalho-Filho, M. A., Carvalheira, J. B., Prada, P. O., Hirabara, S. M., Schenka, A. A., Araújo, E. P., Vassallo, J., Curi, R., Velloso, L. A., & Saad, M. J. (2007). Loss-of-function mutation in toll-like receptor 4 prevents diet-induced obesity and insulin resistance. *Diabetes, 56*(8), 1986–1998. https://doi.org/10.2337/db16-rt04a

Van Poppel, P. C. M., Netea, M. G., Van Asseldonk, E. J. P., Holst, J. J., Vilsbøll, T., & Tack, C. J. (2014). The interleukin-1 receptor antagonist anakinra improves first-phase insulin secretion and insulinogenic index in subjects with impaired glucose tolerance. *Diabetes, Obesity and Metabolism, 16*(12), 1269–1273. https://doi.org/10.1111/dom.12357

Vandanmagsar, B., Youm, Y. H., Ravussin, A., Galgani, J. E., Stadler, K., Mynatt, R. L., Ravussin, E., Stephens, J. M., & Dixit, V. D. (2011). The NLRP3 inflammasome instigates obesity-induced inflammation and insulin resistance. *Nature Medicine, 17*(2), 179–188. https://doi.org/10.1038/nm.2279

Varanasi, V., Avanesyan, L., Schumann, D. M., & Chervonsky, A. V. (2012). Cytotoxic mechanisms employed by mouse T cells to destroy pancreatic β-Cells. *Diabetes, 61*(11), 2862–2870. https://doi.org/10.2337/db11-1784

Velikova, T. V., Kabakchieva, P. P., Assyov, Y. S., & Georgiev, T.A. (2021). Targeting inflammatory cytokines to improve type 2 diabetes control. *BioMed Research International, 2021*, 7297419. https://doi.org/10.1155/2021/7297419

Vivian, E. M. (2014). Sodium-glucose co-transporter 2 (SGLT2) inhibitors: A growing class of antidiabetic agents. *Drugs in Context, 3*, 212264. https://doi.org/10.7573/dic.212264

Vu, T. D., Lin, S. C., Wu, C. C., & Chu, D. T. (2024). RNA therapeutics for metabolic disorders. *Progress in molecular biology and translational science, 203*, 181–196. https://doi.org/10.1016/bs.pmbts.2023.12.014

Wada, T., Hoshino, M., Kimura, Y., Ojima, M., Nakano, T., Koya, D., Tsuneki, H., & Sasaoka, T. (2011). Both type I and II IFN induce insulin resistance by inducing different isoforms of SOCS expression in 3T3-L1 adipocytes. *American Journal of Physiology. Endocrinology and Metabolism, 300*(6), E1112–E1123. https://doi.org/10.1152/ajpendo.00370.2010

Wajchenberg, B. L. (2000). Subcutaneous and visceral adipose tissue: Their relation to the metabolic syndrome. *Endocrine Reviews, 21*(6), 697–738. https://doi.org/10.1210/edrv.21.6.0415

Walter, U., & Santamaria, P. (2005). CD8+ T cells in autoimmunity. *Current Opinion in Immunology, 17* (6), 624–631. https://doi.org/10.1016/j.coi.2005.09.014

Wang, M., Chen, F., Wang, J., Zeng, Z., Yang, Q., & Shao, S. (2018). Th17 and treg lymphocytes in obesity and type 2 diabetic patients. *Clinical immunology, 197*, 77–85. https://doi.org/10.1016/j.clim.2018.09.005

Wang, Z., Ni, X., Zhang, L., Sun, L., Zhu, X., Zhou, Q., Yang, Z., & Yuan, H. (2020). Toll-like receptor 4 and inflammatory micro-environment of pancreatic islets in Type-2 diabetes mellitus: A therapeutic perspective. *Diabetes, Metabolic Syndrome and Obesity: Targets and Therapy, 13*, 4261–4272. https://doi.org/10.2147/DMSO.S279104

Wang, L., Rubinstein, R., Lines, J. L., Wasiuk, A., Ahonen, C., Guo, Y., … Fedorov, A. (2019). VISTA, a novel mouse Ig superfamily ligand that negatively regulates T cell responses. *Journal of Experimental Medicine, 207*(13), 2783–2795. https://doi.org/10.1084/jem.20100619

Wehbe, T. (2024). Advances in stem cell therapy for type 2 diabetes mellitus. *Medical Research Archives, 12*(12). https://doi.org/10.18103/mra.v12i12.6067

Weinberg Sibony, R., Segev, O., Dor, S., & Raz, I. (2024). Overview of oxidative stress and inflammation in diabetes. *Journal of Diabetes, 16*(10). https://doi.org/10.1111/1753-0407.70014

Wen, H., Gris, D., Lei, Y., Jha, S., Zhang, L., Huang, M. T. H., Brickey, W. J., & Ting, J. P. Y. (2011). Fatty acid–induced NLRP3-ASC inflammasome activation interferes with insulin signaling. *Nature Immunology, 12*(5), 408–415. https://doi.org/10.1038/ni.2022

Winer, S., Chan, Y., Paltser, G., Truong, D., Tsui, H., Bahrami, J., Dorfman, R., Wang, Y., Zielenski, J., Mastronardi, F., Maezawa, Y., Drucker, D. J., Engleman, E., Winer, D., & Dosch, H. M. (2009). Normalization of obesity-associated insulin resistance through immunotherapy. *Nature Medicine, 15* (8), 921–929. https://doi.org/10.1038/nm.2001

Winer, D. A., Winer, S., Shen, L., Wadia, P. P., Yantha, J., Paltser, G., Tsui, H., Wu, P., Davidson, M. G., Alonso, M. N., Leong, H. X., Glassford, A., Caimol, M., Kenkel, J. A., Tedder, T. F., McLaughlin, T., Miklos, D. B., Dosch, H. M., & Engleman, E. G. (2011). B cells promote insulin resistance through modulation of T cells and production of pathogenic IgG antibodies. *Nature Medicine, 17*(5), 610–617. https://doi.org/10.1038/nm.2353

Xia, J., Yin, S., Yu, J., Wang, J., Jin, X., Wang, Y., Liu, H., & Sun, G. (2024). Improvement in glycolipid metabolism parameters after supplementing fish oil-derived Omega-3 fatty acids is associated with gut microbiota and lipid metabolites in type 2 diabetes mellitus. *Nutrients, 16*(21), 3755. https://doi.org/10.3390/nu16213755

Xiao, H., Woods, E. C., Vukojicic, P., & Bertozzi, C. R. (2016). Precision glycocalyx editing as a strategy for cancer immunotherapy. *Proceedings of the National Academy of Sciences of the United States of America, 113*(37), 10304–10309. https://doi.org/10.1073/pnas.1608069113

Xie, K., Tang, W., Wang, J., Xu, B., Xia, Y., Huang, Z., Ji, Y., Zhou, K., Chen, M., & Zhang, Y. (2018). A multi-method evaluation of the effects of inflammatory cytokines (IL-1β, IFN-γ, TNF-α) on pancreatic β-cells. *Journal of Cellular Physiology, 233*(12), 9375–9382. https://doi.org/10.1002/jcp.26518

Xu, H., Uysal, K. T., Becherer, J. D., Arner, P., & Hotamisligil, G. S. (2002). Altered tumor necrosis factor-alpha (TNF-alpha) processing in adipocytes and increased expression of transmembrane TNF-alpha in obesity. *Diabetes, 51*(6), 1876–1883. https://doi.org/10.2337/diabetes.51.6.1876

Yang, M., Su, L., Tao, Q., Zhang, C., Wu, Y., & Liu, J. (2018). Depletion of regulatory T cells in visceral adipose tissues contributes to insulin resistance in Hashimoto's thyroiditis. *Frontiers in Physiology, 9*, 136. https://doi.org/10.3389/fphys.2018.00136

Yap, Y. A., & Mariño, E. (2020). Dietary SCFAs immunotherapy: Reshaping the gut microbiota in diabetes. *Advances in Experimental Medicine and Biology, 1307*, 499–519. https://doi.org/10.1007/5584_2020_515

Yoo, J. Y., Groer, M., Dutra, S. V. O., Sarkar, A., & McSkimming, D. I. (2020). Gut microbiota and immune system interactions. *Microorganisms, 8*(10), 1587. https://doi.org/10.3390/microorganisms8101587

Yu, L., Yang, Y. X., Gong, Z., Wan, Q., Du, Y., Zhou, Q., Xiao, Y., Zahr, T., Wang, Z., Yu, Z., Yang, K., Geng, J. , Fried, S. K., Li, J., Haeusler, R. A., Leong, K. W., Bai, L., Wu, Y., Sun, L., ... Qiang, L. (2024). FcRn-dependent IgG accumulation in adipose tissue unmasks obesity pathophysiology. *Cell Metabolism, 37*(3), 656–672.e7. https://doi.org/10.1016/j.cmet.2024.11.001

Zatterale, F., Longo, M., Naderi, J., Raciti, G. A., Desiderio, A., Miele, C., & Beguinot, F. (2020). Chronic adipose tissue inflammation linking obesity to insulin resistance and type 2 diabetes. *Frontiers in Physiology, 10*, 1607. https://doi.org/10.3389/fphys.2019.01607

Zeng, Z., Huang, S. Y., & Sun, T. (2020). Pharmacogenomic studies of current antidiabetic agents and potential new drug targets for precision medicine of diabetes. *Diabetes therapy: Research, Treatment and Education of Diabetes and Related Disorders, 11*(11), 2521–2538. https://doi.org/10.1007/s13300-020-00922-x

Zeng, C., Shi, X., Zhao, Y., Zhang, L., Liu, H., Zhang, B., & Ding, W. (2011). The imbalance of Th17/Th1/Tregs in patients with type 2 diabetes: Relationship with metabolic factors and complications. *Journal of Molecular Medicine, 90*(2), 175–186. https://doi.org/10.1007/s00109-011-0816-5

Zhang, Y. (2023). Role of autoimmunity in development of type 2 diabetes. *Mathews Journal of Immunology & Allergy, 7*(1), 1–7. https://doi.org/10.30654/MJIA.10017

Zhang, L., Chu, J., Hao, W., Zhang, J., Li, H., Yang, C., Yang, J., Chen, X., & Wang, H. (2021). Gut microbiota and type 2 diabetes mellitus: Association, mechanism, and translational applications. *Mediators of Inflammation, 2021*, 5110276. https://doi.org/10.1155/2021/5110276

Zhao, J., & Fang, Z. (2025). Single-cell RNA sequencing reveals the dysfunctional characteristics of PBMCs in patients with type 2 diabetes mellitus. *Frontiers in Immunology, 15*, 1501660. https://doi.org/10.3389/fimmu.2024.1501660

Zhou, Z., Sun, B., Yu, D., & Zhu, C. (2022). Gut microbiota: An important player in type 2 diabetes mellitus. *Frontiers in Cellular and Infection Microbiology, 12*(1). https://doi.org/10.3389/fcimb.2022.834485

Zhou, R., Tardivel, A., Thorens, B., Choi, I., & Tschopp, J. (2010). Thioredoxin-interacting protein links oxidative stress to inflammasome activation. *Nature Immunology, 11*(2), 136–140. https://doi.org/10.1038/ni.1831

Further reading

ElTanbouly, M. A., Croteau, W., Noelle, R. J., & Lines, J. L. (2020). VISTA: A novel immunotherapy target for normalizing innate and adaptive immunity. *Seminars in Immunology, 42,* 101308. https://doi.org/10.1016/j.smim.2019.101308

Gindri Dos Santos, B., & Goedeke, L. (2023). Macrophage immunometabolism in diabetes-associated atherosclerosis. *Immunometabolism, 5*(4), e00032. https://doi.org/10.1097/IN9.0000000000000032

International Diabetes Federation. (2021). *IDF diabetes atlas* (10th ed.). Brussels, Belgium: International Diabetes Federation https://www.idf.org/.

Maruyama, T., Oak, S., Shimada, A., & Hampe, C. S. (2008). GAD65 autoantibody responses in Japanese latent autoimmune diabetes in adult patients. *Diabetes Care, 31*(8), 1602–1607. https://doi.org/10.2337/dc08-0235

Molavi, B., Rassouli, N., Bagwe, S., & Rasouli, N. (2007). A review of thiazolidinediones and metformin in the treatment of type 2 diabetes with focus on cardiovascular complications. *Vascular Health and Risk Management, 3*(6), 967–973.

Santarpia, M., González-Cao, M., Viteri, S., Karachaliou, N., Altavilla, G., & Rosell, R. (2015). Programmed cell death protein-1/programmed cell death ligand-1 pathway inhibition and predictive biomarkers: Understanding transforming growth factor-beta role. *Translational Lung Cancer Research, 4*(6), 728–742. https://doi.org/10.3978/j.issn.2218-6751.2015.12.04

Temelkova-Kurktschiev, T., & Stefanov, T. (2012). Lifestyle and genetics in obesity and type 2 diabetes. *Experimental and Clinical Endocrinology & Diabetes: Official Journal, German Society of Endocrinology [and] German Diabetes Association, 120*(1), 1–6. https://doi.org/10.1055/s-0031-1285832

Templer, S., Abdo, S., & Wong, T. (2024). Preventing diabetes complications. *Internal Medicine Journal, 54*(8), 1264–1274. https://doi.org/10.1111/imj.16455

Wensveen, F. M., Jelenčić, V., & Polić, B. (2021). NKG2D: A master regulator of immune cell responsiveness. *Frontiers in Immunology, 12,* 749. https://doi.org/10.3389/fimmu.2021.707223

Winer, D. A., Winer, S., & Chng, M. H. Y. (2021). Targeting immune checkpoints in metabolic disease. *Nature Reviews Immunology, 21*(3), 162–174. https://doi.org/10.1038/s41577-020-00466-8

Yeoh, J., Huang, J., Cheng, H., & Muir, K. R. (2009). Unusually rapid β-cell failure in a patient newly diagnosed with type 2 diabetes presenting acutely with unprovoked severe hyperglycaemic hyperosmolar state: A case report. *Cases Journal, 2.*

4

Immune cells and T2DM

Rituparna Paul, Lyticia Philabet Sohtun and Kripamoy Aguan
MOLECULAR BIOLOGY LABORATORY, DEPARTMENT OF BIOTECHNOLOGY AND BIOINFORMATICS, NORTH EASTERN HILL UNIVERSITY, SHILLONG, MEGHALAYA, INDIA

1. Introduction

Type 2 diabetes mellitus (T2DM) is a global health problem; about 90% of diabetes cases are type 2 diabetes. It is a metabolic disorder characterized by insufficient insulin or insulin resistance, as well as impaired insulin production by the pancreatic β cells. Insulin, a hormone composed of peptides generated by beta cells in the pancreas, helps maintain correct blood glucose levels by enabling the uptake of cellular glucose in cells and also regulates the metabolism of carbohydrates, fats, and proteins, and supports cellular growth and division through its mitogenic characteristics (Wilcox, 2005). Impaired insulin signaling resistance is characterized by unresponsiveness of tissues such as the skeletal muscles, adipose tissue, and liver. The decreased metabolic response to insulin is also associated with physical inactivity, obesity, and aging. In an insulin resistance condition, the pancreatic β islets increase their cell 4mass and enhance insulin secretion to compensate for the body's insulin demand. However, as the condition progresses, the pancreatic β islets fail to meet the desired degree of insulin, which causes chronically high glucose levels in the blood, and T2DM develops (Donath & Shoelson, 2011; Berbudi et al., 2020). Individuals with T2DM may exhibit varying degrees of beta-cell dysfunction and impaired insulin sensitivity; however, the onset of reduced insulin responsiveness might begin 15 years before clinical diagnosis (Antar et al., 2023). Moreover, 50% of the T2DM patients, after almost 10 years of insulin resistance due to dysfunction of the pancreatic β islet cells, need to undergo insulin therapy (Berbudi et al., 2020).

Individuals with T2DM often exhibit inflammation before the disease onset. Inflammation is a defensive response to injuries, infections, and toxins. It involves the migration of leukocytes from the bloodstream to affected tissues. Cell adhesion molecules, cytokines, and chemokines carefully regulate the process of eliminating damaging stimuli and repairing tissue (Wright & Cooper, 2014). Inflammatory conditions associated with Type 2 diabetes can alter the behavior and recruitment of white blood cells to various tissues (Wu et al., 2011).

Type 2 Diabetes Mellitus. https://doi.org/10.1016/B978-0-443-33590-7.00014-9

Research shows a strong correlation between inflammatory indicators and improper lipid and glucose metabolism, as well as obesity and atherosclerosis. Inflammation in T2DM is predominantly mediated by inflammatory signaling molecules, chemokines, adipokines, and cytokines. Chronic low-grade inflammation is one of the pathogeneses of T2DM (Antar et al., 2023). Due to the inflammation, all the components of the immune cells are altered, particularly in adipose tissue, pancreatic islets, blood vessels, and circulating white blood cells. Cellular stressors such as oxidative stress and lipotoxicity can lead to insulin resistance and pancreatic islet dysfunction, eliciting an inflammatory response and exacerbating local inflammation (Pezhman et al., 2021).

2. Overview of the immune system

The immune system of mammalian species consists of a very complex network of interacting cells, encompassing both antigen-nonspecific (innate) and antigen-specific (adaptive) components. The innate immune system serves as a crucial first response against pathogens through its rapid and nonspecific mechanisms. By utilizing pattern recognition receptors (PRRs), innate immune cells recognize pathogen-associated molecular patterns (PAMPs) such as lipopolysaccharides and viral RNA, triggering immediate responses. These cells, including granulocytes, mononuclear phagocytes, and innate lymphoid cells, play diverse roles in phagocytosis, cytokine production, and immune regulation. Neutrophils and macrophages specialize in engulfing and destroying pathogens, while dendritic cells act as a bridge between innate and adaptive immune responses by presenting antigens to T cells. Other cells, such as eosinophils, natural killer (NK) cells, and mast cells, contribute to inflammation, allergy responses, and antiviral defenses. Whereas the adaptive immune system plays a crucial role in combating infections when the innate immune response is insufficient. Its primary functions include the recognition of specific "nonself" antigens while distinguishing them from "self" antigens, the activation of pathogen-specific effector mechanisms to eliminate infections, and the establishment of immunologic memory to ensure rapid responses to future encounters with the same pathogen. Adaptive immune responses rely on T cells that recognize antigens, which are stimulated by antigen-presenting cells (APCs) to proliferate, and B cells, which mature into plasma cells to produce antibodies. Unlike the innate immune system, which uses germline-encoded pattern recognition receptors (PRRs), adaptive immune cells express receptors generated through random recombination of genetic segments, creating immense receptor diversity. These receptors are further diversified by random nucleotide additions during recombination. Each adaptive immune cell expresses a single, specific receptor, and those recognizing a particular antigen are initially present in low frequency. Upon pathogen recognition, these cells undergo clonal expansion, multiplying to mount an effective response, though this process takes several days. Adaptive immunity, which underpins the effectiveness of immunizations, is slower to develop than innate immunity but provides long-lasting and highly specific protection against pathogens (Leichner & Kambayashi, 2014; Marshall et al., 2018).

T2DM has been associated with immune system disequilibrium. These immunological dysfunction makes people with diabetes more vulnerable to inflammation, infection, and further complications, resulting in higher morbidity and mortality rates due to increased susceptibility to infectious illnesses (Saadh et al., 2025).

3. Innate immune cells

3.1 Neutrophils

Neutrophils are the most abundant leukocytes in humans; these cells serve as the primary response during both chronic and acute inflammation. They constitute the majority of circulating leukocytes and play a crucial role in the innate immune response. During acute inflammation or injury, neutrophils are recruited to the site of injury or inflammation through chemotaxis, initially triggered by complement activation. Neutrophils, upon activation, bind to inflamed endothelial cells through surface receptors, migrate to the tissue, and eliminate pathogens through phagocytosis, reactive oxygen species (ROS),the release of antimicrobial peptides, and, lysosomal enzymes. They contribute to tissue repair and resolution by phagocytosing necrotic cells, releasing growth-promoting mediators and promoting angiogenesis, and producing antiinflammatory substances such asprotectins and resolvins. In a diabetic condition, the reduced scavenging activity and increased proliferation of cytokines initiate the activation of naïve neutrophils (Thimmappa et al., 2023). Conversely, neutrophils contribute to the perpetuation of the inflammatory process by releasing serine proteases, forming neutrophil traps, and stimulating other immune cells. Patients with T2DM have a higher susceptibility to infections, including mycosis, urinary tract infections, diabetic foot ulcers, bloodstream infections, and eye, soft tissue, and skin infections. The severity and the duration of the infections are primarily based on the metabolic well-being of an individual. An imbalance in the immune-metabolic axis is caused by nutritional excess conditions in T2DM, characterized by high glucose levels, increased branched-chain amino acids, and lipids. Due to these imbalances, people are more predisposed to recurring infections that originate from persistent activation, poor mobilization, and hindered development of neutrophil regulatory and effector activities.

3.1.1 Impact of hyperglycemia on neutrophils

Neutrophil recruitment to the site of infection is essential to eliminate the microbes, resolve inflammation, and repair tissue. However, individuals with decreased neutrophil count or those with uncontrolled neutrophil function are more susceptible to recurring infection, tissue damage, or autoimmune conditions. Studies have found that hyperglycemia alters neutrophil function. The generation of Advanced Glycation End products (AGEs) is facilitated by hyperglycemia, which has been found to impede the movement of circulating neutrophils, decrease their viability rate, and promote cell death (Tian et al., 2016). AGEs also increase the synthesis of inflammatory signal molecules and oxidative stress in neutrophils (Thimmappa et al., 2023).

Kuwabara et al. (2018) found that while treating the Bronchoalveolar tissue in Goto Kakizaki and high-fat-diet mice with Lipopolysaccharide, the chemotactic behavior of the neutrophils is impaired, and the number of neutrophils is decreased, as well as a reduction in the secretion of proinflammatory cytokines such as IL-6, IL-β, TNF-α, and the enzyme MPO, produced by the neutrophils during the inflammatory process. An increase in the CXCL3, a chemoattractant for neutrophils, that primarily aids in immune cell recruitment, was reported, demonstrating a dysregulated response. Moreover, a significant decrease in the TLR4 pathway proteins was detected, which are involved in neutrophil activation in response to Lipopolysaccharide. It has been found that the neutrophils in diabetic mice are insensitive to lipopolysaccharide activation, revealing an impaired innate immune response in hyperglycemia (Kuwabara et al., 2018; Thimmappa et al., 2023).

3.1.2 *Impact of T2DM on phagocytosis of neutrophils*

T2DM alters the process of phagocytosis, through which the neutrophils eradicate infectious agents during infection. To eliminate infection, phagocytosis involves several proteins, such as defensin, cathepsin, lactoferrin, and lysozyme (Borregaard, 2010). Neutrophil apoptosis affects the effector function, lifespan, and ROS-mediated damage. Phagocytosis by neutrophils is an efficient immunological response to infection caused by the *Mycobacterium tuberculosis*. The gut microbiota produces short-chain fatty acids as major metabolites such as formate, butyrate, and propionate. The neutrophilic phagocytosis of mycobacteria is decreased due to the increased levels of SCFAs, also leading to the reduced production of hydrogen peroxide, hypochlorous acid, and superoxide. Due to this alteration, the risk of developing tuberculosis increases by around three times in patients with T2DM (Thimmappa et al., 2023).

T2DM is the major risk factor for complications of septic endophthalmitis and liver abscess related to *K. pneumoniae*. It was found that the neutrophil phagocytosis rate of *K. pneumoniae* serotypes K1 and K2 was poorer in individuals with T2DM as compared with healthy individuals. High blood sugar levels in patients with endophthalmitis and meningitis reduce the phagocytosis ability of the neutrophils to consume and kill the *K. pneumoniae,* thus worsening the infection. The phagocytosis rate of neutrophils against *Staphylococcus aureus,* after treatment with nicotinamide for both groups, was also found to be lowered in subjects with diabetes as compared with controls (Lin et al., 2006; Thimmappa et al., 2023).

During inflammation, neutrophils become more glycolytic and produce lactate that stimulates phagocytosis. An individual with T2DM has impaired glucose metabolism, which results in an insufficient supply of energy for the neutrophils to function. This makes the individual with T2DM more susceptible to infections. Finding ways to increase the phagocytosis rate of neutrophils can help balance the innate immune system's homeostasis (Thimmappa et al., 2023).

3.1.3 T2DM neutrophils form constitutive NETs and render to reduced response to infection

Patients with type 2 diabetes have more activated neutrophils as compared with normal healthy individuals, which produces more ROS, increasing the risk of tissue damage, ultimately leading to organ damage. Currently recognized and possibly most damaging weapon of neutrophils is the release of nuclear chromatin lined with toxic protein, called neutrophil extracellular traps (NETs). In diabetic patients, levels of peptidyl arginine deiminase 4 (PAD4) are elevated in neutrophils, along with homocysteine in the bloodstream, leading to the release of neutrophil extracellular traps (NETs) from neutrophils trigger other immune cells and increase inflammation. During this process, the inflammatory cytokines, mitochondrial ROS, and glucose metabolites activate NF-kB, which transcriptionally upregulates the peptidyl arginine deaminase 4 (PAD4), which facilitates histone modification important in NET formation (Bajpai & Tilley, 2018). This process in T2DM is enhanced and may contribute to Diabetic cardiomyopathy (DCM) and impaired wound healing. Increased NET also plays a significant role in atherosclerosis because of its proatherogenic properties. Circulating NET indicators are linked to the severity of cardiovascular disease (CVD) and atherosclerotic lesions. Neutrophils may be involved in recruiting other leukocytes in the atherosclerotic areas because of their depletion during atherogenesis and lower local inflammation and macrophage concentration. It has also been found through demonstration that NETs release histone H4, which causes smooth muscle death, destabilizes plaques, and accelerates the progression of the disease. Furthermore, in hyperglycemic conditions, NET production hinders the improvement of atherosclerotic conditions even after lipid-lowering treatments (Bajpai & Tilley, 2018; Keeter et al., 2021).

Myeloperoxidase (MPO), produced primarily by neutrophils, serves as an early marker of inflammation in diabetic patients. MPO attached to the endothelial cells increases the synthesis of proinflammatory oxidant hypochlorous acid (HOCl) and lengthens the half-life, which damages blood vessels. In T2DM, the migration rate, phagocytosis, and microbial killing activity of neutrophils are impaired, increasing the infection rate. It has also been reported that in animal models of T2DM, neutrophils exhibit defective TLR4 signaling, shorter half-lives, reduced cytokine production, and diminished MPO activity. However, in diabetic patients with coronary heart disease, the MPO levels are elevated in the blood plasma, leading to inflammation and cardiovascular complications (Daryabor et al., 2020).

3.2 Natural killer cells (NK cells)

Natural killer Cells (NK cells), a component of the innate immune system, are formed in the bone marrow, influenced by the interleukins IL-2 and IL-15, as well as bone marrow stromal cells. It exhibits a distinct lineage of lymphoid cells, and upon activation, appears as big granular lymphocytes. NK cells cover only a minor portion of the circulating blood cells and lymphoid cells in the spleen and other secondary lymphoid organs. They lack antigen-specific receptors and interact through the inhibitory receptors present on their surface. Their cytotoxic function is suppressed upon encountering a self-MHC molecule through their inhibitory receptors that detect class 1 HLA molecules (Chaplin, 2010). However, in the absence of or reduced MHC 1expression, NK cells become activated and initiate the damage of the target cells (Chaplin, 2010; Nicholson, 2016).

NK cells can recognize tumors as well as virus-infected or bacterial-infected cells by their intricate network of surface receptors, all of which are more prevalent in individuals associated with type 2 diabetes (Morsink et al., 2020). They exhibit strong antitumor effects and effectively eliminate virally infected cells (Chaplin, 2010). Impairments in NK cell function have been linked to an increased risk of infection and malignancies. NK cell activity is controlled by the activating receptors, such as NKp30, NKp44, NKp46, NKG2c, and NKG2D, which interact with the ligands expressed on the surface of tumor or infected cells.

NK cells are categorized into two main subgroups. One group is primarily involved with cytotoxicity, characterized by CD56dim CD16 bright expression, whereas the other group is involved in the secretion of cytokines, such as TNFα, IFN-γ, IL-8, and IL-10, and expresses CD56 bright CD16dim/negative. Studies have revealed contradictory results regarding the population of NK cells in obese and T2D patients. Some studies have indicated an increase in the number and activation of NK cells in the circulating blood cells or adipose tissue as compared with healthy controls. Some studies also reported a decrease in population or no significant differences in NK cells. However, it is widely accepted that the population of cytotoxic CD56 dim NK cells decreases in number in obesity conditions, and less cytotoxic CD56 bright NK cells increase in number with elevated production of cytokine NKG2D and INF-γ produced by NK cells (Zhou et al., 2018).

Research by Berrou et al. (2013) highlights that T2D patients exhibit a reduced frequency of NK cells expressing NKp46 and NKG2D, alongside functional defects, such as diminished degranulation. Patients with poorly managed diabetes exhibit the lowest expression levels of NKG2D, and an inverse relationship between the frequency of NKG2D-positive NK cells and HbA1c levels. Furthermore, in visceral adipose tissue (VAT) of high-fat diet (HFD)-fed mice, NK cells promote macrophage differentiation into the proinflammatory M1 phenotype, exacerbating inflammation and contributing to obesity-related insulin resistance (Berrou et al., 2013).

3.3 Monocytes

Monocytes originate in the embryonic stage, but the majority develop from the myeloid progenitor cells of hematopoietic stem cells from the bone marrow. These circulating blood cells make up about 10% of human peripheral leukocytes. Monocytes are the precursors of macrophages and dendritic cells, which have physiological functions when recruited to inflamed tissues and play an important role in the overall coordination of immunity. During inflammation, the monocytes that are recruited exhibit different characteristics compared with resident macrophages and conventional dendritic cells. Monocytes, resident macrophages, and conventional dendritic cells (cDC) are constituents of the "mononuclear phagocyte system" (MPS) (Guilliams et al., 2014, 2018).

The primary role of monocytes is to supply tissues with adequate macrophages to induce inflammation, but they also have the ability to acquire regulatory qualities for tissue restoration. It is also necessary for the effective functioning of activated cytotoxic T cells, but they can also have significant tissue-damaging effects. Patrolling monocytes are essential for antitumor immunity; however, in other cases, they contribute to chemotherapy resistance, which promotes tumor growth (Murray, 2018).

3.3.1 Monocytes in T2DM

In response to elevated glucose levels in T2DM, monocytes, endothelial cells, and other cell types release inflammatory mediators (Kolb & Mandrup-Poulsen, 2005). It has been reported that glucose modulates the secretion of proinflammatory cytokines such as TNFα and IL-6, which regulate the intensity of inflammatory processes, in human monocytes and monocytic cell lines (Guha et al., 2000; Morohoshi et al., 1996; Shanmugam et al., 2003).

Monocytes and lymphocytes isolated from T2DM patients exhibit elevated levels of inflammatory mediators in their plasma, including the TNFα system, by expression study of TNFα, TNFR1, TNFR2, and increased cytokines such as IL-6 when compared with nondiabetic individuals. They also effectively reacted to LPS (Lipopolysaccharide) but did not respond to an acute glucose challenge (Chacón et al., 2007; MacEwan, 2002).

Patients with T2DM had higher leukocyte counts and increased expression of activation markers in neutrophils and monocytes when compared with nondiabetic individuals (Van Oostrom et al., 2004). In in vitro studies of T2DM, coronary heart disease, and healthy individuals, activation of circulating monocytes into M1 and M2 macrophages and elevated stimulation of TNF-α and proinflammatory cytokines were reported in diabetic patients in contrast to healthy individuals. TNF-α and HbA1c levels with recently diagnosed diabetes are directly correlated. It is also related to acute oxidative stress in hyperglycemia, as well as in obesity (Kraakman et al., 2014; Nikiforov et al., 2017).

3.3.2 Monocyte polarization in T2DM

Monocyte polarization is an indicator of innate immunity. An imbalance in the monocyte polarization, which enhances the percentage of proinflammatory M1 macrophage comparing it with the percentage of antiinflammatory M2 macrophages, causes chronic inflammation and metabolic dysfunction. The increased monocyte polarization in reaction to proinflammatory stimuli is activated by numerous transcription factors, which trigger pathways for immune and inflammatory responses. The emergence of hyperglycemia and hyperinsulinemia triggers oxidative stress and several inflammatory responses. The increased monocyte polarization when exposed to proinflammatory stimuli is activated by several transcription factors, especially NF-kB, which triggers pathways for immune and inflammatory responses. Oxidative stress is linked to hyperglycemia-induced overproduction of superoxide in mitochondria and NF-kB activation in the pathophysiology of T2DM (Brownlee, 2001; Fernández-Real & Ricart, 2003; Nikiforov et al., 2017; Nedosugova et al., 2022).

3.4 Macrophages

Innate immune cells called macrophages have a tendency to polarize from mononuclear macrophages or naive macrophages (Mφ) to multiple macrophage subtypes. A range of physiological functions, including metabolite and pathogen phagocytosis, antigen presentation, secreting chemokines, inflammatory or antiinflammatory cytokines, and growth factors, are significantly influenced by these immune cells. They significantly influenced pathogenesis for several diseases such as autoimmune and infectious diseases, T2DM and its associated complications, as well as progression of tumors (Sheng et al., 2015; Ye et al., 2025).

In humans, specialized Mφ can typically be categorized into tissue-resident Mφ, including microglial cells in the brain, resident intestinal Mφs, adipose tissue macrophages, and Kupffer cells in the liver. Naïve macrophages (Mφ) can polarize to M1 or M2 subtypes (including M2a, M2b, M2c and M2d) when exposed to various activators (Murray, 2020; Ruytinx et al., 2018; Wu & Hirschi, 2021).

Macrophages are generally classified into two subtypes:

(i) Proinflammatory M1 macrophages: When lipopolysaccharide (LPS) or cytokines such as IFN-γ and GM-CSF activate proinflammatory M1 macrophages, they release proinflammatory cytokines including tumor necrosis factor alpha (TNF-α), interleukin-1β (IL-1β), and IL-6, which are involved in the proinflammatory response (Funes et al., 2018; Shapouri-Moghaddam et al., 2018).

(ii) Antiinflammatory M2 macrophages: When cytokines such as IL-4 and IL-13 produced by TH2 (T-helper 2) cells polarize antiinflammatory M2 macrophages, they release cytokines such as TGF-β and IL-10 to suppress inflammation and repair of tissue (Funes et al., 2018; Shapouri-Moghaddam et al., 2018).

To maintain tissue homeostasis, macrophages are transported throughout the body and reside in different organs. It defends against pathogen invasion, inflammatory response, and repair of tissue (Epelman et al., 2014; Ye et al., 2025; Zhao et al., 2018). Adipocytes and immune cells, especially macrophages release proinflammatory molecules such as TNF-α, interleukin (IL)-1, -6, -8, -12, -23, and MCP-1 as well as adipokines as a result of adipocyte hypertrophy, hypoxia and increased cell death triggered by an increase in lipid accumulation, particularly triglycerides. This leads to more infiltration of circulating monocytes and immune cells into adipose tissue (Taylor, 2021).

3.4.1 Macrophage (M1 vs. M2) polarization

Macrophages are remarkably versatile and flexible as they change from one distinct functional phenotype to another. Macrophage polarization is triggered by the activation of several signaling cascades in reaction to environmental factors in different organs. GM-CSF (granulocyte macrophage colony stimulating factor) and M-CSF (macrophage colony stimulating factor) are two main hematopoietic growth factors that modulates the polarization of monocytes into macrophages. For example, monocytes from the bone marrow cells differentiate into macrophages with antigen-presenting capabilities when GM-CSF is present. Following stimulation, Mφ is activated to M1 macrophages to release proinflammatory responses and M2 macrophages to release antiinflammatory responses (Da Rocha et al., 2014; Hood, 2016; Yang et al., 2014).

3.4.2 M1 polarization

Naive macrophages (Mφ) are polarized to M1 macrophages activated by the lipopolysaccharide (LPS), cytokine interferon-γ (IFN-γ), and GM-CSF. LPS, GM-CSF, through the toll-like receptor (TLR) and IFN-γ regulate macrophage gene expression of cytokine receptors, cell activation, and cell adhesion, promoting M1 polarization. They release proinflammatory molecules such as interleukin IL-1, IL-6, IL-12, IL-23, and tumor necrosis factor (TNF)-α. During acute infections or malignancies, M1 macrophages are significant for the host's resistance against viruses and intracellular microorganisms and also participate in T-helper cell response to infection. However, they can be detrimental to host health and are occasionally linked to persistent inflammation (Lee, 2019; Martinez & Gordon, 2014).

3.4.3 M2 polarization

Naïve macrophages (Mφ) are polarized to M2 macrophages, such as M2a, M2b, M2c, and M2d. M2a polarization is linked to the immune response of T-helper 2 (Th2) cells, triggered by IL-4 and IL-13 or parasitic infections. The production of IL-4 by Th2 cells, macrophages, eosinophils, and basophils is crucial for parasite encapsulation. TLR or IL-1 receptor ligands jointly with immune processes activate M2b polarization, which in turn controls immunological responses. While IL-12 secretion is down-regulated, IL-10 secretion and antigen presentation of MHC II and CD86 are up-regulated. IL-10 and transforming growth factor (TGF)-β activate M2c polarization, which aids in tissue remodeling and the synthesis of extracellular matrix. Additionally, glucocorticoids affect M2c polarization, and adenosine with IL6 activates M2d polarization. These subtypes of M2 macrophages are also crucial in tissue repair despite their involvement in chronic infectious diseases (Lee, 2019; Mantovani et al., 2004; Martinez & Gordon, 2014; Rőszerv, 2015).

3.5 Macrophages in T2DM

Monocytes and macrophages, two essential immune cells, contribute to inflammation in T2DM and its associated complications (Blériot et al., 2023). Monocytes that have been recruited and stimulated by external stimuli differentiate into proinflammatory M1 macrophages, which leads to an imbalance between M1 and M2 macrophages due to increased infiltration of monocytes into the tissue and decreased antiinflammatory activity from M2 macrophages. This leads to increased adipokine and proinflammatory cytokine release, which in turn causes adipose tissue malfunction and reduction in glucose tolerance. T2DM, insulin resistance, and obesity are worsened by prolonged activation of proinflammatory pathways in insulin-sensitive tissues, including the pancreatic islets, liver, muscle, and adipose tissue (Kraakman et al., 2014; Nedosugova et al., 2022; Shoelson et al., 2006).

Proinflammatory cytokines released by macrophage infiltration into adipose tissue activate adipocyte serine kinases such as IKK, S6K, N-terminal c-Jun kinase (JNK), and mTOR and initiate IRS phosphorylation inhibition. The stimulation of inflammatory pathways is achieved by toll-like receptors, specifically TLR4. Research has suggested that in obesity higher levels of free fatty acids (FFA) may stimulate TLR4 signaling, hence contributing to insulin resistance related to obesity and T2DM. In T2DM, activation of inflammatory conditions followed by recruitment of monocytes, activation of macrophages and dendritic cells within the adipose and liver tissue induces the release of TNF-α, IL-6, and IL-1β, highlighting the critical role of monocytes, macrophages, dendritic cells, and other immune cells (Blériot et al., 2023; Ding et al., 2022; Nedosugova et al., 2022).

Insulin sensitivity, resistance, and signaling are mediated by tissue macrophages in response to environmental cues by modifying their functions. Insulin action is specifically linked to serine/threonine phosphorylation, which facilitates insulin receptor signaling. Moreover, proinflammatory cytokines such as TNF, IL-1, and IL-6 released by macrophages can inhibit phosphorylation. These cytokines trigger activation of serine kinases such as IKK (IkappaB kinase), JNK (c-Jun N-terminal kinase), S6K (ribosomal protein S6), and mTOR32 (mammalian target of rapamycin 32). This results in the inhibition of phosphorylation of insulin receptor substrate 1 (IRS1), which contributes to insulin resistance (Ding et al., 2022; Nedosugova et al., 2022).

The pathogenesis of T2DM and its associated complications are influenced by oxidative stress. Hyperglycemia contributes to oxidative stress caused by mitochondrial dysfunction and increased production of ROS (reactive oxygen species). It triggers glucose autoxidation and lowers antioxidant defense activity, resulting in an excess buildup of free radicals (Ding et al., 2022).

3.6 Macrophage polarization in T2DM

In T2DM, macrophage polarization of innate immunity is essential for metabolic inflammation. Modifications to the mononuclear macrophage (Mφ) system promote differentiation to M1 and M2 phenotypes, proinflammatory proliferation, and antiinflammatory recurrence. The increased production of M1 macrophages and down-regulation of M2 macrophages as a result of enhanced monocyte infiltration caused by environmental stressors, followed by elevated release of proinflammatory cytokines. Chronic inflammation is caused by an increased release of a mix of proinflammatory cytokines, including TNF (tumor necrosis factor) α and β, IL (interleukin) 1b, 2, 6, and 17, IFN (interferon) α and γ, and IgG in the bloodstream and glycometabolic tissues, pancreas, muscle, liver, and adipose tissue. This further disrupts metabolism, which leads to pancreatic β-cell dysfunction, glucose intolerance, and insulin resistance (Ding et al., 2022; Donath et al., 2019; Zeyda et al., 2007). M1 polarization of macrophages located in the islets leads to dedifferentiation of the islets and a reduction in glucose-stimulated insulin secretion (GSIS) function in addition to blocking insulin signaling pathways in adipose and liver (Ding et al., 2022).

3.7 Dendritic cells

Dendritic cells are crucial accessory immune cells of the innate and adaptive immunity system. They are specialized antigen-presenting cells (APCs) that stimulate B and T lymphocytes. Unlike other APCs, they have the capacity to activate both memory and naive T cells. Native antigen can be immediately recognized by B cells, which are the progenitors of antibody-secreting cells, through their B-cell receptors. However, an APC is required to digest and present the antigen to T cells, which proceed to the initial injury site to kill viral-infected or tumor cells (Banchereau & Steinman, 1998; Bell et al., 1999; Cabeza-Cabrerizo et al., 2021; Liu & Nussenzweig, 2010).

When MDPs (monocyte and dendritic cell progenitor) differentiate into monocytes and committed DC progenitors (CDPs) in the bone marrow, CDPs trigger migration of predendritic cells (pre-DCs) from the bone marrow to lymphoid and nonlymphoid tissue to generate the two main subgroups of DCs in lymphoid tissue and nonlymphoid tissue (Sato & Fujita, 2007).

Dendritic cells play a crucial role in regulating immunological tolerance, modulating T cell immune responses, and monitoring innate immunity against pathogens. The variability of subtypes and their adaptability in function are crucial for immune regulation. They are part of APC (Antigen-presenting cells) that fragment and present the antigen to T cells. The MHC (major histocompatibility complex) molecules on an APC's surface are attached to antigen fragments that are recognized by TCRs (T-cell antigen receptors). There are two types of peptide-binding proteins: MHC class I, which activates cytotoxic ($CD8^+$) T cells, and MHC class II, which stimulates helper ($CD4^+$) T cells. In the cytosol of the APC, intracellular antigens are broken down into peptides attached to

MHC class I molecules that are identified by cytotoxic T cells, resulting in the ability to destroy a target cell directly once they are activated. After entering the APC endocytic pathway, extracellular antigens are processed and presented to T-helper cells through MHC class II molecules. These cells have significant immune-regulatory effects when activated (Banchereau & Steinman, 1998; Sato & Fujita, 2007).

The extracellular environment, activation signals, receptors, and signaling pathways regulate the initiation of dendritic cells and the generation of proinflammatory cytokines. TNF-α, glucocorticoids, estrogens, bacterial infections, and metabolic control are key factors that affect its function (Kohrgruber et al., 1999; Paharkova-Vatchkova et al., 2004; Piemonti et al., 1999; Seifarth et al., 2008; Serbina et al., 2003).

3.7.1 Dendritic cells in T2DM

In T2DM, innate immune system initiation and chronic low-grade inflammation are linked with its etiology and implications (Pickup, 2004). It is influenced by dendritic cells, which monitor immune cells such as T cells and initiate, coordinate, and regulate immunological responses in T2DM (Banchereau & Steinman, 1998). Patients with T2DM have been reported to have lower circulating dendritic cells in their blood (Seifarth et al., 2008).

When damaged, dying, or infected cells secrete transmit signals, dendritic cells become activated (Matzinger, 1994). For instance, T2DM patients reported having increased levels of circulating soluble CD40L (sCD40L) released from activated T lymphocytes and platelets (Varo et al., 2003, 2005). It is reported that the ligation of the CD40 surface receptors to its ligand CD40L on dendritic cells activates the secretion of proinflammatory cytokines such as TNF-α (Blüml et al., 2005).

Insulin resistance and inflammation are independently influenced by dendritic cells. In visceral adipose tissue, conventional dendritic cells (cDCs) promote immune tolerance by adipocyte-related pathway upregulation. DCs stimulate the production of IL-10 by Wnt/β-catenin pathway activation in cDC1 (conventional type 1 dendritic cells), which stimulates antiinflammatory responses and regulates immune responses. When the pathway of PPARγ is upregulated in cDC2 (conventional type 2 dendritic cells), DCs suppress T cell activation and immunity. Prolonged overnutrition changes adipocyte biology, resulting in PPARγ activation that contributes to chronic low-grade inflammation, which in turn develops insulin resistance. Chronic inflammation is defined by an increased accumulation of immune cells, particularly T lymphocytes and macrophages, in adipose tissue (Macdougall et al., 2018; Murdolo & Smith, 2006).

Diabetes and other inflammatory illnesses are influenced by dendritic cells (DCs). cDC (conventional dendritic cells) may impede these complications by promoting an antiinflammatory response. Dendritic cells are necessary for the recruitment and activation of macrophages, the T cell immune response, and the promotion of immune tolerance. In T2DM, glucose intolerance is influenced by abnormal adipocyte metabolism and altered adipose tissue topography, which results in a decline in the secretion of insulin-sensitizing adipocytokines, such as adiponectin. It also increases the secretion of cytokines such as TNF and ILs, which causes inflammation and insulin resistance. Thus, dendritic cell subsets and adipocytes interact to regulate immunological homeostasis (Hunter & Garvey, 1998; Murdolo & Smith, 2006; Stefanovic et al., 2012).

3.8 Innate lymphoid cells (ILCs)

Innate lymphoid cells (ILCs) are innate immune cells originating from lymphoid lineages. They are essential in regulating tissue immunity and homeostasis, which act as crucial bridges connecting the innate and adaptive immune systems. During the embryonic stages, the progenitors of resident ILCs disperse into peripheral organs. In the adult stage, they originate from progenitors in the bone marrow, including hematopoietic stem cells. The regulatory and effector functions of tissue-resident ILCs respond dynamically to local environmental signals, tissue damage, and infections, thereby modulating the immune response. ILCs lack Ag-specific receptors; hence, they show no antigen specificity, but are highly responsive to environmental and cytokine signals. Notch signaling, IL-7, and IL-33 are essential for ILC2 development. GATA-3 regulates their differentiation and maintenance. Its differentiation is also regulated by the RORα transcription factor (Gasteiger et al., 2015; Nouari & Aribi, 2025; Vivier et al., 2018).

ILCs are generally divided into three subtypes such as:

(i) ILC1: They contribute to antiviral and anticancer immunity by producing type 1 cytokines, mainly tumor necrosis factor (TNF) and IFN-γ, such as $CD4^+$ T helper 1 (Th1) cells.

(ii) ILC2: They are essential in allergic inflammation, type 2 immune response, and tissue repair by producing IL-4,IL-5,IL-9, and IL-13, such as $CD4^+$ T helper 2 (Th2) cells.

(iii) ILC3: They are crucial for gut homeostasis, mucosal immunity, chronic inflammation, and tissue repair by producing IL-17A, IL-17F, IL-22, granulocyte macrophage colony-stimulating factor (GM-CSF), and TNF-like $CD4^+$ T helper 17 (Th17) cells (Artis & Spits, 2015; Vivier et al., 2018; Willinger, 2019).

ILCs and other immune cells play a crucial role in nutrient sensing, metabolic regulation, and the onset of diseases. Alarmins specifically thymic stromal lymphopoietin (TSLP), interleukin (IL)-25, and IL-33 are released by skin and mucosal epithelial cells in reaction to allergens, pathogenic agents, and environmentally toxic compounds. These cytokines stimulate ILC2s and Th2 cells to secrete type 2 cytokines, such as IL-4, IL-5, IL-9, IL-13, and IL-31, thereby stimulating a type 2 immune response (Akdis et al., 2020; Zhang et al., 2025).

3.8.1 Innate lymphoid cells (ILCs) in T2DM

Innate lymphoid cells (ILCs) are crucial innate immune effectors by rapidly producing proinflammatory and regulatory cytokines. The imbalance in the ratio of proinflammatory and antiinflammatory cytokine levels causes chronic, low-grade inflammation, a significant characteristic of T2DM. Inflammation and insulin resistance worsen when innate and adaptive immunity are disrupted in adipose tissue (Artis & Spits, 2015; Asghar & Sheikh, 2017; Ouchi et al., 2011).

Systemic inflammation-related diseases are regulated by ILC1s. In adipose tissues of mice, ILC1s accumulation is linked to systemic insulin resistance and local inflammation. When Rag2−/− Mice, which lack T, B, and NKT cells, were transfected with purified ILC1s from the adipose tissue of HFD (high-fat diet) wild-type mice, they showed glucose intolerance, high levels of fasting blood insulin, and impaired insulin sensitivity (O'Sullivan et al., 2016). In a study that included NGT (normal glucose tolerance) subjects and T2DM patients reported that T2DM patients had significantly higher levels of both circulating and adipose ILC1s. These levels were significantly linked to glycemic irregularities and were also positively correlated with HbA1c and FPG. These patients also reported elevated levels of FFA, Adipo-IR, and HOMA-IR, which correlated with circulating ILC1 levels (Liu et al., 2019).

In metabolic diseases such as T2DM and allergy responses, the role of ILC2s and their protective effects on tissue homeostasis play a crucial role in their pathophysiology. These cells regulate inflammation in adipose tissue and interact with resident cell types, which are influenced by metabolic environment and energy supply (Painter & Akbari, 2021). In T2DM, they reduce detrimental inflammation by producing type 2 cytokines, including IL-5 and IL-13, which in turn trigger eosinophils to produce IL-4, thereby improving glucose homeostasis and inducing macrophages to differentiate into M2 antiinflammatory phenotypes (Molofsky et al., 2013). Insulin resistance and the onset of type 2 diabetes mellitus (T2DM) are facilitated by the accumulation of inflammatory immune cells associated with chronic obesity. ILC2s, which stimulate type 2 or allergic immunity, defend against metabolic dysfunction induced by obesity and T2DM by stimulation of tissue homeostasis, AT browning, and systemic insulin sensitivity (Cautivo & Molofsky, 2016).

4. Adaptive immune cells

4.1 B lymphocyte

B lymphocytes consist of 7% of the circulating leukocytes and are formed in the bone marrow ((Leichner and Kambayashi, 2014)). Upon maturation, B lymphocytes or B cells leave the bone marrow and, on their membrane, express a unique antigen-binding receptor. Mature B cells have functional surface receptors such as sIgs (IgM, IgG, IgA, IgE, and IgD) and MHC complex proteins. An individual B cell has one distinct sIg receptor. Thus, upon activation, individual cell and their lineage create immunoglobulin molecules with a unique specificity and affinity for their antigenic determinant (Lawrence, 2010).

The progression of insulin resistance is markedly influenced by B cells. It produces IgG antibodies, which in turn lead to the stimulation of macrophages and T lymphocytes. It has been found that there is no considerable difference in the number of B cells in peripheral blood mononuclear cells between healthy individuals and those with T2DM or obese individuals. The findings by Beek et al. triggered a controversy, stating that the number of activated CD38 markers on circulating B cells was found to be elevated in obese patients unaffected by T2DM in comparison to obese patients affected with T2DM. DeFuria et al. contended that a high dietary fat intake can lead to a detectable elevation of the B-cell proliferation in visceral adipose tissue (VAT). It was also noted that the decrease in $CD19^+$ cells affects the proliferation of Th17 cells in individuals with T2DM. B cells also alter the proliferation of cytokines in T2DM individuals as compared with healthy individuals. It was observed that both obese and nonobese T2DM individuals exhibit a higher degree of fecal IgG, produced by B-cells, as compared with individuals with similar body mass index (BMI). Additionally, high-fat diets (HFD) lead to an increased proliferation of B cells in visceral adipose tissue (VAT), potentially driven by DNA methylation in obesity and T2DM (Zhou et al., 2018).

Experimental studies in mouse models have shown that those lacking mature B cells had lowered fasting glucose levels and also an improvement in glucose tolerance as compared with wild type (WT) when both the groups were fed with HFD for 8 weeks (Zhou et al., 2018).

Chronic hyperglycemia in T2DM leads to nonenzymatic glycation, resulting in the formation of covalent sugar adducts with proteins. These not only result in structural changes but also affect the function of the antibodies, impairing the humoral immune system in different ways. It has been established that using MALDI mass spectrometry, it is possible to identify the structural difference that occurs in immunoglobulins.

T2DM patients are found to have higher immunoglobulin molecular masses as compared with healthy individuals, resulting in lower vaccine efficacy for antibody secretion in the patients. Studies in mouse models and T2DM patients have highlighted that a defect in antibody production and class switching results in lower levels of total and infection-specific IgG production, despite having increased IgM levels. Although IgM is present in elevated levels, it is unable to prevent infection as it cannot perform phagocytosis directly, which exacerbates the infection (Saadh et al., 2025).

Memory cells, a subgroup of B-cells, produce IgM at the initial stage of infection and prevent the microorganism's growth. In T2DM patients, an increased infection of *Staphylococcus aureus* is presumed to be due to impaired B-cell antibacterial immune response. Similarly, T2DM patients have lower levels of infection-blocking antibodies against *Streptococcus pneumoniae* and also a lowered complement system activation, which can hinder the phagocytosis of the bacteria (Saadh et al., 2025).

Overall, these findings highlight the complex interplay between B cell dysfunction, metabolic disturbances, and immune alterations in T2DM, which collectively contribute to increased infection risks and poor immune responses in affected individuals.

4.2 T lymphocytes

T lymphocytes, also known as T cells, constitute approximately 20% of the peripheral blood leukocytes (Leichner & Kambayashi, 2014). These cells originate in bone marrow from the hematopoietic stem cells. The immature cells from the bone marrow migrate to the thymus, where they undergo maturation. Antigen-binding receptors are formed on the membrane of the T cells, also known as T cell receptors (TCR). Each T cells exhibit a distinct TCR, which is antigen-specific. On receiving a signal, it activates and can proliferate and differentiate. However, for the recognition of the specific antigen, T cells require the assistance of antigen-presenting cells (APCs). APCs have groups of proteins attached to their surface called the major histocompatibility complex (MHC). The TCRs are activated by the binding to MHC-antigen, and the T-cell releases cytokines, which further regulate the immune system. T cells are further stimulated by this antigen presentation pathway to differentiate into T-helper cells ($CD4^+$) and cytotoxic T cells ($CD8^+$) (Marshall et al., 2018).

These cells contribute significantly to T2DM progression. Studies have demonstrated that in T2DM patients, the function of the T cells is impaired. The effector T cells' growth depends on carefully regulated processes that control the synthesis of certain cytokine profiles. However, in people with T2DM, these mechanisms are disrupted, resulting in abnormal T cell differentiation and cytokine production abnormalities. In obese individuals with diabetes compared with nonobese individuals,Th17 cells, $CD4^+$ CD278+ T Helper Cells, and cytotoxic T-cells are activated, and their levels are elevated.

4.2.1 T helper cells

In the past few years, it was detected that $CD4^+$ T cells play a significant role in the pathology of T2DM. In individuals with T2DM, the T-cells differentiate abnormally (Zhou et al., 2018). Based on functions and the types of cytokines secreted, the differentiated $CD4^+$ cells are subdivided into antiinflammatory Th2 cells, Foxp3+ regulatory T cells, also known as Treg, and proinflammatory Th1 and Th17 cells. Th1 cells, on activation, produce proinflammatory tumor necrosis factor β (TNF-β), interferon-γ (IFN-γ), and interleukin-2 (IL-2), and trigger cellular immunity and phagocytosis-mediated inflammation. On the other hand, to control antibody-mediated responses, Th2 cells produce interleukin 4, 5,6, 9, 10, and 13 (IL-4, IL-5, IL-6, IL-9, IL-10, and IL-13) (Xia et al., 2017; Zhou et al., 2018). It was reported that though Th1 and Th2 cells are activated later than the macrophages, they play a key role in regulating inflammatory processes (Xia et al., 2017).

In patients with prediabetes or T2DM, $CD4^+$ T cells preferentially differentiate to proinflammatory Th1 and Th17 cells in the circulating blood and adipocytes; however, a reduction in differentiation of antiinflammatory Th2 was observed. The Th1 and Th2 ratio and cytokine secretion levels were reported to be high, whereas the nuclear factor erythroid 2-related factor (Nrf2) and its subsequent targets, which help in antioxidant protection, maintaining the oxidative balance, and mitochondrial health, are decreased.

It was reported that in the pathophysiology of obesity induced insulin resistance, elevated levels of cytokines such as TNF-α, IL-17, IFN-γ, and T lymphocytes exist (Zhou et al., 2018). Patients with T2DM were shown to have a disproportion of the $CD4^+$ T helper cell subgroups, and on the other hand, it was also noted that naïve $CD4^+$ T cells decrease, which can be linked to persisting inflammation and activation of the adaptive immune system during the disease pathophysiology (Xia et al., 2017).

$CD4^+$ helper T cells have a crucial role to play in T2DM complications. The inflammatory cytokines and activated T lymphocytes are increased in the kidneys of T2DM patients. Diabetes has also been linked with delayed and impaired Th2 cell-mediated immunity. Studies conducted have also found that cytokines associated with Th1 trigger a hyperinflammatory response, which indeed results in the progression of the innate immunity. Studies have shown that T2DM patients have elevated levels of circulating cytokines associated with Th1 in their blood. The increased levels of T-cell-related cytokines, including IL-10 and IL-17, were found, which proves the participation of T-cells in T2DM. Similarly, it was demonstrated that oral administration of anti-CD3 plus glucosylceramide (an NKT cell target antigen) increased IL-10 and TGF-β production, which was linked to improved glucose levels in the fasting state, reduced inflammation of visceral adipose tissue, decreased liver enzyme levels, and hepatic steatosis in ob/ob mice. The observations mentioned above indicate that resistance to insulin and chronic inflammation in T2DM are closely related to the $CD4^+$ subset Th1 and Th2 (Xia et al., 2017).

4.2.2 Th17 cells

The Th17 subset of $CD4^+$ T cells, which secretes IL-17, has always been associated with T2DM. A recent study analyzed the cytokine production by peripheral blood mononuclear cells (PBMCs) to investigate the differentiation of several $CD4^+$ effector subsets in T2DM. According to the results, Th17 cells were higher in the patients with T2DM, which may be related to abnormal lipid metabolism (Garidou et al., 2015). It has also been found that IL-17 may trigger the synthesis of TNF-α, the first cytokine implicated with insulin resistance and obesity. According to reports, intestinal Th17 cells might release AMPs, particularly RegB3b and Reg3g, which would increase intestinal permeability in animals fed with a high-fat diet. Th17 has been linked to an increase in diabetes complications, including nephropathy. Th17 cells play a crucial role in the development of problems associated with T2DM. Diabetes patients, as compared with normal individuals, have higher levels of Th17 cells and a higher Th17/Treg ratio. Adipose tissue (AT)- derived dendritic cells (DCs) obtained from obese individuals and animals were found to promote Th17 cell differentiation in vitro. However, the relation between DCs and Th17 cells has yet to be observed in AT from lean or obese mice. It's unclear whether CD103 DCs can control obesity-associated inflammation in AT by balancing Th17 cell and Treg cell development in vivo. Th17 is responsible for producing IL-22, which comes after IL-6 and IL-23. AT microphages express the IL-22 receptor (IL-22R) and respond to IL-22 by secreting additional IL-1β, which promotes AT inflammation. It is fascinating to see if the metabolic effects related to IL-22 in mice can be applied to people. IL-17 and IL-22 levels suggest that Th17 can play both "protective" and "destructive" roles in T2DM progression (Xia et al., 2017).

4.2.3 Regulatory T cells/treg cells

Regulatory T-cells or Treg cells are a subset of $CD4^+$ cells constituting 5%–20% of T-lymphocytes (Xia et al., 2017; Zhou et al., 2018). The expression of CD4, CD25, and Foxp3, a forkhead family transcription factor, characterizes Treg cells. Treg cells suppress the effector T cells'response by restricting inflammation and impeding autoimmunity. Their immunoregulator functions are mediated through various pathways, including suppressing the responses of the effector T cells by inhibiting the T cell receptor-activated proliferation, secreting antiinflammatory cytokines such as IL-10 and TGF-β, expressing a coinhibitory molecule CTLA-4, inducing transcription factors linked with suppressed $CD4^+$ T cells, and the capacity to translocate glycolytic pathway activation.

In the T2DM condition, Treg cells improve insulin resistance by suppressing the Th1, Th2, and Th17 responses (Xia et al., 2017). To retain the host immune response and to regulate inflammatory damage, it is crucial to maintain an appropriate balance between Treg cells and proinflammatory Th17 or Th1 subsets of T cells. It was found that in patients with T2DM, the percentage of Treg cells decreases, along with a drop in the Treg/Th1 and Treg/Th17 ratios. Additional research indicates that peripherally induced Treg, unlike naturally occurring Treg generated in the thymus, are lowered in T2DM, maybe as a result of low HDL levels and decreased bcl2/bax (Xia et al., 2017). In a nutritionally induced obesity model, elevated insulin levels hindered Tregs' capacity to inhibit inflammatory reactions through the AKT/mTOR signaling cascade, resulting in decreased IL-10 expression and decreased efficiency in suppressing TNF-α production. Moreover, an even lower fraction of Treg cells was seen in obese individuals with type 2 diabetes (Zhou et al., 2018).

Th17 cells are suppressed by $CD39^+$ Treg cells, which are thought to be less prevalent in obese T2DM patients. Additionally, there is a strong association between hyperglycemia and HbA1c expression levels and $CD4^+$ IL-17+ cell levels in T2DM patients with obesity or overweight status (Zhou et al., 2018).

4.2.4 $CD8^+$ cytotoxic cell

The $CD8^+$ cell response is crucial for the adaptive immune system against infections, as it helps in secreting TNFα and IFN-γ cytokines. From research, it has been established that $CD8^+$ cells are present in inflamed tissues and express and synthesize the proinflammatory cytokine IL-17 (Srenathan et al., 2016; Zhou et al., 2018). Studies have found that the accumulation of this cell leads to inflammation and, further, results in insulin resistance (Nishimura et al., 2009; Zhou et al., 2018). $CD8^+$ cells were found to be crucial for the initiation of macrophage migration and activation to adipose tissue (Xia et al., 2017).

Some clinical studies have also reported that the level of $CD8^+$ cells was found to be elevated in patients with T2DM or a mouse model with obesity; however, it was also observed that after 120 min of glucose administration, the ratio of $CD8^+$ cells decreases

(Miya et al., 2018; Zhou et al., 2018). The level of INF-γ cytokines that $CD8^+$ cells secrete was increased in obese individuals as compared with lean individuals. Scientific studies have also reported that the $CD8^+$ cells were found to be higher in the colon and small bowel of some of the obese individuals as compared with a healthy individual (Luck et al., 2015; Xia et al., 2017).

4.3 NKT cells

NKT cells are a diverse type of immune cells that have properties similar to both T lymphocytes and natural killer cells (Lv et al., 2018). They can recognize glycolipids expressed by the CD1d protein, which is presented on the membrane of dendritic cells (DCs) and antigen-presenting cells (APCs). CD1d belongs to the monomorphic MHC class I-like molecule (Tard et al., 2015). NKT cells on their surface can express both NK cell inhibiting as well as NK cell activating receptors (Lv et al., 2018). NKT cells are categorized into three subsets based on their expression of the T cell receptor (TCR) and antigen specificity: NKT-like lymphocytes, iNKT, and type II NKT (Zhou et al., 2018). Surface receptors of NKT cells, such as the NKG2D, NKG2A, NKp44, NKp30, and 158b, are controlled by their specific ligands. When the expression of these receptors is upregulated, the NKT cells are activated and secrete granzyme B and perforin, which kill the targeted cells. NKT cells can also be activated through TCR binding to the ligand, leading to the production of many cytokines, IL-7, IFN-γ, and IL-4, which participate in the subsequent immune reaction and regulate theTh1/Th2 polarization (Lv et al., 2018).

It has been found that the immune cells in diabetic patients exhibit functional abnormalities, including the abnormal activation of NK cells, an imbalance in the ratio of Th1 to Th2 cells, and a role for macrophages in vascular remodeling. Nevertheless, the processes and the role of NKT cells associated with the etiology of diabetes are still unclear. A study by Lv et al. (2018) reported that in type 2 diabetes patients, the ratio of $CD3^+CD56^+$ and $CD3^-CD56^+$ NKT cells in peripheral blood increases significantly. They also found that the expression levels of NKp30, NKG2D, and NKp44 on the surface of NKT cells were significantly upregulated, whereas the NKG2A and 158b expression levels were downregulated. It was also reported that $CD4^+$ and $CD4^-CD8^-$subtypes, as well as $CD8^+$ subtypes, significantly increase in the blood of diabetic patients, and increase the production of cytokines INF-γ and IL-4 (Lv et al., 2018).

5. Conclusion

Immune cells play a significant role in the pathophysiology and development of Type 2 Diabetes Mellitus (T2DM), underscoring the intricate connection between metabolic abnormality and immune dysregulation. Defects in both innate immunity, including impaired neutrophil and macrophage function, and adaptive immunity, characterized by B and T cell imbalances, contribute to chronic inflammation, insulin resistance, and increased susceptibility to infections in individuals with diabetes. Understanding the mechanisms through which hyperglycemia disrupts immune homeostasis is essential for developing innovative therapeutic approaches. Targeting immune cell dysfunction and associated inflammatory pathways offers the potential to mitigate metabolic disturbances, enhance host defense against infections, and improve clinical outcomes in T2DM. Future research focusing on the interplay between immune cells and metabolic regulation could pave the way for personalized immunotherapies that address the systemic complications of diabetes and improve the health status of individuals affected by the condition.

Abbreviations

AGEs Advanced Glycation End products
APCs Antigen-presenting cells
cDC Conventional dendritic cells
CDPs Committed DC progenitors
CVD Cardiovascular disease
DCM Diabetic cardiomyopathy
FFA Free fatty acids
GM-CSF Granulocyte macrophage colony-stimulating factor
GSIS Glucose-stimulated insulin secretion
HFD High-fat diet
HOCl Hypochlorous acid
IFN Interferon
IL Interleukin
ILCs Innate lymphoid cells
IRS1 Insulin receptor substrate 1
JNK N-terminal c-Jun kinase
LPS Lipopolysaccharide
MDPs Monocyte and dendritic cell progenitor
MHC Major histocompatibility complex
MPO Myeloperoxidase
MPS Mononuclear phagocyte system
NETs Neutrophil extracellular traps
NK Natural killer cells
PAD4 Peptidyl arginine deiminase 4
PAMPs Pathogen-associated molecular patterns
PRRs Pattern recognition receptors
ROS Reactive oxygen species
S6K Ribosomal protein S6
SCFAs Short-chain fatty acids
T2DM Type 2 Diabetes mellitus
TCRs T-cell antigen receptors
TGF Transforming growth factor
TLR Toll-like receptor
TNF Tumor necrosis factor
VAT Visceral adipose tissue

References

Akdis, C. A., Arkwright, P. D., Brüggen, M. C., et al. (2020). Type 2 immunity in the skin and lungs. *Allergy, 75*(7), 1582–1605.

Antar, S. A., Ashour, N. A., Sharaky, M., Khattab, M., et al. (2023). Diabetes mellitus: Classification, mediators, and complications; A gate to identify potential targets for the development of new effective treatments. *Biomedicine & Pharmacotherapy = Biomedecine&pharmacotherapie, 168,* Article 115734.

Artis, D., & Spits, H. (2015). The biology of innate lymphoid cells. *Nature, 517*(7534), 293–301.

Asghar, A., & Sheikh, N. (2017). Role of immune cells in obesity induced low grade inflammation and insulin resistance. *Cellular Immunology, 315,* 18–26.

Bajpai, A., & Tilley, D. G. (2018). The role of leukocytes in diabetic cardiomyopathy. *Frontiers in Physiology, 9,* 1547.

Banchereau, J., & Steinman, R. M. (1998). Dendritic cells and the control of immunity. *Nature, 392*(6673), 245–252.

Bell, D., Young, J. W., & Banchereau, J. (1999). Dendritic cells. *Advances in Immunology, 72,* 255–324.

Berbudi, A., Rahmadika, N., Tjahjadi, A. I., et al. (2020). Type 2 diabetes and its impact on the immune system. *Current Diabetes Reviews, 16*(5), 442–449.

Berrou, J., Fougeray, S., Venot, M., Chardiny, V., Gautier, J. F., Dulphy, N., Toubert, A., & Peraldi, M. N. (2013). Natural killer cell function, an important target for infection and tumor protection, is impaired in type 2 diabetes. *PloS One, 8*(4), Article e62418.

Blériot, C., Dalmas, É., Ginhoux, F., et al. (2023). Inflammatory and immune etiology of type 2 diabetes. *Trends in Immunology, 44*(2), 101–109.

Blüml, S., Kirchberger, S., Bochkov, V. N., et al. (2005). Oxidized phospholipids negatively regulate dendritic cell maturation induced by TLRs and CD40. *Journal of Immunology, 175*(1), 501–508.

Borregaard, N. (2010). Neutrophils, from marrow to microbes. *Immunity, 33*(5), 657–670.

Brownlee, M. (2001). Biochemistry and molecular cell biology of diabetic complications. *Nature, 414* (6865), 813–820.

Cabeza-Cabrerizo, M., Cardoso, A., Minutti, C. M., et al. (2021). Dendritic cells revisited. *Annual Review of Immunology, 39*(1), 131–166.

Cautivo, K. M., & Molofsky, A. B. (2016). Regulation of metabolic health and adipose tissue function by group 2 innate lymphoid cells. *European Journal of Immunology, 46*(6), 1315–1325.

Chacón, M. R., Vendrell, J., Miranda, M., et al. (2007). Different TNFα expression elicited by glucose in monocytes from type 2 diabetes mellitus patients. *Atherosclerosis, 194*(2), e18–e25.

Chaplin, D. D. (2010). Overview of the immune response. *Journal of Allergy and Clinical Immunology, 125*(2), S3–S23.

Da Rocha, R. F., De Bastiani, M. A., & Klamt, F. (2014). Bioinformatics approach to evaluate differential gene expression of M1/M2 macrophage phenotypes and antioxidant genes in atherosclerosis. *Cell Biochemistry and Biophysics, 70,* 831–839.

Daryabor, G., Atashzar, M. R., Kabelitz, D., Meri, et al. (2020). The effects of type 2 diabetes mellitus on organ metabolism and the immune system. *Frontiers in Immunology, 11,* 1582.

Ding, Q., Gao, Z., Chen, K., et al. (2022). Inflammation-related epigenetic modification: The bridge between immune and metabolism in type 2 diabetes. *Frontiers in Immunology, 13,* Article 883410.

Donath, M. Y., Dinarello, C. A., & Mandrup-Poulsen, T. (2019). Targeting innate immune mediators in type 1 and type 2 diabetes. *Nature Reviews Immunology, 19*(12), 734–746.

Donath, M. Y., & Shoelson, S. E. (2011). Type 2 diabetes as an inflammatory disease. *Nature Reviews Immunology, 11*(2), 98–107.

Epelman, S., Lavine, K. J., & Randolph, G. J. (2014). Origin and functions of tissue macrophages. *Immunity, 41*(1), 21–35.

Fernández-Real, J. M., & Ricart, W. (2003). Insulin resistance and chronic cardiovascular inflammatory syndrome. *Endocrine Reviews, 24*(3), 278–301.

Funes, S. C., Rios, M., Escobar-Vera, J., et al. (2018). Implications of macrophage polarization in autoimmunity. *Immunology, 154*(2), 186–195.

Garidou, L., Pomié, C., Klopp, P., et al. (2015). The gut microbiota regulates intestinal CD4 T cells expressing RORγt and controls metabolic disease. *Cell Metabolism, 22*(1), 100–112.

Gasteiger, G., Fan, X., Dikiy, S., et al. (2015). Tissue residency of innate lymphoid cells in lymphoid and nonlymphoid organs. *Science, 350*(6263), 981–985.

Guha, M., Bai, W., Nadler, J. L., et al. (2000). Molecular mechanisms of tumor necrosis factor α gene expression in monocytic cells via hyperglycemia-induced oxidant stress-dependent and-independent pathways. *Journal of Biological Chemistry, 275*(23), 17728–17739.

Guilliams, M., Ginhoux, F., Jakubzick, C., et al. (2014). Dendritic cells, monocytes and macrophages: A unified nomenclature based on ontogeny. *Nature Reviews Immunology, 14*(8), 571–578.

Guilliams, M., Mildner, A., & Yona, S. (2018). Developmental and functional heterogeneity of monocytes. *Immunity, 49*(4), 595–613.

Hood, J. L. (2016). Melanoma exosome induction of endothelial cell GM-CSF in pre-metastatic lymph nodes may result in different M1 and M2 macrophage mediated angiogenic processes. *Medical Hypotheses, 94*, 118–122.

Hunter, S. J., & Garvey, W. T. (1998). Insulin action and insulin resistance: Diseases involving defects in insulin receptors, signal transduction, and the glucose transport effector system 1. *The American Journal of Medicine, 105*(4), 331–345.

Keeter, W. C., Moriarty, A. K., & Galkina, E. V. (2021). Role of neutrophils in type 2 diabetes and associated atherosclerosis. *The International Journal of Biochemistry & Cell Biology, 141*, Article 106098.

Kohrgruber, N., Halanek, N., Gröger, M., et al. (1999). Survival, maturation, and function of CD11c− and CD11c+ peripheral blood dendritic cells are differentially regulated by cytokines. *The Journal of Immunology, 163*(6), 3250–3259.

Kolb, H., & Mandrup-Poulsen, T. (2005). An immune origin of type 2 diabetes? *Diabetologia, 48*, 1038–1050.

Kraakman, M. J., Murphy, A. J., Jandeleit-Dahm, K., et al. (2014). Macrophage polarization in obesity and type 2 diabetes: Weighing down our understanding of macrophage function? *Frontiers in Immunology, 5*, 470.

Kuwabara, W. M. T., Yokota, C. N. F., Curi, R., & Alba-Loureiro, T. C. (2018). Obesity and type 2 diabetes mellitus induce lipopolysaccharide tolerance in rat neutrophils. *Scientific Reports, 8*(1), 17534.

Lawrence, D. A. (2010). Overview of the immune system and immunotoxicology. In *Comprehensive toxicology* (Vol. 5, pp. 1–34). Elsevier.

Lee, K. Y. (2019). M1 and M2 polarization of macrophages: A mini-review. *Medical Biological Science and Engineering, 2*(1), 1–5.

Leichner, T., & Kambayashi, T. (2014). White blood cells and lymphoid tissue. In *Encyclopedia of the human brain*. Elsevier Inc.

Lin, J. C., Siu, L. K., Fung, C. P., Tsou, H. H., Wang, J. J., Chen, C. T., Wang, S. C., & Chang, F. Y. (2006). Impaired phagocytosis of capsular serotypes K1 or K2 Klebsiella pneumoniae in type 2 diabetes mellitus patients with poor glycemic control. *The Journal of Clinical Endocrinology and Metabolism, 91*(8), 3084–3087.

Liu, K., & Nussenzweig, M. C. (2010). Origin and development of dendritic cells. *Immunological Reviews, 234*(1), 45–54.

Liu, F., Wang, H., Feng, W., et al. (2019). Type 1 innate lymphoid cells are associated with type 2 diabetes. *Diabetes & Metabolism, 45*(4), 341–346.

Luck, H., Tsai, S., Chung, J., et al. (2015). Regulation of obesity-related insulin resistance with gut anti-inflammatory agents. *Cell Metabolism, 21*(4), 527–542.

Lv, X., Gao, Y., Dong, T., & Yang, L. (2018). Role of natural killer T (NKT) cells in type II diabetes-induced vascular injuries. *Medical Science Monitor: International Medical Journal of Experimental and Clinical Research, 24*, 8322.

Macdougall, C. E., Wood, E. G., Loschko, J., et al. (2018). Visceral adipose tissue immune homeostasis is regulated by the crosstalk between adipocytes and dendritic cell subsets. *Cell Metabolism, 27*(3), 588–601.

MacEwan, D. J. (2002). TNF receptor subtype signalling: Differences and cellular consequences. *Cellular Signalling, 14*(6), 477–492.

Mantovani, A., Sica, A., Sozzani, S., Allavena, P., Vecchi, A., & Locati, M. (2004). The chemokine system in diverse forms of macrophage activation and polarization. *Trends in Immunology, 25*(12), 677–686.

Marshall, J. S., Warrington, R., Watson, W., et al. (2018). An introduction to immunology and immunopathology. *Allergy, Asthma and Clinical Immunology: Official Journal of the Canadian Society of Allergy and Clinical Immunology, 14*(Suppl. 2), 49.

Martinez, F. O., & Gordon, S. (2014). The M1 and M2 paradigm of macrophage activation: Time for reassessment. *F1000Prime Reports, 6*, 13.

Matzinger, P. (1994). Tolerance, danger, and the extended family. *Annual Review of Immunology, 12*(1), 991–1045.

Miya, A., Nakamura, A., Miyoshi, H., et al. (2018). Impact of glucose loading on variations in CD4+ and CD8+ T cells in Japanese participants with or without type 2 diabetes. *Frontiers in Endocrinology, 9*, 81.

Molofsky, A. B., Nussbaum, J. C., Liang, H. E., et al. (2013). Innate lymphoid type 2 cells sustain visceral adipose tissue eosinophils and alternatively activated macrophages. *Journal of Experimental Medicine, 210*(3), 535–549.

Morohoshi, M., Fujisawa, K., Uchimuraa, I., et al. (1996). Glucose-dependent interleukin 6 and tumor necrosis factor production by human peripheral blood monocytes in vitro. *Diabetes, 45*(7), 954–959.

Morsink, M. A. J., Willemen, N. G. A., Leijten, J., Bansal, et al. (2020). Immune organs and immune cells on a chip: An overview of biomedical applications. *Micromachines, 11*(9), 849.

Murdolo, G., & Smith, U. (2006). The dysregulated adipose tissue: A connecting link between insulin resistance, type 2 diabetes mellitus and atherosclerosis. *Nutrition, Metabolism, and Cardiovascular Diseases, 16*, S35–S38.

Murray, P. J. (2018). Immune regulation by monocytes. In *Seminars in immunology* (Vol 35, pp. 12–18). Academic Press.

Murray, P. J. (2020). On macrophage diversity and inflammatory metabolic timers. *Nature Reviews Immunology, 20*(2), 89–90.

Nedosugova, L. V., Markina, Y. V., Bochkareva, L. A., et al. (2022). Inflammatory mechanisms of diabetes and its vascular complications. *Biomedicines, 10*(5), 1168.

Nicholson, L. B. (2016). The immune system. *Essays in Biochemistry, 60*(3), 275–301.

Nikiforov, N. G., Galstyan, K. O., Nedosugova, L. V., et al. (2017). Proinflammatory monocyte polarization in type 2 diabetes mellitus and coronary heart disease. *Vessel Plus, 1*, 192–195.

Nishimura, S., Manabe, I., Nagasaki, M., et al. (2009). CD8+ effector T cells contribute to macrophage recruitment and adipose tissue inflammation in obesity. *Nature Medicine, 15*(8), 914–920.

Nouari, W., & Aribi, M. (2025). Innate lymphoid cells, immune functional dynamics, epithelial parallels, and therapeutic frontiers in infections. *International Reviews of Immunology,* 1–28.

O'Sullivan, T. E., Rapp, M., Fan, X., et al. (2016). Adipose-resident group 1 innate lymphoid cells promote obesity-associated insulin resistance. *Immunity, 45*(2), 428–441.

Ouchi, N., Parker, J. L., Lugus, J. J., et al. (2011). Adipokines in inflammation and metabolic disease. *Nature Reviews Immunology, 11*(2), 85–97.

Paharkova-Vatchkova, V., Maldonado, R., & Kovats, S. (2004). Estrogen preferentially promotes the differentiation of CD11c+ CD11bintermediate dendritic cells from bone marrow precursors. *The Journal of Immunology, 172*(3), 1426–1436.

Painter, J. D., & Akbari, O. (2021). Type 2 innate lymphoid cells: Protectors in type 2 diabetes. *Frontiers in Immunology, 12,* Article 727008.

Pezhman, L., Tahrani, A., & Chimen, M. (2021). Dysregulation of leukocyte trafficking in type 2 diabetes: Mechanisms and potential therapeutic avenues. *Frontiers in Cell and Developmental Biology, 9,* Article 624184.

Pickup, J. C. (2004). Inflammation and activated innate immunity in the pathogenesis of type 2 diabetes. *Diabetes Care, 27*(3), 813–823.

Piemonti, L., Monti, P., Allavena, P., et al. (1999). Glucocorticoids affect human dendritic cell differentiation and maturation. *The Journal of Immunology, 162*(11), 6473–6481.

Rőszer, T. (2015). Understanding the mysterious M2 macrophage through activation markers and effector mechanisms. *Mediators of Inflammation, 2015*(1), Article 816460.

Ruytinx, P., Proost, P., Van Damme, J., et al. (2018). Chemokine-induced macrophage polarization in inflammatory conditions. *Frontiers in Immunology, 9,* 1930.

Saadh, M. J., Allela, O. Q. B., Kareem, R. A., Kyada, A., et al. (2025). Immune cell dysfunction: A critical player in development of diabetes complications. *Current Research in Translational Medicine, 73*(3), Article 103510.

Sato, K., & Fujita, S. (2007). Dendritic cells-nature and classification. *Allergology International, 56*(3), 183–191.

Seifarth, C. C., Hinkmann, C., Hahn, E. G., et al. (2008). Reduced frequency of peripheral dendritic cells in type 2 diabetes. *Experimental and Clinical Endocrinology & Diabetes, 116*(03), 162–166.

Serbina, N. V., Salazar-Mather, T. P., Biron, C. A., et al. (2003). TNF/iNOS-producing dendritic cells mediate innate immune defense against bacterial infection. *Immunity, 19*(1), 59–70.

Shanmugam, N., Reddy, M. A., Guha, M., et al. (2003). High glucose-induced expression of proinflammatory cytokine and chemokine genes in monocytic cells. *Diabetes, 52*(5), 1256–1264.

Shapouri-Moghaddam, A., Mohammadian, S., Vazini, H., et al. (2018). Macrophage plasticity, polarization, and function in health and disease. *Journal of Cellular Physiology, 233*(9), 6425–6440.

Sheng, J., Ruedl, C., & Karjalainen, K. (2015). Most tissue-resident macrophages except microglia are derived from fetal hematopoietic stem cells. *Immunity, 43*(2), 382–393.

Shoelson, S. E., Lee, J., & Goldfine, A. B. (2006). Inflammation and insulin resistance. *The Journal of Clinical Investigation, 116*(7), 1793–1801.

Srenathan, U., Steel, K., & Taams, L. S. (2016). IL-17+ CD8+ T cells: Differentiation, phenotype and role in inflammatory disease. *Immunology Letters, 178,* 20–26.

Stefanovic-Racic, M., Yang, X., Turner, M. S., et al. (2012). Dendritic cells promote macrophage infiltration and comprise a substantial proportion of obesity-associated increases in CD11c+ cells in adipose tissue and liver. *Diabetes, 61*(9), 2330–2339.

Tard, C., Rouxel, O., & Lehuen, A. (2015). Regulatory role of natural killer T cells in diabetes. *Biomedical Journal, 38*(6), 484–495.

Taylor, E. B. (2021). The complex role of adipokines in obesity, inflammation, and autoimmunity. *Clinical Science, 135*(6), 731–752.

Thimmappa, P. Y., Vasishta, S., Ganesh, K., Nair, et al. (2023). Neutrophil (dys)function due to altered immuno-metabolic axis in type 2 diabetes: Implications in combating infections. *Human Cell, 36*(4), 1265–1282.

Tian, M., Qing, C., Niu, Y., Dong, J., Cao, X., Song, F., Ji, X., & Lu, S. (2016). The relationship between inflammation and impaired wound healing in a diabetic rat burn model. *Journal of Burn Care & Research, 37*(2), e115–e124.

Van Oostrom, A. J., Van Wijk, J. P., Sijmonsma, T. P., et al. (2004). Increased expression of activation markers on monocytes and neutrophils in type 2 diabetes. *The Netherlands Journal of Medicine, 62* (9), 320–325.

Varo, N., Libby, P., Nuzzo, R., et al. (2005). Elevated release of sCD40L from platelets of diabetic patients by thrombin, glucose and advanced glycation end products. *Diabetes and Vascular Disease Research, 2*(2), 81–87.

Varo, N., Vicent, D., Libby, P., et al. (2003). Elevated plasma levels of the atherogenic mediator soluble CD40 ligand in diabetic patients: A novel target of thiazolidinediones. *Circulation, 107*(21), 2664–2669.

Vivier, E., Artis, D., Colonna, M., et al. (2018). Innate lymphoid cells: 10 years on. *Cell, 174*(5), 1054–1066.

Wilcox, G. (2005). Insulin and insulin resistance. *Clinical Biochemist Reviews, 26*(2), 19–39.

Willinger, T. (2019). Metabolic control of innate lymphoid cell migration. *Frontiers in Immunology, 10,* 2010.

Wright, R. D., & Cooper, D. (2014). Glycobiology of leukocyte trafficking in inflammation. *Glycobiology, 24*(12), 1242–1251.

Wu, Y., & Hirschi, K. K. (2021). Tissue-resident macrophage development and function. *Frontiers in Cell and Developmental Biology, 8,* Article 617879.

Wu, C. C., Sytwu, H. K., Lu, K. C., et al. (2011). Role of T cells in type 2 diabetic nephropathy. *Journal of Diabetes Research, 2011*(1), Article 514738.

Xia, C., Rao, X., & Zhong, J. (2017). Role of T lymphocytes in type 2 diabetes and diabetes-associated inflammation. *Journal of Diabetes Research, 2017,* Article 6494795.

Yang, Y., Qin, J., Lan, L., et al. (2014). M-CSF cooperating with NFκB induces macrophage transformation from M1 to M2 by upregulating c-Jun. *Cancer Biology & Therapy, 15*(1), 99–107.

Ye, Z., Li, Y., Yang, X., et al. (2025). Targeting regulation of macrophage to treat metabolic disease: Role of phytochemicals. *Cell Proliferation,* Article e70012.

Zeyda, M., Farmer, D., Todoric, J., et al. (2007). Human adipose tissue macrophages are of an anti-inflammatory phenotype but capable of excessive pro-inflammatory mediator production. *International Journal of Obesity, 31*(9), 1420–1428.

Zhang, P., Watari, K., & Karin, M. (2025). Innate immune cells link dietary cues to normal and abnormal metabolic regulation. *Nature Immunology,* 1–13.

Zhao, Y., Zou, W., Du, J., et al. (2018). The origins and homeostasis of monocytes and tissue-resident macrophages in physiological situation. *Journal of Cellular Physiology, 233*(10), 6425–6439.

Zhou, T., Hu, Z., Yang, S., Sun, L., et al. (2018). Role of adaptive and innate immunity in type 2 diabetes mellitus. *Journal of Diabetes Research, 2018,* Article 7457269.

5

Cytokines and insulin sensitivity

Fariya Khan[1], Salman Akhtar[2, 4] and Ajay Kumar[3]

[1]DEPARTMENT OF BIOTECHNOLOGY, KANPUR INSTITUTE OF TECHNOLOGY (KIT), KANPUR, UTTAR PRADESH, INDIA; [2]DEPARTMENT OF BIOENGINEERING, INTEGRAL UNIVERSITY, LUCKNOW, UTTAR PRADESH, INDIA; [3]DEPARTMENT OF BIOTECHNOLOGY, FACULTY OF ENGINEERING AND TECHNOLOGY RAMA UNIVERSITY, MANDHANA, KANPUR, UTTAR PRADESH, INDIA; [4]NOVEL GLOBAL COMMUNITY EDUCATIONAL FOUNDATION, HEBERSHAM, NSW, AUSTRALIA

1. Introduction

Cytokines are tiny proteins that are absolutely necessary for cell-to- cell communication, are especially crucial within the immunosystem, and are responsible for the fine-tuning of lots of physiological processes, especially inflammation, immune response, and cellular communication. Nowadays, their role in metabolic regulation has got much attention, especially on their effect on insulin sensitivity and insulin resistance (Shi et al., 2019). Insulin sensitivity is the degree of the cells' reaction to the insulin hormone, which regulates the levels of glucose in the blood. Thus, when cells are insulin-sensitive, they are able to absorb glucose from the bloodstream, thus energy balance is regulated, and high levels of blood sugar are prevented (Donath & Shoelson, 2011). On the contrary, insulin resistance is a cell's deficiency in reacting to insulin a condition that is very related to the development of type 2 diabetes and metabolic syndrome. The whole issue of cytokines and insulin sensitivity is not an easy one and it includes different mechanisms. Cytokines, such as tumor necrosis factor-alpha (TNF-α), interleukin-6 (IL-6) and interleukin-1 beta (IL-1β)), which play a crucial role in inflammatory processes, have been found to resist insulin signaling, which in turn makes insulin resistance (Rehman et al., 2017). These cytokines mess up the function of the insulin hormone by starting pathways that are inflammatory, such as the nuclear factor-kappa B (NF-κB) pathway. This pathway in turn causes insulin receptor substrates (IRS) to be phosphorylated, which in the end slows down the glucose uptake by cells and at the same time increases insulin resistance.

Additionally, IL-10 (interleukin-10) and adiponectin, both of which are categories of antiinflammatory cytokines, promote glucose-insulin sensitivity by neutralizing the harmful effects of proinflammatory cytokines and training the insulin signaling pathways (Lee et al., 2006). Optimally, the cytokine balance, which can be either proinflammatory or antiinflammatory, is the deciding factor as to whether a person has good

Type 2 Diabetes Mellitus. https://doi.org/10.1016/B978-0-443-33590-7.00008-3

insulin sensitivity and, thus, is healthy. Cytokines are the middlemen between insulin and inflammatory signaling, so the function involves a rather complex interaction between the molecules. Proinflammatory cytokines, namely tumor necrosis factor-alpha (TNF-α), interleukin-6 (IL-6), and interleukin-1 beta (IL-1β), are among the components that have been demonstrated to be the major obstacles to successful insulin signaling (Kataria et al., 2019). These cytokines have the ability of switching on the inflammatory paths among the cells such as the nuclear factor-kappa B (NF-κB) pathway that would then be the parking space for the IRS . The IRS get phosphorylated, thus leading to the abnormal regulation of glucose uptake, which will result in high blood sugar. For instance, TNF-α has been extensively studied for its role in promoting insulin resistance. The Rho group phosphorylates serine on the insulin-receptor substrate one molecule, which, as a result, loses its efficacy in the signal transduction process, thus giving the signal in muscle and adipose tissues weakly. Similarly, IL-6 and IL-1β are also the ones that will be the cause of the pro-inflammatory consequences for a longer time (Pradhan et al., 2001). To assign to cytokines their place as a very important factor in the case of insulin resistance, in fact, this very standpoint should be used to the fullest. New medicines that can repair the insulin signaling problems in the case of type 2 diabetes are born with the help of an enhanced consideration of the functionality of cytokines in the course of insulin sensitivity. Research no sooner than now still puts the immune system and metabolism under the scope, the new fact comes out where the cytokine is, however, the primary target for the treatments of some metabolic illnesses. Insulin sensitivity is the effectiveness of the insulin molecule in signaling cells to absorb sugar from the blood, which in turn keeps blood sugar levels healthy. High insulin sensitivity enables the cells to catabolize (eat) glucose from the blood into energy and helps thus to prevent hyperglycemia, which is an energy imbalance-related condition (Lucas et al., 2012). In the meantime, insulin resistance is a term that is used to express the state when cells do not answer to insulin in the right way thus stopping the entrance of glucose into the cells, which is, as a matter of fact, the main reason for them becoming the tissue insulin improper glucose utilization and insulin resistance conditions, a causal factor, that later metastasizes into the type 2 diabetes and metabolic syndrome, worldwide public health challenges.

The proper pro and antiinflammatory cytokine play a vital part in controlling insulin sensitivity and the entire metabolic health of the body. Insulin sensitivity falls when the body's imbalance shifts to a proinflammatory state, and then metabolic disorders such as obesity and Type 2 diabetes develop (Schenk et al., 2008). However, the predominance of antiinflammatory cytokines contributes to the improvement of insulin action and thus the stabilization of the metabolism, which emphasizes their preventive role in the maintenance of metabolic health. As scientists delve deeper into the convoluted interaction between the immune system and metabolism, cytokines have come to the fore as key players in this interaction. Their acting in both ways, i.e., proinflammatory and antiinflammatory, has brought forth their essentiality for potential therapeutic interventions. By selectively manipulating cytokine activity, it might be possible to not only optimize insulin sensitivity but also, in addition, handle the broader spectrum of metabolic conditions linked with conditions such as obesity and type 2 diabetes. Targeting cytokines through treatment strategies is very important. For example, reducing the levels of particular proinflammatory cytokines could be an excellent way to alleviate the chronic, low-grade inflammation that is usually found in metabolic disorders, thereby leading to the improvement of insulin sensitivity and glucose control. At the same time, stimulating antiinflammatory cytokines may give the body more firepower to prevent metabolic disease issues, not just a new pathway to curb insulin resistance (Mandal.et al., 2010). The ongoing work on the subject of the function of cytokines in the regulation of metabolic syndrome is giving us these kinds of new routes and mechanisms that could be utilized for therapeutic advantage. This ever-broadening learning resource not only further deepens our awareness of the process of the maintenance of metabolic health, but also provides alternatives to the treatments that could remedy insulin resistance and its complications. As we progress with the understanding of cytokine biology, the prospects of better remedies for metabolic diseases that are both more efficient and effective are getting brighter, which also offers the hope of better health for those people who have those diseases.

2. Role of cytokines and insulin sensitivity in the inflammatory system

2.1 Pathogenic role of cytokines leading to diabetes

Cytokines contribute significantly to the inception and evolution of diabetes, especially in both type 1 and type 2 diabetes. These small signaling proteins are integral to the immune system and can trigger inflammatory responses, a common factor that facilitates to the inception and advancement of diabetes.

2.1.1 Cytokines in type 1 diabetes (T1D)

Type 1 diabetes (T1D) is a continuing autoimmune disorder marked by the gradual and often subtle devastation of β cells in the pancreas. This disease arises from a malfunction in the immune system, primarily driven by T helper 1 (Th1) cells (Polychronakos & Li, 2011). The activation and infiltration of immune cells into the islets of the pancreas contribute to the targeted destruction of β cells, ultimately leading to significant hyperglycemia. The pathogenic roles of cytokines in T1D are complicated and not yet fully understood, particularly during disease advancement and inflammation. As the disease progresses, the regulation of cytokines becomes more complex with the rising involvement of numerous cytokines with altered regulation further complicates their interactions (Fig. 5.1). In T1D, cytokines rarely operate solely as proinflammatory or antiinflammatory agents. For the scope of this review, cytokines are grouped into three main categories antiinflammatory cytokines, such as IL-10, TGF-β, and type-2 cytokines; proinflammatory cytokines, including IL-1, IL-6, and TNF-α; and a third category

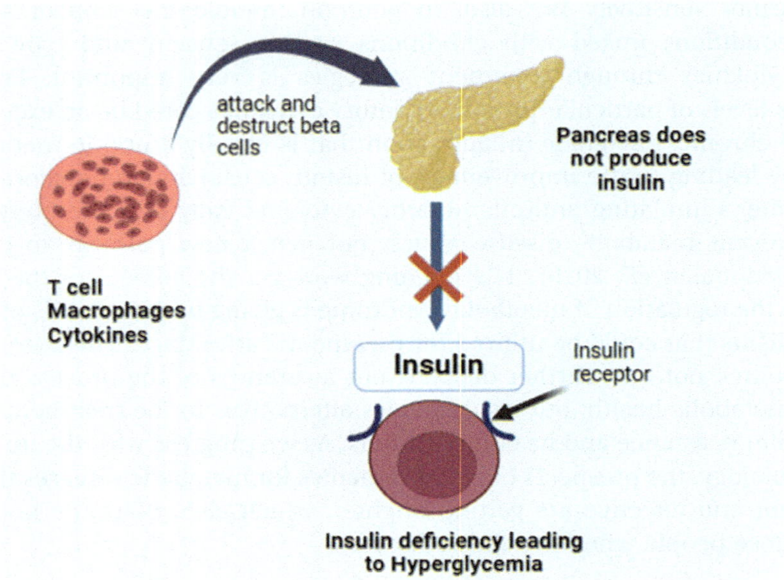

FIGURE 5.1 Role of cytokines and insulin sensitivity in type I diabetes.

comprising cytokines with more recently identified roles, such as members of the IL-12 family, IL-21, and IL-33 (Boshtam et al., 2017).

This categorization highlights the complexity of cytokine functions, as many of these molecules display pleiotropic effects, meaning they can influence the immune response in various ways depending on the context. For example, a single cytokine might be contributing to the initiation and advancement of T1D, determining whether the immune response acts protectively or pathologically (Sprague & Khalil, 2009). These nuanced roles are critical in directing the course of the disease, from the initial immune assault on pancreatic β-cells to their eventual destruction. Furthermore, a deeper understanding of these diverse cytokine activities has important implications for developing innovative immunotherapeutic strategies for T1D. By targeting specific cytokines or modulating their pathways, it may be possible to influence the disease trajectory, potentially preventing the onset of T1D or slowing its progression. This broadened view of cytokine function not only enhances our understanding of T1D pathophysiology but also surfaces the way for new therapeutic approaches aimed at rebalancing the immune system and safeguarding β-cells from autoimmune attack.

2.1.2 Cytokines in type 2 diabetes (T2D)

Insulin resistance and lack of β-cell function, in which cytokines play the necessitating role, are the two creeping mechanisms of type 2 diabetes. Alongside moderating the extent of inflammation through the distribution of proinflammatory versus

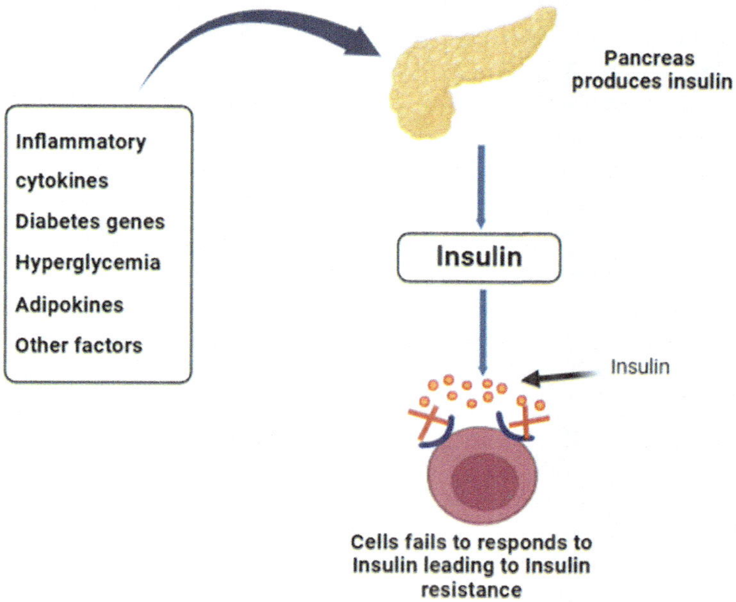

FIGURE 5.2 Role of cytokines and insulin sensitivity in type II diabetes.

antiinflammatory signals, these messenger molecules are also the chief spots in the immunological cure of autoinflammatory and autoimmune diseases (Shi et al., 2019). Recent resources have been devoted to elucidating IL-17's and Th17's role in the inflammatory processes that lead to the development of Type 2 diabetes (T2D). In vitro research has shown that Th17 cells and IL-17A are involved in the destruction of the pancreas, which is connected to diabetes (Kuryłowicz & Koźniewski, 2020). Every bit of note is that when the antiIL-17 neutralizing antibodies were administered, the levels of serum adiponectin were drastically raised, an adipokine whose role is to improve insulin sensitivity (Fig. 5.2). Also, adipocyte proliferation and serum TNF-α levels were downregulated by this therapeutic treatment as well, which shows its potential in the resistance improvement of insulin. These findings bring about the conclusion that IL-17 is a prime culprit in the induction of insulin resistance (IR) and the subsequent Type 2 diabetes (T2D) (Abdel et al., 2018).

Moreover, IL-17 contributes a prominent part in activating the NF-κB pathway, which leads to the upregulation of various inflammatory cytokines. This activation results in the increased production of proinflammatory cytokines such as IL-1β, IL-6, and TNF-α, which are central to the advancement of insulin resistance and the onset of T2D. By amplifying the inflammatory response, IL-17 not only drives the pathogenesis of T2D but also emerges as a promising target for therapeutic intervention in the disease (Ogawa et al., 2004). This highlights the critical involvement of IL-17 in the inflammatory pathways that underlie the pathogenesis of T2D.

2.2 Classification

Cytokines can be categorized into several classes that include tumor necrosis factors (TNFs), Interleukins (ILs), lymphokines, monokines, interferons (IFNs), colony-stimulating factors (CSFs), and transforming growth factors (TGFs). They are classified into type 1 cytokines, those derived from the cells, of which $CD4^+$ T-helper 1 (Th1) cells are the main source, for example: IL-2, IL-12, IFN-γ, and TNF-β; and type 2 cytokines, presented by $CD4^+$ Th2 cells, for instance, IL-4, IL-5, IL-6, IL-10, and IL-13 (Yi et al., 2024). It can be classified based on its function also as either proinflammatory or anti-inflammatory cytokines. Proinflammatory cytokines include IL-1β, IL-6, IL-8, IL-12, TNF-α, and interferons, which initiate inflammatory responses and activate immune cells (Fig. 5.3). Conversely, antiinflammatory cytokines such as IL-4, IL-6, IL-10, IL-11, IL-13, IL-1 receptor antagonist (IL-1RA), and TGF-β suppress inflammation and regulate immune responses. Interestingly, some cytokines, like IL-6, exhibit both proinflammatory and antiinflammatory effects (Propper & Balkwill, 2022).

2.2.1 Proinflammatory cytokines

Proinflammatory cytokines are crucial elements of the immune system, serving as first responders to bacterial and microbial threats. These molecules are essential for mounting an effective defense against external pathogens and managing the body's own microbiota, including those on the skin and in the gut. By activating and guiding immune cells, cytokines like IL-1β, IL-6, IL-8, IL-12, IFN-γ, and TNF-α trigger swift immune

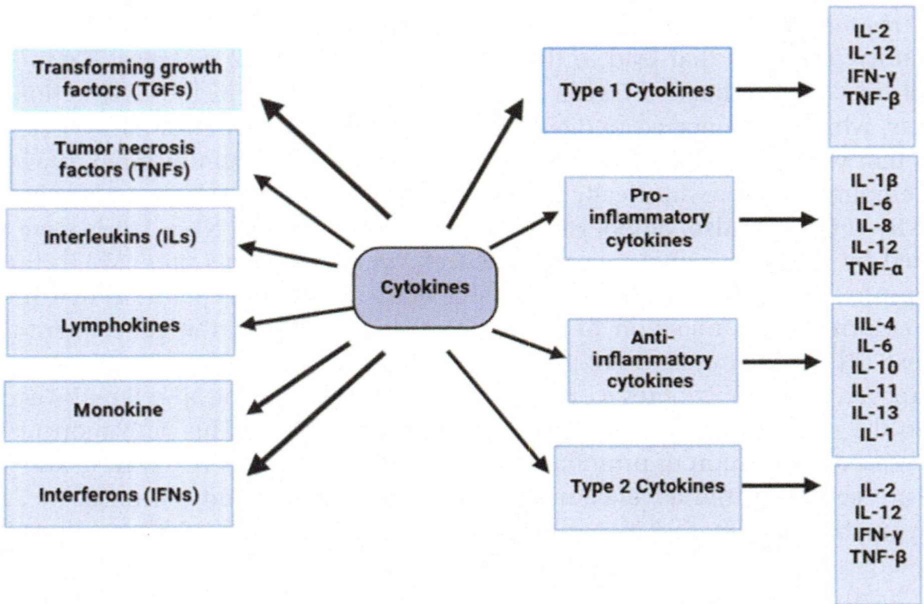

FIGURE 5.3 Classification of cytokines based on their functional and characteristic properties.

responses and maintain a delicate balance between the body and its microbial ecosystem (Kany.et al., 2009). For instance, IL-1 exhibits both cytostatic and cytotoxic effects in lab settings, while IL-6 plays a central role in regulating inflammation. IL-12 enhances T-cell function, and interferons are vital in defending against viral infections. Released from activated macrophages, these cytokines work in concert to coordinate the immune system's response, ensuring harmful microbes are eliminated, and beneficial ones are controlled (Arango & Descoteaux 2014). This dual role highlights their importance not only in immediate immune defense but also in maintaining long-term immune balance.

2.2.2 Antiinflammatory cytokines

Antiinflammatory cytokines, which are the ones that include IL-1 receptor antagonist, IL-4, IL-6, IL-10, IL-11, IL-13, and TGF-β, are pivotal to immune responses modulation by curtailing proinflammatory cytokines. These cytokines work in concert to control the inflammation process and keep the function of the immune system in the proper state. For example, IL-10 is a notable antiinflammatory cytokine with multifaceted immunoregulatory action (Wautier & Wautier, 2023). One crucial element of IL-10 is its ability to inhibit the production of a number of proinflammatory cytokines, which in turn would decrease inflammation. Moreover, IL-10 also is able to control the opiates by a great number of eosinophils, basophils, and mast cells, which are involved in the respiratory allergies and asthma, that is why this is a significant regulator of those. The roles of these antiinflammatory cytokines in addition to merely suppressing inflammation. They are actively affecting the immune cell activities and aiding tissue repair (Scheller et al., 2011). Their normal functions are so important in the context of inflammation, they prevent chronic inflammation and make sure that the immune system is correctly functioning without inflicting damage to the body.

2.3 Significance of cytokines

Cytokines are pivotal signaling molecules that exert significant and wide-ranging effects throughout the body, especially in regulating the immune system and controlling inflammation. Cytokines are the main influential signaling molecules that cause big and multifarious effects on the body, regulating the immune system and controlling inflammation (Zhang & An, 2007). Their influence is in many different diseases and physiological functions, as well as in therapeutic strategies, making it necessary to know them in terms of their involvement in the maintenance of the body balance, the combating of infections, and the management of health conditions. In summary, cytokines are many-sided entities that are essential for the maintenance of health and the thrusting back of disease. They carry out different and important tasks in the body, and new findings on cytokine function and therapy contribute to our understanding and treatment of a wide variety of medical conditions. Taken as an example, their enormous applications in response to inflammation could functionally mirror immune regulation, cell communication, and disease pathogenesis to the extent that our knowledge of human biology can grow, and the steps needed for the appropriate therapeutic actions can be developed. The significance of cytokines are categorized below:

2.3.1 Immune system regulation

Cytokines are fundamental to the immune system, serving as key messengers that facilitate communication between cells. They are crucial in triggering, expanding, and guiding the development of immune cells, ensuring that the immune response is both accurate and effective. In the absence of cytokines, the immune system would be impaired, leaving the body vulnerable to infections and diseases due to its inability to mount an adequate defense against pathogens (Kulbe et al., 2012).

2.3.2 Monitoring inflammation

Inflammation is a crucial response to injury or infection, where cytokines acting as a key drivers of this process. They direct immune cells to the site of damage, aiding in healing and tissue repair. However, when cytokine levels are unstable, it can result in chronic inflammation, which is associated with various diseases such as autoimmune disorders, heart disease, and cancer (Neurath, 2014).

2.3.3 Facilitating physiological functions

Beyond their roles in immunity and inflammation, cytokines play a vital part in a broad range of physiological functions. They are crucial for regulating cell growth, differentiation, and apoptosis (programmed cell death), and are vital for tissue repair. Furthermore, cytokines are critical for nervous system development, the construction of blood cells, and the regulation of metabolic processes.

2.3.4 Role in pathogenesis of disease

Imbalances in cytokine levels or signaling can play a vital part in the onset of several diseases. For instance, excessive fabrication of proinflammatory cytokines can lead to autoimmune disorders, while inadequate cytokine activity may result in immunodeficiencies. A deep understanding of cytokine function is essential for unraveling the complexities of diseases like rheumatoid arthritis, psoriasis, and multiple sclerosis (Pretorius et al., 2015).

2.3.5 Therapeutic applications

Cytokines play a leading role in modern medical therapies and thus, they can be strategically targeted to adjust the immune response therefore enhancing it in cases like cancer immunotherapy, or suppressing it in treatments for autoimmune diseases. The application of synthetic cytokines or inhibitors presents promising avenues for effectively managing a wide range of health conditions (Alexandraki et al., 2006).

3. Insulin sensitivity: Insights into molecular mechanism to therapeutic strategies

Insulin sensitivity defines how effectively the cells of our body react to insulin, the hormone that is responsible for maintaining levels of blood glucose. Insulin resistance is known as a condition when insulin sensitivity is reduced thus leads to various range of metabolic conditions such as obesity, type 2 diabetes and cardiovascular diseases. Gaining vision into the molecular mechanisms of insulin sensitivity and resistance is essential for creating effective therapeutic strategies.

3.1 Characteristics of insulin

Insulin, as a key hormone in the process of human metabolism, is necessary for the maintenance of optimal levels of glucose in the body. This 51-amino-acid anabolic protein is secreted by the β-cells within the Islets of Langerhans in the pancreas and is composed of two polypeptide chains, A and B, connected by disulfide bonds that make up chain A, and chain B, with 21 and 30 residues, respectively. The molecular weight of Insulin is about 5808 Da, and the hormone structure in its free form has been examined extensively and established through power imaging techniques such as NMR spectroscopy and X-ray crystallography (Nakagawa et al., 2000). The mature insulin hormone is derived from its precursor, a single-chain molecule that is known as proinsulin, through posttranslational modification. By means of such advanced techniques, scientists have discerned the molecular anatomy of this hormone in all its depth, elucidating the fine structural details that are indispensable for its biological function. Through the analysis of the exact atomic arrangement and spatial configuration, these methods have made clear how the specific structural components support the hormone to interact with receptors and carry out the functions needed for the body. This profound knowledge of the hormone's structure is an instrumental resource that has improved our perception of its participation in physiological processes and the development of therapeutic strategies for various medical problems.

In β cells, insulin is stored as a Zn^{2+}-stabilized hexamer, which dissociates into a Zn^{2+}-free monomer upon entering the bloodstream to perform its hormonal functions. Research on rare, naturally occurring mutations at positions A3, B24, and B25 has identified key receptor-binding sites (Huang et al., 2004), which are associated with decreased insulin activity and diabetes mellitus. The detailed study of insulin's three-dimensional structure, particularly through the ground-breaking work of D. C. Hodgkin, has been instrumental in developing therapeutic insulin analogs for treating diabetes mellitus (DM). Although mutations in the insulin gene are relatively rare, they have been linked to the onset of DM. These mutations have offered very important findings on the molecular pathways that mediate the production of insulin and the process of insulin binding with its receptor. Most frequent among them are the mutations that cause the inappropriate formation of proinsulin (Edghill et al., 2008). This kind of dysfolding, in turn, triggers the so-called unfolded protein response in the endoplasmic reticulum (ER) of the β-cells, growth of defective cells and earlier onset of diabetes, sometimes in the neonatal period (Wan et al., 2008). Besides the diagnosis of diabetes, these studies concerning molecular mechanisms have also brought about the development of the new healing targeted therapies that will not only reduce the loss of the function of the beta cells and the long run the disease will be prevented protected.

3.2 Pathogenesis of insulin sensitivity

When elevated insulin levels in the bloodstream are required to achieve the glucose-lowering effect to be achieved, the person is called insulin-resistant. Several clinical conditions, such as prediabetes, lipodystrophy, polycystic ovarian syndrome, and nonalcoholic fatty liver disease, are associated with elevated fasting plasma insulin levels. This amplified demand on the endocrine pancreas, leading to β-cell dysfunction, is a key driver in the advancement to overt type 2 diabetes (T2D). Notably, the significance of insulin resistance in T2D development is underscored through longitudinal studies showing it to be the strongest predictor of future T2D diagnosis (Petersen et al., 2002). Since insulin functions vary across diverse cell types, insulin resistance has different effects on numerous insulin-target tissues (Fig. 5.4). The cellular and molecular

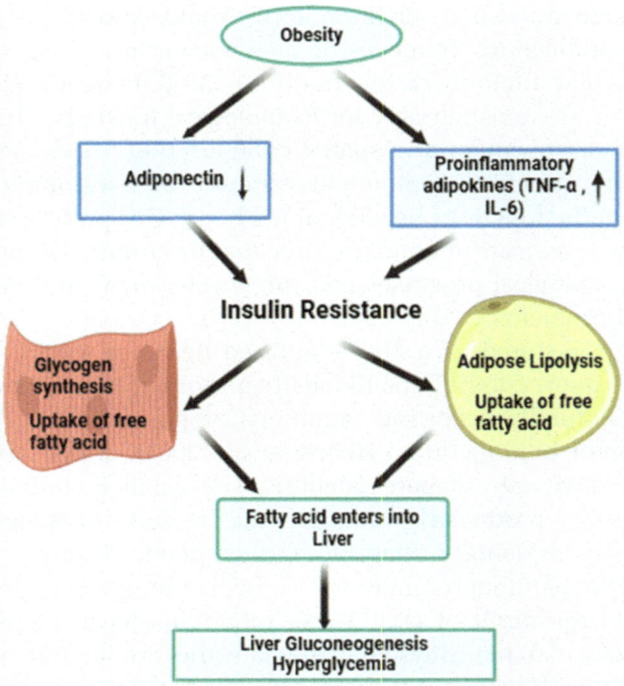

FIGURE 5.4 Pathogenesis of insulin resistance associated with hyperglycemia.

mechanistic background on insulin resistance is intricately connected with the specific molecular blockages, a review of indirect insulin action, and the concept of pathway-selective hepatic insulin resistance where insulin activates several signaling pathways that are activated downstream of the insulin receptor and does not become resistant while the other one does.

Insulin resistance is the result of a combination of reasons, such as the deficiency of receptor binding, the modification of the internal host environment, the alteration of intracellular dynamics, autophagy, and the homeostasis of the intestinal microecology. IR is quite interesting or peculiar since it demonstrates some variability among tissues that are considered insulin sensitive, with the most common place of origination being the adipose tissue before it spreads to other areas. However, these activities can merge and consequently develop to the systemic level more often than not, and this phenomenon was accessed in the case of human subjects (Magkos et al., 2012). A detailed awareness of the diverse sources of IR will be very beneficial and will afford many research options, one of the most unusual and perhaps the most important of which is the determination of turning points for IR and the study of the closely related metabolic diseases.

Insulin resistance (IR) affects multiple tissues, such as skeletal muscle, liver, kidneys, and adipose tissue, each with distinct underlying mechanisms. Notably, bone, is as an endocrine organ that also acts as a target for insulin and thus significantly persuading energy balance by modulating insulin sensitivity. This establishes a mutual relationship between bone and insulin resistance, thereby linking them in a biological partnership. Skeletal muscle acts as a vital insulin-sensitive tissue that plays a significant role in insulin-dependent glucose uptake and insulin sensitivity. Moreover, it also regulates overall glucose levels, supports metabolic health, and acts as an interplay between adipokines and muscle factors that can prompt a negative feedback loop and can worsens muscle loss, obesity, and insulin resistance.

3.3 Relationship between insulin sensitivity and type 2 diabetes

For more than half a century, type 2 diabetes and resistance to insulin have been a couple well navigated. Decrease of insulin sensitivity between impaired insulin productions very often happens as type 2 diabetes continues to evolve. The body routinely does all of the above in very often the case the body tries to keep glucose levels stable by increasing insulin secretion to overtake sensitive period such as reduce and vice versa as well. Investigations on the connection of insulin sensitivity and secretion have largely hiked our accruing knowledge of the evolution of type 2 diabetes. Insulin resistance is the primary factor contributing to the development of type 2 diabetes and the major treatment target with the onset of high blood sugar (Kawamori & Kulkarni, 2009). Additionally to its important part in diabetes and a number of other physiological functions, such as bone health, the recent studies that have been revealed are the effects of insulin on critical structures like the brain, heart, and bone, as well as the skin and hair follicles and the enhanced bone formation, decreased osteoporosis-related inflammation, impact on the central nervous system, and the activities of the pro and anti-atherogenicn in the vascular system. In type 2 diabetes, disorders in the feedback mechanisms of insulin affect insulin action and secretion. In such a case of β-cells failure decreases insulin secretion, thereby the body cannot regulate glucose properly thus, hyperinsulinemia (IR) begets glucose overproduction in the liver and impaired glucose uptake in liver, muscle and adipose tissue. Albeit the two are involved in the onset, β-cell dysfunction, nevertheless, is most commonly seen and so the disease progresses.

3.4 Consequences of insulin sensitivity

Insulin sensitivity is the endogenic sort of insulin, and it is a very important component of the glucose homeostasis process, because it affects both the pancreas function and insulin resistance. Insulin sensitivity is the ability of the cells in the body to respond to insulin, and the level of insulin sensitivity affects a variety of physiological processes and is associated with both beneficial and harmful health outcomes (Fig. 5.5). High insulin sensitivity is generally good as it enables more efficient glucose uptake and use, while decreased insulin sensitivity can lead to many metabolic disorders (Estall. et al., 2009). Persons with reduced insulin sensitivity show a decline in the ability of insulin to

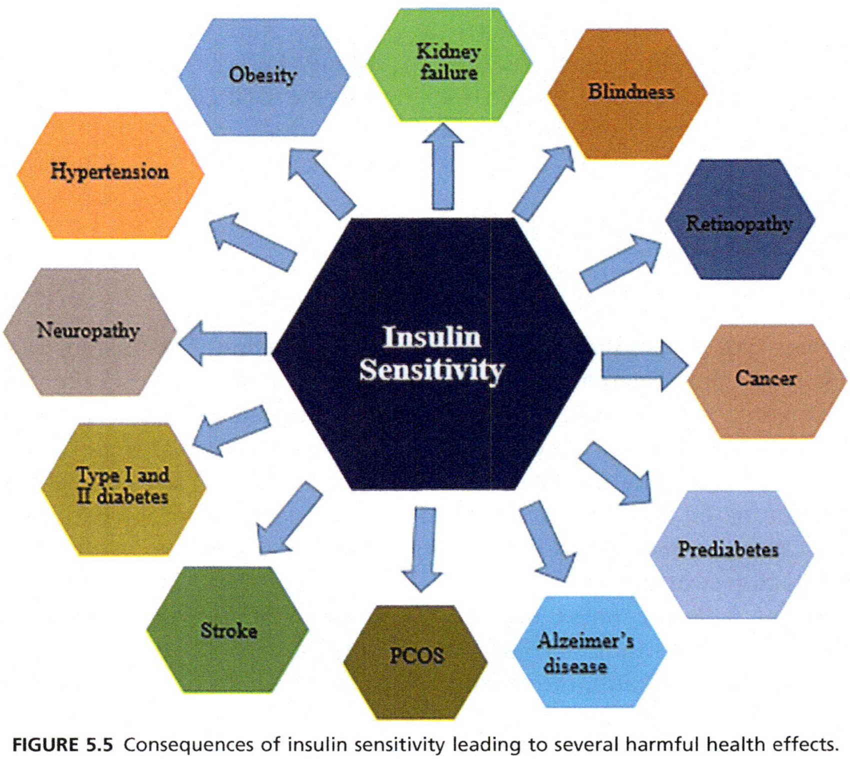

FIGURE 5.5 Consequences of insulin sensitivity leading to several harmful health effects.

regulate glucose transport in the whole. Therefore, the level of blood sugar goes up, leading to poor glycemic control. Thereafter, the increased demand on the pancreas might cause β-cell dysfunction, which contributes to type 2 diabetes.

Long-term exposure to high levels of blood sugar in the body, along with the continuous metabolic strain due to insulin resistance, is the main culprit in the many health problems that accompany it. One of the health problems is the development of cardiovascular conditions such as hypertension, atherosclerosis, and heart disease, but chronic inflammation as well, has also been the major culprit which, little by little, can damage tissues and organs (Palmer et al., 2015). Moreover, the persistent strain metabolic systems experience can lead to disorders such as kidney dysfunction and nonalcoholic fatty liver disease (NAFLD). The aftermath caused by the weakened glycemic control and insulin resistance, therefore, can cause no less than severe short and long-term health damage.

4. Targeting cytokines to act as antiinflammatory signals in type II diabetes

Cytokines are important in regulating the inflammatory responses by balancing proinflammatory and antiinflammatory signals that could offer a potential treatment option for diabetes patients. Nowadays, several cytokines are the focus of biological therapies aimed at treating auto inflammatory and autoimmune conditions, with anticytokine treatments along with disease-modifying therapies for patients with rheumatic conditions. Certain cytokines are directly involved in glucose metabolism and play a significant role in the onset and progression of insulin resistance as well (Velikova. et al., 2021). Proinflammatory cytokines such as TNF-α, IL-6, and IL-1β, are elevated in individuals with type 2 diabetes and thus contributes to the inflammatory environment that worsens metabolic dysfunction. Targeting these proinflammatory cytokines, while boosting antiinflammatory cytokines like IL-10 and IL-4, has become a promising approach to improving insulin sensitivity (Fig. 5.6).

TNF-α is a major proinflammatory cytokine and is often referred to have critical role in triggering the inflammatory response as it has been proven to demonstrate in numerous noninfectious processes, including angiogenesis, morphogenesis, metastasis, allergy, and glucose regulation. Produced by adipocytes and inflammatory cells during chronic inflammation, TNF-α level are strongly associated with obesity in individuals with type 2 diabetes (Burska et al., 2015). The therapeutic potential extends across a range of autoimmune and immune-mediated conditions that includes rheumatoid arthritis, spondylitis, inflammatory bowel disease, refractory asthma and hidradenitis suppurativa. Additionally, confirmation supports that targeting the TNF-α pathway in patients with inflammatory rheumatic diseases and T2D can improve insulin sensitivity and lead to moderate reductions in HbA1c levels.

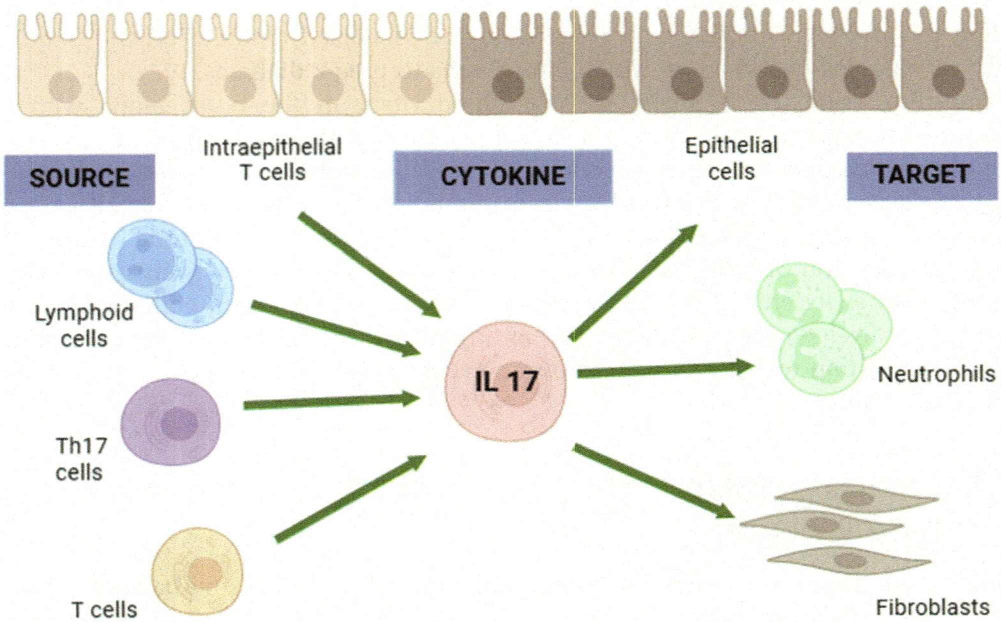

FIGURE 5.6 Targeting Cytokine pathways to offer potential treatment in inflammation-related diseases.

IL-6 plays a complex role in maintaining the glucose homeostasis and metabolism by affecting various cell types such as adipocytes, skeletal muscle cells, hepatocytes and pancreatic beta cells. Its major role in the immune system is to enhance the effects of other cytokines and acts as a crucial predictor and biomarker for the development and progression of type 2 diabetes. Elevated IL-6 levels are closely tied to metabolic issues as well as insulin resistance and the application of beta-cell apoptosis, the reduction of insulin secretion and impairment of metabolic dysfunction in T2D (Tsalamandris et al., 2019). Growing evidence of IL-6, serving a second integral function of immune regulation, and metabolic processes, is a recognized novel pharmacological option for T2D management and prevention. The IL-1 family of cytokines play an important part in the development of some inflammation-related diseases and are prominent proinflammatory mediators. IL-1β has been associated with the insulin secretion reduction and beta-cell apoptosis by which it increases metabolic dysfunction thus the progression of diabetes. Therapies directed at IL-1 like anakinra, which Interleukin-1 receptor antagonist inhibits the actions of both IL-1α and IL-1β, are also on the course of metabolic health. In patients with T2D, IR-1 blocking has perceived significant improvements in glucose metabolism and the attenuation in systemic inflammation markers (Spranger et al., 2003). The data also indicates that activation of the IL-1 pathway could be a successful therapy not only for autoimmune diseases but also for metabolic-related disorders like T2D, where chronic inflammation is a key factor in disease development.

5. Factors leading to impaired insulin sensitivity

5.1 Inadequate insulin secretion

Insulin secretion must be carefully regulated to match metabolic demands, which is why maintaining the integrity of the islets is crucial. This allows β-cells to effectively respond to the body's changing metabolic needs. Shortcomings in the synthesis of insulin and their disturbance of the secretion pathway, can results in insulin secretory dysfunction, the primary driver of β-cell failure, and a foundation of T2D (Christensen & Gannon, 2019). Insulin Resistance mentions to a reduction of insulin-sensitive cells to insulin can be affected by systemic factors, leading to a reduced or impaired reaction to circulating insulin as reflected by glucose levels in blood (Wilcox, 2005). There are three main types of inadequate insulin conditions: reduced insulin secretion from β-cells, the occurrence of insulin antagonists in the bloodstream due to counterregulatory hormones or other nonhormonal factors that interrupt insulin receptor function or signaling, and impaired insulin response in target tissues. Under pathogenic conditions, the mechanism of insulin production can disrupt islet integrity, hindering effective cell-to-cell communication within the pancreatic islets. As a result, it can result to poor regulation of insulin and glucagon release, ultimately worsening hyperglycaemia (Fig. 5.7).

5.2 Defect in the insulin gene

Defects in the insulin gene can significantly influence insulin production and function and it is essential for encoding the insulin precursor, playing a crucial role in both the synthesis and secretion of the hormone. Mutations or abnormalities in the insulin gene can disrupt the production of important insulin precursors, such as preproinsulin and proinsulin, or interfere with the maturation process that converts these precursors into active insulin (Stoy et al., 2021). Such disruptions can result in inadequate insulin production and contribute to metabolic imbalances. Mutations in the insulin gene can produce a variety of clinical manifestations and thus changes that influence receptor binding or postGolgi processing might lead to increased levels of insulin, proinsulin, or proinsulin split products in the blood, but may not necessarily cause hyperglycemia. Conversely, mutations that impair insulin processing within the endoplasmic reticulum (ER) typically result in β-cell apoptosis and a reduction in β-cell mass. The severity of these defects, combined with the β-cell's capacity to manage ER stress, determines the rate of β-cell loss and thus influences the age of onset and severity of the resulting clinical condition.

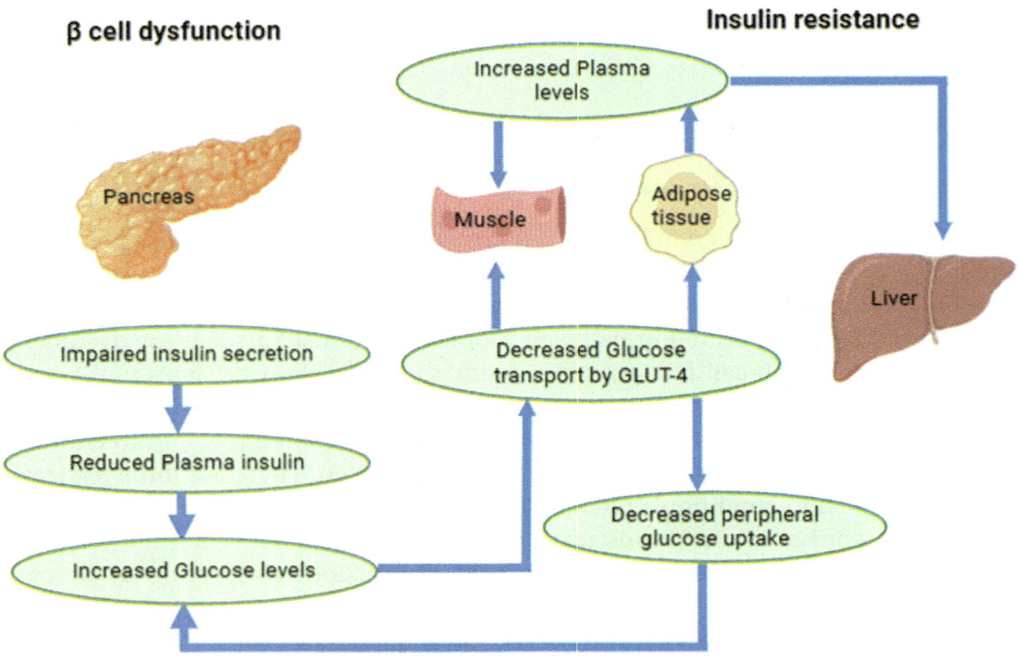

FIGURE 5.7 Impaired insulin secretion leading to hyperglycemia.

5.3 Insulin resistance syndrome

Rare disorders include a variety of advanced insulin resistance syndromes, which can be characterized by extreme insulin resistance, pathological changes to the metabolism and a wide array of clinical symptoms and complications. These conditions can stem from both genetic and environmental factors, highlighting a complex interaction of underlying causes. Insulin resistance, which is caused by mutations in the INSR gene, is a rare disease that runs in families and occurs at the same time as other types of diabetes such as Donohue's syndrome, Rabson-Mendenhall's syndrome, and type A insulin resistance syndrome (Grasso et al., 2013).

5.3.1 Donohue syndrome

Donohue syndrome, also known as leprechaunism, is an exceedingly rare autosomal recessive disorder caused by mutations in the INSR gene (Falik et al., 2014). Diagnosis is typically made through a combination of genetic, biochemical, and clinical evaluations. Functional analyses aim to uncover potential correlations between genotype and phenotype, as well as between the structural features of the mutations and their impact on disease severity (Takeuchi et al., 2020).

5.3.2 Rabson-Mendenhall syndrome

Rabson-Mendenhall syndrome is one of the rare autosomal recessive disorders arising from INSR gene mutations (Longo et al., 1999). It is characterized by elevated insulin levels, fasting hypoglycaemia, and inadequate responses in patients. This condition leads to refractory diabetes mellitus, severe ketoacidosis, and microvascular complications associated with diabetes. The symptoms of this syndrome usually appear early in life and sometimes it may occur later in their age. Diagnosis includes clinical manifestations and laboratory results and is confirmed through genetic testing.

5.3.3 Type A insulin resistance syndrome

Type A insulin resistance syndrome is a rare and severe condition caused by mutations in the INSR gene (Takasawa et al., 2019). These mutations, which can be either heterozygous or, in some cases, homozygous, impair the function of the insulin receptor and disrupt signal transduction. Despite the severity of the syndrome, individuals may live beyond middle age. Diagnosing type A insulin resistance syndrome can be challenging, but early and accurate identification is crucial for implementing targeted treatments.

5.3.4 Type B insulin resistance syndrome

Type B insulin resistance syndrome is a rare autoimmune disorder characterized by the presence of polyclonal autoantibodies, typically of the IgG type, that target insulin receptors (Willard et al., 2016). Elevated levels of these auto antibodies may inhibit insulin receptor function, leading to insulin resistance and hyperglycemia. In contrast, lower levels of auto antibodies can partially activate the receptor, which may result in hypoglycemia. Consequently, patients generally experience pronounced insulin resistance and hyperglycemia, with hypoglycemia being less common (Malek et al., 2010).

6. Recent advances in molecular biomarkers of cytokines and insulin sensitivity

When it comes to type II diabetes (T2DM), relations between molecular biomarkers which are connected to diseases such as cytokines and insulin sensitivity express our more profound knowledge in pathophysiology. These newly discovered pieces of information provide crucial insights into the complicated interaction between chronic inflammation, insulin resistance, and overall metabolism, which in turn guides a new perspective for refining diagnostic, monitoring, and treatment methods (Li et al., 2022). By taking these biomarkers as their main target, doctors can improve diagnostic accuracy, make predictions of disease outcomes much more precise, and design treatments based on the genetic features of every patient—a major step toward personalized medicine and elevated clinical outcomes.

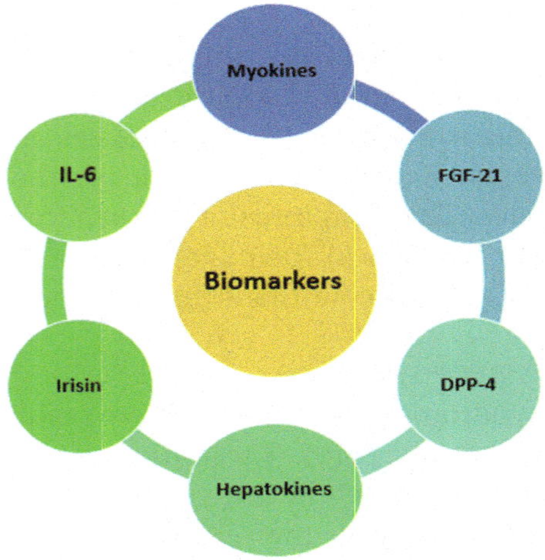

FIGURE 5.8 Recent advancement of different molecular biomarkers of cytokines and insulin sensitivity.

The finding of ideal biomarkers is expected to be an unprecedented development in which treatments for metabolic disorders will be more directed and efficient. This could be in the form of less unnecessary treatments, decreased occurrences of the associated side effects, and of course the overall reduced healthcare costs. The escalating attention in adipokines, and recently also in myokines and hepatokines, as potential indicators of insulin sensitivity, signals a very promising and easy to pursue line of research. The adipose tissue (AT) is the one that secretes numerous bioactive substances that are getting into the regulation of chronic inflammation and insulin resistance, which together with genetic factors conducive to its emergence and progression, are considered as the most principal factors for T2DM. The research on adipokines which act as both antiinflammatory and proinflammatory agents is opening revealing them as a new molecule in adipo-tissue inflammation in the context of obese states (Pei et al., 2022). Here, we present the up-to-date news of these biomarkers, underlining their fundamental roles in triggering the inflammatory processes linked to metabolic malfunctions, with the aspiration of developing therapeutic strategies that are more specific and more working in the fight against insulin resistance and T2DM (Fig. 5.8).

6.1 Hepatokines

Fetuin-A (FetA), the protein, happens to be the main contributor to the inflammation in the adipose tissue (AT) at issue with obesity. FetA excites the arrival of proinflammatory cytokines from both adipocytes and macrophages, resulting in the boom of inflammatory environment typical of obesity (Song et al., 2011). Also, FetA has been determined to decrease adiponectin levels in human adipocytes, a hormone that takes part in protecting the body in its metabolic processes by stimulating insulin sensitiveness and induction of antiinflammatory effects. Its engagement in provoking swelling and downplay of adiponectin gives support to its claim in the induction of some metabolic disorders such as Type II diabetes (T2DM).

Since the gutkin Fet-A impacts the earlier stages of inflammation process and lowers insulin responsiveness, it seems to be quite an appropriate target in developing a novel approach for obesity-induced inflexion and the abiding T2DM. FetA may be the object of treatment that commonly directs toward the long-term or lasting stage of this type of inflammation in the AT, so at the same time insulin treatment and improved metabolic health were also achieved. Half of the problem of obesity-related inflammation would be solved by the activations of these treatments by giving a chance for the treatment and avoidance of T2DM, and as well correcting metabolic conditions in some of the affected individuals. The activation of research will further delve likely impacts of FetA blocking on causing a therapeutic strategy, which in turn sets the stage for the initiation of novel therapeutic approaches for the metabolic disorders that stem from obesity.

6.2 DPP4

Dipeptidyl peptidase 4 (DPP4), which can be used in reference to the T cell surface marker CD26, is participants the membrane protein transferring of about 110 kDa and establishment of the membrane surface it. It is mainly found in various cell types, which are endothelial cells, immune cells, and adipocytes, etc. (Klemann et al., 2016). The main biological task of DPP4 is to cut N-terminal dipeptides from the peptides. It is most well-known for its influx of nucleine hormones like GLP-1 and GIP.DPP4, through the action of its proteolytic activity, is doing a regulation in the process that marks the stimulus of insulin secretion by pancreatic islets. The decrease in insulin secretion levels as a result of breaking down of glucose causes the formation of a condition wherein glucose does not get equally distributed in the blood vessels due to the glucose homeostasis. In this manner, DPP4 functions as an essential factor in the metabolism of insulin and glucose which makes it the main player in the pathological process of Type II diabetes (T2DM).

For quite some time now, the blockage of DPP4 has been a means of treating T2DM. DPP4 inhibitors, a family of products designed to keep the performance of GLP-1 and GIP, which in return, the secretion of insulin, proper glucose regulation, and suppression of glucose rises that commonly happen in diabetic individuals (Anderluh et al., 2016). As they prevent the degradation of the incretins, DPP4 inhibitors are a very important part of the toolset that is used to defeat diabetes. Given its participation in multiple pathways and its expression in many different cell types, DPP4 is still the area of research in developing new drugs to stabilize glycemic levels and help with insulin resistance in metabolic diseases.

6.3 FGF-21

The fibroblast growth factor-21 (FGF-21) is a ~22-kDa protein which is a member of the fibroblast growth factor (FGF) family but acts in a unique endocrine manner proving to be a significant regulator of various metabolic processes. Unlike other cellular signaling factors for instance, this type of protein functions all over the whole body by doing things for example affecting the energy balance in the body, lipid metabolism and glucose regulation (Geng et al., 2020). FGF21 is a new candidate that can cure metabolic diseases and the research done on this theme attracts many researchers leading to gene therapies and various FGF21 analogs. These alternative approaches are very potential especially when they are used in the treatment of dyslipidemia; they manage to do that by improving the lipid profile and decreasing the triglycerides levels. However, FGF21's hypoglycemic effect is not that impressive which shows the multifaceted role of FGF21 in glucose metabolism.

FGF21 not only influences lipid and glucose metabolism but also participates in the regulation of inflammation in the brain and pancreas. It shields the hypothalamus against obesity-associated inflammation, a disease usually linked to metabolic disorders. Decreased expression of FGF21 has been related to enhance hypothalamic inflammation, a condition that aids in the advancement of obesity and its difficulties. Moreover, FGF21 has been revealed to be antiinflammatory in the pancreas of high-fat diet (HFD)-induced obesity models making it a promising therapeutic agent for metabolic unhealthy conditions.

6.4 Myokines

6.4.1 Irisin

Irisin, a newly discovered myokine that is created when muscles are used and then divided from the fibronectin type III domain including protein five (FNDC5) in the muscle. This 112-amino-acid fragment with a molecular weight of 12 kDa shows high genetic similarity between humans and mice. Irisin, in addition to its muscle presence, can also be found in adipose tissue (AT), thus, its role in metabolic regulation is more extensive (Bernardes et al., 2024). The most significant contribution of Irisin is its capability to stimulate the browning of white adipose tissue by means of fostering the transition of white fat cells to beige fat cells, which leads to the process of thermogenesis through the elevation of uncoupling protein-1 (UCP-1). This thermogenic action reinforces irisin's role as a major player in energy production and weight control.

New researches have also emphasized the strong antiinflammatory effects of irisin. It was observed to be of benefit from the control of inflammation in a wide range of cell types which include adipocytes, macrophages, hepatocytes, pancreatic β-cells, and endothelial cells. These impacts are triggered by certain main pathways such as TLR4/MyD88 being necessary for NF-κB activation and the NLRP3 inflammasome, which are crucial for the body's inflammatory response. This dual function in metabolic regulation and inflammation suggests that irisin could be formulated as a drug to treat obesity and related diseases.

6.4.2 IL-6

Interleukin-6 (IL-6) is a cytokine with a molecular weight of approximately 24 kDa that belongs to the gp130 cytokine superfamily. IL-6 has long been identified as a proinflammatory cytokine, the main producers of which are immune cells such as macrophages and T-cells. Nevertheless, it is secreted not only by these cells but also by other somatic cells, when an injury has occurred or an infection has developed. Its release marks the beginning of the body's response to inflammation and thus, it seems to play a central role in the immunity at the infection site. Meanwhile, IL-6 presents a clear-cut duality pattern, as it not only behaves as a proinflammatory mediator, but it also acts as antiinflammatory ones working in the repair process of the damaged tissues when the body context is different. Upon the activation of the classical signaling route of IL-6, the cytokine becomes bound to the IL-6 receptors that are attached to the membrane of the cells, thus the downstream signaling cascades are unregulated and the inflammation occurs. This way is the most prevalent in their activation in immune cells and it is connected to the acute -phase responses to infections or injuries.

Due to its participation in both inflammation and metabolism, IL-6 still is the main candidate for therapeutic intervention. Modulating its signal pathways is likely to lead to new therapies in the treatment of the diseases of inflammation, and at the same time saving the metabolic effects of positive. The implication of the dual roles that cytokines play in inflammation and the immune system is a key determinant in the development of successful therapies.

7. Perspectives of new approach to improve insulin sensitivity and inflammatory cytokines

7.1 Drug based therapy

A metabolic disorder like Type II diabetes (T2DM) and inflammation are treated with drug which regulates the inflammatory cytokines and enhances insulin sensitivity is the healthcare habit that needs to be adapted. Such treatments not only deal with insulin resistance but also aim for prolonged low-grade chronic inflammation that is the main disease-progression factor. There are different categories of drugs that are of great importance for both the improvement of insulin sensitivity and the regulation of inflammatory cytokines. Regarding the glucose lowering effect, drugs such as thiazolidinedione exhibited the best performance of reducing the markers of inflammation as opposed to the other therapies (Goltsman et al., 2016). This consequence could have arisen through the inhibition by peroxisome proliferator-activated receptor-γ (PPAR-γ) trans repression of inflammatory-response genes. In other words, the drug set-up a decrease in the inflammation reaction that is the reason for the positive effects. The drugs, due to their antiinflammatory effects, do not have any added benefit to their glucose level modulation observed; therefore it is a direct effect free from any glucose influence.

Statins are another group of drugs that are commonly used in diabetes mellitus and also cause antiinflammatory action. Statins block the action of HMG-CoA reductase, thus, resulting in a marked reduction in cholesterol levels (Castro et al., 2016).

Furthermore, research has already established the potential use of statins for the purposes of reducing the levels of CRP (C-reactive protein, acute-phase reactant) by 25%–30%. This effect does not depend on the dose and does not produce any dose-related changes. The lower CRP levels do not reflect the lipid-decreasing levels, suggesting that the action is a direct effect of statins. CRP is a predictor of nonischemic myocardial dysfunction.

DPP-4 inhibitors are the mainstay of vascular protection by ensuring the bioavailability of GLP-1 and subsequently its action.GLP-1 augments insulin release not only through increasing the insulin secretion but also by the numerous mechanisms that help maintain low glucose levels (Rosenstock et al., 2006). It involves reducing the glucagon production, the retardation of gastric emptying, and probably the suppression of hunger. In fact, the contribution of GLP-1 to beta-cell health might be mainly realized by the proliferation and the elimination of indigenous cases of apoptosis. This in turn would be able to give further boost to glucose management.However, the part of DPP-4 inhibitors in the regulation of inflammatory cytokines and vasotropic actions yet to be explored and leaving a space for further trials.

7.2 Gene-based therapy

Gene therapy approaches are designed to enhance insulin sensitivity and regulate inflammatory cytokines offer promising solutions for treating metabolic disorders like Type II diabetes (T2DM) and obesity-related inflammation (Yue et al., 2019). These therapies target specific genetic pathways involved in insulin signaling, glucose metabolism, and the body's inflammatory response, providing a novel strategy for addressing both insulin resistance and chronic inflammation.

7.2.1 Glucose transporters (GLUTs) and sodium-glucose cotransporters (SGLTs)

Regulation of glucose flux in muscle and liver tissues is significantly influenced by glucose transporters (GLUTs). GLUT4, encoded by the Slc2a4 gene, and GLUT2, encoded by the Slc2a2 gene, are presenting the results on gene therapy in the treatment of Type II diabetes (T2DM), as their reexpression together with muscle and liver can fraudulently increase blood sugar. Sodium-glucose cotransporters (SGLTs) are involved in the transport of reabsorbed glucose from the glomerulus to the blood (Wang et al., 2020). In patients with T2DM, expression of SGLT1 increases by 3.5 times, which is one of the reasons between higher blood glucose levels mainly during the fasting interval and after meals, as well as HbA1c rise. On the other hand, the expression levels of SGLT2 and GLUT2 are reduced in diabetic individuals. Therefore, inhibiting SGLT1 and/or increasing SGLT2 expression could be a possible approach to reduce hyperglycemia in T2DM patients.

7.2.2 Sirtuin 6 (SIRT6)

Recent studies suggested that SIRT6 is an important regulator in the onset and progression of metabolic diseases such as Type II diabetes (T2DM). SIRT6 has been found to stimulate insulin release in the pancreas thus suppressing gluconeogenesis and synthesis of triglycerides in the liver as well as inhibiting obesity. In knockout mice models, the inhibition of SIRT6 has also demonstrated that it improved glucose tolerance, glycolysis and the expression of glucose transporters GLUT1 and GLUT4 in skeletal muscle were unregulated (Khan et al., 2018). However, muscle-specific knockout of SIRT6 induced impaired glucose regulation and insulin resistance. Under these conditions, the expression of glucose and lipid uptake genes, fatty acid oxidation, and mitochondrial oxidative phosphorylation were decreased because of down-regulated AMPK activity. In contrast, overexpression of SIRT6 in C2C12 myotubes led to the activation of AMPK, which in turn, maintained metabolic balance (Zhong et al., 2010).

7.2.3 Fibroblast growth factors (FGFs)

Fibroblast growth factors are a class of promising targets being explored for gene therapy in relation to T2DM. Some of the family members of FGFs including FGF1, FGF19 and FGF21 are the most important in this family and they have a dominant role mobilizing the glucose level. There is evidence that FGF1 knockout mice showed symptoms of diabetes, including increased blood glucose levels and insulin resistance. Beyond this, a single intra cerebroventricular (ICV) injection of FGF1 normalized glucose levels in diabetic mice for at least 18 weeks, without side effects such as hypoglycemia or weight gain. In contrast, FGF19 primarily regulates glycogen metabolism, and its antidiabetic effects are closely linked to the central nervous system (Beenken & Mohammadi, 2012). ICV injection of FGF19 improves glycemic control and enhances insulin sensitivity by suppressing hypothalamic activity. Additionally, FGF21 plays a role in regulating glucose and lipid homeostasis and is notably elevated in individuals with impaired glucose tolerance, increasing further in patients with overt type 2 diabetes mellitus (T2DM) (Fazeli et al., 2015).

7.3 Combinational therapy

Combination therapy, which is the use of two or more drugs to control hyperglycemia, is a treatment process that offers the patient multiple advantages, one of these being the ability to attack various pathophysiological processes that lead to hyperglycemia. In clinical studies, initial combination therapy appeared to be more effective in controlling blood sugar than monotherapy or a stepwise approach to treatment. Some preliminary evidence has proposed that initial combination therapy keeps β-cell function intact and is most prone to T2D complications (Xie et al., 2023). From the perspective of glycemic control alone, use of agents with a significant glucose-lowering effect would be appropriate for patients with initial elevated HbA1c levels. The VERIFY (Vildagliptin Efficacy in Combination with Metformin for Early Treatment of Type 2 Diabetes) study is an exception to the general evidence in the area it has been observed that continued dual therapy shows long-term (5-year) patient benefits (Ding. et al., 2022). The usage of SGLT2 inhibitors in combination with metformin together could result in the two medications not just controlling the glucose level but also lessening the occurrences of heart failure and cardiovascular complications. It would therefore be even higher treatment quality, for example, as evidenced by the reduction of heart-related deaths and invalidity, and it could be considered as an excellent choice for those diabetic patients with the heart problems. Additionally, the combination therapy that is being analyzed is exclusive to the metabolic and cardiovascular elements of the disease and therefore, it offers a more elaborate mode of treatment.

7.4 Immunotherapy

Research over past few years aimed at preventing and treating the disease has concentrated on immunotherapy for Type 1 diabetes (T1D). A cure that would keep autoimmunity at bay on a long-term basis is still not available now, but science shows that developments in the prediction of T1D onset, immunological mechanisms involved, and β cell decline progression suppression have been made (Nera et al., 2015). With these great changes, closer interventions for T1D management are now possible. Regulatory T cells are essential in the development of the autoimmune disease of NOD mouse and mensurative measures have been to identify and mark the autoreactive ones in T1D individuals, along with the ablation of the newly generated memory T cells to be affected to T1D. Moreover, our dual antiCD20 antibody (ublituximab) and abatacept are also evaluated in TrialNet's second-line secondary prevention trials at-risk relatives and are already showing promise. Here, the response in each of these studies is modeled in an individual format and depicted (Fox et al., 2020). Nonetheless, using T cell-based therapies that work earlier with lessings of T cell traffic might be the issue at stake in the recent clinical scenario of the β cells.

8. Conclusion

In conclusion, cytokines are fundamental in regulating insulin sensitivity, serving as both mediators and regulators of various metabolic processes. They function within a delicate balance that influences the body's response to insulin and its ability to maintain glucose homeostasis. Proinflammatory cytokines such as TNF-α, IL-1β, and IL-6 are prominent in promoting insulin resistance. These cytokines trigger inflammatory responses that disrupt insulin signaling pathways, particularly by interfering with insulin receptor function and downstream signaling molecules, such as IRS-1 and Akt. This disruption impairs glucose uptake in key tissues, including skeletal muscle, liver, and adipose tissue, contributing to the development of insulin resistance.

Conversely, antiinflammatory cytokines, such as IL-10 and IL-13, work to mitigate the harmful effects of inflammation by promoting an antiinflammatory environment that preserves insulin sensitivity. They help restore proper signaling in insulin target tissues and maintain metabolic homeostasis by suppressing the inflammatory cascades that lead to insulin resistance. Additionally, some cytokines, like IL-6, exhibit dual roles, functioning as both proinflammatory and antiinflammatory, depending on the context and signaling environment.

The interplay between proinflammatory and antiinflammatory cytokines is critical in determining the overall impact on insulin sensitivity. Disruptions in this balance, often observed in conditions like obesity and metabolic syndrome, lead to chronic low-grade inflammation, which perpetuates insulin resistance. The accumulation of visceral fat in obesity is particularly significant, as adipose tissue acts as a major source of proinflammatory cytokines, driving systemic inflammation and impairing insulin action.

This chronic inflammatory state is a central mechanism in the pathogenesis of type 2 diabetes (T2D), where long-term insulin resistance leads to compensatory hyperinsulinemia and eventual β-cell dysfunction. As the pancreas becomes unable to meet the increased demand for insulin, blood glucose levels rise, resulting in hyperglycemia and the progression to overt T2D.

Given the pivotal role of cytokines in insulin sensitivity and resistance, understanding the complex interactions between these signaling molecules provides valuable insights into the development of therapeutic strategies. Targeting specific cytokines or modulating the pro and antiinflammatory balance may offer novel approaches to enhance insulin sensitivity and prevent or treat insulin resistance and diabetes. Therapies that inhibit proinflammatory cytokines or enhance antiinflammatory signaling could potentially alleviate insulin resistance, improve metabolic outcomes, and reduce the burden of T2D.

References

Abdel-Moneim, A., Bakery, H. H., & Allam, G. (2018). The potential pathogenic role of IL-17/Th17 cells in both type 1 and type 2 diabetes mellitus. *Biomedicine & Pharmacotherapy, 101*, 287–292.

Alexandraki, K., Piperi, C., Kalofoutis, C., Singh, J., Alaveras, A., & Kalofoutis, A. (2006). Inflammatory process in type 2 diabetes: The role of cytokines. *Annals of the New York Academy of Sciences, 1084*, 89–117.

Anderluh, M., Kocic, G., Tomovic, K., Kocic, R., Deljanin-Ilic, M., & Smelcerovic, A. (2016). Cross-talk between the dipeptidyl Peptidase-4 and stromal cell-derived Factor-1 in stem cell homing and myocardial repair: Potential impact of dipeptidyl Peptidase-4 inhibitors. *Pharmacology & Therapeutics, 167*, 100–107.

Arango Duque, G., & Descoteaux, A. (October 7, 2014). Macrophage cytokines: Involvement in immunity and infectious diseases. *Frontiers in Immunology, 5*, 491.

Beenken, A., & Mohammadi, M. (2012). The structural biology of the FGF19 subfamily. *Advances in Experimental Medicine & Biology, 728*, 1–24.

Bernardes-Ribeiro, M., Patrone, L. G. A., Cristina-Silva, C., et al. (2024). Exercise derived myokine irisin as mediator of cardiorespiratory, metabolic and thermal adjustments during central and peripheral chemoreflex activation. *Scientific Reports, 14*, Article 12262.

Boshtam, M., Asgary, S., Kouhpayeh, S., Shariati, L., & Khanahmad, H. (2017). *Inflammation, 40*, 340.

Burska, A. N., Sakthiswary, R., & Sattar, N. (2015). Effects of tumour necrosis factor antagonists on insulin sensitivity/resistance in rheumatoid arthritis: A systematic review and meta-analysis. *PLoS One, 25; 10*(6), Article e0128889.

Castro, M. R., Simon, G., Cha, S. S., et al. (2016). Statin use, diabetes incidence and overall mortality in normoglycemic and impaired fasting glucose patients. *Journal of General Internal Medicine, 31*(5), 502–508.

Christensen, A. A., & Gannon, M. (2019). The beta cell in type 2 diabetes. *Current Diabetes Reports, 19*, 81.

Ding, Y., Liu, Y., Qu, Y., Lin, M., Dong, F., Li, Y., et al. (2022). Efficacy and safety of combination therapy with vildagliptin and metformin vs. metformin monotherapy for type 2 diabetes mellitus therapy: A meta-analysis. *European Review for Medical and Pharmacological Sciences, 26*(8), 2802–2817.

Donath, M. Y., & Shoelson, S. E. (2011). Type 2 diabetes as an inflammatory disease. *Immunology, 11*(2), 98–107.

Edghill, E. L., Flanagan, S. E., Patch, A. M., Boustred, C., Parrish, A., Shields, B., Shepherd, M. H., Hussain, K., Kapoor, R. R., Malecki, M., MacDonald, M. J., & Stoy, J. (2008). Neonatal diabetes international collaborative group insulin mutation screening in 1044 patients with diabetes: Mutations in the INS gene are a common cause of neonatal diabetes but a rare cause of diabetes diagnosed in childhood or adulthood. *Diabetes, 57*, 1034–1042.

Estall, J. L., Kahn, M., Cooper, M. P., Fisher, F. M., Wu, M. K., Laznik, D., Qu, L., Cohen, D. E., Shulman, G. I., & Spiegelman, B. M. (2009). Sensitivity of lipid metabolism and insulin signaling to genetic alterations in hepatic peroxisome proliferator-activated receptor-gamma coactivator-1alpha expression. *Diabetes, 58*, 1499–1508.

Falik Zaccai, T. C., et al. (2014). Two novel mutations identified in familial cases with donohue syndrome. *Molecular Genetics & Genomic Medicine, 2*(1), 64–72.

Fazeli, P. K., Lun, M., Kim, S. M., Bredella, M. A., Wright, S., et al. (2015). FGF21 and the late adaptive response to starvation in humans. *The Journal of Clinical Investigation, 125*, 4601–4611.

Fox, E., Lovett-Racke, A. E., Gormley, M., Liu, Y., Petracca, M., Cocozza, S., Shubin, R., Wray, S., Weiss, M. S., Bosco, J. A., Power, S. A., Mok, K., & Inglese, M. (2020). A phase 2 multicenter study of ublituximab, a novel glycoengineered anti-CD20 monoclonal antibody, in patients with relapsing forms of multiple sclerosis. *Multiple Sclerosis*, Article 1352458520918375.

Geng, L., Lam, K. S. L., & Xu, A. (2020). The therapeutic potential of FGF21 in metabolic diseases: From bench to clinic. *Nature Reviews Endocrinology, 16*, 654–667.

Goltsman, I., Khoury, E. E., Joseph, W., & Zaid, A. (2016). Does thiazolidinedione therapy exacerbate fluid retention in congestive heart failure? *Pharmacology & Therapeutics, 168*, 75–97.

Grasso, V., et al. (2013). Six cases with severe insulin resistance (SIR) associated with mutations of insulin receptor: Is a Bartter-like syndrome a feature of congenital SIR? *Acta Diabetologica, 50*(6), 951–957.

Huang, K., Xu, B., Hu, S. Q., Chu, Y. C., Hua, Q. X., Qu, Y., Li, B., Wang, S., Wang, R. Y., Nakagawa, S. H., Theede, A. M., Whittaker, J., et al. (2004). How insulin binds: The B-chain α-helix contacts the L1 β-helix of the insulin receptor. *Journal of Molecular Biology, 341*, 529–550.

Kany, S., Vollrath, J. T., & Relja, B. (November 28, 2019). Cytokines in inflammatory disease. *International Journal of Molecular Sciences, 20*(23), 6008.

Kataria, Y., Ellervik, C., & Mandrup-Poulsen, T. (2019). Treatment of type 2 diabetes by targeting interleukin-1: A meta-analysis of 2921 patients. *Seminars in Immunopathology, 41*(4), 413–425.

Kawamori, D., & Kulkarni, R. N. (2009). Insulin modulation of glucagon secretion: The role of insulin and other factors in the regulation of glucagon secretion. *Islets, 1*, 276–279.

Khan, R. I., Nirzhor, S. S. R., & Akter, R. (2018). A review of the recent advances made with SIRT6 and its implications on aging related processes, major human diseases, and possible therapeutic targets. *Biomolecules, 8*(3), 44.

Klemann, C., Wagner, L., Stephan, M., & von Horsten, S. (2016). Cut to the chase: A review of CD26/dipeptidyl peptidase-4's (DPP4) entanglement in the immune system. *Clinical and Experimental Immunology, 185*(1), 1–21.

Kulbe, H., Chakravarty, P., Leinster, D. A., Charles, K. A., Kwong, J., Thompson, R. G., Coward, J., Schioppa, T., Robinson, S. C., & Gallagher, W. M. (2012). *Cancer Research, 72,* 66.

Kuryłowicz, A., & Koźniewski, K. (2020). Anti-inflammatory strategies targeting metaflammation in type 2 diabetes. *Molecules, 25*(9), 2224.

Lee, M., Park, H., Youn, J., Oh, E. T., Ko, K., Kim, S., & Park, Y. (2006). Interleukin-10 plasmid construction and delivery for the prevention of type 1 diabetes. *Annals of the New York Academy of Sciences, 1079,* 313–319.

Li, M., Chi, X., Wang, Y., et al. (2022). Trends in insulin resistance: Insights into mechanisms and therapeutic strategy. *Signal Transduction and Targeted Therapy, 7,* 216.

Longo, N., et al. (1999). Progressive decline in insulin levels in Rabson-Mendenhall syndrome. *Journal of Clinical Endocrinology & Metabolism, 84*(8), 2623–2629.

Lucas, S., Taront, S., Magnan, C., Fauconnier, L., Delacre, M., Macia, L., Delanoye, A., Verwaerde, C., Spriet, C., Saule, P., et al. (2012). Interleukin-7 regulates adipose tissue mass and insulin sensitivity in high-fat diet-fed mice through lymphocyte-dependent and independent mechanisms. *PLoS One, 7,* Article e40351.

Magkos, F., Su, X., Bradley, D., Fabbrini, E., Conte, C., Eagon, J. C., Varela, J. E., Brunt, E. M., Patterson, B. W., & Klein, S. (2012). Intrahepatic diacylglycerol content is associated with hepatic insulin resistance in obese subjects. *Gastroenterology, 142,* 1444–1446.e2.

Malek, R., et al. (2010). Treatment of type B insulin resistance: A novel approach to reduce insulin receptor autoantibodies. *Journal of Clinical Endocrinology & Metabolism, 95*(8), 3641–3647.

Mandal, P., Park, P. H., McMullen, M. R., Pratt, B. T., & Nagy, L. E. (2010). The anti-inflammatory effects of adiponectin are mediated via a heme oxygenase-1-dependent pathway in rat Kupffer cells. *Hepatology, 51*(4), 1420–1429. https://doi.org/10.1002/hep.23427

Nakagawa, S. H., Tager, H. S., & Steiner, D. F. (2000). Mutational analysis of invariant valine B12 in insulin: Implications for receptor binding. *Biochemistry, 39,* 15826–15835.

Nera, K. P., Kylaniemi, M. K., & Lassila, O. (2015). Regulation of B cell to plasma cell transition within the follicular B cell response. *Scandinavian Journal of Immunology, 82,* 225–234.

Neurath, M. F. (2014). Cytokines in inflammatory bowel disease. *Nature Reviews Immunology, 14*(5), 329–342.

Ogawa, A., Andoh, A., Araki, Y., Bamba, T., & Fujiyama, Y. (2004). Neutralization of interleukin-17 aggravates dextran sulfate sodium-induced colitis in mice. *Clinical Immunology, 110,* 55–62.

Palmer, N. D., Stevens, R. D., Antinozzi, P. A., Anderson, A., Bergman, R. N., Wagenknecht, L. E., Newgard, C. B., & Bowden, D. W. (2015). Metabolomic profile associated with insulin resistance and conversion to diabetes in the insulin resistance atherosclerosis study. *Journal of Clinical Endocrinology & Metabolism, 100,* E463–E468.

Pei, J., Wang, B., & Wang, D. (2022). Current studies on molecular mechanisms of insulin resistance. *Journal of Diabetes Research,* Article 1863429.

Petersen, K. F., Oral, E. A., Dufour, S., Befroy, D., Ariyan, C., Yu, C., Cline, G. W., DePaoli, A. M., Taylor, S. I., Gorden, P., & Shulman, G. I. (2002). Leptin reverses insulin resistance and hepatic steatosis in patients with severe lipodystrophy. *Journal of Clinical Investigation, 109,* 1345–1350.

Polychronakos, C., & Li, Q. (2011). Understanding type 1 diabetes through genetics: Advances and prospects. *Nature Reviews Genetics, 12,* 781–792.

Pradhan, A. D., Manson, J. E., Rifai, N., Buring, J. E., & Ridker, P. M. (2001). C-reactive protein, interleukin 6, and risk of developing type 2 diabetes mellitus. *JAMA, 286*(3), 327–334.

Pretorius, E., Bester, J., Vermeulen, N., Alummoottil, S., Soma, P., Buys, A. V., & Kell, D. B. (2015). Poorly controlled type 2 diabetes is accompanied by significant morphological and ultrastructural changes in both erythrocytes and in thrombin-generated fibrin: Implications for diagnostics. *Cardiovascular Diabetology, 14,* 30.

Propper, D. J., & Balkwill, F. R. (2022). Harnessing cytokines and chemokines for cancer therapy. *Nature Reviews Clinical Oncology, 19,* 237–253.

Rehman, K., Akash, M. S. H., Liaqat, A., Kamal, S., Qadir, M. I., & Rasul, A. (2017). Role of Interleukin-6 in development of insulin resistance and type 2 diabetes mellitus. *Critical Reviews in Eukaryotic Gene Expression, 27*(3), 229–236.

Rosenstock, J., Brazg, R., Andryuk, P. J., et al. (2006). Efficacy and safety of the dipeptidyl peptidase-4 inhibitor sitagliptin added to ongoing pioglitazone therapy in patients with type 2 diabetes: A 24-week, multicenter, randomized, double-blind, placebo-controlled, parallel-group study. *Clinical Therapeutics, 28,* 1556–1568.

Scheller, J., Chalaris, A., Schmidt-Arras, D., & Rose-John, S. (2011). The pro- and anti-inflammatory properties of the cytokine interleukin-6. *Biochimica et Biophysica Acta, 1813,* 878–888.

Schenk, S., Saberi, M., & Olefsky, J. M. (2008). Insulin sensitivity: Modulation by nutrients and inflammation. *Journal of Clinical Investigation, 118*(9), 2992–3002.

Shi, J., Fan, J., Su, Q., & Yang, Z. (2019). Cytokines and abnormal glucose and lipid metabolism. *Frontiers in Endocrinology, 10,* 703.

Song, A., Xu, M., Bi, Y., Xu, Y., Huang, Y., Li, M., et al. (2011). Serum fetuin-A associates with type 2 diabetes and insulin resistance in Chinese adults. *PLoS One, 6*(4), Article e19228.

Sprague, A. H., & Khalil, R. A. (2009). *Biochemical Pharmacology, 78,* 539.

Spranger, J., Kroke, A., Möhlig, M., et al. (2003). Inflammatory cytokines and the risk to develop type 2 diabetes: Results of the prospective population-based European prospective investigation into cancer and nutrition (EPIC)-potsdam study. *Diabetes, 52*(3), 812–817.

Stoy, J., De Franco, E., Ye, H., Park, S. Y., Bell, G. I., & Hattersley, A. T. (2021). In celebration of a century with insulin - Update of insulin gene mutations in diabetes. *Molecular Metabolism, 52,* Article 101280.

Takasawa, K., et al. (2019). Clinical characteristics of adolescent cases with type A insulin resistance syndrome caused by heterozygous mutations in the β-subunit of the insulin receptor (INSR) gene. *Journal of Diabetes, 11*(1), 46–54.

Takeuchi, T., et al. (2020). Clinical characteristics of insulin resistance syndromes: A nationwide survey in Japan. *Journal of Diabetes Investigation, 11*(3), 603–616.

Tsalamandris, S., Antonopoulos, A. S., Oikonomou, E., et al. (2019). The role of inflammation in diabetes: Current concepts and future perspectives. *European Cardiology, 14*(1), 50–59.

Velikova, T. V., Kabakchieva, P. P., Assyov, Y. S., & Georgiev, T.A. (2021). Targeting inflammatory cytokines to improve type 2 diabetes control. *BioMed Research International,* Article 7297419.

Wan, Z., Huang, K., Whittaker, J., & Weiss, M. A. (2008). The structure of a mutant insulin uncouples receptor binding from protein allostery. An electrostatic block to the TR transition. *Journal of Biological Chemistry, 283,* 21198–21210.

Wang, T., Wang, J., Hu, X., Huang, X. J., & Chen, G. X. (2020). Current understanding of glucose transporter 4 expression and functional mechanisms. *World Journal of Biological Chemistry, 11*(3), 76–98.

Wautier, J. L., & Wautier, M. P. (June 1, 2023). Pro- and anti-inflammatory prostaglandins and cytokines in humans: *A mini review. International Journal of Molecular Sciences, 24*(11), 9647.

Wilcox, G. (2005). Insulin and insulin resistance. *Clinical Biochemist Reviews, 26,* 19–39.

Willard, D. L., et al. (2016). Type B insulin resistance syndrome. *Current Opinion in Endocrinology Diabetes and Obesity, 23*(4), 318–323.

Xie, X., Wu, C., Hao, Y., Wang, T., Yang, Y., Cai, P., Zhang, Y., Huang, J., Deng, K., Yan, D., & Lin, H. (2023). Benefits and risks of drug combination therapy for diabetes mellitus and its complications: A comprehensive review. *Frontiers in Endocrinology, 14,* Article 1301093.

Yi, M., Li, T., Niu, M., et al. (2024). Targeting cytokine and chemokine signaling pathways for cancer therapy. *Signal Transduction and Targeted Therapy, 9,* 176.

Yue, Z., Zhang, L., Li, C., Chen, Y., Tai, Y., Shen, Y., & Sun, Z. (2019). Advances and potential of gene therapy for type 2 diabetes mellitus. *Biotechnology & Biotechnological Equipment, 33*(1), 1150–1157.

Zhang, J. M., & An, J. (2007). Cytokines, inflammation, and pain. *International Anesthesiology Clinics, 45* (2), 27–37. Spring.

Zhong, L., D'Urso, A., Toiber, D., Sebastian, C., Henry, R. E., Vadysirisack, D. D., Guimaraes, A., Marinelli, B., Wikstrom, J. D., Nir, T., et al. (2010). The histone deacetylase Sirt6 regulates glucose homeostasis via Hif1α. *Cell, 140,* 280–293.

6

Genetic variations influencing immune response

Showkat Hussain

FACULTY OF ALLIED AND HEALTHCARE, GURU KASHI UNIVERSITY, BATHINDA, PUNJAB, INDIA

1. Introduction

The immune system's main function is to protect the body from invasive pathogens. The innate immune system is destined for immediate, nonspecific, responses and the adaptive for late, specific, responses and memory. Individual differences exist in the timing and degree of the programmed responses of each of these immune system arms. The genome of the individual and the epigenetic transcriptional regulation of the genome are presumably accountable for at least some of that inter-individual diversity. The capability of the immune system to differentiate between self and non-self molecules is indispensable for both innate and adaptive immunity. In the context of immunology, self molecules are components of an organism's body that the immune system can differentiate from foreign substances (Alberts 2002). On the other hand, molecules that are identified as foreign are known as non-self molecules. Antigens are a class of non-self molecules that attach to particular immune receptors and trigger an immunological response.Infact these were initially known for their ability to generate antibodies (Sompayrac, 2019).

The macrophages and neutrophils of the innate immune system are indispensable first line of defense against many common microorganisms and are very important for the control of common bacterial infections. Nevertheless, they are not always able to wipe out infectious organisms, and they are unable to identify certain infections. The adaptive immune system's lymphocytes have developed into a more adaptable defense mechanism that also offers better defense against recurrent infections with the same pathogen.

Nonetheless, the innate immune system's cells are pivotal for both triggering and coordinating adaptive immune responses. They also help eradicate infections that an adaptive immune response has targeted. Moreover, because there is a delay of 4–7 days before the initial adaptive immune response takes effect, the innate immune response has a critical role in controlling infections during this period (Janeway 2001).

Type 2 Diabetes Mellitus. https://doi.org/10.1016/B978-0-443-33590-7.00005-8

The specificity of innate and adaptive immunity is often used to differentiate between the two. The adaptive immune system's antigen receptors mediate highly specific responses, whereas the innate immune system's receptors recognize pathogens in a more promiscuous and hence less specific manner. Innate immune receptors recognize a small number of molecules, some of which are evolutionarily conserved and are shared by many infectious agents (Janeway & Medzhitov, 2002). Although their expression may be limited to specific cell types, these germline-encoded receptors are not clonally dispersed. The Toll-like receptor (TLR) family is one of the several innate recognition sensors known as pattern-recognition receptors (Medzhitov et al., 1997). The genes encoding the innate receptors exhibit varying degrees of polymorphism within a species. The genetic basis of immune responses involves several prominent gene families: MHC genes for antigen presentation, cytokine genes for synchronizing immune cell activity, TLR genes for innate immune recognition, and Fc receptor genes for antibody-mediated responses (Jin & Wang, 2003a).

One of the main goals of human genetics is to clarify the mechanisms by which genome variations lead to phenotypic differences, primarily to individual differences in susceptibility to diseases and in sensitivity to drugs. SNPs, or single-nucleotide polymorphisms, are the most prevalent kind of variation in the genome (Chanock, 2001). Nowadays, over 950 million SNPs of the human genome are listed in the dbSNP database thanks to advancements in next-generation sequencing (NGS) technology.Additionally, almost 90% of all SNPs are rare SNPs with a frequency (prevalence in the population) of less than 1% (Sherry, 2001).

Cytokines are an essential secreted signaling molecules that pave the way for communication between cells of the immune system during both innate and acquired immune responses (Graham et al., 2007). Cytokines are indispensable and critical in the polarization, amplification and modulation of immune responses and help to infer which effector mechanisms are executed in response to a given immune challenge (Kourilsky, 2001). Various studies in humans and domesticated animals have shown associated genetic variants at cytokine loci with susceptibility to specific pathogens or with host immunopathology (Bayley et al., 2004). These associations arise due to different cytokine alleles vary in their immune responsiveness, with consequent downstream effects on the development of immune effector functions (Kelso, 1998). In natural populations too, genetic variation at cytokine loci could therefore underlie important differences between individuals in their immune responses or resistance to pathogens. For example, the balance between cytokines promoting Th1- and Th2-type immune responses and, in turn, the modulation of these responses by regulatory T cells, is a major factor in the outcome of the host response to infection (Allen & Maizels, 2011). When bacteria are detected, the innate immune system starts processes to get rid of potentially contagious dangers. Germline-encoded pattern-recognition receptors (PRRs) are used to identify microorganisms by searching the extracellular and intracellular spaces for conserved microbial determinants that act as infection markers (Kumar et al., 2011). The body's capacity to determine and destroy pathogens is substantially affected by variations in the genes encoding Human Leukocyte Antigens (HLA) and T-cell receptors, which also affect the immune response to infections and the vulnerability to different diseases. T-cell receptors are the molecules on T cells that are able to recognize the antigens that are presented to them by HLA molecules, which are a component of the major histocompatibility complex (MHC) (Hudson & Allen, 2016).

Advances in genomic technologies like Genome-Wide Association Studies (GWAS) and Next-Generation Sequencing (NGS) have indeed paved the way for new genes and pathways involved in regulating the immune system. GWAS are potent tools for identifying common genetic variants associated with complex traits or diseases, including those related to the immune system. They can pinpoint specific regions of the genome that are linked to increased susceptibility to certain diseases (Ciani et al., 2019). NGS offers a more comprehensive approach to understanding the genome, including noncoding regions and structural variations. This has made it possible for the identification of rare variants with significant impact on immune function and the discovery of novel genes and pathways. By combining GWAS and NGS, researchers can better comprehend the interplay of common and rare variants in shaping immune responses and disease risk (Ciani et al., 2019).

2. Genetic basis of immune response

The genetic basis of the immune response refers to the way genes influence how the body reacts to foreign invaders and other threats. This includes variations in genes involved in immune cell development, receptor function, and signaling pathways, impacting individual susceptibility to diseases and effectiveness of treatments. Innate and adaptive immune responses are the two ways the immune system responds. The innate immune system provides immediate, nonspecific defense. Its response is affected by genes that control the activity of immune cells like macrophages and neutrophils, which engulf pathogens. The adaptive immune system develops specific responses to pathogens, with T and B cells playing key roles.The adaptive immune response is potent but takes time as depicted in Fig. 6.1. Genetic variations can affect T cell receptor diversity, antibody production, and memory cell formation (Justiz Vaillant, Sabir, and Jan 2025). The immune response is orchestrated by both innate and adaptive immune systems, which rely mainly on genes of Major Histocompatibility Complex (MHC), Cytokinegenes, Toll-Like Receptor (TLR) and Fc Receptor complex for their functionality.

2.1 Major histocompatibility complex (MHC) genes

The Major Histocompatibility Complex (MHC) genes, also known as the human leukocyte antigens (HLA) in humans, are a group of genes that encode proteins involved in antigen presentation to T cells. These genes are located on chromosome 6. The MHC is essential for immune function, playing a cardinal role in recognizing foreign

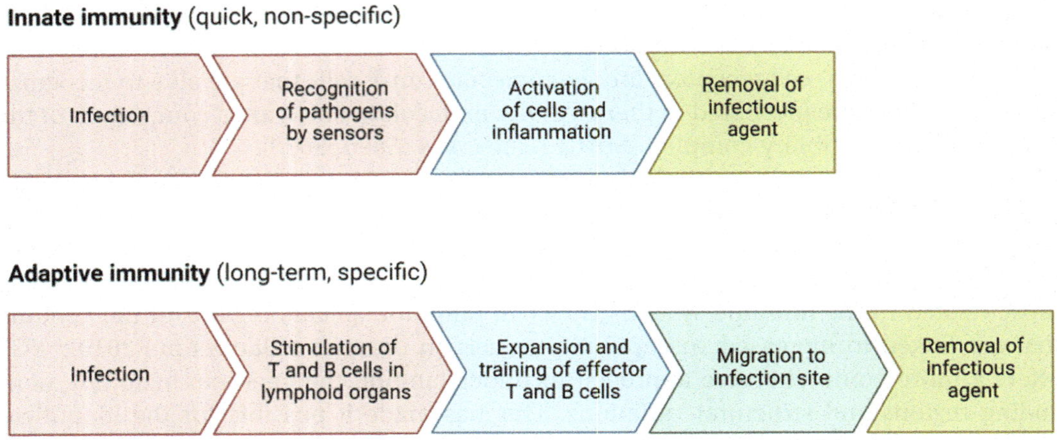

FIGURE 6.1 Basic mechanism of immune response.

substances and initiating immune responses. The Key Functions of the Major Histocompatibility Complex (MHC) are Antigen Presentation, Immune System Recognition, Transplant Rejection and Disease Association (Kelly & Trowsdale, 2017). These MHC molecules are found in all nucleated cells and are involved in antigen presentation to T cells.The T cell has to bind to the antigen-presenting cell (APC) and the antigen-bound MHC molecule in order for them to interact and trigger an immune response. These MHC molecules are produced by a group of genes known as a major histocompatibility complex. Multiple genes code for different parts of the molecules, and several possible combinations of gene products exist.Because of this, it is extremely unlikely that two people will express the same MHC molecules. Since MHC molecules are the main mediators of transplant rejection, they are essential from a clinical standpoint (Alvaro-Benito et al., 2016).

2.1.1 *Role of major histocompatibility complex (MHC) genes in immunity*

MHC molecules are comprised of over 200 genes, encoding for several different molecules involved in immune defense. Class I and class II MHC molecules are the two main types of MHC molecules that are involved in antigen presentation and in eliciting immune response. Both classes of MHC I and MHC II share the task of presenting peptides on the cell surface for recognition by T cells. MHC class I genes (e.g., HLA-A, HLA-B, HLA-C) are expressed on nearly all nucleated cells and present peptides to cytotoxic $CD8^{+}$ T cells. MHC class II genes (e.g., HLA-DPA1, HLA-DPB1, HLA-DQA1, HLA-DQB1, HLA-DRA, HLA-DRB1) are primarily expressed on antigen-presenting cells (APCs) and present peptides to $CD4^{+}$ T cells (Kamal et al., 2025). Pathogens find it challenging to circumvent immune responses in this manner due to two distinct characteristics of the MHC. First, each person has a unique set of MHC molecules with varying ranges of peptide-binding specificities due to the polygenic nature of the MHC, which is made up of several MHC class I and class II genes. Second, the MHC is highly polymorphic, meaning that each gene has several variations in the entire population. The MHC genes are, in fact, the most polymorphic genes known (Janeway, 2001). All the MHC class I and class II molecules can present peptides to T cells, but each protein binds a different range of peptides. Therefore, a single individual can display a far wider variety of peptides when many genes from each MHC class are present, as opposed to when only one MHC molecule from each class is expressed at the cell surface. While the tapasin gene, which binds to both TAP and empty MHC class I molecules, is located at the border of the MHC closest to the centromere, the two TAP genes are located in the MHC class II region, closely grouped with the LMP genes that encode proteasome components. The entire MHC has likely been selected for antigen processing and presentation during evolution due to the genetic linkage between the MHC class I genes, whose products deliver cytosolic peptides to the cell surface, and the TAP, tapasin, and proteasome genes, which encode the molecules that generate peptides in the cytosol and transport them into the endoplasmic reticulum. The genetic organization, diversity, and regulation of MHC molecules along with their role in antigen presentation is shown in Fig. 6.2 (Becar & Kasi, 2025). The transcription of the genes for the proteasome, tapasin, and TAP as well as the MHC class I α-chain and β2-microglobulin is significantly increased when cells are exposed to the interferons IFN-α, -β, or -γ. Early in viral infections, the innate immune response produces interferons.Consequently, this impact improves the cells' capacity to digest viral proteins and display the peptides that are produced at the cell surface. This aids in starting the adaptive immune response against the virus and activating the right T cells. Many of these genes are linked in the MHC, which may help to coordinate the regulation of the genes encoding these components (Janeway, 2001).

2.1.2 Major histocompatibility complex (MHC) genes and polymorphisms

The human major histocompatibility complex or human leukocyte antigen system exhibits polymorphism. Genes encoding Class I MHC molecules, designated A, B, and C, are found at three distinct loci. The loci known as DR, DQ, and DP are linked to class II MHC genes. Each of these loci may have more than one allele, and a person may be homozygous or heterozygous for each gene, resulting in polymorphism. Due to the codominance of the MHC system's genes, all inherited alleles code for the expression of particular MHC molecules on the cell surface. Consequently, a collection of genes for A, B, C, DR, DP, and DQ are inherited by every individual. Because of the remarkable variety, each person's MHC type is special (Meyer et al., 2018). Another distinguishing feature of the HLA molecule is polymorphism. Multiple antigen or allele variations are made possible via polymorphism. Because the structural genes of the HLA class I and class II antigens are the most widely polymorphic in humans, the amino acids in each particular HLA molecule can differ slightly between individuals. In addition to producing different HLA types, this variance results in allograft rejection during tissue transplantation (Tiercy, 2002). To broaden their repertoire of antigen presentation, HLA molecules, which are responsible for presenting intracellular antigens on cell surfaces to

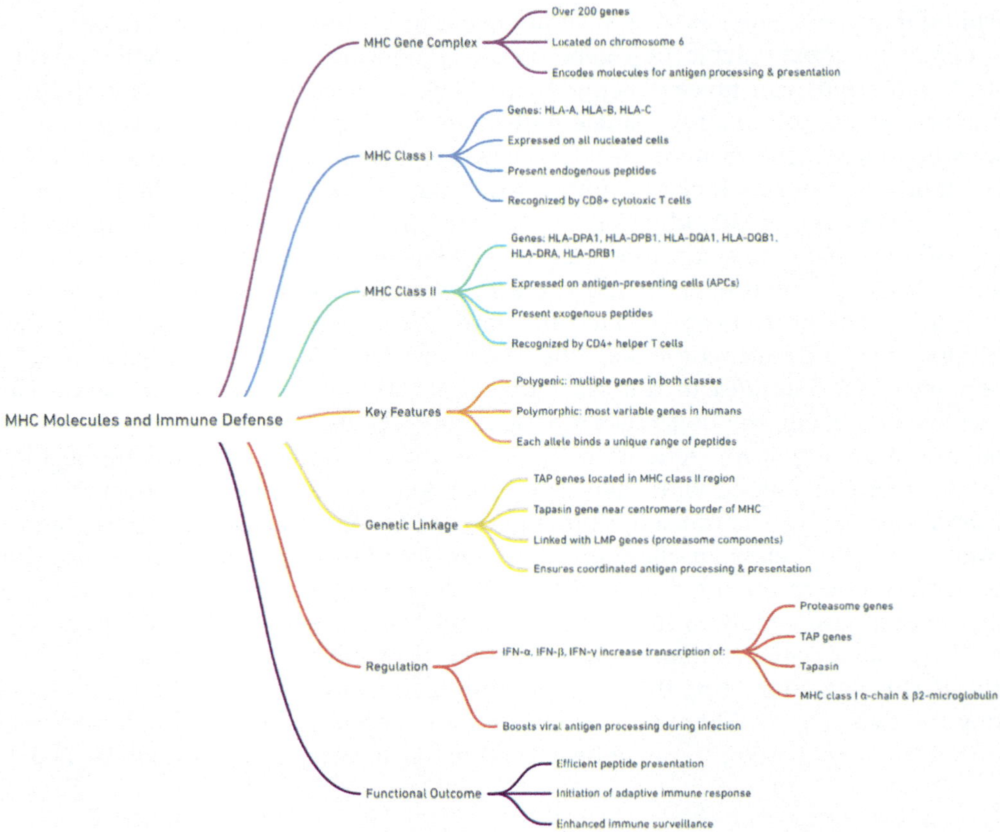
MHC Molecules and Immune Defense
MHC Gene Complex
Over 200 genes
Located on chromosome 6
Encodes molecules for antigen processing & presentation
MHC Class I
Genes: HLA-A, HLA-B, HLA-C
Expressed on all nucleated cells
Present endogenous peptides
Recognized by CD8+ cytotoxic T cells
MHC Class II
Genes: HLA-DPA1, HLA-DPB1, HLA-DQA1, HLA-DQB1, HLA-DRA, HLA-DRB1
Expressed on antigen-presenting cells (APCs)
Present exogenous peptides
Recognized by CD4+ helper T cells
Key Features
Polygenic: multiple genes in both classes
Polymorphic: most variable genes in humans
Each allele binds a unique range of peptides
Genetic Linkage
TAP genes located in MHC class II region
Tapasin gene near centromere border of MHC
Linked with LMP genes (proteasome components)
Ensures coordinated antigen processing & presentation
Regulation
IFN-α, IFN-β, IFN-γ increase transcription of:
Proteasome genes
TAP genes
Tapasin
MHC class I α-chain & β2-microglobulin
Boosts viral antigen processing during infection
Functional Outcome
Efficient peptide presentation
Initiation of adaptive immune response
Enhanced immune surveillance

FIGURE 6.2 MHC molecules and immune defense.

cytotoxic and helper T lymphocytes, have taken up a different approach. This tactic involved a large number of genes that performed duplicate functions but differed slightly in how they were carried out. Small amounts of antigenic proteins, or epitopes, are presented to T cells by all traditional HLA molecules; however, the selection of these epitopic determinants differs significantly amongst the HLA genes and their alleles. Therefore, HLA molecules exhibit broad polymorphism in domains responsible for antigen binding and interactions in variable regions of T cell receptors, while being generally conserved in domains of the protein that interact with conserved components of T cell receptors and their co-receptors (such as CD8 molecules) (Jin & Wang, 2003b). A molecule's functional domains may exhibit selective polymorphism, which can have a significant impact on the presentation and selection of epitopes (Bjorkman & Parham, 1990).

The key benefit of the widespread MHC polymorphism is thought to be the higher probability that members of a particular species will be heterozygous, meaning they will carry two distinct MHC alleles for each HLA locus. Heterozygosity may double an ethnic group's ability to deliver antigens since MHC polymorphism(s) occur in regions that are responsible for epitope binding. Most significantly, because members of the same ethnic group are likely to exhibit distinct HLA phenotypes, the presence of widespread polymorphism greatly expands the group's overall repertoire and increases the species' chances of surviving a wide range of infections (Dawkins et al., 1991). Even though it is challenging to establish a direct link between HLA phenotype and disease susceptibility, it is well established at the molecular level that a single amino acid alteration in the HLA gene sequence can significantly alter the antigen binding affinity and, as a result, the effectiveness of inducing T cell reactivity both in vitro and in vivo (Rivoltini et al., 1996). This can in turn regulate the immune dominance of individual antigens according to the HLA haplotype bore by different individuals.Furthermore, it is worth noting that associations have been observed between HLA phenotype and diseases that may or may not be caused by pathogen (Kozuch & Mayer, 1975). It's interesting to note that in these situations, the significance of the structural alterations brought about by the polymorphism site for the etiology and pathophysiology is still unknown. Polymorphisms can occur in functional sections of molecules, have functional significance, and may have clinical relevance, as we have seen from HLA (Ehrlich & Lemonnier, 2000).

2.2 Cytokine genes

The immune system is essentially a network supersystem utilizing specialized languages for communication between cells.To defend an organism against disease and outside invaders, the immune system is able to communicate effectively and is built to react swiftly,and precisely. The cytokine superfamily of proteins plays a crucial role in the development and control of the immune system and is a vital component of the cell-to-cell signaling network. Cytokines are tiny soluble factors with pleiotropic properties that are produced by many cell types as part of a gene expression pattern that can impact and regulate the function of the immune system (Cohen et al., 1974).

2.2.1 Role of cytokine genes in immunity

Cytokines are essential proteins that are part of a bigger immune program, e.g., T cell subset differentiation.Mature CD4 and CD8 T cells secrete a range of cytokines and migrate out of the thymus with a naive phenotype. Upon encountering antigen-presenting cells (APCs) in the periphery, these T cells come into contact with either major histocompatibility complex (MHC) class I molecules, which present cytosolically generated peptides to CD8 T cells, or MHC class II molecules, which present intracellularly degraded peptides to CD4 T cells. Following activation, CD4 T helper (Th) cells in mice and humans can be divided into two main subpopulations based on their distinctive cytokine and chemokine secretion characteristics (Paul & Seder, 1994). While

Th2 cells primarily produce IL-4, IL-5, IL-6, IL-10, and IL-13, Th1 cells primarily secrete IL-2, interferon-γ (IFN-γ), and tumor necrosis factor-β (TNF-β). Th1 cells induce inflammation, cytotoxicity, and delayed-type hypersensitivity (DTH) via supporting cell-mediated immunity. Th2 cells reduce Th1 cells' inflammatory responses while promoting humoral immunity. This paradigm is a nice example of an integrated biological network and is very useful in simplifying our understanding of typical immune responses and those that turn pathogenic.For instance, the failure to communicate "self" can lead to a loss of tolerance to our own antigens and prompt destructive immune responses to self-tissues and autoimmune disease (Mosmann et al., 1986).

Th2 cytokines, such as IL-4, IL-5, IL-10, IL-13, and IL-6, are essential for immunological responses, especially when it comes to controlling allergic reactions and fighting parasite infections. Th2 cells and other immune cells produce them, and they have the ability to control B-cell responses, promote tissue repair, and modulate inflammation (Copray, 2001). A vital cytokine in Th2 cell growth, IL-4 is essential for the type 2 immune response. IL-4 promotes B-cell development, activation, and antibody isotype switching, especially for IgG and IgE. Because of its well-known anti-inflammatory qualities, IL-4 aids in tissue healing and inflammation reduction (Lebman & Coffman, 1988). Eosinophils, which are crucial in the battle against allergic reactions and parasitic infections, are recruited and activated in large part by IL-5. In order to help produce antibodies, IL-5 promotes the proliferation and differentiation of B-cells (Chaplin, 2010). A versatile cytokine, IL-6 has the ability to mediate inflammation in both pro- and anti-inflammatory ways. By encouraging Th2 responses and suppressing Th1 responses, IL-6 affects the development of T helper cells. IL-6 has the ability to promote B-cell differentiation and proliferation. A strong anti-inflammatory cytokine, IL-10 aids in reducing inflammation and avoiding tissue damage. In order to maintain immunological homeostasis, IL-10 controls the activity of other immune cells, including dendritic and macrophage cells. B cell survival can be improved by IL-10, especially in germinal centers (Tanaka et al., 2014). Goblet cells produce mucus in response to IL-13, which aids in the removal of allergens and pathogens from epithelial surfaces. By promoting the synthesis of collagen and other extracellular matrix constituents, IL-13 can aid in tissue repair. IL-13 has the ability to alter B-cell responses, such as class switching and antibody production (Siddiqui et al., 2021). Several different cell types coordinate their efforts as part of the immune system via a variety of cytokines as shown in Fig. 6.3.

Th1 cells are essential for cell-mediated immunity, especially in the fight against some cancers and intracellular infections. They generate cytokines such as IL-2, IFN-γ, and TNF-β, which stimulate macrophages, neutrophils and improve the function of T cells and natural killer (NK) cells, and encourage the production of opsonizing and complement-fixing antibodies. A T cell growth factor called IL-2 encourages T cells, especially Th1 cells, to proliferate and differentiate. It is a crucial cytokine in the initial phases of T cell reactions. Macrophages are strongly activated by IFN-γ, which improves their capacity to phagocytose and eliminate intracellular infections. Additionally, it promotes antigen presentation and inflammation by upregulating MHC molecules and

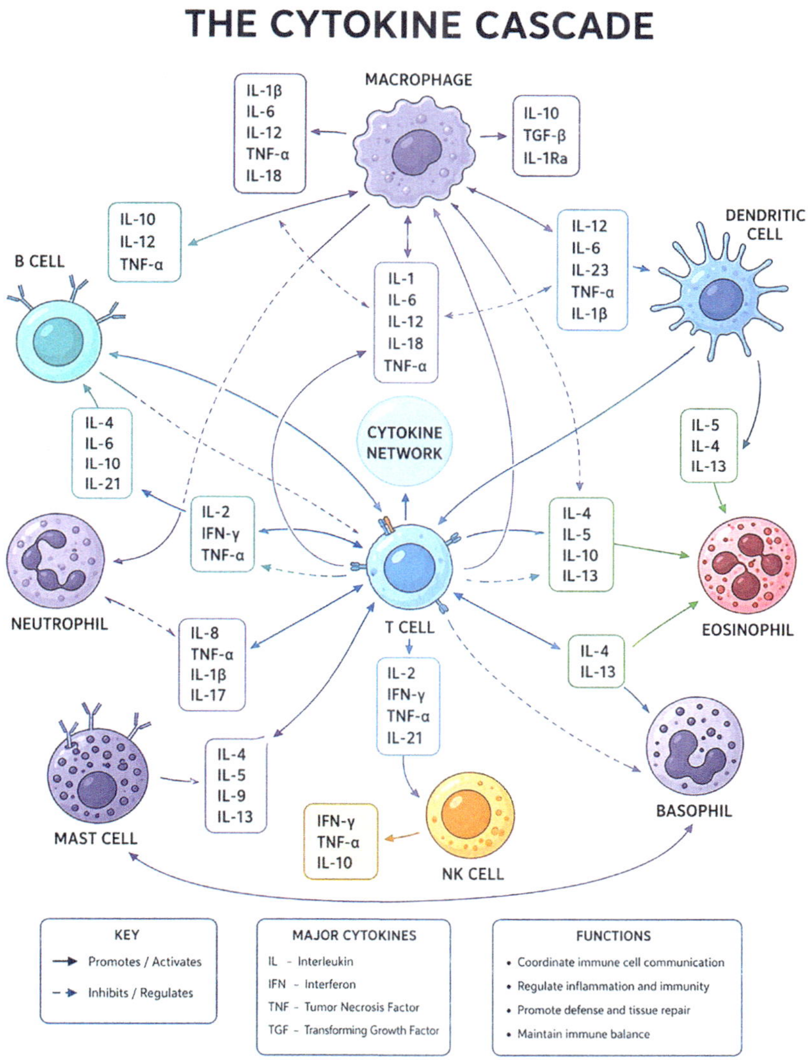

FIGURE 6.3 Showing cytokine cascade.

ICAM-1 on different cells (Viallard et al., 2001). IFN-γ can also alter immune responses, such as preventing anti-tumor immunity, and cause tumor cells to undergo apoptosis. Together with TNF-α, TNF-β regulates the differentiation and proliferation of immune cells. It also has a role in tissue injury and inflammation. Macrophages are activated by IFN-γ and TNF-β, which increases their capacity to phagocytose and eliminate infections (Fig. 6.3). T cells and NK cells, which are crucial for destroying intracellular infections and tumor cells, proliferate and become activated when IL-2 and IFN-γ are present. Th1 cells aid in the synthesis of antibodies that improve phagocytosis and neutralize infections. In order to promote a balanced immune response, Th1 cell cytokines can also alter the functions and kinds of other immune cells (Torre et al., 2002).

2.2.2 Cytokine genes and polymorphisms

Genes that code for cytokines such as IL-6, IL-10, and TNF-α can have variations (polymorphisms) that change how these signaling molecules are produced, which can affect immune responses and disease susceptibility. Conditions like inflammatory bowel disease, asthma, and sepsis are associated with these alterations. Signaling molecules called cytokines are essential to the immune system because they mediate cell-to-cell communication and affect inflammation. Changes in the amount or activity of the cytokine that is encoded can result from genetic variations (polymorphisms) in cytokine genes. A higher risk of contracting or worsening conditions like sepsis, asthma, and inflammatory bowel disease (IBD) has been connected to these changed cytokine production patterns (Chaudhry et al., 2013). Increased vulnerability to inflammatory diseases and sepsis has been linked to polymorphisms in the IL-6 gene. The balance between pro- and anti-inflammatory responses can be impacted by mutations in the gene for IL-10, a crucial anti-inflammatory cytokine that may make people more vulnerable to infections or autoimmune disorders. TNF-α is a cytokine that promotes inflammation, and variations in its gene can affect how severe inflammatory diseases like sepsis and IBD are (Segbefia et al. 2024).

Cytokine polymorphisms are increasingly being studied in order to better understand a number of disorders (Vandenbroeck & Goris, 2003). Cytokines are mostly secreted chemicals that provide cell-to-cell signaling, which affects the surrounding microenvironment. The majority of them are not constitutively expressed, and their expression is strictly controlled due to the signaling function. Remarkably, majority of the polymorphic sites found in cytokine genes thus far have been found in non-coding areas that contain regulatory sequences. The clinical progression of numerous immunological disorders and organ transplantation may be affected by disruptions in the equilibrium between various cytokines (Keen, 2002). The promoter, intronic, and 3′ untranslated regions contain a significant portion of the polymorphisms in cytokine genes and their receptors. By changing the stability of RNA molecules, SNPs in 3′ untranslated regions can still have an impact on gene expression and function. Furthermore, promoter polymorphism may interfere with transcription factors including NF-κB, Jak, STAT, and IRF's ability to bind to regulatory areas. It's interesting to note that a number of transcription and signaling factors essential for controlling cytokine production are also polymorphic (Knight, 2003).

2.3 Toll-like receptor (TLR) genes

Both innate and adaptive immune responses are shaped and initiated by Toll-Like Receptors (TLRs), which are essential pattern recognition receptors. Pathogen-associated molecular patterns (PAMPs) are recognized by TLRs, which sets off signaling cascades that result in the activation of genes that regulate immune responses. These pathways have the ability to affect immune cell formation, stimulate T and B cells, and increase the synthesis of cytokines and other chemicals involved in defense and inflammation (Knight, 2003).

2.3.1 Role of toll-like receptor (TLR) genes in immunity

Toll-like receptors (TLRs) are distinct pattern recognition receptors that are in control of identifying pathogens and triggering innate immune reactions. Since their discovery, TLRs have transformed immunology by bridging the gap between innate immunity cells' initial identification of pathogens and the adaptive immune response's activation. By controlling the activation of antigen-presenting cells and important cytokines, TLRs play a crucial role in connecting innate immunity to adaptive immunity.TLRs are members of the Type I integral membrane glycoprotein family, which is distinguished by the presence of a cytoplasmic Toll/interleukin 1 (IL-1) receptor (TIR) homology domain and extracellular domains with varying numbers of leucine-rich-repeat (LRR) motifs (Fitzgerald & Kagan, 2020). Ten TLRs in humans (TLR1–TLR10) and 12 in mice (TLR1–TLR9 and TLR11–TLR13) have been discovered so far. While TLR11–TLR13 are expressed only in mice and not in humans, TLR1–TLR10 are conserved across mice and humans, however mouse TLR10 is not functional. These receptors can be found in internal compartments including the endoplasmic reticulum, endosome, lysosome, or endolysosome (TLR3, TLR7, TLR8, and TLR9) or on the cell surface (TLR1, TLR2, TLR4, and TLR5) (Kawasaki & Kawai, 2014). The distribution of importantTLRs and their functions in the immune system is shown in Table 6.1.

Cell surface TLRs primarily identify the lipids, lipoproteins, and proteins that make up an organism's membrane. For instance, lipopolysaccharide (LPS) is recognized by TLR4. TLR2 detects many pathogen PAMPs, such as lipoproteins, peptidoglycans, lipoteichoic acids, zymosan, mannan, and glycosylphosphatidylinositol-anchored mucin-like glycoproteins from Trypanosomacruzitrypomastigotes. It can form a heterodimer

Table 6.1 Cellular distribution and function of human TLRs.

Cells	TLR expression	Roles
Neutrophils(PMN)	1,2,4,6,8	Pattern recognition
Mast cells	2,4	Pattern recognition
Monocytes	1,2,4,5,6,8	Pattern recognition
Macrophages	1,2,3,4,6,7,9	Pattern recognition
NK cells	1,(7,9)	Pattern recognition
Resting B cells	(1,4),6,7,(8)9,10	Pattern recognition
iDC (CD11c + iDC)	1,2,3,(5,6,8,10)	Pattern recognition Ag presentation (Ag cross presentation)

with either TLR1 or TLR6 (Kawai & Akira, 2010). All innate immune cells and the vast majority of non-hematopoietic cells, including mast cells, basophils, eosinophils, DCs, neutrophils, macrophages, and epithelial cells, express TLRs. In addition, adaptive immune cells, such as T and B cells, may also have TLRs (Hua & Hou, 2013). Adaptive immunity constitute of humoral immunity and cell-mediated immunity, which are mainly mediated by B lymphocytes and T lymphocytes, respectively. A cluster of differentiation 8 (CD8) + cytotoxic T-lymphocytes (CTLs) and an antigen-specific cluster of differentiation 4 (CD4) + T helper (Th) cells are produced by cell-mediated immunity, also known as cellular immunity, and facilitate B cells in producing antibodies. CTLs recognize and produce molecules that directly kill infected host cells. On the otherhand, Th cells release various cytokines that affect the function of other cells involved in both adaptive and innate immune responses (Bhagavan & Ha, 2011). Antigen-presenting cells (APCs) must simultaneously provide T cells with co-stimulatory signaling and antigen presentation in order to effectively activate and clonally expand antigen-specific T cells. Crucially, microbe-derived adjuvants induce or enhance the production of cytokines, expression of costimulatory molecules, and antigen-presenting activity in APCs. These adjuvants are recognized by TLRs expressed on APCs and enhance APC signaling to promote T cell immune response activation.As a result, TLRs are essential for connecting cell-mediated immunity with innate immunity (Bhagavan & Ha, 2011).

2.3.2 Toll-like receptor (TLR) genes and polymorphisms

In the innate immune response, Toll-Like Receptor (TLR) genes are essential for identifying different pathogens and triggering immunological responses. The operation of the immune system and vulnerability to specific diseases, especially autoimmune and infectious ailments, might be affected by genetic changes or polymorphisms in TLR genes. It is unclear how TLR polymorphisms alter TLR functions, however recent research indicates that SNPs influence receptor function via influencing TLR expression, localization, trafficking, and signaling. For instance, the common TLR1 SNP I602S is linked to abnormal receptor trafficking to the cell surface (Bhagavan & Ha, 2011). Additionally, it has been demonstrated that the R753Q polymorphism modifies the TIR domain's electrostatic potential, which prevents TLR2-TLR6 dimerization, NF-kB activation, and cytokine production.The TLR4 D299G polymorphism suppresses the activation of the transcription factor NF-kB by preventing mutant receptors from interacting with adapters MyD88 and TRIF (Johnson et al., 2007). Type I diabetes (T1D) is an organ-specific autoimmune disease in which pancreatic beta cells are specifically destroyed by Th1 lymphocytes. In 2004, a Korean population was the subject of one of the first investigations concentrating on the identification of SNPs linked to T1D in the TLR2 gene. In this study, SNP rs3804100 (S450S, +1350) was found. Furthermore, a comparable study carried out in Norway produced same findings. Nevertheless, the Spanish sample population showed no such association (Ciesielska et al., 2021).

An overactive and enlarged thyroid gland (Graves' hyperthyroidism), abnormalities of the eyes (Graves' orbitopathy; GO), and localized dermatosis (anterior tibial myxedema;

PTM) are the hallmarks of Graves' disease (GD), a hyperthyroidism linked to organ-specific autoimmune inflammation. A Chinese Cantonese population was used to investigate the relationship between TLR gene polymorphisms and GD. Three SNPs were examined in 331 unrelated controls and 332 GD patients: rs179010 for TLR7, rs5744174 for TLR5, and rs5743565 for TLR1 (Xiao et al., 2014). Numerous hypotheses have been put out to explain the protective function of these polymorphisms. Adapter proteins with TIR domains first trigger adaptive immune responses by altering TLR signaling and releasing a series of signals. Second, the flagellin response to cytokines is attenuated by SNP rs5744174, which decreases vulnerability to bacterial infection. Third, the existence of these particular gene variants may lower the risk of GD because these three SNPs can influence translation, lower TLR protein expression, lower autoantibody or cytokine synthesis, and control the immunological response to ligands (Dvornikova et al., 2020).

The autoimmune condition known as systemic lupus erythematosus affects several systems and is typified by the development of immune complexes, nuclear autoantigens, and a loss of self-tolerance. SNPs of TLRs have also been linked to SLE in other studies. In Asian populations, SNPs of TLR7 (rs3853839), TLR8 (rs3764880), and TLR9 (rs351240) raise the risk of SLE. SNPs for TLR3 (rs3775291), TLR8 (rs3764879), and TLR9 (rs352143) were linked to SLE in Danish samples. These findings imply that genetic variations in specific TLRs are linked to the pathophysiology of SLE and are connected to the clinical phenotype and susceptibility of SLE (Laska et al., 2014).

Rheumatoid arthritis is a prevalent inflammatory systemic autoimmune disease that affects around 1% of adults worldwide. It is characterized by swollen and painful joints that significantly impair quality of life and motor function.In comparison to healthy controls, RA patients' synovial tissue had increased expression levels of several TLR isoforms. RA patients' blood and synovial joints are also rich in TLR3 (host-derived RNA) and TLR4 (HSPB8) ligands. Further evidence of a dysregulated TLR response in RA comes from the fact that TLR4-mediated dendritic cell stimulation led to noticeably greater cytokine concentrations in RA patients compared to controls (Enevold et al., 2010).

2.4 Fc receptor genes

Fc Receptors (FcRs) serve as a link between the effector activities of innate immune cells and antibody-mediated adaptive immunity, making them crucial for both innate and adaptive immune responses. Numerous immune cells contain FcRs, which are able to identify the Fc component of antibodies that have already attached to antigens. They facilitate a variety of processes, such as B cell activation, degranulation, antibody-dependent cell-mediated cytotoxicity (ADCC), and phagocytosis. By immediately identifying and reacting to pathogens without the aid of antibodies, FcRscontribute to innate immunity. Certain FcRs, such as FcαRI, have the ability to connect directly with bacteria and cause their removal. Additionally, FcRs may have a role in the early phases of infection by inducing innate immune responses such as cytokine secretion and inflammation. Pathogen clearance can be aided by ITAM-bearing FcRs, such as FcγRIIA and FcγRIII, which can start signaling pathways that activate innate immune cells. The effector activities of adaptive immunity, especially antibody-mediated responses, depend on FcRs.

They make it possible for effector cells to react to antigens that certain antibodies have identified and bound. Antibody-antigen complexes can activate FcRs on innate immune cells, such as natural killer cells and macrophages, resulting in ADCC and the phagocytosis of infected cells.

Additionally, FcRs control B cell activation and aid in dendritic cell maturation and activation, both of which are critical for the start of adaptive immune responses. The immune response is balanced by FcRs, which comprise both activating and inhibitory receptors. Inflammatory cytokines and other effector molecules are released when FcRs are activated, whereas inhibition can help control immune responses and avoid excessive inflammation. FcRs are involved in tolerance, and if their function is dysregulated, it may lead to the onset of autoimmune disorders.

The type of FcR and the particular Igisotype (IgA, IgD, IgE, IgG, and IgM) affect how immune responses turn out (Pincetic et al., 2014).

2.4.1 Role of Fc receptor genes in immunity

Fc receptor genes are indispensable in the immune system by encoding proteins that bind to the Fc region of antibodies, linking the adaptive and innate immune responses. These receptors, which are present on a variety of immune cells, set off a series of events that have the potential to either activate or modify immune responses, impacting processes such as antibody-mediated cytotoxicity, inflammation, and phagocytosis. Dysregulation of Fc receptor genes can pave the way for autoimmune diseases and other immune-related disorders. FcR are in fact third-type immunoreceptors. They "recognize" antigen–antibody complexes rather than natural antigens like B-cell receptors (BCR) or the binding of antigen-derived peptides to major histocompatibility complex components like T-cell receptors (TCR). When the Fab and Fc components of antibodies attach to particular antigen epitopes and to the cell membrane's FcR, respectively, they act as extracellular adapter molecules. The three ways that an antigen can connect with and communicate with immune system cells are through receptors for BCR, TCR, and FcR. Additionally, FcR produces intracellular signals that alter the biological activity of cells that express them, just like other immunoreceptors do when activated by particular ligands. While some FcR activate cellular responses, others suppress them (Mancardi & Daëron, 2014). The affinity with which antibodies attach to FcR varies. The mass action law governs the reversible binding of antibodies to FcR.A proportion of high-affinity FcR, which can bind monomeric immunoglobulins in the absence of antigen, are occupied in vivo whereas low-affinity FcR, which can bind antibodies as multivalent immune complexes only, are not in spite of the high concentration of circulating immunoglobulins. The dissociation of bound antibodies, however, can release occupied high-affinity FcR. Therefore, the availability of high-affinity FcR is highly dependent on the dissociation constant. In contrast, immune complexes can typically access low-affinity FcR whenever they approach sufficiently (Hulett & Hogarth, 1994).

Antibodies have strong adjuvant properties. These characteristics rely on FcR being expressed by various cell types under various circumstances via various pathways. It is possible that dendritic cell FcR-mediated absorption of antigen–IgG antibody complexes contributes to both cross presentation andthe MHC class II presentation of antigen to T cells (Heyman, 1990). It has been demonstrated that antigen–antibody complexes can activate and mature dendritic cells by binding to activating FcγR on dendritic cells and to fascilitate antigen-specific CD8 responses in vivo (Schuurhuis et al., 2002). It is true that dendritic cells lacking activating FcR cannot cause MHC class I and class II presentation, which in turn prevents an effective antitumor response. IgG-induced immune response improvement is believed to increase efficient memory responses rather than initial responses since it necessitates the production of particular IgG antibodies previously (Desai et al., 2007).

2.4.2 Fc receptor genes and polymorphisms

Significant variation exists in the Fc receptor (FcR) genes, which may affect an individual's susceptibility to certain diseases as well as the way Fc receptors function. Numerous immunological effects can result from these polymorphisms, especially single nucleotide polymorphisms (SNPs), which can change intracellular signaling, expression levels, and receptor affinity for antibodies. The great majority of the genes that code for the Fc receptor exhibit genetic variation, either in the form of copy number changes or SNPs. Despite the fact that numerous SNPs have been found for Fc receptors, it is still unclear how exactly these SNPs affect receptor function for the majority of them. The R131H allelic variant for the low-affinity Fcγ receptor FcγRIIa was one of the first functional SNPs for Fc receptors to be discovered. The extracellular region's membrane proximal Ig-like domain contains position 131, where this point mutation (519G > A) causes an amino acid substitution [arginine (R) to histidine (H)](Clark et al., 1989). According to recent crystallographic research and earlier mutational analysis, this area interacts with the Fc component of IgG through the receptor interface, and the R131H variation controls the affinity of FcγRIIa for human IgG2. In particular, H131 has been demonstrated to bind and facilitate the phagocytosis of hIgG2-coated particles, but the R131 variation is unable to engage with hIgG2. Due to its potential to improve leukocyte activation by IgG2 and increase the ability to remove circulating IgG2 complexes, the H131 variation may be especially significant in circumstances with large IgG2 antibody responses (Warmerdam et al., 1990). For FcγRIII, SNPs influencing the binding affinity for IgG subclasses have also been identified. Two allelic variants of FcγRIIIa that are co-dominantly expressed have either a phenylalanine (F) or a valine (V) at position 158. It has been shown that this one amino acid change increases the V158 allotype's affinity for IgG1 and IgG3 in comparison to F158 and induces the ability to bind IgG4. Additionally, it has been discovered that 158V/V, as opposed to 158F/F, have much higher IgG-induced NK cell activity.Apart from polymorphisms that increase receptor affinity for

IgG subclasses, SNPs that significantly affect Fc receptor functional effector responses after immunoglobulin binding have also been identified. For instance, it has been shown that altering a non-polar isoleucine to a polar threonine at position 232 (I232T) in the transmembrane region may impact receptor function in the inhibitory Fcγ receptor FcγRIIb. It has been demonstrated that the T232 variation translocates less effectively to membrane areas known as lipid rafts that are high in sphingolipids and cholesterol. Consequently, the T232 showed decreased inhibitory activity, which may have been caused by a poorer ability to interact with protein kinases that preferentially dwell in lipid raft membrane regions (Floto et al., 2005).

The substitution of tryptophan (W) for arginine (R) at position 62 (R62W) is a recently discovered functional polymorphism in FcεRII. The W62 variant, as opposed to the R62 version, is resistant to proteolytic shedding after being treated with a variety of different proteases, which may have an impact on the mitogenic activity and receptor function (Meng et al., 2007). Finally, a quite common polymorphism found in the FcαRI coding area is linked to a decreased ability to initiate processes like cytokine release.This polymorphism (844A > G) involves the change of serine 248 to glycine (S248G) within the cytoplasmic domain of the receptor's α chain (Jasek et al., 2004). Compared to equal cross-linking of the receptor on neutrophils from donors homozygous for the S248 variant, IgA-mediated cross-linking of FcαRI on neutrophils from people homozygous for the G248 variant resulted in a considerably higher release of IL-6. In actuality, the G248 form can trigger cytokine release without the FcRγ chain, in contrast to the S248 variation. This ability is thought to be caused, at least in part, by its direct interaction with Lyn, a member of the Src family and a crucial part of the FcαRI signaling cascade.A variety of SNPs that regulate the expression of certain Fcγ and Fcε receptors have been identified. For instance, in exon 3 of the FCGR2C gene, a glutamine residue is changed to a stop codon at position 57 (Q57X) by a single nucleotide substitution at position 202, producing a shortened, non-functional protein. Additionally, homozygous 57X/X donors showed no expression of NK cell surface receptors, whereas NK cells from heterozygous 57Q/X donors showed decreased expression in comparison to 57Q/Q donors (Breunis et al., 2008).

Similarly, it has been demonstrated that certain SNPs, such as −66T > C, −315)C > T, and −335)C > T, inside the promoter of the gene coding for the α chain of the FcεRI (FCER1A), control receptor production by differentially binding and transactivating transcription regulatory factors. For instance, because the −66T variant had an extra GATA-1 binding motif, it showed higher in vitro transcriptional activity than the −66C form (Hasegawa et al., 2003). Similarly, the binding of the Sp1 transcriptional regulator was thought to be responsible for the much greater promoter activity linked to the C to T alteration at position −315 (also known as −344). Comparable SNPs have been found in the promoter regions of the gene that codes for the FcεRI receptor's beta chain. Compared to the −426T and −654C haplotypes, the −426C and −654T haplotypes have been found to have stronger promoter activity and increased YY-1 binding (Nishiyama et al., 2004). Moreover, it has been demonstrated that Fc receptor polymorphisms are closely linked to pathogen susceptibility, making them a significant genetic risk factor for a variety of infectious disorders (Forthal et al., 2007).

2.5 Advances in genomic technologies

Our understanding of genetics and its role in health and disease is being revolutionized by recent developments in genomic technologies such as Genome-Wide Association Studies (GWAS), CRISPR-Cas9 andNext-Generation Sequencing (NGS). Researchers can now precisely alter DNA sequences, examine gene expression at the single-cell level, and analyze the entire genome thanks to these technologies, which could lead to advances in personalized medicine, disease diagnosis, and medical treatment.

2.5.1 Genome-wide association studies (GWAS)

Indeed, GWAS has greatly improved our knowledge of the genetic foundations of the immune system by identifying a large number of genetic loci connected to immune-related features and illnesses. These studies identify genetic variants linked to particular qualities or disorders by comparing the genomes of people with and without those traits or diseases. Insights into disease causes and possible treatment targets are provided by the identified loci, which frequently highlight genes implicated in inflammatory pathways, cytokine signaling, and immune cell activity. Genetic association studies have discovered causative amino-acid variations of HLA genes that contribute to various autoimmune reactions, in addition to hundreds of susceptibility loci to immune-mediated illnesses. The non-coding regulatory region contains the majority of non-HLA genetic variations. According to expression QTL research, these variations mostly impact disease by controlling gene expression.Many regions found by GWAS are extremely large and contain several genes, which is a direct result of significant linkage disequilibrium (LD), despite the fact that GWAS has been very successful in identifying risk loci. The immunochip, a specialized genotyping array made to hone association signals in autoimmune disorders, was thus used to fine-map the GWAS-associated autoimmune loci. Ankylosing spondylitis, autoimmune thyroid disease, celiac disease (CeD), Crohn's disease (CD), immunoglobulin A deficiency, multiple sclerosis, primary biliary cirrhosis, psoriasis, rheumatoid arthritis (RA), systemic lupus erythematosus (SLE), type 1 diabetes, and ulcerative colitis were the first 12 immune-mediated diseases that the consortium that informed the immunochip's design initially targeted (Hou & Zhao, 2013). Numerous pre-GWAS candidate gene association studies have identified the human leukocyte antigen (HLA) alleles in the major histocompatibility complex (MHC) on chromosome 6p21 as susceptibility alleles for a number of immune-mediated illnesses (Ricaño-Ponce & Wijmenga, 2013a). The substantial and noticeable genetic correlation between specific HLA alleles and a number of immune-mediated illnesses was validated by GWAS. This was expected since numerous HLA alleles are necessary to transmit self-antigens to T cells, which subsequently trigger autoimmune reactions, and the MHC area is enriched for genes with immunological functions (Horton et al., 2004).

Post-GWAS efforts were prompted by this work in order to identify the causative amino acid variations of HLA genes that contribute to autoimmune reactions as well as to validate the connections to HLA alleles. HLA-DRB1 alleles, for instance, have long been thought to be RA risk alleles. By utilizing RA GWAS data for haplotype and conditional analyses, Raychaudhuri et al. extended these findings and discovered five amino acid polymorphisms (three in HLA-DRB1, one in HLA-B, and one in HLA-DPB1) that all localize to peptide-binding grooves, indicating effects on auto-antigen presentation (Han et al., 2014).

The second significant finding was that over 90% of SNPs linked to immune-mediated diseases are found in the genome's non-coding regions, indicating that these variants may have a regulatory role. Using Encyclopedia of DNA Elements (ENCODE) data, functional annotation of GWAS SNPs linked to immune-mediated diseases showed that 14.4% of the variants map to protein-binding regions, 32.1% are in DNase-hypersensitive sites, 42.3% are SNPs that alter motifs, 7.6% map to promoter histone marks, and 18.8% map to enhancer histone marks (Ricaño-Ponce & Wijmenga, 2013b). More than 93% of SNPs among variations found in GWAS for non-immune diseases match with gene regulatory areas, confirming this finding.It is evident from this regulatory function of the majority of SNPs linked to immune-mediated disorders that they may contribute to disease by altering gene expression levels (Maurano et al., 2012).

2.5.2 CRISPR-Cas9 technology

Clustered Regularly Interspaced Short Palindromic Repeats (CRISPR) and CRISPR-associated (Cas) proteins constitute an RNA-guided adaptive immune system found in several bacteria and most archaea (Murugan et al., 2017). The precise editing of genes, particularly those involved in immune function, is made possible by CRISPR-Cas9 technology, which provides important insights into the function of genes and possible therapeutic uses. It's an effective tool for both comprehending the activity of genes and creating unique disease treatments.It consists of a collection of CRISPR-associated (cas) genes that encode Cas proteins with endonuclease activity, as well as CRISPR repeat-spacer arrays that can be further translated into CRISPR RNA (crRNA) and trans-activating CRISPR RNA (tracrRNA) (Koonin & Makarova, 2009). Originally identified as bacterial immune systems, CRISPR-Cas systems have developed into effective instruments for functional genomics research, especially when it comes to the investigation of immune-related genes. Researchers can examine gene function, pinpoint important participants in immune responses, and create novel treatment approaches for immune-related illnesses by using CRISPR-Cas to enable precise gene editing (Ford et al., 2019).

Three primary steps make up the process by which bacteria fend off the invasion of foreign nucleic acids: interference, expression, and adaptability. When a virus initially infects a bacterium, the bacteria will recognize its unique PAM sequences and incorporate them into its CRISPR spacer region, allowing the bacteria to memorize the invading virus and digest its DNA into spacer sequences of the right sizes (Ford et al.,

2019). The bacteria can identify the virus and convert the spacer sequences into pre-crRNA when it infects them again. With the aid of CnsI and RNaseIII, the pre-crRNA will be coupled with tracrRNA and transformed into mature crRNA (Deltcheva et al., 2011). Guide RNA (gRNA) is another name for crRNA, which uses complementary sequences to identify and bind foreign DNA. Although Cas nuclease cannot break foreign DNA on its own, when it forms a ribonucleoprotein complex with a mature tracrRNA and crRNA, the Cas protein can be directed by the crRNA to cleave the invading DNA by identifying its PAM site, destroying the foreign DNA and achieving self-defense (Cong et al., 2013).

CRISPR-Cas9 Technology allows precise manipulation of immune-related genes, providing insights into gene function and therapeutic potential.Immunotherapy fights a variety of illnesses, including cancer, autoimmunity, and neurological disorders, by utilizing the immune system. Because of their strong and target-specific cytotoxic potential, quick growth, and long-term in vivo persistence, T cell-based cancer therapies have proven to be the most effective. Checkpoint inhibitors, bi-specific T-cell engagers, and ex vivo-expanded endogenous and genetically modified T cells are a few examples of antibodies that interact with T cells (Guedan et al., 2019). The primary goal of T cell genetic engineering is to reroute bulk T lymphocytes against certain cancer antigens by transferring extra receptors. These can be either chimeric antigen receptors (CAR), which are created by combining cytoplasmic signaling domains with an antigen-specific protein domain (often scFv), or recombinant tumor-reactive T-cell receptors (TCR). Particularly effective in treating recurrent and refractory hematological malignancies, CAR-T cells can be directed to any surface-bound tumor-associated antigen and do not require MHC-peptide recognition (Schuster et al., 2017).

T cell efficacy has been increased through the use of CRISPR/Cas9-based gene disruption to increase T cell activity. Genes implicated in T-cell fatigue, a dysfunctional state brought on by repeated and prolonged exposure to target antigens and frequently observed in cancer and many chronic viral infections, have been among the targeted genes (Blank et al., 2019). The prolonged expression of inhibitory checkpoint receptors, such as PD-1, CTLA-4, LAG-3, and TIGIT, which suppress T cell activation upon ligation with their respective ligands expressed on cancer cells or antigen-presenting cells, is one significant phenotypic alteration in exhausted T cells. In fact, many malignancies have responded well to PD-1 blocking antibody therapy in the clinic. Therefore, CRISPR/Cas9 deletion of PD-1 has been tried and has demonstrated enhanced CAR-T cell activity in preclinical models. It is also being evaluated clinically. Similarly, TCR T treatment is being researched to disrupt it (Stadtmauer et al., 2020).

2.5.3 Next-generation sequencing (NGS)

NGS technologies provide high-throughput, rapid, and accurate methods for determining the order of nucleotides in DNA and RNA molecules, enabling comprehensive genome sequencing, transcriptomics, and epigenomics studies. Because next-generation sequencing (NGS) makes it possible to analyze DNA and RNA quickly and affordably, it is completely changing our understanding of genetics and how it affects health and illness. Millions of DNA fragments may be sequenced simultaneously thanks to this technology, which offers thorough insights into gene expression, genome structure, genetic variants, and epigenetic changes. Comprehensive genome sequencing has been made possible by NGS, which has also made transcriptomics, epigenomics, metagenomics, and other omicsresearch easier. By enabling the parallel sequencing of millions to billions of DNA fragments, the introduction of sophisticated NGS systems like Oxford Nanopore, Pacific Biosciences, and Illumina has revolutionized the study of genomics (Vaser et al., 2017). This capability has paved the way for new opportunities for comprehending genetic variation, gene expression, epigenetic modifications, and microbial diversity. NGS has been pivotal in identifying disease-causing variants, uncovering novel drug targets, and shedding light on complex biological phenomena, including the heterogeneity of tumors and developmental processes (Amarasinghe et al., 2020).

Genomics studies using NGS profoundly analyze DNA using various approaches such as whole-genome sequencing, whole-exome sequencing, and targeted sequencing. Finding the entire DNA sequence of a person's genome is the goal of whole-genome sequencing (WGS), a potent and thorough genomic analysis method. It offers a comprehensive genetic blueprint of a person, including all of the genes, regulatory areas, and non-coding components found in their genome. Research on plants and animals, cancer, unusual genetic illnesses, patients with complex disease symptoms, population genetics, and novel genome assembly of eukaryotes and prokaryotes are among the areas in which it is primarily used in discovery science (Costain et al., 2021). WGS makes it possible to identify genetic differences, from single-nucleotide polymorphisms (SNPs) to more significant structural alterations like insertions, deletions, and rearrangements, by sequencing every DNA molecule in an organism's genome. There are numerous uses in a variety of sectors for this abundance of data acquired through WGS.Based on genome size, WGS offers two different sequencing approaches: (1) big whole-genome sequencing, which decodes larger genomes (>5 Mb), such those of eukaryotes, and (2) small whole-genome sequencing, which decodes smaller genomes (<5 Mb), mostly of prokaryotes. While long-read sequencing is preferable for genome assemblies, short-read sequencing is preferred for mutation calling. Accurate genome assembly without a reference sequence has been achieved by successfully combining short and long-read sequencing for novel genome sequencing (Logsdon et al., 2020).

The other sequencing technique known as whole-exome sequencing (WES) aims to identify and sequence the exome, or the parts of the genome that code for proteins. The bulk of known disease-causing variations are found in the exome, which makes up 1%–2% of the whole genome. WES makes it possible to identify genetic variations in protein-coding genes, such as single-nucleotide variants (SNVs), insertions, deletions, and copy number variations (CNVs), by sequencing the exome (Iglesias et al., 2014). WES is a cost-effective option to WGS for rare clinical diseases with clusters of symptoms, as well as in identifying variants for population and cancer genetics (Van Dijk et al., 2014).

Targeted sequencing, as the name indicates, has less exploratory power than WGS or WES as it targets specific regions of the gene and is able to pick up various types of genetic variations from SNVs to small gene deletions, duplications, insertions, or gene rearrangements associated with disease phenotypes. However, advantages include cost-effectiveness and manageable data for clinicians, making clinical decisions easier with more specific disease-relevant information. It can give much deeper coverage up to 5000× for rare alleles in genetic diseases, as well as for low-abundant evolving mutant clones arising as a result of tumor heterogeneity or disease evolution in cancer (Williams et al., 2019).

2.6 Conclusion

In conclusion genetic variations play a cardinal role in shaping the human immune response by influencing both innate and adaptive immunity. The expression and function of genes involved in pathogen identification, cytokine generation, antigen presentation, and immune cell signaling can be altered by these changes, which include single nucleotide polymorphisms (SNPs), insertions, deletions, and copy number variations. Thus, they play a role in the significant inter-individual variations in immune responses to cancer, autoimmune disorders, infections, vaccines, and allergies. Thus genetic variations are central to the diversity and regulation of immune responses across individuals.

References

Alberts, B. (Ed.). (2002). *Molecular biology of the cell* (4th ed.). New York: Garland Science.

Allen, J. E., & Maizels, R. M. (2011). Diversity and dialogue in immunity to helminths. *Nature Reviews Immunology, 11*(6), 375–388. https://doi.org/10.1038/nri2992

Alvaro-Benito, M., Morrison, E., Wieczorek, M., Sticht, J., & Freund, C. (2016). Human leukocyte Antigen-DM polymorphisms in autoimmune diseases. *Open Biology, 6*(8), Article 160165. https://doi.org/10.1098/rsob.160165

Amarasinghe, S. L., Su, S., Dong, X., Zappia, L., Ritchie, M. E., & Gouil, Q. (2020). Opportunities and challenges in long-read sequencing data analysis. *Genome Biology, 21*(1). https://doi.org/10.1186/s13059-020-1935-5

Bayley, J.-P., Ottenhoff, T. H. M., & Verweij, C. L. (2004). Is there a future for TNF promoter polymorphisms? *Genes and Immunity, 5*(5), 315–329. https://doi.org/10.1038/sj.gene.6364055

Becar, M., & Kasi, A. (2025). In *Physiology, MHC class I*. StatPearls Publishing. http://www.ncbi.nlm.nih.gov/books/NBK556022/.

Bhagavan, N. V., & Ha, C.-E. (2011). Immunology. In *Essentials of medical biochemistry* (pp. 449–472). Elsevier. https://doi.org/10.1016/B978-0-12-095461-2.00033-3

Bjorkman, P. J., & Parham, P. (1990). Structure, function, and diversity of class I major histocompatibility complex molecules. *Annual Review of Biochemistry, 59*(1), 253–288. https://doi.org/10.1146/annurev.bi.59.070190.001345

Blank, C. U., Nicholas Haining, W., Held, W., Hogan, P. G., Kallies, A., Lugli, E., Lynn, R. C., et al. (2019). Defining 'T cell exhaustion. *Nature Reviews Immunology, 19*(11), 665–674. https://doi.org/10.1038/s41577-019-0221-9

Breunis, W. B., Van Mirre, E., Bruin, M., Geissler, J., De Boer, M., Peters, M., Roos, D., De Haas, M., Koene, H. R., & Kuijpers, T. W. (2008). Copy number variation of the activating FCGR2C gene predisposes to idiopathic thrombocytopenic purpura. *Blood, 111*(3), 1029–1038. https://doi.org/10.1182/blood-2007-03-079913

Chanock, S. (2001). Candidate genes and single nucleotide polymorphisms (SNPs) in the study of human disease. *Disease Markers, 17*(2), 89–98. https://doi.org/10.1155/2001/858760

Chaplin, D. D. (2010). Overview of the immune response. *Journal of Allergy and Clinical Immunology, 125*(2), S3–S23. https://doi.org/10.1016/j.jaci.2009.12.980

Chaudhry, H., Zhou, J., Zhong, Y., Ali, M. M., McGuire, F., Nagarkatti, P. S., & Nagarkatti, M. (2013). Role of cytokines as a double-edged sword in sepsis. *In Vivo (Athens, Greece), 27*(6), 669–684.

Ciani, M., Benussi, L., Bonvicini, C., & Ghidoni, R. (2019). Genome wide association study and next generation sequencing: A glimmer of light toward new possible Horizons in frontotemporal dementia research. *Frontiers in Neuroscience, 13*(May), 506. https://doi.org/10.3389/fnins.2019.00506

Ciesielska, A., Matyjek, M., & Kwiatkowska, K. (2021). TLR4 and CD14 trafficking and its influence on LPS-induced pro-inflammatory signaling. *Cellular and Molecular Life Sciences, 78*(4), 1233–1261. https://doi.org/10.1007/s00018-020-03656-y

Clark, M. R., Clarkson, S. B., Ory, P. A., Stollman, N., & Goldstein, I. M. (1989). Molecular basis for a polymorphism involving Fc receptor II on human monocytes. *Journal of Immunology, 143*(5), 1731–1734.

Cohen, S., Bigazzi, P. E., & Yoshida, T. (1974). Similarities of T cell function in cell-mediated immunity and antibody production. *Cellular Immunology, 12*(1), 150–159. https://doi.org/10.1016/0008-8749(74)90066-5

Cong, Le, Ann Ran, F., Cox, D., Lin, S., Barretto, R., Habib, N., Hsu, P. D., et al. (2013). Multiplex genome engineering using CRISPR/cas systems. *Science, 339*(6121), 819–823. https://doi.org/10.1126/science.1231143

Copray, J. (2001). Expression of Interleukin-1 beta in rat dorsal root ganglia. *Journal of Neuroimmunology, 118*(2), 203–211. https://doi.org/10.1016/S0165-5728(01)00324-1

Costain, G., Cohn, R. D., Scherer, S. W., & Marshall, C. R. (2021). Genome sequencing as a diagnostic test. *Canadian Medical Association Journal, 193*(42), E1626–E1629. https://doi.org/10.1503/cmaj.210549

Dawkins, R. L., Degli-Esposti, M. P., Abraham, L. J., Zhang, W., & Christiansen, F. T. (1991). Conservation versus polymorphism of the MHC in relation to transplantation, immune responses and autoimmune disease. In J. Klein, & D. Klein (Eds.), *Molecular evolution of the major histocompatibility complex* (pp. 391–402). Berlin, Heidelberg: Springer Berlin Heidelberg. https://doi.org/10.1007/978-3-642-84622-9_32

Deltcheva, E., Chylinski, K., Sharma, C. M., Gonzales, K., Chao, Y., Pirzada, Z. A., Eckert, M. R., Vogel, J., & Charpentier, E. (2011). CRISPR RNA maturation by trans-encoded small RNA and host factor RNase III. *Nature, 471*(7340), 602–607. https://doi.org/10.1038/nature09886

Desai, D. D., Harbers, S. O., Flores, M., Colonna, L., Downie, M. P., Bergtold, A., Jung, S., & Clynes, R. (2007). Fcγ receptor IIB on dendritic cells enforces peripheral tolerance by inhibiting effector T cell responses. *The Journal of Immunology, 178*(10), 6217–6226. https://doi.org/10.4049/jimmunol.178.10.6217

Dvornikova, K. A., Bystrova, E. Y., Platonova, O. N., & Churilov, L. P. (2020). Polymorphism of toll-like receptor genes and autoimmune endocrine diseases. *Autoimmunity Reviews, 19*(4), Article 102496. https://doi.org/10.1016/j.autrev.2020.102496

Ehrlich, R., & Lemonnier, F. A. (2000). HFE—A novel nonclassical class I molecule that is involved in iron metabolism. *Immunity, 13*(5), 585–588. https://doi.org/10.1016/S1074-7613(00)00058-3

Enevold, C., Radstake, T. R. D., Coenen, M. J. H., Fransen, J., Toonen, E. J. M., Bendtzen, K., & Van Riel, P. L. C. M. (2010). Multiplex screening of 22 single-nucleotide polymorphisms in 7 toll-like receptors: An association study in rheumatoid arthritis. *Journal of Rheumatology, 37*(5), 905–910. https://doi.org/10.3899/jrheum.090775

Fitzgerald, K. A., & Kagan, J. C. (2020). Toll-like receptors and the control of immunity. *Cell, 180*(6), 1044–1066. https://doi.org/10.1016/j.cell.2020.02.041

Floto, R. A., Clatworthy, M. R., Heilbronn, K. R., Rosner, D. R., MacAry, P. A., Rankin, A., Lehner, P. J., et al. (2005). Loss of function of a lupus-associated FcγRIIb polymorphism through exclusion from lipid rafts. *Nature Medicine, 11*(10), 1056–1058. https://doi.org/10.1038/nm1288

Ford, K., McDonald, D., & Mali, P. (2019). Functional genomics via CRISPR–cas. *Journal of Molecular Biology, 431*(1), 48–65. https://doi.org/10.1016/j.jmb.2018.06.034

Forthal, D. N., Gary, L., Jay, B., Jacobson, L. P., Phan, T. B., & Benjamin, M. (2007). FcγRIIa genotype predicts progression of HIV infection. *The Journal of Immunology, 179*(11), 7916–7923. https://doi.org/10.4049/jimmunol.179.11.7916

Graham, A. L., Cattadori, I. M., Lloyd-Smith, J. O., Ferrari, M. J., & Bjørnstad, O. N. (2007). Transmission consequences of coinfection: Cytokines writ large? *Trends in Parasitology, 23*(6), 284–291. https://doi.org/10.1016/j.pt.2007.04.005

Guedan, S., Ruella, M., & June, C. H. (2019). Emerging cellular therapies for cancer. *Annual Review of Immunology, 37*(1), 145–171. https://doi.org/10.1146/annurev-immunol-042718-041407

Han, B., Diogo, D., Eyre, S., Kallberg, H., Zhernakova, A., Bowes, J., Padyukov, L., et al. (2014). Fine mapping seronegative and seropositive rheumatoid arthritis to shared and distinct HLA alleles by adjusting for the effects of heterogeneity. *The American Journal of Human Genetics, 94*(4), 522–532. https://doi.org/10.1016/j.ajhg.2014.02.013

Hasegawa, M., Nishiyama, C., Nishiyama, M., Akizawa, Y., Mitsuishi, K., Ito, T., Kawada, H., et al. (2003). A novel −66T/C polymorphism in FcεRI α-Chain promoter affecting the transcription activity: Possible relationship to allergic diseases. *The Journal of Immunology, 171*(4), 1927–1933. https://doi.org/10.4049/jimmunol.171.4.1927

Heyman, B. (1990). The immune complex: Possible ways of regulating the antibody response. *Immunology Today, 11*(January), 310–313. https://doi.org/10.1016/0167-5699(90)90126-T

Horton, R., Wilming, L., Rand, V., Lovering, R. C., Bruford, E. A., Khodiyar, V. K., Lush, M. J., et al. (2004). Gene map of the extended humanMHC. *Nature Reviews Genetics, 5*(12), 889–899. https://doi.org/10.1038/nrg1489

Hou, L., & Zhao, H. (2013). A review of Post-GWAS prioritization approaches. *Frontiers in Genetics, 4*. https://doi.org/10.3389/fgene.2013.00280

Hua, Z., & Hou, B. (2013). TLR signaling in B-Cell development and activation. *Cellular and Molecular Immunology, 10*(2), 103–106. https://doi.org/10.1038/cmi.2012.61

Hudson, L. E., & Allen, R. L. (2016). Leukocyte Ig-Like receptors – A model for MHC class I disease associations. *Frontiers in Immunology, 7*(July). https://doi.org/10.3389/fimmu.2016.00281

Hulett, M. D., & Hogarth, P. M. (1994). Molecular basis of Fc receptor function. *Advances in Immunology, 57*, 1–127. https://doi.org/10.1016/S0065-2776(08)60671-9

Iglesias, A., Anyane-Yeboa, K., Wynn, J., Wilson, A., Cho, M. T., Guzman, E., Sisson, R., Egan, C., & Chung, W. K. (2014). The usefulness of whole-exome sequencing in routine clinical practice. *Genetics in Medicine, 16*(12), 922–931. https://doi.org/10.1038/gim.2014.58

Janeway, C. (Ed.). (2001). *Immunobiology 5: The immune system in health and disease* (5th ed.). New York: Garland Pub.

Janeway, C. A., & Medzhitov, R. (2002). Innate immune recognition. *Annual Review of Immunology, 20,* 197–216. https://doi.org/10.1146/annurev.immunol.20.083001.084359

Jasek, M., Mańczak, M., Sawaryn, A., Obojski, A., Wiśniewski, A., Łuszczek, W., & Kuśnierczyk, P. (2004). A novel polymorphism in the cytoplasmic region of the human immunoglobulin A Fc receptor gene. *European Journal of Immunogenetics, 31*(2), 59–62. https://doi.org/10.1111/j.1365-2370.2004.00445.x

Jin, P., & Wang, E. (2003a). Polymorphism in clinical immunology - From HLA typing to immunogenetic profiling. *Journal of Translational Medicine, 1*(1), 8. https://doi.org/10.1186/1479-5876-1-8

Jin, P., & Wang, E. (2003b). Polymorphism in clinical immunology – From HLA typing to immunogenetic profiling. *Journal of Translational Medicine, 1*(1), 8. https://doi.org/10.1186/1479-5876-1-8

Johnson, C. M., Lyle, E. A., Omueti, K. O., Stepensky, V. A., Yegin, O., Alpsoy, E., Hamann, L., Schumann, R. R., & Tapping, R. I. (2007). Cutting edge: A common polymorphism impairs cell surface trafficking and functional responses of TLR1 but protects against leprosy. *The Journal of Immunology, 178*(12), 7520–7524. https://doi.org/10.4049/jimmunol.178.12.7520

Justiz, V., Angel, A., Sabir, S., & Jan, A. (2025). In *Physiology, immune response.* StatPearls Publishing. http://www.ncbi.nlm.nih.gov/books/NBK539801/.

Kamal, S., Kerndt, C. C., & Lappin, S. L. (2025). In *Genetics, histocompatibility antigen.* StatPearls Publishing. http://www.ncbi.nlm.nih.gov/books/NBK541023/.

Kawai, T., & Akira, S. (2010). The role of pattern-recognition receptors in innate immunity: Update on toll-like receptors. *Nature Immunology, 11*(5), 373–384. https://doi.org/10.1038/ni.1863

Kawasaki, T., & Kawai, T. (2014). Toll-like receptor signaling pathways. *Frontiers in Immunology, 5* (September). https://doi.org/10.3389/fimmu.2014.00461

Keen, L. J. (2002). The extent and analysis of cytokine and cytokine receptor gene polymorphism. *Transplant Immunology, 10*(2–3), 143–146. https://doi.org/10.1016/S0966-3274(02)00061-8

Kelly, A., & Trowsdale, J. (2017). Introduction: MHC/KIR and governance of specificity. *Immunogenetics, 69*(8–9), 481–488. https://doi.org/10.1007/s00251-017-0986-6

Kelso, A. (1998). Cytokines: Principles and prospects. *Immunology & Cell Biology, 76*(4), 300–317. https://doi.org/10.1046/j.1440-1711.1998.00757.x

Knight, J. C. (2003). Functional implications of genetic variation in non-coding DNA for disease susceptibility and gene regulation. *Clinical Science, 104*(5), 493–501. https://doi.org/10.1042/CS20020304

Koonin, E. V., & Makarova, K. S. (2009). CRISPR-Cas: An adaptive immunity system in prokaryotes. *F1000 Biology Reports, 1*(December). https://doi.org/10.3410/B1-95

Kourilsky, P. (2001). Cytokine fields and the polarization of the immune response. *Trends in Immunology, 22*(9), 502–509. https://doi.org/10.1016/s1471-4906(01)02012-9

Kozuch, O., & Mayer, V. (1975). Pig kidney epithelial (PS) cells: A perfect tool for the study of flaviviruses and some other arboviruses. *Acta Virologica, 19*(6), 498.

Kumar, H., Kawai, T., & Akira, S. (2011). Pathogen recognition by the innate immune system. *International Reviews of Immunology, 30*(1), 16–34. https://doi.org/10.3109/08830185.2010.529976

Laska, M. J., Troldborg, A., Hansen, B., Stengaard-Pedersen, K., Junker, P., Andersen Nexø, B., & Voss, A. (2014). Polymorphisms within toll-like receptors are associated with systemic lupus erythematosus in a cohort of Danish females. *Rheumatology, 53*(1), 48–55. https://doi.org/10.1093/rheumatology/ket316

Lebman, D. A., & Coffman, R. L. (1988). Interleukin 4 causes isotype switching to IgE in T cell-stimulated clonal B cell cultures. *Journal of Experimental Medicine, 168*(3), 853–862. https://doi.org/10.1084/jem.168.3.853

Logsdon, G. A., Vollger, M. R., & Eichler, E. E. (2020). Long-read human genome sequencing and its applications. *Nature Reviews Genetics, 21*(10), 597–614. https://doi.org/10.1038/s41576-020-0236-x

Mancardi, D., & Daëron, M. (2014). Fc receptors in immune responses. In *Reference module in biomedical sciences*. Elsevier. https://doi.org/10.1016/B978-0-12-801238-3.00119-7

Maurano, M. T., Humbert, R., Rynes, E., Thurman, R. E., Haugen, E., Wang, H., Reynolds, A. P., et al. (2012). Systematic localization of common disease-associated variation in regulatory DNA. *Science, 337*(6099), 1190–1195. https://doi.org/10.1126/science.1222794

Medzhitov, R., Preston-Hurlburt, P., & Janeway, C. A. (1997). A human homologue of the drosophila toll protein signals activation of adaptive immunity. *Nature, 388*(6640), 394–397. https://doi.org/10.1038/41131

Meng, J.-F., McFall, C., & Rosenwasser, L. J. (2007). Polymorphism R62W results in resistance of CD23 to enzymatic cleavage in cultured cells. *Genes and Immunity, 8*(3), 215–223. https://doi.org/10.1038/sj.gene.6364376

Meyer, D., Vitor, R., Aguiar, C., Bitarello, B. D., Brandt, D. Y. C., & Nunes, K. (2018). A genomic perspective on HLA evolution. *Immunogenetics, 70*(1), 5–27. https://doi.org/10.1007/s00251-017-1017-3

Mosmann, T. R., Cherwinski, H., Bond, M. W., Giedlin, M. A., & Coffman, R. L. (1986). Two types of Murine helper T cell clone. I. Definition according to profiles of lymphokine activities and secreted proteins. *Journal of Immunology, 136*(7), 2348–2357.

Murugan, K., Babu, K., Sundaresan, R., Rajan, R., & Sashital, D. G. (2017). The revolution continues: Newly discovered systems expand the CRISPR-Cas toolkit. *Molecular Cell, 68*(1), 15–25. https://doi.org/10.1016/j.molcel.2017.09.007

Nishiyama, C., Akizawa, Y., Nishiyama, M., Tokura, T., Kawada, H., Mitsuishi, K., Hasegawa, M., et al. (2004). Polymorphisms in the FcεRI β promoter region affecting transcription activity: A possible promoter-dependent mechanism for association between FcεRI β and atopy. *The Journal of Immunology, 173*(10), 6458–6464. https://doi.org/10.4049/jimmunol.173.10.6458

Paul, W. E., & Seder, R. A. (1994). Lymphocyte responses and cytokines. *Cell, 76*(2), 241–251. https://doi.org/10.1016/0092-8674(94)90332-8

Pincetic, A., Bournazos, S., DiLillo, D. J., Maamary, J., Wang, T. T., Dahan, R., Fiebiger, B.-M., & Ravetch, J. V. (2014). Type I and type II Fc receptors regulate innate and adaptive immunity. *Nature Immunology, 15*(8), 707–716. https://doi.org/10.1038/ni.2939

Ricaño-Ponce, I., & Wijmenga, C. (2013a). Mapping of immune-mediated disease genes. *Annual Review of Genomics and Human Genetics, 14*(1), 325–353. https://doi.org/10.1146/annurev-genom-091212-153450

Ricaño-Ponce, I., & Wijmenga, C. (2013b). Mapping of immune-mediated disease genes. *Annual Review of Genomics and Human Genetics, 14*(1), 325–353. https://doi.org/10.1146/annurev-genom-091212-153450

Rivoltini, L., Loftus, D. J., Barracchini, K., Arienti, F., Mazzocchi, A., Biddison, W. E., Salgaller, M. L., Appella, E., Parmiani, G., & Marincola, F. M. (1996). Binding and presentation of peptides derived from melanoma antigens MART-1 and Glycoprotein-100 by HLA-A2 subtypes. Implications for peptide-based immunotherapy. *Journal of Immunology, 156*(10), 3882–3891.

Schuster, S. J., Svoboda, J., Chong, E. A., Nasta, S. D., Mato, A. R., Anak, Ö., Brogdon, J. L., et al. (2017). Chimeric antigen receptor T cells in refractory B-Cell lymphomas. *New England Journal of Medicine, 377*(26), 2545–2554. https://doi.org/10.1056/NEJMoa1708566

Schuurhuis, D. H., Ioan-Facsinay, A., Nagelkerken, B., Van Schip, J. J., Sedlik, C., Melief, C. J. M., Verbeek, J. S., & Ossendorp, F. (2002). Antigen-antibody immune complexes empower dendritic cells to efficiently prime specific CD8+ CTL responses in vivo. *The Journal of Immunology, 168*(5), 2240–2246. https://doi.org/10.4049/jimmunol.168.5.2240

Segbefia, S. P., Asandem, D. A., Amoah, L. E., & Kusi, K. A. (2024). Cytokine gene polymorphisms implicated in the pathogenesis of Plasmodium Falciparum infection outcome. *Frontiers in Immunology, 15*(February), Article 1285411. https://doi.org/10.3389/fimmu.2024.1285411

Sherry, S. T. (2001). dbSNP: The NCBI database of genetic variation. *Nucleic Acids Research, 29*(1), 308–311. https://doi.org/10.1093/nar/29.1.308

Siddiqui, S., Johansson, K., Joo, A., Bonser, L. R., Koh, K. D., Le Tonqueze, O., Bolourchi, S., et al. (2021). Epithelial miR-141 regulates IL-13–Induced airway mucus production. *JCI Insight, 6*(5), Article e139019. https://doi.org/10.1172/jci.insight.139019

Sompayrac, L. M. (2019). How the immune system works. In *The how it works* (6th ed.). Newark: John Wiley & Sons, Incorporated.

Stadtmauer, E. A., Fraietta, J. A., Davis, M. M., Cohen, A. D., Weber, K. L., Lancaster, E., Mangan, P. A., et al. (2020). CRISPR-engineered T cells in patients with refractory cancer. *Science, 367*(6481), Article eaba7365. https://doi.org/10.1126/science.aba7365

Tanaka, T., Narazaki, M., & Kishimoto, T. (2014). IL-6 in inflammation, immunity, and disease. *Cold Spring Harbor Perspectives in Biology, 6*(10), a016295. https://doi.org/10.1101/cshperspect.a016295

Tiercy, J.-M. (2002). Molecular basis of HLA polymorphism: Implications in clinical transplantation. *Transplant Immunology, 9*(2–4), 173–180. https://doi.org/10.1016/S0966-3274(02)00007-2

Torre, D., Speranza, F., Giola, M., Matteelli, A., Tambini, R., & Biondi, G. (2002). Role of Th1 and Th2 cytokines in immune response to uncomplicated Plasmodium falciparum malaria. *Clinical and Vaccine Immunology, 9*(2), 348–351. https://doi.org/10.1128/CDLI.9.2.348-351.2002

Van Dijk, Erwin, L., Auger, H., Jaszczyszyn, Y., & Thermes, C. (2014). Ten years of next-generation sequencing technology. *Trends in Genetics, 30*(9), 418–426. https://doi.org/10.1016/j.tig.2014.07.001

Vandenbroeck, K., & Goris, A. (2003). Cytokine gene polymorphisms in multifactorial diseases: Gateways to novel targets for immunotherapy? *Trends in Pharmacological Sciences, 24*(6), 284–289. https://doi.org/10.1016/S0165-6147(03)00131-7

Vaser, R., Sović, I., Nagarajan, N., & Šikić, M. (2017). Fast and Accurate de Novo Genome Assembly from Long Uncorrected Reads. *Genome Research, 27*(5), 737–746. https://doi.org/10.1101/gr.214270.116

Viallard, J. F., Pellegrin, J. L., Ranchin, V., Schaeverbeke, T., Dehais, J., Longy-Boursier, M., Ragnaud, J. M. , Leng, B., & Moreau, J. F. (2001). Th1 (IL-2, interferon-gamma (IFN-γ)) and Th2 (IL-10, IL-4) cytokine production by peripheral blood mononuclear cells (PBMC) from patients with systemic Lupus Erythematosus (SLE). *Clinical and Experimental Immunology, 115*(1), 189–195. https://doi.org/10.1046/j.1365-2249.1999.00766.x

Warmerdam, P. A., Van De Winkel, J. G., Gosselin, E. J., & Capel, P. J. (1990). Molecular basis for a polymorphism of human Fc gamma receptor II (CD32). *Journal of Experimental Medicine, 172*(1), 19–25. https://doi.org/10.1084/jem.172.1.19

Williams, M. J., Sottoriva, A., & Graham, T. A. (2019). Measuring clonal evolution in cancer with genomics. *Annual Review of Genomics and Human Genetics, 20*(1), 309–329. https://doi.org/10.1146/annurev-genom-083117-021712

Xiao, W. J., Liu, Z. L., Lin, J. H., Xiong, C. J., Li, J. B., Wu, K. J., Ma, Y., Gong, Y. X., & Liu, Z. H. (2014). Association of TLR4 and TLR5 gene polymorphisms with graves' disease in Chinese Cantonese population. *Human Immunology, 75*(7), 609–613. https://doi.org/10.1016/j.humimm.2014.05.001

7

Gene-environment interaction in type 2 diabetes mellitus (T2DM)

Lyticia Philabet Sohtun and Kripamoy Aguan

DEPARTMENT OF BIOTECHNOLOGY AND BIOINFORMATICS, NORTH EASTERN HILL UNIVERSITY, SHILLONG, MEGHALAYA, INDIA

1. Introduction

The increased prevalence of type 1 diabetes mellitus (T1DM), type 2 diabetes mellitus (T2DM), liver lipid disorders, obesity, and other related metabolic diseases are major global health problems. It is defined by insulin resistance, hyperglycemia, dyslipidemia, hypertension, and abdominal obesity, which are risk factors for T2DM, cardiovascular disease, stroke, kidney disease, and other chronic diseases (Cole & Florez, 2020; Heindel et al., 2017; Priyadarshini et al., 2024).

A metabolic condition like diabetes mellitus is complex and characterized by hyperglycemia resulting from defects either in the release of a peptide hormone, insulin, by the pancreatic β-islets or in insulin action in adipose tissue, skeletal muscles, and liver. It is classified into three categories: Type 1 Diabetes Mellitus (T1DM), Type 2 Diabetes Mellitus (T2DM), and Gestational DM (GDM). T1DM accounts for about 5%–10%, while T2DM accounts for 90%–95% of the total cases of diabetes (Forouhi & Wareham, 2019; Priyadarshini et al., 2024).

The World Health Organization (WHO, 2024) estimates that 830 million people worldwide have diabetes, with the majority residing in low- and middle-income nations, and it directly contributes to 1.5 million deaths annually. Over the past few decades, there has been a gradual increase in both the number of individuals with diabetes and a steady rise in the number of people with untreated diabetes [WHO 2024].

2. Type 2 diabetes mellitus

The two primary causes of type 2 diabetes mellitus (T2DM) are defective insulin production by pancreatic β-cells and inadequate reaction to insulin by insulin-sensitive tissues. The complementary actions of insulin and glucagon tightly regulate metabolic homeostasis in mammals. Blood glucose homeostasis is dependent on the release of these hormones from pancreatic β-cells and α-cells, respectively, which are regulated by

Type 2 Diabetes Mellitus. https://doi.org/10.1016/B978-0-443-33590-7.00017-4

metabolic, endocrine, and paracrine processes. The disease may occur as a result of a metabolic imbalance brought on by the dysregulation of the systems underlying these activities (Campbell & Newgard, 2021; Galicia-Garcia et al., 2020).

The glucose transporter GLUT2 transports glucose in the blood into pancreatic β-cells, where it participates in the process of glycolysis to generate adenosine triphosphate (ATP). The cell membrane depolarizes and voltage-gated calcium channels open when the ATP/ADP ratio increases in hyperglycemic states, closing ATP-operated potassium channels. Insulin is released by pancreatic β-cell secretory granules in response to calcium influx, which modulates blood glucose levels under physiological circumstances (Galicia-Garcia et al., 2020) (Fig. 7.1).

White adipose tissue, liver, and skeletal muscle are the three key target tissues in which insulin receptors (INSR) are present, and insulin molecules bind to these receptors, resulting in a cascade of phosphorylation processes. First, the insulin receptor IRS1/2 is phosphorylated, which initiates the two main pathways, PI3K/Akt and MAPK. The PI3K/Akt pathway activates glucose transporters 4 (GLUT4), glycogen synthase kinase 3 (GSK3), the mammalian target of rapamycin complex 1 (mTORC1), and transcription factor forkhead box O1 (FoxO1) to facilitate insulin activity for metabolic homeostasis. Cell growth, proliferation, differentiation, survival, and death are all

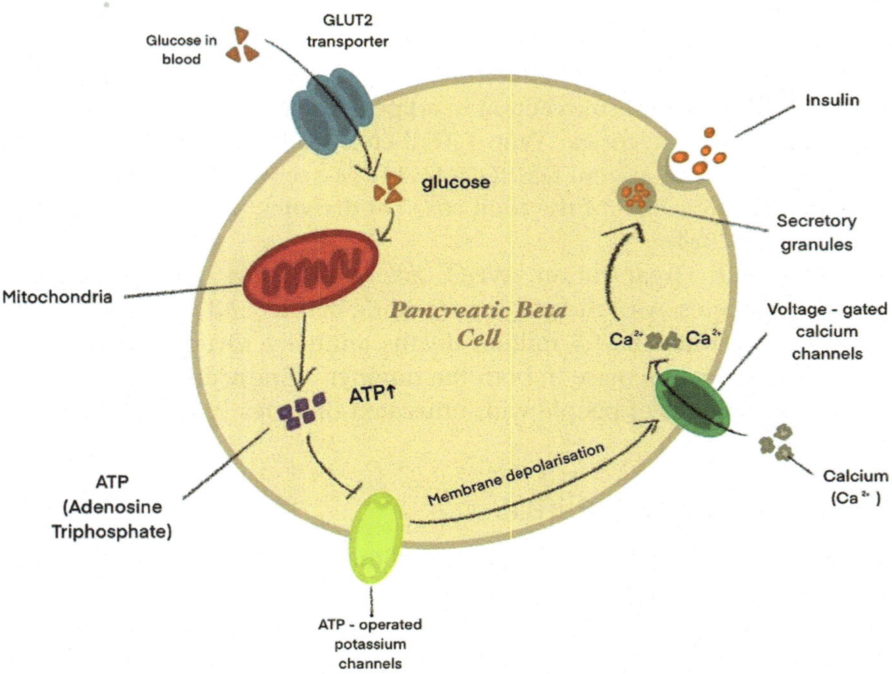

FIGURE 7.1 Glucose-stimulated insulin secretion (GSIS) in pancreatic β cells.

regulated by the MAPK pathway (Ersahin et al., 2015; Huang et al., 2018; Klimczak et al., 2024).

3. T2DM pathogenesis

The basis of T2DM pathogenesis is β-cell dysfunction and insulin resistance (IR), resulting in lowered insulin secretion. Determining the pathophysiology of T2DM requires an understanding of the numerous pathways that contribute to beta cell homeostasis and dysregulation (Galicia-Garcia et al., 2020). It is modulated by a combination of genetics, environmental factors, and different epigenetic modifications (Ding et al., 2022) (Fig. 7.2).

3.1 Insulin resistance (IR)

A pathophysiological condition known as insulin resistance (IR) occurs when there is an inadequate physiological concentration of insulin. It stimulates the liver to release more glucose and reduces glucose absorption in the muscle, liver, and adipose tissue. In IR, the proximal insulin signaling pathway process, such as INSR, IRS1/2, PI3K, or Akt stage, and the distal part pathway can be impaired in these target tissues (Ersahin et al., 2015; Galicia-Garcia et al., 2020).

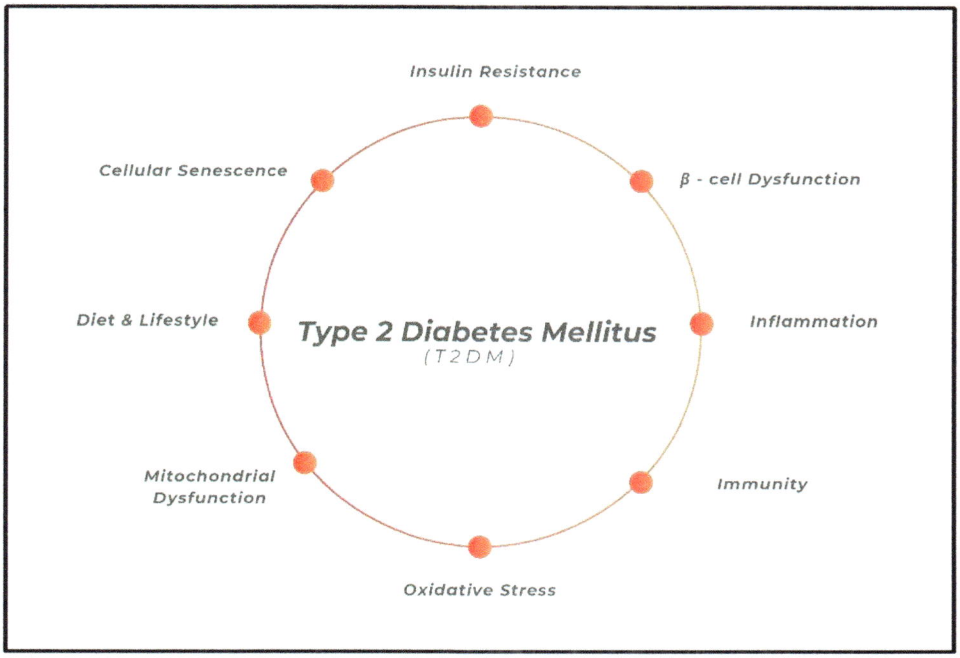

FIGURE 7.2 Type 2 diabetes mellitus (T2DM) pathogenesis.

Adipose tissue, especially visceral adipose tissue, produces adipokines, which are a group of hormones, cytokines, and chemokines that lower insulin sensitivity. TNF-α, an inflammatory cytokine, contributes to the IR by increasing the serine phosphorylation of the IRS1/2 substrate and decreasing GLUT4 expression. Insulin signaling is also inhibited by IRS-phosphorylating protein kinases, such as NF-kB, jun kinase (JNK), and PCK of free fatty acids. For example, nuclear factor kinase-kB (NF-kB) expression affects another insulin target tissue, skeletal muscle, by lipid accumulation and dysfunction of GLUT4 translocation (Ding et al., 2022; Klimczak et al., 2024).

Improper lifestyle, stress, and unbalanced diets are the main problems of the progression of IR. High-calorie intake causes obesity, followed by chronic inflammation, another factor for IR. Adipose tissue expands in obesity, resulting in increased production of proinflammatory adipokines like leptin, and decreased levels of anti-inflammatory adipokines like adiponectin have been reported to cause chronic inflammation and exacerbate IR (Jazieh et al., 2024; Klimczak et al., 2024).

An epigenome-wide association study of cross-ancestry DNA methylation reported three CpG sites in TXNIP, one in SLC7A11, and one in ZSCAN26 were inversely correlated with IR (Fragoso-Bargas et al., 2023). Thioredoxin-interacting protein (TXNIP), which is encoded by TXNIP, stimulates β-cell apoptosis in hyperglycemic conditions. Its depletion protects mice against T2DM by promoting Akt/Bcl-xL pathways and β-cell mass (Cha-Molstad et al., 2009; Chen et al., 2008).

3.2 β-cell dysfunction

β-cells of the pancreas synthesize insulin, which regulates glucose levels in biological conditions, and an imbalance or an increased secretion of insulin ultimately results in β-cell failure and advancement of T2DM. β-cell homeostasis, imbalances, and understanding various pathways contributing to these processes in the pathophysiology of T2DM are essential. The loss of cellular function and disruption of β-cell formation pathways or increased β-cell death further progress such conditions. Insulin production is decreased in β-cell dysfunction, which affects the body's ability to maintain normal blood glucose levels. A complicated network of interactions between several molecular pathways and the environment may be the result of this dysfunction. β-cell dysfunction is usually more severe than IR, and the rate of progression of T2DM due to hyperglycemia increases when both β-cell dysfunction and IR occur (Jazieh et al., 2024).

Type 2 diabetes mellitus (T2DM) is associated with various pathophysiological processes such as immunity, oxidative stress, inflammation, senescence, mitochondrial dysfunction, and cell death (Nedosugova et al., 2022).

3.3 Inflammation

A complicated physiological reaction to undesirable factors like pathogens, irritants, and damaged cells is called inflammation. Leukocyte migration from blood to affected areas is the first reaction in acute inflammation. Inflammatory cytokines, which are signaling proteins that modulate and impact the inflammatory process, are then synthesized and released. On the other hand, cytokine production and inflammatory signaling pathway activation are altered in chronic inflammation. The interaction between the genome, environmental factors, and inflammatory signaling pathways accompanying metabolic disorders serves as the primary connection of the pathogenesis of such diseases. Research studies conducted in T2DM patients reported that the NF-kB, STAT, FOXP3, and IRF transcription factors with epigenetic modifications have significance in inflammatory gene regulation. For instance, TNF-α, IL-1β, and IL-6 play major roles in the occurrence of IR and T2DM (Klimczak et al., 2024; Roshanzamir & Hassan-Zadeh, 2020; Zatterale et al., 2022).

3.4 Immunity

The crucial components of immunity, such as monocytes and macrophages, play a part in inflammation in diabetic complications. In T2DM, activation of inflammatory conditions followed by activation of macrophages within the adipose and liver tissue induces the secretion of TNF-α, IL-6, and IL-1β, highlighting the critical role of macrophages and other immune cells. Pro-inflammatory cytokines released by macrophage infiltration into adipose tissue activate adipocyte serine kinases such as IKK, N-terminal c-Jun kinase (JNK), S6K, and mTOR and initiate IRS phosphorylation inhibition. The stimulation of inflammatory pathways is achieved by toll-like receptors, specifically TLR4. Research has suggested that higher levels of free fatty acids (FFA) in obesity may stimulate TLR4 signaling, hence contributing to insulin resistance related to obesity. Chronic inflammation and metabolic dysfunction result from an imbalance in the M1/M2 macrophage ratio, which increases the proportion of pro-inflammatory M1 macrophages relative to anti-inflammatory M2 macrophages (Blériot et al., 2023; Ding et al., 2022; Nedosugova et al., 2022).

3.5 Oxidative stress

In diabetic complications, oxidative stress caused by an imbalance between oxidative and antioxidative processes triggers lipid accumulation, inflammation, and fibrosis (Zhang, Li, et al., 2020). Oxidative stress generates reactive oxygen species (ROS), such as superoxide anions, hydroxyl and peroxyl radicals, and other free radicals. It can reduce insulin secretion and predispose patients to T2DM. The main intracellular source of ROS is mitochondria, and its dysfunction is intimately linked to oxidative stress (Cojocaru et al., 2023). The integral mechanism of metabolic memory in diabetic complications and its progression is associated with oxidative stress and mitochondrial dysfunction. It also relates to other organelle dysfunctions such as endoplasmic reticulum (ER) dysfunction, lysosomal stress, and Golgi apparatus homeostasis. The imbalance in mitochondrial fission, mitophagy, new mitochondrial formation, and other organelle dysfunctions caused by hyperglycemia progresses oxidative stress in diabetic-related complications (Newsholme et al., 2007; Yang et al., 2024).

3.6 Mitochondrial dysfunction

Mitochondrial dysfunction is a condition marked by a decreased ratio of energy generation to respiration resulting from an imbalance between energy intake and usage in mitochondria. It involves an inhibition in mitochondrial biogenesis as well as mitochondrial oxidative protein expression, such as ETC complexes, which contributes to decreased substrate oxidation. The primary role of mitochondria is ATP synthesis via oxidative phosphorylation in response to metabolic demand, while preserving ion homeostasis, eliminating ROS, stress response, and coordinating several signaling pathways. Additionally, it takes part in the synthesis of numerous metabolites that serve as constituents of macromolecules such as DNA, lipids, and proteins. High levels of oxidative stress cause damage to the mitochondria, which triggers mitophagic processes to remove damaged mitochondria or, in the event of extreme cellular stress, cellular senescence, and reduced nutrition oxidation efficiency implies a lower ATP synthesis/oxygen consumption ratio and an increase in O_2 production. A possible association of IR and mitochondrial dysfunction is the accumulation of ROS in the mitochondria. The development of T2DM is tightly linked to oxidative stress, impaired mitochondrial biogenesis, mitochondrial integrity, and aging, all of which contribute to mitochondrial dysfunction (Newsholme et al., 2007; Rautenberg et al., 2022; Yang et al., 2024).

3.7 Cellular senescence

Cellular senescence is closely similar to programmed cell death (PCD), a form of persistent proliferative arrest without cell death. It is categorized into DNA damage-senescence, oxidative stress-senescence, and epigenetically induced senescence. To repair macromolecular degradation and restore cellular activities, cells are subjected to relatively minor disorders of their microenvironment, which trigger the activation of stress-responsive pathways. The same pathways activate signaling modules that influence cellular death, a process called PCD due to prolonged damage by stressful stimuli. Cells can restore physiological functioning and homeostasis when damage is effectively recovered (Galluzzi & Myint, 2023; Hernandez-Segura et al., 2018).

Senescent cells are distinguished by enhanced cell size, glucose absorption, mitochondrial activity, and resistance to apoptosis (Kumari & Jat, 2021). Epigenetic modification interacts with senescence and cell death in hyperglycemic memory, causing aging and age-related diseases such as T2DM (Anaraki et al., 2024; Khosla et al., 2020). Senescent cell clearance enhances insulin sensitivity and glucose tolerance, which in turn reduces inflammatory markers. Thus, senomorphics (compounds that affect intercellular communication and regulate senescent cell activity) and senolytics (compounds that specifically remove senescent cells) as potential therapeutics in cellular senescence and understanding its role in the progression of T2DM are essential (Iwasaki et al., 2023; Zheng et al., 2024).

3.8 Diet and lifestyle

Dietary factors significantly influence the management and severity of T2DM. Insulin resistance and obesity are related to impaired glucose absorption in T2DM; therefore, carbohydrate restriction aids in maintaining weight loss and optimizing metabolic benefits. Remission of T2DM is significantly affected by calorie restriction, weight loss, physical activity, and fitness (Forouhi et al., 2018; Gal et al., 2024; Magkos et al., 2020). Several environmental factors, dietary habits, and gut microbiota composition contribute to epigenetic modification and act as modulators of the development of T2DM (Jazieh et al., 2024; Lin et al., 2024).

4. Gene-environment interaction or epigenetic modifications

The study of functional modifications to the genome that disregard changes to the deoxyribonucleic acid (DNA) nucleotide sequences is known as epigenetics. It refers to a wide range of processes that control chromatin-level gene expression and also allow cells to function in a reversible and stable manner in response to environmental stimuli throughout life. The potential role of gene-environment interactions or epigenetics, such as changes in diet, exercise, and aging, acts as a mediator between the genome, environment, and epigenome, relating it to metabolic disorder (Capparelli & Iannelli, 2021; Ling et al., 2019). Furthermore, the early onset of T2DM and its related complications can be significantly affected by epigenetic biomarkers that are impacted by genetics, environment, diet, obesity, and stress. DNA methylation (DNAme), histone post-translational modifications (PTMs) or non-coding RNAs like microRNAs (miRNAs) and long non-coding RNAs (lncRNAs), and regulatory elements such as enhancers/super-enhancers are some examples of such modifications (Ding et al., 2022; Heindel et al., 2017; Priyadarshini et al., 2024) (Fig. 7.3).

4.1 DNA methylation

DNA methylation, a crucial epigenetic modification and commonly studied mechanism, mainly modulates gene expression by the addition of methyl groups to cytosine residues in DNA. This frequently results in gene silencing through the recruitment of transcriptional repressors and disruption of transcription factor binding to the DNA. This process primarily occurs in CpG-rich regions (i.e., CpG islands) at gene promoters, where 70% of methylation events occur. It regulates cellular differentiation, cellular development, cellular functions and plays an essential part in disease pathogenesis. DNMT1, DNMT3A, and DNMT3B are DNA methyltransferases that regulate the addition of a methyl group, 5-methylcytosine (5 mC), covalently at the CpG sites on cytosine. It can be reversed by ten-eleven translocation (TET) proteins, namely TET1, TET2, and TET3, that

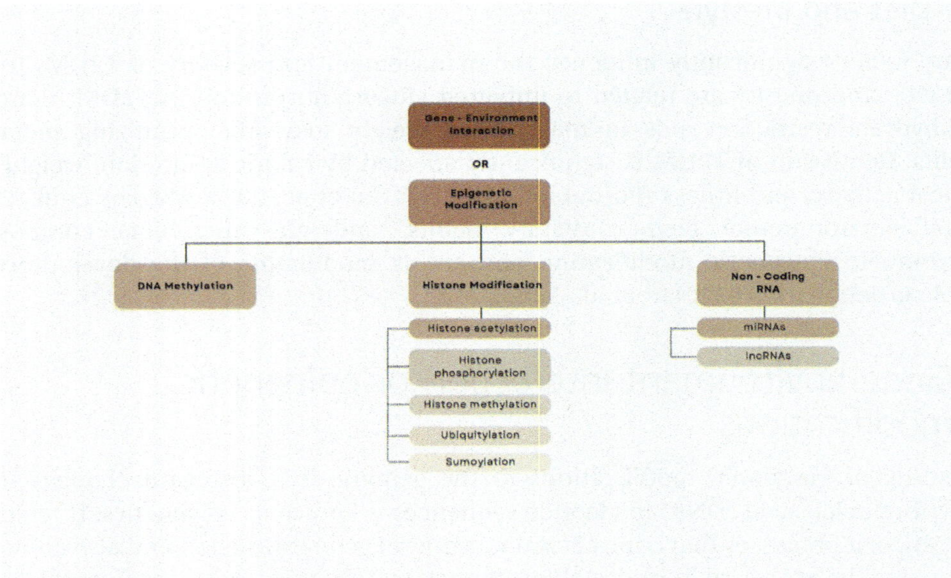

FIGURE 7.3 Flowchart for the different epigenetic modifications, such as DNA methylation, histone modification, and non-coding RNAs (ncRNAs).

modify 5-methylcytosine to 5-hydroxymethylcytosine, which catalyzes the active demethylation process (Jazieh et al., 2024; Zatterale et al., 2022).

4.2 Histone modification

Histones are involved in the formation of nucleosomes alongside DNA, and histone epigenetic modifying enzymes modify the N-terminal end of histones. V.G. Allfrey, R. Faulkner, and A.E. Mirsky were the first to report about histone acetylation in 1964. They stated that modification of histone-chromatin structure through the addition or removal of acetyl or methyl groups by certain specific enzymes is vital in nuclear function and that acetylation inhibits ribonucleic acid formation in vivo (Allfrey et al., 1964). Histone acetylation, which is a primary aspect of histone modification, is the process by which enzymes called lysine acetyltransferases add an acetyl group to the lysine residues of histone proteins. It is essential for regulating chromatin accessibility, which affects gene transcription (Jazieh et al., 2024; Shvedunova & Akhtar, 2022).

Histone acetylation is a process for the regulation of a highly regulated process, i.e., eukaryotic transcription, and a group of acetyltransferases called histone acetyltransferases (HATs), which interact on particular lysine side chains of histone proteins, regulates the transcription of many genes by modifying chromatin proteins, transcription-related factors, and other non-histone proteins involved (Sterner & Berger,

2000). The process of lysine acetylation is regulated by two enzyme families with different modes of action:

1) HATs or histone acetyltransferases: These acetyltransferases act as catalysts for transferring an acetyl group to the ε (epsilon)-amino group of lysine side chains in the histone tails, neutralizing the positive charge of lysine and weakening bonds between histones (positively charged by lysine residues) and DNA (negatively charged by phosphate groups), resulting in less compact chromatin and increased accessibility to the transcriptional machinery. HATs are categorized as type-A located in the nucleus linked to transcription (e.g., GNAT, MYST and CBP/p300 families), and type-B located in the cytoplasm possessing housekeeping role in the cell (Yang & Seto, 2007).

2) HDACs or histone deacetylases: In both histone and non-histone proteins, HDACs facilitate the removal of the acetyl group from acetyllysine (Ac-Lys), restoring the ε-amino group, and release an acetate molecule that regenerates the lysine's positive charge. They significantly act as transcriptional repressors and can stabilize the local chromatin structure. They are classified into four classes: Class I (HDAC 1, 2, 3, and 8), Class IIa (HDAC 4, 5, 7, and 9), Class IIb (HDAC 6 and 10), Class III (Sirtuins 1–7), and Class IV (HDAC 11). The HDAC bromodomain functions as an acetyllysine-recognizing module, and its inhibitors have been actively known as potential anticancer agents and evaluated as drug targets in clinical trials for the treatment of many diseases (Seto & Yoshida, 2014).

Histone post-translational modifications such as phosphorylation, methylation, ubiquitylation, sumoylation, ADP (adenosine diphosphate) ribosylation, and glycosylation also regulate gene transcription (Bannister & Kouzarides, 2011; Singh et al., 2020).

4.3 Histone phosphorylation

Histone phosphorylation is highly effective and mainly takes place on serines, threonines, and tyrosines. This modification is regulated by kinases and phosphatases that add and remove phosphate groups, respectively. Histone kinases add a negative charge to the histone by relocating a phosphate group from ATP to the hydroxyl group of the targeted amino acid side chain and significantly affect the chromatin structure. The intrinsic DNA-binding domain of kinase enzyme MAPK1 associates with a chromatin-bound factor before it directly attaches to DNA for stabilizing the overall reactions (Bannister & Kouzarides, 2011).

4.4 Histone methylation

Histone methylation is a stable and static modification that primarily occurs on the lysine side chains (lysine methylation) and arginines (arginine methylation) by not altering the histone protein's charge. It also involves the methylation of RNA molecules that significantly impact RNA stability, localization, and translation without altering their primary sequence. Since these RNA alterations reversibly control gene expression post-transcriptionally, they are associated with epigenetic modifications. The CpG methylation stimulates lysine 9 methylation on H3, or histone 3, promoting DNA methylation. Such modifications are essential for genetic regulation and have been increasingly linked to the pathogenesis of T2DM (Geng et al., 2022).

4.5 Ubiquitination

Ubiquitylation is highly dynamic by transferring ubiquitin, a 76-amino acid polypeptide, to histone lysines by the sequential activity of three enzymes: E1-activating, E2-conjugating, and E3-ligating enzymes, and involves significant covalent modification. The substrate selectivity (i.e., which lysine is targeted) as well as ubiquitylation degree (i.e., whether mono- or polyubiquitylated) are regulated by these enzyme complexes. Mono-ubiquitylation appears to be the most significant for histones, while the specific sites are still mostly unidentified. H2A and H2B sites, however, have been thoroughly studied, where H2AK119ub1 is implicated in gene silencing and H2BK123ub1 in transcriptional initiation and elongation. The de-ubiquitin enzyme, an isopeptidases reduces these modification and their activity is crucial for both gene activation and silencing (Bannister & Kouzarides, 2011).

4.6 Sumoylation

Sumoylation is a ubiquitylation-related modification that enables small ubiquitin-like modifier molecules to covalently attach to histone lysine by the E1, E2, and E3 enzymes. All four core histones have been reported with this modification, and it functions by inhibiting acetylation and ubiquitylation that might coexist on the same lysine side chain. Although it has primarily been related to repressive roles, knowledge of its molecular mechanism is crucial to comprehending how it affects chromatin (Bannister & Kouzarides, 2011).

4.7 Non-coding RNAs (ncRNAs)

Non-coding RNAs (ncRNAs) are RNA molecules that are transcribed but not translated into protein, but they modify RNA, DNA, and protein molecules, affecting gene expression. They are involved in genetic silencing and affect epigenetic modifications, such as DNA methylation and histone modification.

They are classified into two categories: ordering non-coding RNAs and regulatory non-coding RNAs. Based on their size, the regulatory ncRNAs are further divided into two types:

(i) With fewer than 30 nucleotides, which are short-chain molecules like short interfering RNAs (siRNAs) and microRNAs (miRNAs). Through complete and incomplete base complementary pairing with mRNA, miRNA suppresses translation, creating a miRNA-mRNA system that silences the target genes (Klimczak et al., 2024; Long et al., 2024)

(ii) With a minimum of 200 nucleotides, which are long-chain molecules such as long non-coding RNAs (lncRNAs). They affect cell proliferation, differentiation, apoptosis, and carcinogenic pathways. There are five different types of lncRNA, including sense, antisense, bidirectional, intronic, and intergenic (Guo et al., 2023; Zhang, Lu, & Chang, 2020).

In the development and progression of T2DM, microRNA (miRNA) and long noncoding RNA (lncRNA) have been shown to play a significant role (Guo et al., 2023).

5. Gene-environment interaction or epigenetics in type 2 diabetes

The gene-environment interaction, or epigenetics, is essential to the initiation and progression of numerous diseases (Zhang, Lu, & Chang, 2020). Recent epigenetic research has focused on the role of epigenetic modifications in the pathophysiology of T2DM. Environment and lifestyle act as diabetic stimuli by modifying epigenetic processes, including DNA methylation, histone post-translational modifications, and long non-coding RNAs, all of which modulate chromatin structure and gene expression, facilitating the development of T2DM. These mechanisms are studied for predicting the risk of T2DM and as potential therapeutic targets (Dhawan & Natarajan, 2019; Singh et al., 2020; Zhang, Lu, & Chang, 2020). The development, management, and progression of diabetes and associated complications are significantly affected by epigenetic factors and mechanisms that modify genes through upstream signal transduction pathways and other processes. Major genes for β-cell differentiation, including PDX1, PAX4, and GLP1 receptors, are regulated by epigenetic modifications. Consequently, the development of diabetes and associated consequences may be decreased by preventing and reversing the epigenetic changes (Singh et al., 2020).

5.1 DNA methylation in T2DM

DNA methylation is a biological process that has been studied extensively to identify diagnostics and therapeutics concerning T2DM (Nadiger et al., 2024). In T2DM patients, the methylation of the insulin promoter gene in human pancreatic islet cells and several CpG sites resulting in glycated hemoglobin (HbA1c) level increases have been reported (Yang et al., 2011). The association of differential methylation in blood samples of T2DM patients was reported in five CpG sites, namely *ABCG1*, *LOXL2*, *SLC1A5*, *SREBF1*, and *TXNIP* (Walaszczyk et al., 2018). Moreover, it was also reported in relation to *FTO*,

KCNQ1, *SLC30A8*, *TCF7L2*, and *PHOSPHO1* (Willmer et al., 2018) in patient samples with T2DM.

The CpG sites of ABCG1, LGALS3BP, SREBF1, and TXNIP genes are potential targets for T2DM diagnosis. The increased methylation of ABCG1 and SREBF1 results in downregulation of gene expression of these two genes, associated with T2DM. The reduced methylation of the TXNIP gene, a crucial oxidative stress regulator, is associated with inflammation, and its overexpression promotes NLRP3-inflammasome activation. It results in releasing LGALS3BP, an inflammatory mediator encoding a secretory glycoprotein modulated by the NF-kB pathway, which is linked with prevalent T2DM (Ding et al., 2022; Nadiger et al., 2024).

Hypermethylation of the hepcidin antimicrobial peptide (HAMP) gene promoter in the livers of mice predisposed to T2DM. It can serve as a candidate gene for assessing susceptibility to T2DM and potentially mitigating excessive insulin secretion. The absorption of fatty acids and lipid metabolism regulation are both influenced by CD36. Hypermethylation and polymorphism of the CD3 may be linked to the progression of obesity and T2DM (Yin et al., 2021). Compared to individuals without diabetes, T2DM patients reported nearly double DNA methylation in the PPARg and PPARGC1A gene promoter in islet cells (Ling et al., 2008). Furthermore, DNA methylation has been reported to be modified in the pancreatic islets of diabetic patients, which regulates insulin secretion, insulin resistance, and β cell development, which impacts the pathogenesis of T2DM (Volkov et al., 2017).

5.2 Histone acetylation in T2DM

Histone acetylation and deacetylation have garnered significant attention as possible targets for the development of anti-diabetic medications in diabetes. It was the first known post-translational histone modification triggered by histone acetyltransferases (HATs) and histone deacetylases (HDACs) (Ding et al., 2022).

In HFD-fed mice, histone H3 K27 acetylation (H3K27ac) activated a number of genes in adipose tissue, primarily those involved in the MAPK signaling cascade (Ding et al., 2022). Under low glucose conditions, the PDX1 gene is linked to HDACs like HDAC1 and HDAC2, inhibiting insulin gene transcription (Ding et al., 2020).

TNF-*a* and COX-2 promoters have been detected with increased levels of histone acetylation upon treatment of monocytes with HDAC inhibitors. HDACs have been actively used as therapeutic targets due to their conserved catalytic domains. HDACi (HDAC inhibitor) has been studied extensively in modulating inflammatory processes, rendering it crucial for understanding therapeutic targets for T2DM (Wang et al., 2019).

The development of IR (insulin resistance), a major contributor in T2DM pathogenesis, is dependent on various metabolic processes regulated by the sirtuin (SIRT) family of deacetylases, particularly SIRT1. These processes include inflammatory responses, adiponectin secretion, and reactive oxygen species (ROS) levels (Zatterale et al., 2022).

5.3 ncRNAs in T2DM

The pathophysiology of T2DM is significantly influenced by noncoding RNA (ncRNA), including microRNA (miRNA) and long noncoding RNA (lncRNA). Targeting these pathways with small molecules or RNA-based therapeutics offers a more accurate and efficient method of treating diabetes. It has been shown that miRNA-223 modulates glucose absorption by targeting the glucose transporter protein GLUT4, while miRNA-29 modulates insulin signaling by targeting the insulin receptor substrate-1 (*IRS-1*) gene. Dysregulation of miRNA expression binds to the 3-untranslated region of target mRNAs, causing translation suppression and/or mRNA destruction, leading to impaired glucose metabolism and insulin resistance. It influences other epigenetic modifications, like DNA methylation and histone modification, and is linked to chronic inflammation in T2DM. For instance, miR-146a is downregulated in serum samples, while miR-375 is overexpressed in pancreatic β-cells in T2DM patients. It can be considered a potential prognostic indicator for T2DM (Ding et al., 2022; Hashimoto & Tanaka, 2017; Long et al., 2024).

LncRNAs having a length greater than 200 nucleotides and lacking open reading frames affect cell proliferation, differentiation, apoptosis, and carcinogenic pathways. The lncRNA MEG3 regulates the expression of genes involved in the production and release of insulin. In diabetic individuals, transcriptional markers of impaired glucose regulation, IR, and aging are linked with the dysregulated lncRNAs. Several lncRNAs, namely *ANRIL, MALAT1, MIAT, HOTAIR, MEG3*, and *Kcnq10t1* from in silico studies, are reported to be consistently dysregulated in DM patients and participate in different metabolic pathways (Dieter et al., 2021). ANRIL, an extensively researched lncRNA linked with diabetes, has been proposed as an ideal biomarker. MALAT1 causes endothelial lesions in the microvasculature linked to increased production of proinflammatory cytokines and reactive oxygen species. In animal models and renal tissues from diabetic patients, MIAT and MALAT1 were found to be overregulated. Similar outcomes were seen in newly diagnosed diabetes individuals, suggesting that dysregulated lncRNAs regulate inflammation and insulin resistance, which eventually contributes to disruption of glucose homeostasis. Insulin synthesis is carried out by pancreatic cells whose proliferation and differentiation are regulated by lncRNA taurine upregulated gene 1. It was demonstrated that T2DM patients with worsened neuralgia symptoms had higher NONRATT021972 together with higher levels of tumor necrosis factor (TNF)-α (Guo et al., 2023; Priyadarshini et al., 2024).

6. Treatment of T2DM

Multiple medications and treatments have been researched and developed to treat diabetes and its related complications since the discovery of insulin in 1922. Oral antihyperglycemic drugs, insulin therapy, and non-insulin injectables are the initial treatments recommended for pharmacological management of diabetes. A few examples are biguanides (metformin), which reduce glucose production by the liver; glucosidase inhibitors (acarbose, miglitol, and voglibose), which prevent glucose absorption in the intestine; sulfonylurea preparations (glibenclamide, glipizide, gliclazide, and glimepiride) promote pancreatic islets to release insulin; sodium–glucose cotransporter inhibitors (canagliflozin, dapagliflozin, empagliflozin, ertugliflozin, and sotagliflozin) and thiazolidinediones (pioglitazone and rosiglitazone) enhance the action of insulin. In addition to pharmaceutical treatment, changes in lifestyle and exercise are suggested for diabetes management and for the prevention of associated complications (Chaudhury et al., 2017; Padhi et al., 2020; Priyadarshini et al., 2024).

7. Potential therapeutic targets for treatment of T2DM

7.1 PDX-1 (pancreatic duodenal homeobox-1) transcription factor

Epigenetic modifications of transcription factor pancreatic duodenal homeobox-1 (PDX-1) in pancreatic cells have been thoroughly investigated in T2DM. The early development of the endocrine and exocrine pancreas is significantly influenced by the PDX1 transcription factor. Additionally, it controls the physiology of mature islet cells and is essential for pancreatic development (Ashizawa et al., 2004). A significant finding was that out of 1749 genes analyzed, PDX-1 (one of only 15) contains methylation-susceptible CpG islands in the promoter caused by overexpression of a DNA methyltransferase. When the PDX-1 gene is knocked out, mice die from hyperglycemia resulting from failure of pancreatic bud generation. Following high glucose, PDX-1 methylation rapidly increased in pancreatic islet cells while PDX1 expression declined in T2DM patients (Yang et al., 2012). Epigenetic modifications eventually impact gene expression by altering genes crucial for pancreatic development (Pinney & Simmons, 2010).

7.2 FOXO1 (forkhead box O1) transcription factor

A transcription factor, FOXO1 (forkhead box O1), is regulated through the MAPK, Akt, and Pdx1 pathways, and its activation induces stress and apoptosis in pancreatic cells. It is responsible for β-cell dysfunction in the pancreas. FOXO1 expression is increased in rats with T2DM. It is activated in the liver under circumstances similar to oxidative stress and can enhance the activation of several gluconeogenesis genes. Insulin resistance (IR) and blood glucose levels during an oral glucose tolerance test were both decreased in transgenic mice's adipose tissue when *the FOXO1* gene was inhibited. In conclusion, IR can be decreased by targeting FOXO1 expression in adipose tissue. It is a promising target in preventing the onset of insulin resistance and obesity in T2DM (Borozdina et al., 2024). Such promising and potential targets of transcription factors and understanding epigenetic modification involved in its expression are essential for the therapeutic management of T2DM.

7.3 SLCs (solute carriers)

The most prominent superfamily of membrane transporter proteins is comprised of solute carriers (SLCs), which play a vital role in promoting the transport of glucose, fatty acids, amino acids, nucleotides, and ions, which aids in energy metabolism. Based on their roles, they are classified as passive transporters, which transport diverse molecules across the membrane without consuming active energy, and active transporters transfer substances by movement of a second solute, consuming active energy against electrochemical or chemical gradients. They play an essential role in glucose metabolism homeostasis, such as SLC2A4/GLUT4 (glucose uptake), SLC5A2/SGLT2 (glucose reabsorption), SLC25A7/UCP-1 (thermogenesis) SLC25A4/ANT1 and SLC25A5/ANT2 (*e.g.*, amino acid and ATP production). The SLC2 family glucose transporters (GLUT1, GLUT2, GLUT3, GLUT4) facilitate glucose uptake by peripheral tissues. In the intestine and kidney, the SLC5 family, such as SLC5A1 (SGLT1) and SLC5A2 (SGLT2), facilitates glucose absorption and reabsorption (Le et al., 2024).

7.3.1 GLUT2

GLUT2 plays a role in glucose uptake for energy metabolism and glucose sensing. It is mostly expressed in the brain, intestine, liver, kidney, and pancreatic islet β cells. When blood glucose levels increase, glucose is transported into the cytosol of pancreatic β cells by GLUT2, followed by glucose-stimulated insulin secretion (GSIS). The inhibition of GLUT2 suppresses insulin production and helps control hyperinsulinemia in T2DM (Ogawa et al., 1995). GLUT2 is responsible for glucose uptake by liver hepatocytes in the fed state but not in fasting conditions. In T2DM, its inhibition reduces hepatocyte glucose absorption, which is followed by lipogenesis to maintain energy homeostasis (Hosokawa & Thorens, 2002). GLUT2 facilitates glucose transport into the bloodstream of epithelial cells; it is necessary for second glucose reabsorption, which follows the first glucose reabsorption in the kidney (Ghezzi et al., 2018).

In T2DM, reduced expression of GLUT2 is linked to β-cell dysfunction, as it is necessary for GSIS in pancreatic β-cells. According to genome-wide association studies (GWASs), multiple GLUT2 genetic loci linked to insulin resistance, impaired pancreatic islet β-cell function, and hyperglycemia have emerged as a potential target for treating T2DM (Le et al., 2024; Ono & Kataoka, 2024; Schumann et al., 2020).

7.3.2 GLUT4

GLUT4 is a glucose transporter that is highly insulin-sensitive, and insulin production activates its membrane translocation. In skeletal muscles, adipose tissue, and cardiac muscles, GLUT4 is highly expressed. Upon activation by an insulin signal, GLUT4, which is located in the cytosol, is translocated to the cell surface. Fasting hyperglycemia and glucose intolerance were reported in mice with GLUT4 gene knockout. Insulin sensitization in adipose tissue is observed by overactivation of GLUT4, and its increased density in the cell surface is followed by glucose uptake, muscle glucose clearance, and systemic glucose utilization. In T2DM, impaired glucose uptake stimulated by insulin is related to the dysfunction in GLUT4 translocation in the mechanism of insulin resistance. Thus, indicating that GLUT4 activation by drugs could regulate hyperglycemia in T2DM (Borozdina et al., 2024; Le et al., 2024).

7.3.3 GLUT1 and GLUT3

In red blood cells, GLUT1 is the primary glucose transporter. It is also expressed in adipocytes, the blood-brain barrier, and kidney cortex mesangial cells. It mediates glucose uptake under stress conditions like hypoxia. The primary glucose transporter in the placenta and central nervous system, GLUT3, facilitates the uptake of glucose. Patients with T2DM have been reported as having lower levels of *GLUT1* and *GLUT3* expression, which may lead to hyperglycemia, as well as elevated HbA1c levels. The applications of glucose transporters GLUT1 and GLUT3 in T2DM treatment must be extensively researched. The potential applications of SLCs and enhancing our understanding of their roles influencing energy metabolism in T2DM as potential targets in maintaining T2DM or other diabetic complications (Le et al., 2024).

7.4 Histone acetyltransferase p300

The coactivator p300/CBP is essential in gene regulation by acetylating histones and various factors essential in facilitating the assembly of transcriptional machinery (Ma et al., 2021). It interacts directly or through cofactors with nuclear hormone receptor coactivators, promoter-binding transcription factors, tumor-suppressor proteins, oncoprotein-related activators, and non-histone chromosomal proteins (Sterner & Berger, 2000). Eckner et al. first isolated human p300 that contains a bromodomain in its center and three cysteine/histidine-rich (C/H) regions, with the carboxy-terminal region interacting exclusively with the adenoviral E1A oncoprotein (Eckner et al., 1994). Both p300 and CBP (CREB-binding protein) are recognized as structural and functional homologs; their interactions have been referred to as a single entity (p300/CBP) (Lundblad et al., 1995). p300 (also referred to as EP300 or KAT3B) contains at least four main domains, including a bromodomain, the HAT domain, TAZ, and ZZ putative zinc fingers, including various motifs that bind with different DNA-binding transcriptional factors. It is a well-characterized coactivator of multicellular eukaryotes and acts as a histone acetyltransferase, or HAT (Bannister & Kouzarides, 2011).

The inhibition of CBP/p300 HAT by A-485, a selective inhibitor of CBP/p300 HAT activity, highlighted the dominant role of CBP/p300 HAT activity in the maintenance of β cell identity and function. This results in decreased expressions of islet cell identity genes and impaired islet function. The CBP/p300 gene shows a substantial reduction in essential β cell function genes in the islets of prediabetic mice. It acetylates H3K27 and the transcription factors Hnf1α and Foxo1, as well as creating a hierarchical transcription network (Zhang et al., 2021). The islets of the pancreas produce hormones that trigger adaptive cellular and systemic reactions in response to metabolic and inflammatory stress. β-cell identity and function are maintained by intracellular Ca2+ and ROS signals produced by high glucose, and cytokine-induced ER stress activates calcineurin

(CN)/NFATc2 and PI3K/AKT genes. This was explained by direct stimulation of the endocrine differentiation gene RFX6 and inhibition of several β-cell genes such as MCT1. To stimulate and suppress gene transcription, CN/NFATc2 targeted p300 and HDAC1 to the promoter of RFX6 and MCT1, respectively (Darden et al., 2022). Histone acetyltransferase (HAT) p300 is crucial for activating NF-kB target genes, which in turn inhibits inflammatory processes (Zatterale et al., 2022).

7.5 Histone deacetylase sirtuin (SIRT)

Acetyl groups on histones and other protein regulatory factors are removed by conserved enzymes called histone deacetylases (HDACs), which have functional implications for gene expression and chromatin remodeling (Milazzo et al., 2020). The sirtuin (SIRT) family of deacetylases are nicotinamide adenine dinucleotide (NAD+)-dependent enzymes and have an ADP-ribosyltransferase activity (Yamamoto et al., 2007). SIRT1 modulates numerous metabolic processes, including the release of adiponectin, inflammatory reactions, and reactive oxygen species levels. Hyperglycemic memory, oxidative stress, and mitochondrial dysfunction are all linked to SIRT1-related dysfunction in diabetes (Letonja et al., 2021). It modulates energy metabolism, organelle homeostasis, and antioxidant defense, making it a key target in numerous disease treatments (Nandave et al., 2023). SIRT1 is found in the nucleus, and SIRT3 is found in the mitochondria. This plays a prominent role in regulating abnormal metabolic diseases such as T2DM and obesity. This suggests that sirtuins could constitute therapeutic targets to combat metabolic diseases like T2DM (Mihanfar et al., 2024).

7.6 ncRNAs

ncRNAs such as miRNAs and lncRNAs have been correlated with the maintenance of insulin sensitivity and glucose homeostasis. It has been demonstrated that miRNA-107 and miRNA-103 stimulate IR by targeting the GLUT4 and insulin receptor, respectively. The treatment of T2DM may be more accurate and efficient if small molecules or RNA-based therapeutics are used to target these mechanisms. Preclinical models of DM have already been tested with miRNA-based therapies with positive findings. lncRNAs are newly emerging and promising biomarkers for understanding the pathogenesis and prevention of T2DM (Guo et al., 2023).

The clinical trials of some histone acetyltransferase (HAT), HDAC, and miRNA inhibitors have shown favorable results in T2DM progression and prevention.

8. Treatment of epigenetic modifications in T2DM

To prevent the progression of T2DM, oral anti-hyperglycemic drugs, insulin therapy, and non-insulin injectables are standard treatment prescribed to patients, but long-term use of such treatment has many adverse side effects, suggesting the need for further therapeutic approaches. Since epigenetic modifications are frequently reversible, making them potential therapeutic targets (Singh et al., 2020). Diet is an epigenetic regulator that can reverse defects or alter gene expression correlated to metabolic homeostasis, as well as have a substantial impact on genome stability. In the era of precision medicine, epigenetics and nutrigenomics research have substantial prospects to enhance the prevention of disorders like T2DM. Numerous bioactive compounds have the ability to induce or reverse epigenetic risk markers; an epigenetic diet, which translates into dietary practices, can be used in disease management (Priyadarshini et al., 2024; Zhang, Lu, & Chang, 2020). Based on literature, they influenced numerous biological processes, such as DNA methylation, histone modifications, and expression of noncoding microRNA, which impacts the expression of epigenetically altered genes (Zhang, Lu, & Chang, 2020). Thus, an effective method for identifying antidiabetic medications based on natural compounds that can modulate glucose metabolism and reverting the action mechanism of several chromatin modifiers in the management of T2DM complications are essential (Borozdina et al., 2024).

9. Natural compound with antidiabetic properties

9.1 Curcumin

Turmeric has a polyphenolic compound called curcumin, which is used in renowned traditional herbal remedies. It comprises 80% of the curcuminoid complex, with demethoxycurcumin (17%) and bisdemethoxycurcumin (3%) as the remaining components (Ammon & Wahl, 1991). It possesses antidiabetic, anti-inflammatory, antioxidant, and antifibrotic properties. It also improves inflammatory disorders by CpG demethylation (Deng et al., 2014). Its anti-diabetic activity lowers the activity of α-amylase and α-glycosidase, which helps control hyperglycemia. In addition, it also helps to regulate insulin in tissues like skeletal muscle, adipose tissue, and liver (Wojcik et al., 2018).

Under hyperglycemic conditions in THP-1 monocytes, curcumin (p300/CBP inhibitor) inhibits the transcriptional activity and acetylation of NF-kB p65, reduces the activation of the inflammatory gene promoters, and lowers pro-inflammatory mediators such as TNF and IL-6 (Yun et al., 2011). In T2DM patients, it improves glycemic management, peripheral neuropathy, and vision (Chous et al., 2016). In diabetes therapy studies with T2DM, it was reported that curcumin-zinc oxide nanoparticles (10 mg/kg) over 21 days are more effective in the production of serum insulin, lowering blood glucose, and activating GLUT-2 and glucokinase (GCK) in the rat pancreas and liver (Raslan et al., 2018). Curcumin and its analogs having anti-diabetic properties play an essential role in preventing and treating T2DM (Tang et al., 2024; Thirumalaisamy et al., 2022).

9.2 Resveratrol

Resveratrol exerts glucose-lowering effects in humans through the restoration of normal insulin levels, insulin-like growth factors (IGFs), AMP-dependent protein kinase (AMPK), and sirtuin (SIRT) regulating blood glucose (Liu, Zhang, et al., 2016). It has successfully completed clinical trials (clinical trial number NCT01354977), and it is used for treating T2DM in nations like the United States. The daily oral intake of 5 mg-5g resveratrol for 1 year lowered the levels of blood glucose and increased insulin sensitivity in diabetic patients (Öztürk et al., 2017).

The regulators SIRT1 and NAD + -dependent deacetylase, which influence T2DM development with treatment of resveratrol, are shown to activate SIRT1 pathways (Lagouge et al., 2006). Resveratrol-activated SIRT1 and SIRT3 can further improve mitochondrial metabolism, which in turn reduces ROS production (de Kreutzenberg et al., 2010). In mouse hepatocytes, resveratrol significantly increases levels of SIRT1 protein and AMPK phosphorylation, restoring the over-activation of the NF-kB pathway. With its HDAC inhibitor properties, it suppresses expression of pro-inflammatory genes, which enhances glucose regulation and insulin sensitivity in T2DM patients. When taken as a supplement, it reduces systemic inflammation markers, including IL-6 and TNF-a, and increases insulin sensitivity in obese individuals, with no side effects. When doses of 1, 5, and 10 mg/kg resveratrol were administered orally for 30 days in rats with modeled diabetes mellitus, it reduced FOXO1 expression and decreased insulin resistance and glucose levels (Thirumalaisamy et al., 2022). A significant improvement relating to glucose absorption and sensitivity to insulin in T2DM patients by administering resveratrol may be accomplished by integrating antioxidant enzymes such as catalase, superoxide dismutase, and glutathione transferase, followed by reinstatement of cytokines. It also helps in managing the blood pressure of diabetic patients (Zhu et al., 2017).

9.3 Flavonoids

Flavonoids modulate glucose homeostasis by pancreatic β-cell proliferation and the activation of insulin-sensitive PI3K/Akt signaling as well as insulin-independent AMPK, SIRT-1, and mTOR pathways, all of which enhance the expression of GLUT4. It alters DNA methylation, histone modifications, and non-coding RNA expression, among other aspects of epigenetic networks (Han, Luo, Liu, et al., 2022; Lv et al., 2021). According to research on human and animal models, flavonoids could prevent and treat diabetes by modifying intracellular signaling pathways and gene expression by lowering hyperglycemia. As natural epigenetic modulators, dietary flavonoids aid in the identification of biomarkers for the prevention of diabetes and the development of alternative treatment (Han et al., 2022a, 2022b).

Epigallocatechin-3-gallate (EGCG) controls the activity of histone acetyltransferases and DNA methyltransferases, so acting as an epigenetic modulator. Vascular toxicity caused by polychlorinated biphenyl (PCB) can be lowered by EGCG-induced H3 hypoacetylation (Khan et al., 2015; Liu, Perkins, & Hennig, 2016). According to the findings, isorhamnetin protects the kidneys by suppressing the autophagy gene miRNA regulation (Matboli et al., 2021).

9.3.1 Flavonols

Flavonols (3-hydroxyflavonoids), which are prevalent flavonoids abundant in many fruits and vegetables, have been linked to diabetes (Han, Luo, Liu, et al., 2022). Quercetin has anti-diabetic properties and is commonly integrated into the diet (Shi et al., 2019). It reverses detrimental epigenetic profiles regulating transcription factors through histone modification by interacting with cell signaling pathways, modulating gene expression, and chromatin remodeling, which are linked to the etiology of obesity (Cione et al., 2019; Nettore et al., 2019). Combination therapy of fisetin (flavonol) and luteolin (flavones) may be used to treat and prevent diabetes and its related disorders by decreasing histone acetyltransferase activity and activating the expression of sirtuin (SIRT)1 and forkhead box O3a (FOXO3a) (Kim & Yun, 2017). Isorhamnetin (IHN) reduces insulin resistance linked to T2DM in skeletal muscle and adipose tissue by upregulating AKT2 mRNA, miR-1, and miR-3163 and downregulating lncRNA-RP11-773H22.4 expression (Matboli et al., 2021).

9.3.2 Flavones

Flavones, which include luteolin, apigenin, baicalein, and chrysin, are flavonoids having a 2-phenyl-1-benzopyran-4-one backbone and possess anti-diabetic properties (Hostetler et al., 2017). For instance, apigenin (4,5,7-trihydroxyflavones) improves glucose and lipid homeostasis in obese mice by lowering total protein acetylation and enhancing nicotinamide adenine dinucleotide (NAD^+) levels, thereby contributing to the prevention of chronic disorders (Escande et al., 2013). NF-κB activity and cytokine production in endothelial cells and peripheral blood cells are inhibited by luteolin, a flavonoid extracted from celery, peppers, perilla leaves, and chamomile tea. It substantially decreases CREB binding protein/p300 (CBP/p300) acetylation levels and employs epigenetic modifications involving NF-κB to prevent cytokine production by hyperglycemia in monocytes (Kim et al., 2014). In HepG2 tumors, baicalein possesses hypoglycemic and antioxidant properties that hinder HKDC1 (DNA 5 mC and RNA m6A) from being epigenetically modified (Jiang et al., 2022). Such studies suggest that flavonoids having antioxidant and antidiabetic properties act as epigenetic modulators in controlling gene expression and are involved in T2DM (Han, Luo, Liu, et al., 2022).

9.3.3 Flavan-3-ols

Flavan-3-ols, including catechins, epicatechin gallate, procyanidins, theaflavins, and thearubigins, are the most prominent flavonoids in a variety of beverages, whole and processed foods, herbal medications, and supplements (Han, Luo, Liu, et al., 2022). For treating diabetes, epicatechin (EC) is considered a drug or adjunctive medication present in tea, fruits, vegetables, grains, and cocoa (Fu et al., 2013). It decreased the dimethylation of H3K9 stimulated by glucose and the release of TNF-α and HDAC4 levels by high glucose (Cordero-Herrera et al., 2017). Under high glucose, it has anti-inflammatory and antidiabetic properties by controlling chromatin remodeling through epigenetic modifications. DNA methylation and histone acetylation are regulated by EGCG (epigallocatechin gallate), which has antidiabetic properties. According to these findings, flavan-3-ols taken as a dietary supplement may help prevent complications from hyperglycemia of T2DM (Han, Luo, Liu, et al., 2022).

9.3.4 Flavanones

Flavanones are polyphenolic compounds, some of which have sugar moieties, including hesperidin and naringin (flavanone-O-glycosides), and some of which lack sugar moieties, like hesperetin and naringenin (flavone aglycones), prevalent in citrus fruits such as lemons, oranges, grapefruit, and bergamot (Saini et al., 2022). Diabetes risk was reduced with the intake of flavonoid-rich foods (Guo et al., 2019), and by modulating AMPK-mediated p300 inactivation, naringenin and hesperetin exerted an inhibitory effect that prolonged the onset and progression of diabetes (Wang et al., 2021).

Naringenin decreases blood glucose level activity (Ortiz-Andrade et al., 2008), and 50 mg/kg of naringenin improves insulin resistance, tyrosine phosphorylation, and reduced oxidative stress (Kannappan & Anuradha, 2010). It inhibits glucose intake via the Na + -GLUT co-transporter, GLUT4 translocation (Harmon & Patel, 2003), and intestinal alpha-glucosidase inhibition (Priscilla et al., 2014), lowering glucose levels.

In type 2 diabetic rats, naringenin enhances glucose metabolism by stimulating the release of insulin by the pancreas, ameliorating pathological modification in diabetic mice organs, and improving vascular dysfunction by lowering oxidative stress and inflammation (Bhattacharya et al., 2014; Ren et al., 2016; Sirovina et al., 2016). Hyperglycemia and oxidative stress in diabetic rats are reduced when treated with naringenin encapsulated with core-shell polymeric nanoparticles (Han, Luo, Liu, et al., 2022; Thirumalaisamy et al., 2022).

9.3.5 Isoflavones

Isoflavones such as genistein and puerarin, mainly found in beans, soybeans, and soy foods, induce various physiological effects in living organisms and are used in alternative medicine to treat T2DM (Gómez-Zorita et al., 2020; Kuryłowicz, 2020). They are proposed as epigenetic regulators of epigenetic modifications affecting gene expression through metabolic pathways, including direct impacts on proliferation of β-cells and insulin secretion (Smeriglio et al., 2019; Weng et al., 2019). Puerarin is an isoflavone glycoside used for the development of puerarin injection for diseases such as cardiovascular disease (Zhou et al., 2014). Genistein has been suggested as a potential alternative for the treatment of diabetes, and it is the most bioactive isoflavone in soybeans (Guevara-Cruz et al., 2020). It maintains lipid metabolism in the adipose tissue of obese mice through in vitro and in vivo studies, regulating miR-222 and its expression of target genes BTG family, BTG2, and adiponectin receptor protein 1 (adipor1) (Gan et al., 2020). For the treatment of diabetes, these studies can provide important references.

Dietary flavonoids function as epigenetic regulators to regulate the expression of genes and potential therapeutic agents in the progression of T2DM (Han, Luo, Liu, et al., 2022).

9.4 γ-polyglutamic acid (γ-PGA)

L-glutamic acid and D-glutamic acid monomers are linked together by peptide bonds between γ-carboxylic groups and α-amino groups to generate γ-polyglutamic acid (γ-PGA), a homopolyamino acid derived from food. It has hypoglycemic, lipid-lowering properties and is present in abundance in traditional fermented food. It improves insulin resistance and lipid metabolism, lowering fasting blood glucose levels in diabetic mice. High-throughput sequencing of mouse gut microbiota using 16S rRNA revealed that γ-PGA enhanced the diversity and uniformity of beneficial bacteria in diabetic mice's intestines, which hindered pathogenic bacteria's proliferation. It can exert hypoglycemic effects, modulating and improving relevant metabolic pathways associated with diabetes symptoms. It significantly increased INSR, IRS-1, Akt, and PI3K expression in diabetic mice, corresponding to the insulin signaling pathway improving insulin resistance and insulin sensitivity to modulate glucose metabolism. These novel discoveries highlight the significant potential of γ-PGA in the treatment and management of T2DM (Li et al., 2024).

10. Conclusion and perspective

Type 2 Diabetes Mellitus (T2DM) is a complex polygenic disorder regulated by genetics and environmental factors such as lifestyle, stress, diet, and age, which are controlled by endocrine, paracrine, and metabolic pathways. The dysfunction of these pathways leads to the progression and severity of T2DM and the development of other related chronic diseases (Galicia-Garcia et al., 2020).

The pathogenesis of T2DM is linked to insulin resistance, β-cell dysfunction, inflammation, immunity, oxidative stress, mitochondrial dysfunction, cellular senescence, diet and lifestyle. Gene-environment interactions, or epigenetics, regulate these processes by DNA methylation, histone modification, and non-coding RNAs (Galicia-Garcia et al., 2020; Heindel et al., 2017; Jazieh et al., 2024). Understanding these processes and their regulators in T2DM is essential for finding potential targets and alternative therapeutic. A few targets are referred to in this chapter, such as transcription factors (PDX1 and FOXO1), glucose transporters (GLUT 1, 2, 3, and 4), histone acetyltransferase (p300), histone deacetylase (SIRT), and non-coding RNAs (miRNAs and lncRNAs).

Prolonged use of hypoglycemic medications has been associated with serious adverse effects, indicating the need for alternative therapeutics as a foundation for treatment of T2DM (Singh et al., 2020). Numerous molecular compounds modulate mechanisms such as epigenetic modifications, inflammation, and senescence. Curcuma, cinnamon, and ginseng are common sources of compounds that have significant effects against AMPK/SIRT1/PGC-1α, Nrf2, and PTP1β, in T2DM treatment. Resveratrol shows antidiabetic activity against the following relatively novel therapeutic targets for the treatment of T2DM: AMPK/SIRT1/PGC-1α, FOXO1, CCN3, and PI3K/Akt/mTOR. Flavonoids from plant extracts are effective against Akt/Erk1/2/p38MAPK GLUT4, PI3K/Akt/mTOR, and PPAR-γ, expression (Borozdina et al., 2024). These natural compounds have been proposed to be essential for the management of T2DM, which indicates further research of natural compounds and their properties in the prevention and progression of T2DM.

References

Allfrey, V. G., Faulkner, R., & Mirsky, A. (1964). Acetylation and methylation of histones and their possible role in the regulation of RNA synthesis. *Proceedings of the National Academy of Sciences, 51*(5), 786–794.

Ammon, H. P., & Wahl, M. A. (1991). Pharmacology of Curcuma longa. *Planta Medica, 57*(01), 1–7.

Anaraki, S., Kheirandish, M., Mousavi, P., Tamandegani, A. E., Mohammadi, S., & Shekari, M. (2024). Cellular senescence molecules expression in type 2 diabetes mellitus: CDKN2A, CDKN2B, and lncRNA ANRIL. *Gene, 911*, Article 148319.

Ashizawa, S., Brunicardi, F. C., & Wang, X. P. (2004). PDX-1 and the pancreas. *Pancreas, 28*(2), 109–120.

Bannister, A. J., & Kouzarides, T. (2011). Regulation of chromatin by histone modifications. *Cell Research, 21*(3), 381–395.

Bhattacharya, S., Oksbjerg, N., Young, J. F., & Jeppesen, P. B. (2014). Caffeic acid, naringenin and quercetin enhance glucose-stimulated insulin secretion and glucose sensitivity in INS-1E cells. *Diabetes, Obesity and Metabolism, 16*(7), 602–612.

Blériot, C., Dalmas, É., Ginhoux, F., & Venteclef, N. (2023). Inflammatory and immune etiology of type 2 diabetes. *Trends in Immunology, 44*(2), 101–109.

Borozdina, N. A., Dyachenko, I. A., & Popkova, D. V. (2024). Promising directions for regulating signaling pathways involved in the type 2 diabetes mellitus development (A review). *Russian Journal of Bioorganic Chemistry, 50*(4), 1263–1284.

Campbell, J. E., & Newgard, C. B. (2021). Mechanisms controlling pancreatic islet cell function in insulin secretion. *Nature Reviews Molecular Cell Biology, 22*(2), 142–158.

Capparelli, R., & Iannelli, D. (2021). Role of epigenetics in type 2 diabetes and obesity. *Biomedicines, 9*(8), 977.

Cha-Molstad, H., Saxena, G., Chen, J., & Shalev, A. (2009). Glucose-stimulated expression of Txnip is mediated by carbohydrate response element-binding protein, p300, and histone H4 acetylation in pancreatic beta cells. *Journal of Biological Chemistry, 284*(25), 16898–16905.

Chaudhury, A., Duvoor, C., Reddy Dendi, V. S., Kraleti, S., Chada, A., et al. (2017). Clinical review of antidiabetic drugs: Implications for type 2 diabetes mellitus management. *Frontiers in Endocrinology, 8*, 6.

Chen, J., Hui, S. T., Couto, F. M., Mungrue, I. N., Davis, D. B., et al. (2008). Thioredoxin-interacting protein deficiency induces Akt/Bcl-xL signaling and pancreatic beta-cell mass and protects against diabetes. *The FASEB Journal, 22*(10), 3581.

Chous, A. P., Richer, S. P., Gerson, J. D., & Kowluru, R. A. (2016). The diabetes visual function supplement study (DiVFuSS). *British Journal of Ophthalmology, 100*(2), 227–234.

Cione, E., La Torre, C., Cannataro, R., Caroleo, M. C., Plastina, P., & Gallelli, L. (2019). Quercetin, epigallocatechin gallate, curcumin, and resveratrol: From dietary sources to human microRNA modulation. *Molecules, 25*(1), 63.

Cojocaru, K. A., Luchian, I., Goriuc, A., Antoci, L. M., Ciobanu, C. G., et al. (2023). Mitochondrial dysfunction, oxidative stress, and therapeutic strategies in diabetes, obesity, and cardiovascular disease. *Antioxidants, 12*(3), 658.

Cole, J. B., & Florez, J. C. (2020). Genetics of diabetes mellitus and diabetes complications. *Nature Reviews Nephrology, 16*(7), 377–390.

Cordero-Herrera, I., Chen, X., Ramos, S., & Devaraj, S. (2017). Epicatechin attenuates high-glucose-induced inflammation by epigenetic modulation in human monocytes. *European Journal of Nutrition, 56*, 1369–1373.

Darden, C. M., Vasu, S., Mattke, J., Liu, Y., Rhodes, C. J., et al. (2022). Calcineurin/NFATc2 and PI3K/AKT signaling maintains β-cell identity and function during metabolic and inflammatory stress. *iScience, 25*(4).

de Kreutzenberg, S. V., Ceolotto, G., Papparella, I., Bortoluzzi, A., Semplicini, A., et al. (2010). Downregulation of the longevity-associated protein sirtuin 1 in insulin resistance and metabolic syndrome: Potential biochemical mechanisms. *Diabetes, 59*(4), 1006–1015.

Deng, Y., Lu, X., Wang, L., Li, T., Ding, Y., et al. (2014). Curcumin inhibits the AKT/NF-κB signaling via CpG demethylation of the promoter and restoration of NEP in the N2a cell line. *The AAPS Journal, 16*, 649–657.

Dhawan, S., & Natarajan, R. (2019). Epigenetics and type 2 diabetes risk. *Current Diabetes Reports, 19*, 1–14.

Dieter, C., Lemos, N. E., Corrêa, N. R. D. F., Assmann, T. S., & Crispim, D. (2021). The impact of lncRNAs in diabetes mellitus: A systematic review and in silico analyses. *Frontiers in Endocrinology, 12*, Article 602597.

Ding, Q., Gao, Z., Chen, K., Zhang, Q., Hu, S., & Zhao, L. (2022). Inflammation-related epigenetic modification: The bridge between immune and metabolism in type 2 diabetes. *Frontiers in Immunology, 13*, Article 883410.

Ding, H., Wang, F., Shi, X., Ma, H., Du, Y., et al. (2020). LncRNA MALAT1 induces the dysfunction of β cells via reducing the histone acetylation of the PDX-1 promoter in type 1 diabetes. *Experimental and Molecular Pathology, 114*, Article 104432.

Eckner, R., Ewen, M. E., Newsome, D., Gerdes, M., DeCaprio, J. A., et al. (1994). Molecular cloning and functional analysis of the adenovirus E1A-associated 300-kD protein (p300) reveals a protein with properties of a transcriptional adaptor. *Genes & Development, 8*(8), 869–884.

Ersahin, T., Tuncbag, N., & Cetin-Atalay, R. (2015). The PI3K/AKT/mTOR interactive pathway. *Molecular BioSystems, 11*(7), 1946–1954.

Escande, C., Nin, V., Price, N. L., Capellini, V., Gomes, A. P., et al. (2013). Flavonoid apigenin is an inhibitor of the NAD+ ase CD38: Implications for cellular NAD+ metabolism, protein acetylation, and treatment of metabolic syndrome. *Diabetes, 62*(4), 1084–1093.

Forouhi, N. G., Misra, A., Mohan, V., Taylor, R., & Yancy, W. (2018). Dietary and nutritional approaches for prevention and management of type 2 diabetes. *BMJ, 361*.

Forouhi, N. G., & Wareham, N. J. (2019). Epidemiology of diabetes. *Medicine, 47*(1), 22–27.

Fragoso-Bargas, N., Elliott, H. R., Lee-Ødegård, S., Opsahl, J. O., Sletner, L., et al. (2023). Cross-ancestry DNA methylation marks of insulin resistance in pregnancy: An integrative epigenome-wide association study. *Diabetes, 72*(3), 415–426.

Fu, Z., Yuskavage, J., & Liu, D. (2013). Dietary flavonol epicatechin prevents the onset of type 1 diabetes in nonobese diabetic mice. *Journal of Agricultural and Food Chemistry, 61*(18), 4303–4309.

Gómez-Zorita, S., González-Arceo, M., Fernández-Quintela, A., Eseberri, I., Trepiana, J., & Portillo, M. P. (2020). Scientific evidence supporting the beneficial effects of isoflavones on human health. *Nutrients, 12*(12), 3853.

Gal, A. M., Iatcu, C. O., Popa, A. D., Arhire, L. I., Mihalache, L., et al. (2024). Understanding the interplay of dietary intake and eating behavior in type 2 diabetes. *Nutrients, 16*(6), 771.

Galicia-Garcia, U., Benito-Vicente, A., Jebari, S., Larrea-Sebal, A., Siddiqi, H., Uribe, K. B., et al. (2020). Pathophysiology of type 2 diabetes mellitus. *International Journal of Molecular Sciences, 21*(17), 6275.

Galluzzi, L., & Myint, M. (2023). Cell death and senescence. *Journal of Translational Medicine, 21*(1), 425.

Gan, M., Shen, L., Wang, S., Guo, Z., Zheng, T., et al. (2020). Genistein inhibits high fat diet-induced obesity through miR-222 by targeting BTG2 and adipor1. *Food & Function, 11*(3), 2418–2426.

Geng, X., Li, Z., & Yang, Y. (2022). Emerging role of epitranscriptomics in diabetes mellitus and its complications. *Frontiers in Endocrinology, 13*, Article 907060.

Ghezzi, C., Loo, D. D., & Wright, E. M. (2018). Physiology of renal glucose handling via SGLT1, SGLT2 and GLUT2. *Diabetologia, 61*, 2087–2097.

Guevara-Cruz, M., Godinez-Salas, E. T., Sanchez-Tapia, M., Torres-Villalobos, G., Pichardo-Ontiveros, E., et al. (2020). Genistein stimulates insulin sensitivity through gut microbiota reshaping and skeletal muscle AMPK activation in obese subjects. *BMJ Open Diabetes Research and Care, 8*(1), Article e000948.

Guo, Y. C., Cao, H. D., Lian, X. F., Wu, P. X., Zhang, F., et al. (2023). Molecular mechanisms of noncoding RNA and epigenetic regulation in obesity with consequent diabetes mellitus development. *World Journal of Diabetes, 14*(11), 1621.

Guo, X. F., Ruan, Y., Li, Z. H., & Li, D. (2019). Flavonoid subclasses and type 2 diabetes mellitus risk: A meta-analysis of prospective cohort studies. *Critical Reviews in Food Science and Nutrition, 59*(17), 2850–2862.

Han, S., Luo, Y., Hu, Z., Qin, D., & Luo, F. (2022). Targeting gut microbiota in type 2 diabetes mellitus: Potential roles of dietary flavonoids. *Food Bioscience, 45*, Article 101500.

Han, S., Luo, Y., Liu, B., Guo, T., Qin, D., & Luo, F. (2022). Dietary flavonoids prevent diabetes through epigenetic regulation: Advance and challenge. *Critical Reviews in Food Science and Nutrition, 63*(33), 11925–11941. https://doi.org/10.1080/10408398.2022.2097637

Harmon, A. W., & Patel, Y. M. (2003). Naringenin inhibits phosphoinositide 3-kinase activity and glucose uptake in 3T3-L1 adipocytes. *Biochemical and Biophysical Research Communications, 305*(2), 229–234.

Hashimoto, N., & Tanaka, T. (2017). Role of miRNAs in the pathogenesis and susceptibility of diabetes mellitus. *Journal of Human Genetics, 62*(2), 141–150.

Heindel, J. J., Blumberg, B., Cave, M., Machtinger, R., Mantovani, A., et al. (2017). Metabolism disrupting chemicals and metabolic disorders. *Reproductive Toxicology, 68*, 3–33.

Hernandez-Segura, A., Nehme, J., & Demaria, M. (2018). Hallmarks of cellular senescence. *Trends in Cell Biology, 28*(6), 436–453.

Hosokawa, M., & Thorens, B. (2002). Glucose release from GLUT2-null hepatocytes: Characterization of a major and a minor pathway. *American Journal of Physiology - Endocrinology And Metabolism, 282*(4), E794–E801.

Hostetler, G. L., Ralston, R. A., & Schwartz, S. J. (2017). Flavones: Food sources, bioavailability, metabolism, and bioactivity. *Advances in Nutrition, 8*(3), 423–435.

Huang, X., Liu, G., Guo, J., & Su, Z. (2018). The PI3K/AKT pathway in obesity and type 2 diabetes. *International Journal of Biological Sciences, 14*(11), 1483.

Iwasaki, K., Abarca, C., & Aguayo-Mazzucato, C. (2023). Regulation of cellular senescence in type 2 diabetes mellitus: From mechanisms to clinical applications. *Diabetes & Metabolism Journal, 47*(4), 441–453.

Jazieh, C., Arabi, T. Z., Asim, Z., Sabbah, B. N., Alsaud, A. W., et al. (2024). Unraveling the epigenetic fabric of type 2 diabetes mellitus: Pathogenic mechanisms and therapeutic implications. *Frontiers in Endocrinology, 15*, 1295967.11.

Jiang, H., Yao, Q., An, Y., Fan, L., Wang, J., & Li, H. (2022). Baicalin suppresses the progression of Type 2 diabetes-induced liver tumor through regulating METTL3/m6A/HKDC1 axis and downstream p-JAK2/STAT1/clevaged Capase3 pathway. *Phytomedicine, 94*, Article 153823.

Kannappan, S., & Anuradha, C. V. (2010). Naringenin enhances insulin-stimulated tyrosine phosphorylation and improves the cellular actions of insulin in a dietary model of metabolic syndrome. *European Journal of Nutrition, 49*, 101–109.

Khan, M. A., Hussain, A., Sundaram, M. K., Alalami, U., Gunasekera, D., et al. (2015). (-)-Epigallocatechin-3-gallate reverses the expression of various tumor-suppressor genes by inhibiting DNA methyltransferases and histone deacetylases in human cervical cancer cells. *Oncology Reports, 33*(4), 1976–1984.

Khosla, S., Farr, J. N., Tchkonia, T., & Kirkland, J. L. (2020). The role of cellular senescence in ageing and endocrine disease. *Nature Reviews Endocrinology, 16*(5), 263–275.

Kim, H. J., Lee, W., & Yun, J. M. (2014). Luteolin inhibits hyperglycemia-induced proinflammatory cytokine production and its epigenetic mechanism in human monocytes. *Phytotherapy Research, 28* (9), 1383–1391.

Kim, A., & Yun, J. M. (2017). Combination treatments with luteolin and fisetin enhance anti-inflammatory effects in high glucose-treated THP-1 cells through histone acetyltransferase/histone deacetylase regulation. *Journal of Medicinal Food, 20*(8), 782–789.

Klimczak, S., & Śliwińska, A. (2024). Epigenetic regulation of inflammation in insulin resistance. *Seminars in Cell & Developmental Biology, 154*, 185–192.

Kumari, R., & Jat, P. (2021). Mechanisms of cellular senescence: Cell cycle arrest and senescence associated secretory phenotype. *Frontiers in Cell and Developmental Biology, 9*, Article 645593.

Kuryłowicz, A. (2020). The role of isoflavones in type 2 diabetes prevention and treatment—A narrative review. *International Journal of Molecular Sciences, 22*(1), 218.

Lagouge, M., Argmann, C., Gerhart-Hines, Z., Meziane, H., Lerin, C., et al. (2006). Resveratrol improves mitochondrial function and protects against metabolic disease by activating SIRT1 and PGC-1α. *Cell, 127*(6), 1109–1122.

Le, J., Chen, Y., Yang, W., Chen, L., & Ye, J. (2024). Metabolic basis of solute carrier transporters in treatment of type 2 diabetes mellitus. *Acta Pharmaceutica Sinica B, 14*(2), 437–454.

Letonja, J., Završnik, M., Makuc, J., Šeruga, M., Peterlin, A., et al. (2021). Sirtuin 1 rs7069102 polymorphism is associated with diabetic nephropathy in patients with type 2 diabetes mellitus. *Bosnian Journal of Basic Medical Sciences, 21*(5), 642.

Li, Y., Zhang, W., Tang, C., Wang, C., Liu, C., et al. (2024). Antidiabetic effects and mechanism of γ-polyglutamic acid on type II diabetes mice. *International Journal of Biological Macromolecules, 261*, Article 129809.

Lin, X., Han, H., Wang, N., Wang, C., Qi, M., et al. (2024). The gut microbial regulation of epigenetic modification from a metabolic perspective. *International Journal of Molecular Sciences, 25*(13), 7175.

Ling, C., Del Guerra, S., Lupi, R., Rönn, T., Granhall, C., et al. (2008). Epigenetic regulation of PPARGC1A in human type 2 diabetic islets and effect on insulin secretion. *Diabetologia, 51*, 615–622.

Ling, C., & Rönn, T. (2019). Epigenetics in human obesity and type 2 diabetes. *Cell Metabolism, 29*(5), 1028–1044.

Liu, D., Perkins, J. T., & Hennig, B. (2016). EGCG prevents PCB-126-induced endothelial cell inflammation via epigenetic modifications of NF-κB target genes in human endothelial cells. *The Journal of Nutritional Biochemistry, 28*, 164–170.

Liu, L., Zhang, Q., Cai, Y., Sun, D., He, X., et al. (2016). Resveratrol counteracts lipopolysaccharide-induced depressive-like behaviors via enhanced hippocampal neurogenesis. *Oncotarget, 7*(35), Article 56045.

Long, Y., Mao, C., Liu, S., Tao, Y., & Xiao, D. (2024). Epigenetic modifications in obesity-associated diseases. *MedComm, 5*(2), Article e496.

Lundblad, J. R., Kwok, R. P., Laurance, M. E., Harter, M. L., & Goodman, R. H. (1995). Adenoviral ElA-associated protein p300 as a functional homologue of the transcriptional co-activator CBP. *Nature, 374*(6517), 85–88.

Lv, Y., Zhao, P., Pang, K., Ma, Y., Huang, H., et al. (2021). Antidiabetic effect of a flavonoid-rich extract from Sophora alopecuroides L. in HFD-and STZ-induced diabetic mice through PKC/GLUT4 pathway and regulating PPARα and PPARγ expression. *Journal of Ethnopharmacology, 268*, Article 113654.

Ma, L., Gao, Z., Wu, J., Zhong, B., Xie, Y., et al. (2021). Co-condensation between transcription factor and coactivator p300 modulates transcriptional bursting kinetics. *Molecular Cell, 81*(8), 1682–1697.

Magkos, F., Hjorth, M. F., & Astrup, A. (2020). Diet and exercise in the prevention and treatment of type 2 diabetes mellitus. *Nature Reviews Endocrinology, 16*(10), 545–555.

Matboli, M., Ibrahim, D., Hasanin, A. H., Hassan, M. K., Habib, E. K., et al. (2021). Epigenetic modulation of autophagy genes linked to diabetic nephropathy by administration of isorhamnetin in Type 2 diabetes mellitus rats. *Epigenomics, 13*(03), 187–202.

Mihanfar, A., Akbarzadeh, M., Ghazizadeh Darband, S., Sadighparvar, S., & Majidinia, M. (2024). SIRT1: A promising therapeutic target in type 2 diabetes mellitus. *Archives of Physiology and Biochemistry, 130*(1), 13–28.

Milazzo, G., Mercatelli, D., Di Muzio, G., Triboli, L., De Rosa, P., et al. (2020). Histone deacetylases (HDACs): Evolution, specificity, role in transcriptional complexes, and pharmacological actionability. *Genes, 11*(5), 556.

Nadiger, N., Veed, J. K., Chinya Nataraj, P., & Mukhopadhyay, A. (2024). DNA methylation and type 2 diabetes: A systematic review. *Clinical Epigenetics, 16*(1), 67.

Nandave, M., Acharjee, R., Bhaduri, K., Upadhyay, J., Rupanagunta, G. P., & Ansari, M. N. (2023). A pharmacological review on SIRT 1 and SIRT 2 proteins, activators, and inhibitors: Call for further research. *International Journal of Biological Macromolecules, 242*, Article 124581.

Nedosugova, L. V., Markina, Y. V., Bochkareva, L. A., Kuzina, I. A., Petunina, N. A., et al. (2022). Inflammatory mechanisms of diabetes and its vascular complications. *Biomedicines, 10*(5), 1168.

Nettore, I. C., Rocca, C., Mancino, G., Albano, L., Amelio, D., et al. (2019). Quercetin and its derivative Q2 modulate chromatin dynamics in adipogenesis and Q2 prevents obesity and metabolic disorders in rats. *The Journal of Nutritional Biochemistry, 69*, 151–162.

Newsholme, P., Haber, E. P., Hirabara, S. M., Rebelato, E. L. O., Procopio, J., et al. (2007). Diabetes associated cell stress and dysfunction: Role of mitochondrial and non-mitochondrial ROS production and activity. *The Journal of Physiology, 583*(1), 9–24.

Öztürk, E., Arslan, A. K. K., Yerer, M. B., & Bishayee, A. (2017). Resveratrol and diabetes: A critical review of clinical studies. *Biomedicine & Pharmacotherapy, 95*, 230–234.

Ogawa, Y., Noma, Y., Davalli, A. M., Wu, Y. J., Thorens, B., et al. (1995). Loss of glucose-induced insulin secretion and GLUT2 expression in transplanted β-cells. *Diabetes, 44*(1), 75–79.

Ono, Y., & Kataoka, K. (2024). Glucocorticoids reduce Slc2a2 (GLUT2) gene expression through HNF1 in pancreatic β-cells. *Journal of Molecular Endocrinology, 1*(aop).

Ortiz-Andrade, R. R., Sánchez-Salgado, J. C., Navarrete-Vázquez, G., Webster, S. P., Binnie, M., et al. (2008). Antidiabetic and toxicological evaluations of naringenin in normoglycaemic and NIDDM rat models and its implications on extra-pancreatic glucose regulation. *Diabetes, Obesity and Metabolism, 10*(11), 1097–1104.

Padhi, S., Nayak, A. K., & Behera, A. (2020). Type II diabetes mellitus: A review on recent drug based therapeutics. *Biomedicine & Pharmacotherapy, 131*, Article 110708.

Pinney, S. E., & Simmons, R. A. (2010). Epigenetic mechanisms in the development of type 2 diabetes. *Trends in Endocrinology and Metabolism, 21*(4), 223–229.

Priscilla, D. H., Roy, D., Suresh, A., Kumar, V., & Thirumurugan, K. (2014). Naringenin inhibits α-glucosidase activity: A promising strategy for the regulation of postprandial hyperglycemia in high fat diet fed streptozotocin induced diabetic rats. *Chemico-Biological Interactions, 210*, 77–85.

Priyadarshini, A., Madan, R., & Das, S. (2024). Genetics and epigenetics of diabetes and its complications in India. *Human Genetics, 143*(1), 1–17.

Raslan, M. M., Mohamed, S., Abd El Maksoud, M. D. E., & El Nesr, K. (2018). Role of curcumin-zinc oxide composite nanoparticles on streptozotocin-induced diabetic rats. *Journal of Biotechnology & Biomaterials, 8*, 55.

Rautenberg, E. K., Hamzaoui, Y., & Coletta, D. K. (2022). Mini-review: Mitochondrial DNA methylation in type 2 diabetes and obesity. *Frontiers in Endocrinology, 13*, Article 968268.

Ren, B., Qin, W., Wu, F., Wang, S., Pan, C., et al. (2016). Apigenin and naringenin regulate glucose and lipid metabolism, and ameliorate vascular dysfunction in type 2 diabetic rats. *European Journal of Pharmacology, 773*, 13–23.

Roshanzamir, N., & Hassan-Zadeh, V. (2020). Methylation of specific CpG sites in IL-1β and IL1R1 genes is affected by hyperglycaemia in type 2 diabetic patients. *Immunological Investigations, 49*(3), 287–298.

Saini, R. K., Ranjit, A., Sharma, K., Prasad, P., Shang, X., et al. (2022). Bioactive compounds of citrus fruits: A review of composition and health benefits of carotenoids, flavonoids, limonoids, and terpenes. *Antioxidants, 11*(2), 239.

Schumann, T., König, J., Henke, C., Willmes, D. M., Bornstein, S. R., et al. (2020). Solute carrier transporters as potential targets for the treatment of metabolic disease. *Pharmacological Reviews, 72*(1), 343–379.

Seto, E., & Yoshida, M. (2014). Erasers of histone acetylation: The histone deacetylase enzymes. *Cold Spring Harbor Perspectives in Biology, 6*(4), Article a018713.

Shi, G. J., Li, Y., Cao, Q. H., Wu, H. X., Tang, X. Y., et al. (2019). In vitro and in vivo evidence that quercetin protects against diabetes and its complications: A systematic review of the literature. *Biomedicine & Pharmacotherapy, 109*, 1085–1099.

Shvedunova, M., & Akhtar, A. (2022). Modulation of cellular processes by histone and non-histone protein acetylation. *Nature Reviews Molecular Cell Biology, 23*(5), 329–349.

Singh, R., Chandel, S., Dey, D., Ghosh, A., Roy, S., et al. (2020). Epigenetic modification and therapeutic targets of diabetes mellitus. *Bioscience Reports, 40*(9), Article BSR20202160.

Sirovina, D., Oršolić, N., Gregorović, G., & Končić, M. Z. (2016). Naringenin ameliorates pathological changes in liver and kidney of diabetic mice: A preliminary study/naringenin reducira histopatološke promjene u jetri i bubregu miševa s dijabetesom. *Archives of Industrial Hygiene and Toxicology, 67*(1), 19–24.

Smeriglio, A., Calderaro, A., Denaro, M., Laganà, G., & Bellocco, E. (2019). Effects of isolated isoflavones intake on health. *Current Medicinal Chemistry, 26*(27), 5094–5107.

Sterner, D. E., & Berger, S. L. (2000). Acetylation of histones and transcription-related factors. *Microbiology and Molecular Biology Reviews, 64*(2), 435–459.

Tang, C., Liu, Y., Liu, S., Yang, C., Chen, L., et al. (2024). *Curcumin and analogues as potential epigenetic modulators: Prevention of metabolic diseases.*

Thirumalaisamy, R., Bhuvaneswari, M., Haritha, S., Jeevarathna, S., Janani, K. S., & Suresh, K. (2022). Curcumin, naringenin and resveratrol from natural plant products hold promising solutions for modern world diseases–A recent review. *South African Journal of Botany, 151*, 567–580.

Volkov, P., Bacos, K., Ofori, J. K., Esguerra, J. L. S., Eliasson, L., et al. (2017). Whole-genome bisulfite sequencing of human pancreatic islets reveals novel differentially methylated regions in type 2 diabetes pathogenesis. *Diabetes, 66*(4), 1074–1085.

Walaszczyk, E., Luijten, M., Spijkerman, A. M., Bonder, M. J., Lutgers, H. L., et al. (2018). DNA methylation markers associated with type 2 diabetes, fasting glucose and HbA1c levels: A systematic review and replication in a case–control sample of the lifelines study. *Diabetologia, 61*(2), 354–368.

Wang, Y., Hou, C., Wisler, J., Singh, K., Wu, C., et al. (2019). Elevated histone H3 acetylation is associated with genes involved in T lymphocyte activation and glutamate decarboxylase antibody production in patients with type 1 diabetes. *Journal of Diabetes Investigation, 10*(1), 51–61.

Wang, S. W., Sheng, H., Bai, Y. F., Weng, Y. Y., Fan, X. Y., et al. (2021). Inhibition of histone acetyltransferase by naringenin and hesperetin suppresses Txnip expression and protects pancreatic β cells in diabetic mice. *Phytomedicine, 88*, Article 153454.

Weng, L., Zhang, F., Wang, R., Ma, W., & Song, Y. (2019). A review on protective role of genistein against oxidative stress in diabetes and related complications. *Chemico-Biological Interactions, 310*, Article 108665.

Willmer, T., Johnson, R., Louw, J., & Pheiffer, C. (2018). Blood-based DNA methylation biomarkers for type 2 diabetes: Potential for clinical applications. *Frontiers in Endocrinology, 9*, 744.

Wojcik, M., Krawczyk, M., Wojcik, P., Cypryk, K., & Wozniak, L. A. (2018). Molecular mechanisms underlying curcumin-mediated therapeutic effects in type 2 diabetes and cancer. *Oxidative Medicine and Cellular Longevity, 2018*(1), Article 9698258.

Yamamoto, H., Schoonjans, K., & Auwerx, J. (2007). Sirtuin functions in health and disease. *Molecular Endocrinology, 21*(8), 1745–1755.

Yang, B. T., Dayeh, T. A., Kirkpatrick, C. L., Taneera, J., Kumar, R., et al. (2011). Insulin promoter DNA methylation correlates negatively with insulin gene expression and positively with HbA 1c levels in human pancreatic islets. *Diabetologia, 54*, 360–367.

Yang, B. T., Dayeh, T. A., Volkov, P. A., Kirkpatrick, C. L., Malmgren, S., et al. (2012). Increased DNA methylation and decreased expression of PDX-1 in pancreatic islets from patients with type 2 diabetes. *Molecular Endocrinology, 26*(7), 1203–1212.

Yang, T., Qi, F., Guo, F., Shao, M., Song, Y., et al. (2024). An update on chronic complications of diabetes mellitus: From molecular mechanisms to therapeutic strategies with a focus on metabolic memory. *Molecular Medicine, 30*(1), 71.

Yang, X. J., & Seto, E. H. A. T. (2007). HATs and HDACs: From structure, function and regulation to novel strategies for therapy and prevention. *Oncogene, 26*(37), 5310-5310.

Yin, L., Zhu, X., Novák, P., Zhou, L., Gao, L., et al. (2021). The epitranscriptome of long noncoding RNAs in metabolic diseases. *Clinica Chimica Acta, 515*, 80–89.

Yun, J. M., Jialal, I., & Devaraj, S. (2011). Epigenetic regulation of high glucose-induced proinflammatory cytokine production in monocytes by curcumin. *The Journal of Nutritional Biochemistry, 22*(5), 450–458.

Zatterale, F., Raciti, G. A., Prevenzano, I., Leone, A., Campitelli, M., De Rosa, V., et al. (2022). Epigenetic reprogramming of the inflammatory response in obesity and type 2 diabetes. *Biomolecules, 12*(7), 982.

Zhang, P., Li, T., Wu, X., Nice, E. C., Huang, C., & Zhang, Y. (2020). Oxidative stress and diabetes: Antioxidative strategies. *Frontiers of Medicine, 14*, 583–600.

Zhang, L., Lu, Q., & Chang, C. (2020). Epigenetics in health and disease. *Epigenetics in Allergy and Autoimmunity*, 3–55.

Zhang, L., Sheng, C., Zhou, F., Zhu, K., Wang, S., et al. (2021). CBP/p300 HAT maintains the gene network critical for β cell identity and functional maturity. *Cell Death & Disease, 12*(5), 476.

Zheng, L., He, S., Wang, H., Li, J., Liu, Y., & Liu, S. (2024). Targeting cellular senescence in aging and age-related diseases: Challenges, considerations, and the emerging role of senolytic and senomorphic therapies. *Aging and Disease, 15*(6), 2554–2594.

Zhou, Y. X., Zhang, H., & Peng, C. (2014). Puerarin: A review of pharmacological effects. *Phytotherapy Research, 28*(7), 961–975.

Zhu, X., Wu, C., Qiu, S., Yuan, X., & Li, L. (2017). Effects of resveratrol on glucose control and insulin sensitivity in subjects with type 2 diabetes: Systematic review and meta-analysis. *Nutrition & Metabolism, 14*, 1–10.

8

HLA associations in T2DM susceptibility

Shweta Arya[1], Annanya Antal[1], Khushi Negi[1], Harshit Devtalla[2], Priyanka Yadav[1], Prachi Chauhan[1], Shalini Mani[1], Manisha Singh[1], Shazia Haider[3] and R. Rachana[1]

[1]*DEPARTMENT OF BIOTECHNOLOGY, JAYPEE INSTITUTE OF INFORMATION TECHNOLOGY, NOIDA, UTTAR PRADESH, INDIA;* [2]*DEPARTMENT OF BIOCHEMISTRY, POST GRADUATE INSTITUTE OF MEDICAL EDUCATION AND RESEARCH, CHANDIGARH, INDIA;* [3]*DEPARTMENT OF BIOSCIENCES, FACULTY OF NATURAL SCIENCES, JAMIA MILLIA UNIVERSITY, DELHI, NEW DELHI, INDIA*

1. Overview of T2DM

Diabetes is widely categorized into type 1 (insulin dependent) and type 2 (non-insulin independent), which is a chronic disorder with high blood sugar level. Type 2 diabetes accounts for approximately 90% of the cases worldwide (Ahmad et al., 2022). While diabetes mellitus type 1 (type 1 DM) is a noncommunicable endocrine disorder wherein the pancreatic β-cells fail to produce insulin (Kahanovitz et al., 2017), type 2 diabetes mellitus (type 2 DM/T2D) is a chronic condition where the cells utilizing glucose become resistant to insulin or β-cells do not produce insulin in sufficient amounts, leading to an increase in blood glucose levels (Galicia-Garcia et al., 2020). The symptoms for "type 2 diabetes mellitus" (T2DM) could be mild and appear similar to type 1 diabetes at the initial stage. It may not be diagnosed easily and could take years to be noticed by an individual (World Health Organization, 2024). The elevated demand for insulin in the targeted tissues is caused by insulin resistance, which could not be completed due to β-cell dysfunctioning (Młynarska et al., 2025). T2DM generally arises due to the combination of genetic predisposition and environment related factors such as unhealthy diet, obesity, lack of exercises, and stress (Dendup et al., 2018) (Fig. 8.1). With time, insulin-resistant conditions rise in the body, and the pancreas becomes incapable of making the excess amount of insulin to overcome the condition (Institute of Health Metrics and Evaluation, 2021).

Type 2 Diabetes Mellitus. https://doi.org/10.1016/B978-0-443-33590-7.00009-5

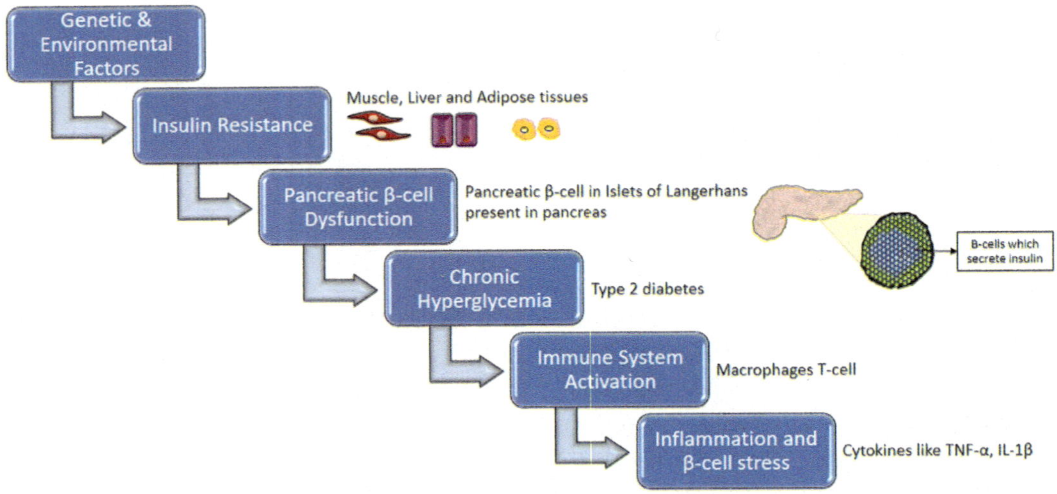

FIGURE 8.1 Pathogenesis of type 2 diabetes Mellitus: The diagram illustrates the pathogenesis of type 2 diabetes Mellitus, showing influence of genetic and environmental factors contributing to insulin resistance primarily affecting muscle, liver, and adipose tissues. This leads to pancreatic β-cell dysfunctioning, reducing the insulin secretion. Chronic hyperglycemia, triggering immune system activation involving macrophages and T cells. This response leads to inflammation and β-cell stress with cytokines such as TNF-α and IL-1β further worsening the condition.

2. Global prevalence and burden of T2D

Over the past few decades, type 2 diabetes and its prevalence and burden have increased dramatically worldwide suggesting these projections will further increase. According to estimates, the prevalence of adult diabetes was 4% in 1995, rising to 5.4% by 2025 with the number of adults with diabetes increasing from 135 million to 300 million during this time (King et al., 1998). By 2023, approximately 529 million individuals were badly affected with diabetes, comprising a prevalence rate of 6.1% (Liane et al., 2023). Diabetic cases are expected to increase 1.3 billion by 2050, with influential prevalence likely in the Middle East, Latin America, and North Africa (Liane et al., 2023). Greater rates of prevalence are found in the Middle East and North Africa (Bai & Ameyaw, 2024). Maximum of the type 2 diabetes cases, which constituted 96% and 95% cases, are associated with diabetes-related disability-adjusted life years (DALYs) (Safiri et al., 2022).

Developing countries report alarmingly high prevalence rates, with over 80% of cases occurring in these regions (Alam et al., 2021). Greater BMI is found to be highly responsible for over half of the world's type 2 diabetes DALYs, and its impact has been found to be increasing (Tandon et al., 2018). The highest rates of diabetes are currently found in China, India, Pakistan, United States, and Indonesia (Magliano et al., 2021). By 2045, it is estimated that Pakistan will surpass the United States in the number of diabetes cases, moving from the fourth to the third position globally. As of now, there are 19.4 million people with diabetes in Pakistan, a significant increase from 5.5 million in

2000 (Azeem et al., 2022). Managing the rise in diabetes due to various internal and external factors needed highly targeted strategies to resolve and prevent the disease (Sun et al., 2022).

3. Effect of heritability and environmental factors

The genetic architecture of a complex phenotype, such as type 2 diabetes (T2D), is influenced by the number, frequency, and effect size of causal alleles. Various hypothesis have been proposed to explain the genetic basis of T2D. One hypothesis suggested unexplained heritability may arise from many common genetic variants with small effects, and the disease represents the extreme end of a normal distribution (Manolio et al., 2009). Another hypothesis posits that rare alleles could account for the effects seen with common variants through synthetic associations, potentially explaining much of the heritability. However, an argument against both common and rare variants is that they would have been eliminated by natural selection (Gibson, 2012). This argument, though, does not hold for T2D, as the disease's genetic effects are heavily influenced by environmental interactions, particularly in the context of recent lifestyle changes, where genetic variants might have been neutral or advantageous in the past (Prasad & Groop, 2015). In a study, DeForest and Majithia (2022) have concluded that there could be more than 700 risk loci found in T2D. Using WGS (whole-genome sequencing) and large-scale exome within a population could introduce biobanks that enable rare-variant studies by identifying novel T2D loci. Therefore, genetic mapping to enhance novel locus findings can lead to new treatments for T2D (DeForest & Majithia, 2022); for example, α-1 antitrypsin (AAT) therapy and C-peptide preservation therapy are one of the cost-effective and viable options for the treatment of type 1 diabetes (Chopra & Rachana, 2024). In a plant-based traditional system, Basu et al. (2013) have described that the bark of the *Salacia* genus has the ability to lower blood sugar. Its compounds such as mangiferin and salacinol help lower blood sugar, along with antioxidant and pancreatic lipase inhibitory activities, making it a potential natural remedy for diabetes (Basu et al., 2013).

4. HLA association with other diseases

HLAs (human leukocyte antigen) association with diseases normally shows a strong link between the specific variations in the HLA genes with increased susceptibility to various autoimmune diseases, for example, type 1 diabetes, celiac disease, multiple sclerosis, and rheumatoid arthritis (Table 8.1). HLA plays an important role in antigen presentation, leading to abnormal immune responses against the self-antigens that allow cells to recognize the foreign substances (Crux & Elahi, 2017). In this way, variations in different HLA genes (alleles) can affect the ability of the immune system to recognize and respond to antigens, which results in disease susceptibility (Medhasi & Chantratita, 2022). Type 1

Table 8.1 Association of HLA allele with diseases, their mechanism, and references.

S. no.	HLA allele	Associated disease	Mechanism involved	References
1	HLA-DR	Type 1 diabetes, rheumatoid arthritis	Autoimmune destruction of pancreatic β-cells due to abnormal antigen presentation	Nguyen et al. (2013)
2	HLA-DR1	Type 1 diabetes mellitus	Alters antigen presentation, leading to autoreactive T cell activation and β-cell destruction	Jacobi et al. (2020)
3	HLA-DR6	Type 1 diabetes mellitus	Strongly associated with onset of type 1 diabetes and enhances the β-cell autoimmunity	Jacobi et al. (2020)
4	HLA-DR9	Type 2 diabetes mellitus	Contributes to impaired immune dysregulation and chronic inflammation	Jacobi et al. (2020)
5	HLA-DQA1*0301, DQB106:02	Type 2 diabetes mellitus	Insulin resistance and β-cell dysregulation	Ma et al. (2013); Guo et al. (2016)
6	HLA-A*03:01:01:01*, HLA-C01:02:01:01	Type 2 diabetes	Antigen presentation and β-cell vulnerability	Jan et al. (2021)
7	HLA-A*68*	Protective allele in type 1 diabetes and type 2 diabetes mellitus, HIV infection	Influence immune responses, leading to autoimmune β-cell destruction (T1D) or inflammation-related insulin dysfunction (T2D)	Jan et al. (2021)
8	HLA-DRB108, HLA-DRB103, HLA-DRB104	Type 1 diabetes	Activation of cytotoxic T cells that target and destroy insulin-producing β-cells, resulting in impaired insulin secretion characteristic of T1D	Altobelli et al. (2005); Williams et al. (2011)
9	HLA-DQ8	Type 1 diabetes, celiac disease	Inflammation caused by abnormal T cell activation	Pugliese (2017)
10	HLA-DQ2	Type 1 diabetes	Triggers immune destruction of β-cells in T1D	Pugliese (2017)
11	HLA-DQB103*:02*, HLA-DRB105:01	Type 2 diabetes	Immune dysregulation	Ma et al. (2013)
12	HLA-DRB1	Type 1 diabetes, celiac disease	Improper immune recognition, triggering autoimmunity	Lee and Lam (2019)
13	HLA-DQA1	Type 2 diabetes mellitus	Increased inflammation and insulin resistance in type 2 diabetes	Scott et al. (2017)
14	HLA-DRB107:01	Type 2 diabetes mellitus	Immune-mediated destruction of pancreatic β-cells	Jacobi et al. (2020)
15	HLA-DQA102:01, DRB 501:01, DQA 01:02, DRB115:01, DQB 06:02, DQB1*03:03	Type 2 diabetes mellitus	Increases the risk of non–insulin-treated diabetes by promoting β-cell dysfunction but delaying insulin treatment	Jacobi et al. (2020)

Table 8.1 Association of HLA allele with diseases, their mechanism, and references.—cont'd

S. no.	HLA allele	Associated disease	Mechanism involved	References
16	HLA-DRB1*0701, 1501, 1502, 1301, 1001, 0403, and 1404 and HLA-DRB1*0101, 0301, 0401, 0803, 1101, 1202, and 1302	Type 1 diabetes and type 2 diabetes mellitus	Linked to T1D through autoimmune β-cell destruction and contributing to insulin resistance in T2D	Weiskopf et al. (2016)
17	HLA-C1C1	Type 2 diabetes mellitus	Increased NK cell activation affecting immune response	Caselli et al. (2013)

diabetes is one of the examples of such HLA-associated diseases; it shows strong association with HLA-DR and HLA-DQ2 alleles (Nguyen et al., 2013). Similarly, the disease rheumatoid arthritis is shown to be linked to the specific HLA-DRB1 alleles, particularly the "shared epitope." Celiac disease is primarily shown to be associated with HLA-DQ2 and HLA-DQ8. Certain HLA-DR alleles are considered risk factors (Koning et al., 2015). The following is a description of association of HLA types and their associated roles in causing diabetes.

5. HLA association with diabetes (T1DM and T2DM)

Similar to many other diseases, HLA-related genetic predispositions have been noted in T2DM, however, less frequently than in T1DM, although the exact HLA associations vary greatly between these two conditions. Various HLA variants such as HLA-DQA1*0301 and HLA-DQA1*0501 were found to be susceptibility markers for type 2 diabetes (Ma et al., 2013) (Table 8.1). In another study, other HLA variants, including HLA-DRB1 and HLA-DQB1, were shown to be linked to type 2 diabetes in Bahraini populations; some of these alleles confer vulnerability, while others had protective effects as well such as HLA-DQB1*0501 (Table 8.2). This implies that HLA alleles may affect the risk of complications from type 2 diabetes as well as susceptibility to the disease (Ma et al., 2013).

5.1 HLA associations in diabetes mellitus in different ethnic groups

The HLA system has been shown to be associated with type 2 diabetes in different ethnic groups. Variants such as HLA-A*03:01:01:01 and HLA-C*01:02:01:01 are associated with T2DM in populations such as Mexicans, where hypervariable regions influence antigen presentation and β-cell vulnerability (Fig. 8.2). Protective alleles, such as HLA-A*68* and *A*11, identified in South Indian and Mexican American populations, mitigate disease risk. Variants such as rs2308655 in HLA-B, observed in the Pashtun ethnic group, alter peptide-binding regions, affecting immune recognition and increasing β-cell vulnerability under hyperglycemic conditions (Jan et al., 2021).

Table 8.2 HLA alleles having protective association with T1D and T2D along with its mechanism and their references.

S. no.	HLA Allele	Associated disease	Mechanism	References
1	HLA-DR2	Protective in type 1 diabetes	Protective against T1D by promoting immune tolerance and reducing autoimmune responses.	Rich et al. (2018)
2	HLA-DR3 (DRB103:01)	Protective in type 1 diabetes	Protective against T1D by promoting immune tolerance and reducing autoimmune responses.	Rich et al. (2018)
3	HLA-DR4 (DRB104:01)	Protective in type 1 diabetes	Protective against T1D by promoting immune tolerance and reducing autoimmune responses.	Rich et al. (2018)
4	HLA DRB1*15:01	Protective in type 1 diabetes	Protective against T1D by promoting immune tolerance and reducing autoimmune responses.	Rich et al. (2018)
5	HLA-DRB 102	Protective against T2DM	Enhanced self-tolerance and reduced risk of autoimmune-mediated impairment of insulin secretion.	Božič (2002)

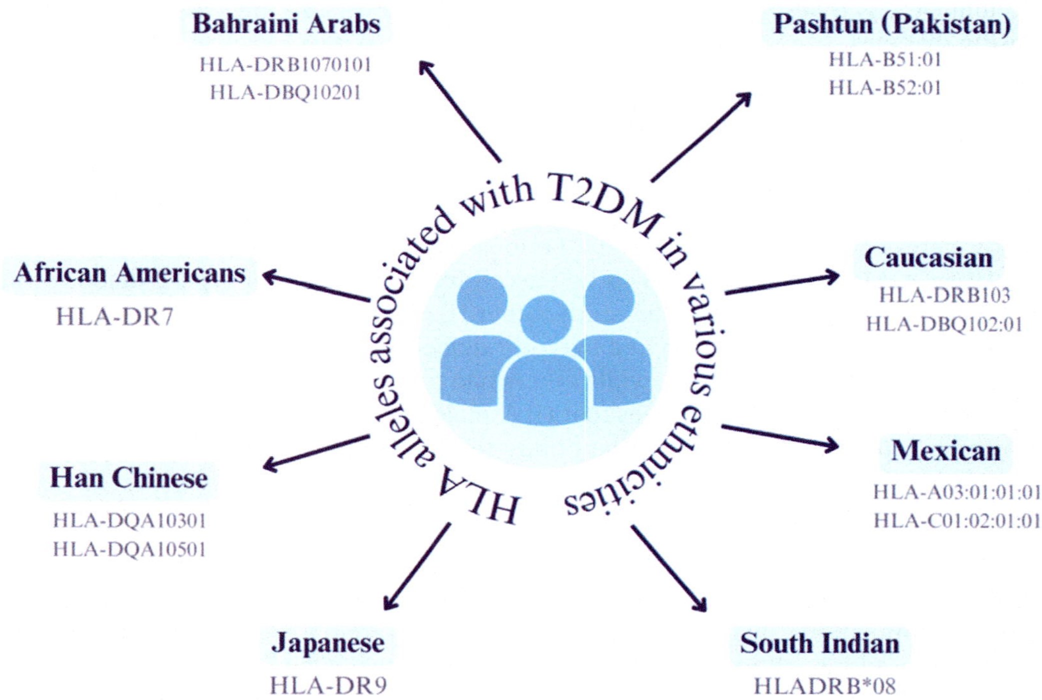

FIGURE 8.2 Susceptible HLA alleles associated with type 2 diabetes mellitus (T2DM) across various ethnic groups: The diagram illustrates the association of specific HLA alleles withT2DM across various ethnic groups. The central icon represents human populations, with arrows pointing toward different ethnic groups, each labeled with the corresponding HLA alleles linked to T2DM susceptibility. These ethnic groups include Bahraini Arabs, Pashtun (Pakistan), Caucasian, Mexican, South Indian, Japanese, Han Chinese, and African Americans. The identified HLA alleles vary among populations, highlighting genetic diversity in T2DM predisposition.

HLA-DQA10301 and HLA-DQA10501 alleles are linked to an increased susceptibility to type 2 diabetes in the Han Chinese population (Ma et al., 2013) (Fig. 8.2). According to studies conducted on Pakistan's Pashtun ethnic group, the HLA-B gene variant rs2308655 is linked to an elevated risk of type 2 diabetes, suggesting that certain HLA class I gene variations also play a role in the condition (Medhasi & Chantratita, 2022).

The HLA-DRB 102 (1602) allele has been found to be beneficial among the Pima Indian community because it enhances insulin secretion and HLA-DRB1 mRNA expression (Božič, 2002) (Fig. 8.2). By promoting immunological tolerance and avoiding autoimmune damage to insulin-producing β-cells, this lowers the risk of type 2 diabetes (Burrack et al., 2017).

Research on children in Mexico revealed that HLA-DRB108 was more than 10 times more common in T2DM than in T1DM, suggesting that it may serve as a differentiator. Remarkably, HLA-DRB1 04, a significant risk factor for type 1 diabetes, seems to offer protection against type 2 diabetes (Fig. 8.2) (Williams et al., 2011).

Saxena et al. (2012) in his study reported that new genetic risk and its association with type 2 diabetes can be identified using a dense gene-centric approach for multiethnic metaanalysis for large scale. Three new European T2DM loci (GATAD2A/CILP2/PBX4, SREBF1, AND TH/INS), one African American locus (HMGA2), and one multiethnic locus (BCL2) have been identified as new risk loci. T2DM loci were associated with genetic influence across different ethnicities (Fig. 8.2) (Saxena et al., 2012).

5.2 Mechanism responsible for diabetes

Diabetes mellitus is a chronic metabolic disorder characterized by persistent hyperglycemia, resulting from either insufficient insulin production due to pancreatic β-cell dysfunction, i.e., type I or impaired insulin utilization by peripheral tissues such as the liver, skeletal muscles, and adipocytes, i.e., type II (Rachana & Sharma, 2024). Recent researches have highlighted the involvement of the human leukocyte antigen (HLA) system in modulating the immune responses that contribute to T2D. This system is central to antigen presentation and immune regulation (Jacobi et al., 2020). This way there are two major categories of the mechanisms causing diabetes, which include HLA molecules. The first one is related to the antigens expression causing autoimmunity to be provoked, and another one is majorly related to modulation of the immune system and increase in inflammatory responses. The first one is majorly known to be responsible for type 1 diabetes.

T2DM is a multifactorial metabolic disorder characterized by insulin resistance and progressive pancreatic β-cell dysfunction. Genetic factors, including variations in the human leukocyte antigen (HLA) system, have been implicated in immune dysregulation and chronic low-grade inflammation, contributing to disease progression (Hameed et al., 2015). Environmental factors such as high-caloric intake and a sedentary lifestyle further promote insulin resistance in peripheral tissues such as the liver, muscles, and adipose tissue, leading to hyperglycemia. Chronic inflammation, driven by cytokines such as IL-6 and TNF-α, plays a key role in worsening insulin sensitivity and β-cell dysfunction, highlighting the immune-metabolic interface in T2DM pathogenesis (Donath & Shoelson, 2011). Addressing both genetic susceptibility and modifiable lifestyle factors is crucial for effective prevention and management of T2DM (Fig. 8.3).

5.2.1 Antigen expression, autoantibodies and β-cell destruction

As mentioned before, this mechanism is majorly responsible for type 1 diabetes and can distinguish the two types of diabetes on the basis of their underlying genetic and immunological mechanisms, and these are reflected in their HLA connections (Li et al., 2025). It has been shown that heterozygous combinations such as HLA-DR3/DR4 greatly increase susceptibility to diabetes as they play a role in autoimmune β-cell destruction (Fig. 8.4). T1DM is reported to be highly linked to the HLA-DRB103 and HLA-DRB104 alleles (Altobelli et al., 2005).

Certain HLA molecules, such HLA-DQ8 and HLA-DQ2, express β-cell antigens, such as insulin to $CD4^+$ T cells in diabetes. This leads to autoreactive T cell activation, which

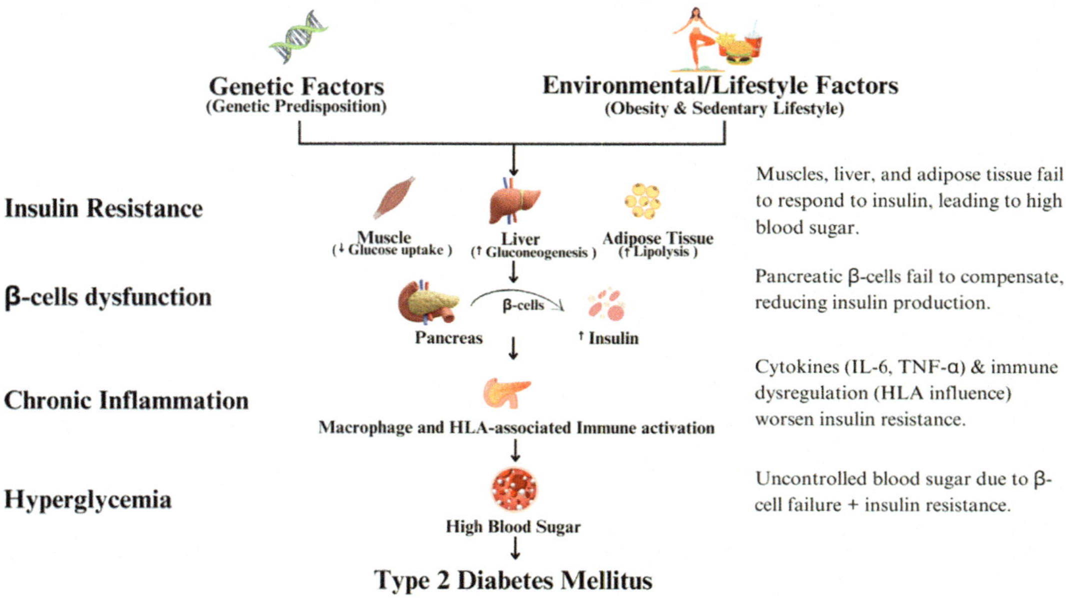

FIGURE 8.3 A schematic representation of the factors contributing to type 2 diabetes mellitus (T2DM): genetic factors (genetic predisposition) and environmental/lifestyle factors (obesity and sedentary lifestyle) lead to insulin resistance, β-cell dysfunction, chronic inflammation, and hyperglycemia. Insulin resistance occurs as muscles, the liver, and adipose tissue fail to respond to insulin, leading to high blood sugar. β-cell dysfunction results in inadequate insulin production. Chronic inflammation, mediated by cytokines (IL-6, TNF-α) and HLA-associated immune activation, worsens insulin resistance. These combined effects lead to persistent hyperglycemia, ultimately resulting in type 2 diabetes mellitus.

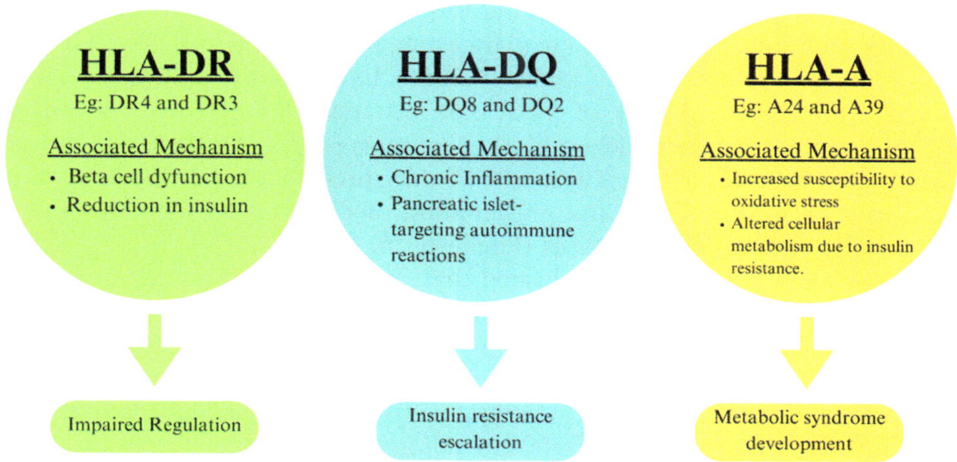

FIGURE 8.4 Role of HLA alleles and its associated mechanism with type 2 diabetes mellitus with outcome.

results in the death of β-cells, decreased insulin production, and the advancement of diabetes (Pugliese, 2017). High expression of HLA class I genes such as HLA-A24 and HLA-B39 raises the risk of developing autoimmune diabetes by upregulating β-cell antigens presented to CD^{8+} T cells, targeting them for cell mediated cytotoxic destruction (Yeo et al., 2020) (Table 8.1).

HLA class I molecules (HLA-A, HLA-B, HLA-C) present intracellular peptides of β-cells to $CD8^{+}$ cytotoxic T cells, increasing their susceptibility to immune-mediated damage (Cruz-Tapias et al., 2013).

Type 1 diabetes has also been shown to have clear association with several HLA class II alleles such as HLA-DR and HLA-DQ alleles: Research in this field has demonstrated that HLA-DR3 (DRB103:01) and HLA-DR4 (DRB104:01) alleles have a positive association with increasing the risk for T1DM (Fig. 8.4). A homozygous combination of such alleles is still at an even higher risk of developing T1DM. Some alleles even show protective effects against T1DM such as HLA-DR2, or DRB1*15:01 (Rich et al., 2018). Mclaughlin et al. (2014) in a study investigated the interactions between T cell and B cell, and if IA-2-specific autoantibodies correlate with T cell responses to IA-2 peptides presented by HLA-DR4. To quantify the T cells secreting interferon-γ (IFN-γ) and interleukin-10 (IL10) with response to seven IA-2 peptides in HLA-T1D patients, cytokine ELISPOT was used. T cell responses to peptide 841–860 correlated with antibodies targeting IA-2 juxtamembrane epitopes, which appear early in prediabetes. This suggested the HLA association of IA-2 autoantibodies serving as a promising target for preventing type 1 diabetes through its immune interventions (Mclaughlin et at., 2014).

Type 2 diabetes is also reported to be caused by HLA-mediated antigen expression (Popoviciu et al., 2023). As HLA II has also been found to be involved in the regulation of immune responses that lead to β-cell damage, especially in latent autoimmune diabetes in adults (LADA), these autoimmune processes based on the production of β-cell autoantibodies and autoreactive T cell activity establish a genetic link between T1D and T2DM. Genome-wide association studies (GWAS) have identified several HLA alleles associated with increased risk of T2D. For instance, HLA-DQB1*03:02 and HLA-DRB1*05:01 are significantly enriched in T2D patients, suggesting their role in immune dysregulation (Ma et al., 2013). These alleles may predispose individuals to a proinflammatory state by facilitating the presentation of diabetogenic peptides to T cells, thereby amplifying immune responses (Pugliese, 2017).

Study by Williams et al. (2011) indicated that certain HLA haplotypes may influence susceptibility to T2D by modulating immune responses to pancreatic β cell antigens or by altering interactions with inflammatory cytokines. For instance, HLA-DRB1 alleles have been associated with the progression of insulin resistance through inflammatory pathways (Williams et al., 2011). On the other hand, dysregulated HLA-mediated antigen presentation may trigger inappropriate activation of autoreactive T cells, exacerbating systemic inflammation—a hallmark of T2D (Girard & Vandiedonck, 2022).

5.2.2 HLA-mediated inflammatory mechanism causing T2D

The study by de Bakker et al. (2006) demonstrates a genetic map of the HLA locus. This achievement has significantly advanced the field of HLA genotyping. By enabling the imputation of HLA genotypes from SNP data, this map has facilitated the identification of numerous alleles and their associations with various diseases, including T2D. A metaanalysis conducted by Guo et al. (2016) represents a significant association between the specific HLA alleles including DQB102, DQB106:02, and DRB1*13:02 and the risk of gestational diabetes. It is reported that gestational diabetes increases the lifetime risk of developing type 2 diabetes. This outcome holds a potential role of certain HLA alleles in increasing susceptibility to both gestational diabetes and subsequently T2D (Guo et al., 2016).

T2DM is a multifactorial metabolic disorder characterized by insulin resistance and progressive pancreatic β-cell dysfunction. Genetic factors, including variations in the human leukocyte antigen (HLA) system, have been implicated in immune dysregulation and chronic low-grade inflammation, contributing to disease progression (Arora et al., 2011). Environmental factors such as high-caloric intake and a sedentary lifestyle further promote insulin resistance in peripheral tissues such as the liver, muscles, and adipose tissue, leading to hyperglycemia. In a study, Donath and Shoelson (2011) reported that chronic inflammation, driven by cytokines such as IL-6 and TNF-α, plays a key role in worsening insulin sensitivity and β-cell dysfunction, highlighting the immune–metabolic interface in T2DM pathogenesis (Donath & Shoelson, 2011). Addressing both genetic susceptibility and modifiable lifestyle factors is crucial for effective prevention and management of T2DM (Fig. 8.4).

As mentioned before, HLA has a significant role in immune responses related to self-antigens and damage-associated molecular patterns, and so in diabetes-related inflammation as well (Bodis et al., 2018). Certain HLA polymorphisms may contribute to prolonged low-grade inflammation (metaflammation) in T2DM by increasing the production of cytokines (such as IL-6 and TNF-α) and interacting with dysbiosis of the gut microbiota (Campbell et al., 2017) (Fig. 8.5).

This way HLA-mediated immune dysregulation influences various pathways in T2D, including chronic inflammation and improper function of immune cells, making the HLA system a crucial factor in understanding the immunological underpinnings of this disease (Naito et al., 2021) (Fig. 8.4).

Chronic inflammation is a key driver of β-cell dysfunction and insulin resistance in T2D. HLA-mediated immune dysregulation contributes to this process by perpetuating inflammatory signaling pathways. For example, aberrant HLA expression on antigen-presenting cells (APCs) can enhance T cell activation, leading to sustained production of proinflammatory cytokines such as IL-1β, TNF-α, and IFN-γ (Donath & Shoelson, 2011). These cytokines not only impair insulin signaling in peripheral tissues but also induce β-cell apoptosis.

Jacobi et al. (2020) in their study highlight the role that inflammatory cytokines such as IL-6, TNF-α, and IL-1β play in the development of metabolic dysregulation, insulin resistance, and inflammation in disorders including obesity, diabetes, and metabolic syndrome. This research also gives some possible therapeutic strategies targeting these cytokines to slow down disease progression. This study gives a great insight into cytokine-mediated inflammation in metabolic disorders and, eventually, sets the platform for a novel therapeutic intervention (Jacobi et al., 2020).

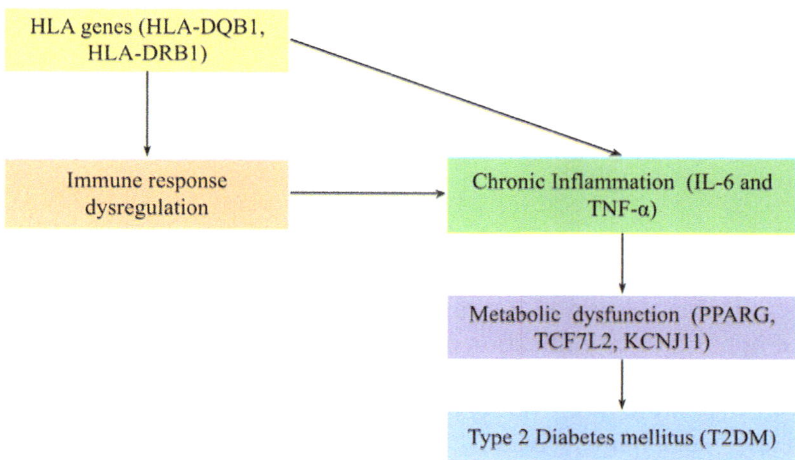

FIGURE 8.5 The role of HLA genes in type 2 diabetes mellitus (T2DM) development. This diagram depicts the interaction between HLA genes (HLA-DQB1, HLA-DRB1) and other genetic factors associated with T2DM. HLA polymorphisms contribute to immune response dysregulation, which can lead to chronic inflammation mediated by cytokines such as IL-6 and TNF-α. Chronic inflammation further influences metabolic dysfunction, involving key T2DM susceptibility genes (PPARG, TCF7L2, KCNJ11), ultimately leading to β-cell dysfunction, insulin resistance, and the development of T2DM. Arrows indicate the direction of influence between these factors.

Additionally, studies suggest that HLA-DR expression on monocytes correlates with systemic inflammation and metabolic dysfunction in T2D. Increased HLA-DR expression has been linked to higher levels of C-reactive protein (CRP), an established marker of inflammation and cardiovascular risk in T2D patients (Quirant-Sanchez et al., 2023).

Study by Al-Daghri et al. (2012) finds that in the patients with T2DM, HLA DRB104 is significantly associated with certain polymorphisms in the vitamin D receptor (VDR) gene, specifically rs731236 (TaqI) and rs1544410 (BsmI), which influence VDR expression and function. The vitamin D response element (VDRE) in the HLA-DRB1 promoter may mechanistically mediate this relationship, allowing for a synergistic effect on autoimmune processes for enhancing the inflammatory response. Additionally, the study found that those with these VDR polymorphisms had greater levels of VDR expression and IL-12 production, suggesting a proinflammatory Th1 response that could be a contributing factor to the autoimmune characteristics of type 2 diabetes. It is also linked to higher cholesterol and lower HDL concentrations when they raise the risk of cardiovascular disease in people with type 2 diabetes; these metabolic alterations that are a hallmark of dyslipidemia are especially worrisome. This genetic interaction highlights the part the HLA/VDR axis plays in both autoimmune regulation and the metabolic dysfunction linked to type 2 diabetes (Al-Daghri et al., 2012).

In 2022, Alvarado et al. in his study reported that blood of type 2 diabetes patients has elevated presence of CD14+HLA-DR-/low cells, which increasingly appears to be influenced by glycemic control and age rather than obesity, suggesting a hyperglycemia-related effect independent of body weight. With increased susceptibility to infections and certain types of cancers, type 2 diabetes patients face alterations in their immune responses. Regardless of weight, T2DM patients have elevated levels of immunosuppressive monocytes such as CD14+HLA-DR-/low monocytes. Higher levels of CD14+HLA-DR-/low monocytes are found in T2DM patients with poor glycemic control (HbA1c $> 9\%$) compared with those with better control. These monocytes correlate with the factor of the patient's age, years since T2DM was diagnosed and glycemic index (Valtierra-Alvarado et al., 2022).

5.2.3 How HLA associations may interact with other genetic loci linked to T2DM?

There are various studies exploring the links between HLA class II gene variants and T2DM, proposing that these links may interact with additional genetic regions associated with T2DM emphasizing identification of various HLA alleles, which are related to T2DM as a part of a wider genetic framework, encompassing various single nucleotide polymorphisms (SNPs) throughout the genome. It was identified that there are 13 novel T2DM-associated loci namely ACSL1, HLA-DQA1, SLC35D3, MNX1, ABO, PLEKHA1, HSD17B12, MAP3K11, NRXN3, CMIP, ZZEF1, GLP2R, and GIP found from the combination of 1000G-imputed GWAS metaanalysis (stage 1) and Metabochip follow-up (stage 2) (Scott et al., 2017).

A study by Scott et al. highlights advancements made through GWAS, which have detected numerous SNPs in the HLA region and other genetic loci related to T2DM.

These observations imply that the genetic makeup of T2DM is intricate and involves multiple loci, including those situated outside the HLA region, potentially working in concert to influence disease risk (Scott et al., 2017).

Specific HLA alleles, such as HLA-DQB105:01 and HLA-DRB101:01, have been correlated with metabolic characteristics such as fasting plasma glucose levels and insulin resistance (HOMA-IR). This suggests that HLA associations may not function independently but could engage with other genetic components that impact glucose metabolism and insulin sensitivity (Jacobi et al., 2020).

In a study, Chen et al. (2021) reported that HLA haplotypes such as HLA-DQA-DQB, DRB-DQB, and latent autoimmune diabetes in adults or LADA have been found to be correlated. It has been significantly found that ethnic variations in genetic predisposition to LADA may enhance susceptibility (Chinese population: DQA105-DQB10201, DQA103-DQB10401, DQA103-DQB10303*$P < .001$, and Caucasian population: DRB1-3DRB103-DQB10201, DR104-DQB10302($P < .001$) and decreases risk in Japanese population: *DRB*103-*DQB*10201, DRB*104-DQB10302* ($P < .001$) and no risk associations (*DRB*10405-*DQB*10401* ($P = .136$)). Hence, it can be concluded that the study on HLA associations with LADA risks highlights the significance of personalized medicine using HLA typing for LADA (Chen et al., 2021).

5.2.4 Protective association of HLA from T2D

It is interesting to note that HLA class II genotypes have been found to have both protective and risk-enhancing effects on type 2 diabetes (Jacobi et al., 2020). Specific alleles, such as HLA-DR2 and DR9, are linked to increased T2DM risk, whereas DR1 and DR6 are protective factors.

In 2020, Jacobi et al. found out several alleles associated with reduced risk as well as increased risk. The allele with increased risk identified as namely DRB 501:01, DQA 01:02, DQB 06:02, and DRB115:01, and the alleles associated with the increased risk of non–insulin-treated type 2 diabetes were DRB107:01, DQA102:01, DQB1*03:03. These protective alleles are known to enhance the proinsulin binding for diabetes development (Jacobi et al., 2020).

Weiskopf et al. (2016) investigated the association between HLA-DRB1 allele with the dengue virus epitopes in patients who had prior DENV exposure to analyze the specificity of $CD4^+$ T cell responses. In HLA typing in Sri Lankan cohort, it was found that allelic variants that were most frequent with phenotypic frequencies of $\geq$10% were DRB1*0701, 1501, 1502, 1301, 1001, 0403, and 1404. and low response alleles were DRB1*0101, 0301, 0401, 0803, 1101, 1202, and 1302. The 15 DRB1 alleles covered at least one DRB1 gene in 95% of cases and both genes in 60% of cases. Hence, it can be concluded that HLA alleles influence the immune responses among the population variably (Weiskopf et al., 2016).

In a study, De Groot et al. (2021) found few alleles such as HLA-DRB1*0101, *0301, *0401, *0701, *1101, *1301, and *1501, which appear to modulate regulatory T cell (Treg) activity, promoting immune tolerance. The balance between protective and risk alleles is a critical determinant of immune homeostasis in T2D (De Groot et al., 2021).

5.2.5 HLA associated with T2D and its effect on transplantation and other treatments

HLA has majorly to deal with transplantations of tissue and organs. Studies have been conducted to study if HLA association with diabetes 2 also affects transplantation reactions in T2D patients. It is well known that certain HLA alleles may make people more susceptible to immunological reactions, which could worsen inflammation and the rejection of grafts (Valenzuela & Reed, 2013). Moreover, it has also been observed that immunosuppressive treatment adapted to HLA compatibility helps lessen immunological dysregulation associated with diabetes, and HLA matching enhances transplant outcomes by lowering alloimmune reactions.

In diabetics receiving organ transplants, especially kidney transplants, HLA molecules are found to be important to be responsible for immunological responses and disease risk. HLA mismatches affect the risk of graft rejection and immune-mediated problems in patients with T2DM or posttransplant diabetes mellitus (PTDM) (Lawrence et al., 2023). Even in case of tumor surveillance inhibitors in diabetics, HLA dysregulation on immunosuppressive CD14+HLA-DR-/low monocytes (M-MDSCs) affects tumor immunity. These cells, which are increased in type 2 diabetes because of inflammation and persistent hyperglycemia, raise the risk and progression of cancer.

Immunotherapy for diabetic patients may benefit from an understanding of HLA's function in this process (Valtierra-Alvarado et al., 2022). According to a Sardinian study, T2DM patients had substantially greater HHV8 infection rates. T2DM and HHV8 infection were substantially correlated with KIR2DL2/DS2 and its ligand HLA-C1C1 (62% vs. 15%, $P < .0001$, OR = 8.64). These results point to an immune-mediated aspect of T2DM and point to HHV8 as a possible cofactor in the development of the illness in genetically predisposed people (Caselli et al., 2013).

In a study by Soltani et al. (2020), the association between HLA-C1C1 and Kir genes (KIR2DS2, KIR2DL2 and KIR2DL3) were reported. The homozygosity of C1C1 genotype has implicated genetic predisposition leading to onset of type 1 diabetes. The study also shows significant associations with KIR2DL1 (OR = 0.42, 95% CI = 0.23–0.77; $P = .005$), KIR2DL2 (OR = 1.15, 95% CI = 1.00–1.32; $P = .048$), and KIR2DL5 (OR = 0.86, 95% CI = 0.75–0.98; $P = .03$) with type 1 diabetes susceptibility. Hence, it was concluded that HLA C1C1-KIR interactions have a significant role in emphasizing type 1 diabetes and its disease pathogenesis (Soltani et al., 2020).

6. Conclusion

HLA molecules play an important role in immune regulation by presenting antigens to T cells and determining immune tolerance or activation. There are various haplotypes of

HLA that raises the likelihood of autoimmunity and so impairs insulin secretion. Some HLA haplotypes, such HLA-DRB1*02, are even protective in type 2 diabetes because they retain immunological tolerance to self-antigens and increase insulin production. The elevated risk for diabetes arises from the possibility that nonprotective HLA haplotypes could more successfully expose T cells to self-antigens originating from β-cells or adipocytes, which could set off an autoimmune reaction. The ensuing loss of self-tolerance may result in autoreactive T cell activation and further autoantibody formation, which target pancreatic β-cells and worsen β-cell dysfunction while lowering insulin secretion. Additionally various HLA variants are known to be prone to easily dysregulated and cause inflammation. High levels of certain cytokines and cells have been shown to raise the risk of T2D in various studies. Because of this, immunological dysregulation brought on by particular HLA backgrounds causes T2DM patients to be more susceptible to autoimmunity (Chang et al., 2015).

Many metaanalysis conducted sought to evaluate the connections between HLA alleles and T2DM across various populations. It discovered that although specific HLA alleles exhibited significant associations, the overall genetic risk for T2DM is likely due to a combination of HLA-related elements and other genetic variants identified in earlier research (Jacobi et al., 2020). Also, the interaction between HLA associations and additional genetic loci related to T2DM indicates a multifactorial framework for disease susceptibility, wherein both HLA and non-HLA genetic components play a role in the risk and pathophysiology of T2DM.

While understanding genetic susceptibility offers numerous benefits, it also raises ethical and psychological considerations. Individuals who learn about their genetic risk for T2DM may experience anxiety or stress. Therefore, it is important to provide genetic counseling and support to help individuals understand their risk and make informed decisions about their health (Nielsen & Cummings, 2016). Additionally, ensuring the confidentiality and appropriate use of genetic information is essential to address privacy concerns and prevent genetic discrimination.

Current research efforts are increasingly focused on identifying specific HLA alleles associated with T2D risk, elucidating their molecular mechanisms, and exploring their interactions with environmental and lifestyle factors. Emerging studies highlight specific HLA polymorphisms as risk or protective factors for T2D, influencing immune responses and β-cell resilience. Moreover, the interplay between HLA and inflammatory cytokines amplifies islet dysfunction. Recent advances in transcriptomics, proteomics, and single-cell analyses have provided deeper insights into the islet microenvironment, revealing the nuanced role of HLA-restricted T cells and innate immune cells in T2D pathophysiology. Current research emphasizes the translational potential of targeting HLA-mediated pathways for therapeutic interventions. Precision medicine approaches, such as HLA genotyping, could stratify patients based on genetic susceptibility, enabling tailored interventions to preserve β-cell function. Immunomodulatory therapies targeting HLA–T cell interactions and inflammatory mediators are being explored as strategies to mitigate immune-mediated β-cell damage.

It is observed by the authors that there are very few studies that have been conducted to establish. In conclusion, additional studies are required to clarify these intricate interactions and their significance in diabetes genetics (Scott et al., 2017).

References

Ahmad, E., Lim, S., Lamptey, R., Webb, D. R., & Davies, M. J. (2022). Type 2 diabetes. *The Lancet, 400* (10365), 1803–1820. https://doi.org/10.1016/S0140-6736(22)01655-5

Al-Daghri, N. M., Al-Attas, O., Alokail, M. S., Alkharfy, K. M., Draz, H. M., Agliardi, C., Mohammed, A. K., Guerini, F. R., & Clerici, M. (2012). Vitamin D receptor gene polymorphisms and HLA DRB1*04 cosegregation in Saudi type 2 diabetes patients. *Journal of immunology (Baltimore, Md.: 1950), 188* (3), 1325–1332. https://doi.org/10.4049/jimmunol.1101954

Alam, S., Hasan, M. K., Neaz, S., Hussain, N., Hossain, M. F., & Rahman, T. (2021). Diabetes mellitus: Insights from epidemiology, biochemistry, risk factors, diagnosis, complications and comprehensive management. *Diabetology, 2*(2), 36–50. https://doi.org/10.3390/diabetology2020004

Altobelli, E., Blasetti, A., Petrocelli, R., et al. (2005). HLA DR/DQ alleles and risk of type I diabetes in childhood: A population-based case–control study. *Clinical and Experimental Medicine, 5*, 72–79. https://doi.org/10.1007/s10238-005-0069-0

Arora, P., Garcia-Bailo, B., Dastani, Z., et al. (2011). Genetic polymorphisms of innate immunity-related inflammatory pathways and their association with factors related to type 2 diabetes. *BMC Medical Genetics, 12*, 95. https://doi.org/10.1186/1471-2350-12-95

Azeem, S., Khan, U., & Liaquat, A. (2022). The increasing rate of diabetes in Pakistan: A silent killer. *Annals of Medicine and Surgery, 79*. https://doi.org/10.1016/j.amsu.2022.103901

Bai, W., & Ameyaw, E. K. (2024). Global, regional and national trends in tuberculosis incidence and main risk factors: A study using data from 2000 to 2021. *BMC Public Health, 24*, 12. https://doi.org/10.1186/s12889-023-17495-6

Basu, S., Yoffe, P., Hills, N., & Lustig, R. H. (2013). The relationship of sugar to population-level diabetes prevalence: An econometric analysis of repeated cross-sectional data. *PLoS ONE, 8*(2), Article e57873. https://doi.org/10.1371/journal.pone.0057873

Bodis, G., Toth, V., & Schwarting, A. (2018). Role of human leukocyte antigens (HLA) in autoimmune diseases. *Rheumatology and Therapy, 5*, 5–20. https://doi.org/10.1007/s40744-018-0100-z

Božič, B. (2002). Diabetes and autoimmunity. *Electronic Journal of the International Federation of Clinical Chemistry and Laboratory Medicine, 13*(5), 164–169.

Burrack, A. L., Martinov, T., & Fife, B. T. (2017). T-cell mediated beta cell destruction: Autoimmunity and alloimmunity in the context of type 1 diabetes. *Frontiers in Endocrinology, 8*, 343. https://doi.org/10.3389/fendo.2017.00343

Campbell, J. M., Bellman, S. M., Stephenson, M. D., & Lisy, K. (2017). Metformin reduces all-cause mortality and diseases of ageing independent of its effect on diabetes control: A systematic review and meta-analysis. *Ageing Research Reviews, 40*, 31–44. https://doi.org/10.1016/j.arr.2017.10.003

Caselli, E., Rizzo, R., Ingianni, A., Contini, P., Pompei, R., & Di Luca, D. (2013). High prevalence of HHV8 infection and specific killer cell immunoglobulin-like receptors allotypes in Sardinian patients with type 2 diabetes mellitus. *Journal of Medical Virology, 86*(10), 1745–1751. https://doi.org/10.1002/jmv.23771

Chang, D. C., Piaggi, P., Hanson, R. L., Knowler, W. C., Bucci, J., Thio, G., Hohenadel, M. G., Bogardus, C., & Krakoff, J. (2015). Use of a high-density protein microarray to identify autoantibodies in subjects with type 2 diabetes mellitus and an HLA background associated with reduced insulin secretion. *PLoS One, 10*(11), Article e0143551. https://doi.org/10.1371/journal.pone.0143551

Chen, W., Chen, X., Zhang, M., & Huang, Z. (2021). The association of human leukocyte antigen class II (HLA II) haplotypes with the risk of latent autoimmune diabetes of adults (LADA): Evidence based on available data. *Gene, 767,* Article 145177. https://doi.org/10.1016/j.gene.2020.145177

Chopra, I., & Rachana, R. (2024). Rethinking Type-1 diabetes treatment: Emerging medicines based on AAT therapy and C-peptide preservation therapy. *Research & Reviews: A Journal of Life Sciences, 14* (03), 19–29.

Crux, N. B., & Elahi, S. (2017). Human leukocyte antigen (HLA) and immune regulation: How do classical and non-classical HLA alleles modulate immune response to human immunodeficiency virus and hepatitis C virus infection? *Frontiers in Immunology, 8.* https://doi.org/10.3389/fimmu.2017.00832

Cruz-Tapias, P., Castiblanco, J., & Anaya, J. M. (2013). Major histocompatibility complex: Antigen processing and presentation. In J. M. Anaya, Y. Shoenfeld, A. Rojas-Villarraga, et al. (Eds.), Autoimmunity: From bench to bedside *(chap. 10).* El Rosario University Press. https://www.ncbi.nlm.nih.gov/books/NBK459467/.

de Bakker, P. I. W, McVean, G., Sabeti, P. C., Miretti, M. M., Green, T., Marchini, J., Ke, X., Monsuur, A. J., Whittaker, P., Delgado, M., Morrison, J., Richardson, A., Walsh, E. C., Gao, X., Galver, L., Hart, J., Hafler, D. A., Pericak-Vance, M., Todd, J. A., ... Rioux, J. D. (2006). A high-resolution HLA and SNP haplotype map for disease association studies in the extended human MHC. *Nature Genetics, 38*(10), 1166–1172. https://doi.org/10.1038/ng1885

De Groot, A. S., Rosenberg, A. S., Miah, S. M. S., Skowron, G., Roberts, B. J., Lélias, S., Terry, F. E., & Martin, W. D. (2021). Identification of a potent regulatory T cell epitope in factor V that modulates CD4+ and CD8+ memory T cell responses. *Clinical Immunology, 224,* Article 108661. https://doi.org/10.1016/j.clim.2020.108661

DeForest, N., & Majithia, A. R. (2022). Genetics of type 2 diabetes: Implications from large-scale studies. *Current Diabetes Reports, 22,* 227–235. https://doi.org/10.1007/s11892-022-01462-3

Dendup, T., Feng, X., Clingan, S., & Astell-Burt, T. (2018). Environmental risk factors for developing type 2 diabetes mellitus: A systematic review. *International Journal of Environmental Research and Public Health, 15*(1), 78. https://doi.org/10.3390/ijerph15010078

Donath, M., & Shoelson, S. (2011). Type 2 diabetes as an inflammatory disease. *Nature Reviews Immunology, 11,* 98–107. https://doi.org/10.1038/nri2925

Galicia-Garcia, U., Benito-Vicente, A., Jebari, S., Larrea-Sebal, A., Siddiqi, H., Uribe, K. B., Ostolaza, H., & Martín, C. (2020). Pathophysiology of type 2 diabetes mellitus. *International Journal of Molecular Sciences, 21*(17), 6275. https://doi.org/10.3390/ijms21176275

Gibson, G. (2012). Rare and common variants: Twenty arguments. *Nature Reviews Genetics, 13,* 135–145. https://doi.org/10.1038/nrg3118

Girard, D., & Vandiedonck, C. (2022). How dysregulation of the immune system promotes diabetes mellitus and cardiovascular risk complications. *Frontiers in Cardiovascular Medicine, 9,* Article 991716. https://doi.org/10.3389/fcvm.2022.991716

Guo, C., Jin, Y., Lee, K. K. H., Yang, G., Jing, C., & Yang, X. (2016). The relationships between HLA class II alleles and antigens with gestational diabetes mellitus: A meta-analysis. *Scientific Reports, 6*(1), 35005. https://doi.org/10.1038/srep35005

Hameed, I., Masoodi, S. R., Mir, S. A., Nabi, M., Ghazanfar, K., & Ganai, B. A. (2015). Type 2 diabetes mellitus: From a metabolic disorder to an inflammatory condition. *World Journal of Diabetes, 6*(4), 598. https://doi.org/10.4239/wjd.v6.i4.598

Institute for Health Metrics and Evaluation. (2021). *GBD results.* University of Washington. https://vizhub.healthdata.org/gbd-results/.

Jacobi, T., Massier, L., Klöting, N., Horn, K., Schuch, A., Ahnert, P., Engel, C., Löffler, M., Burkhardt, R., Thiery, J., Tönjes, A., Stumvoll, M., Blüher, M., Doxiadis, I., Scholz, M., & Kovacs, P. (2020). HLA class II allele analyses implicate common genetic components in type 1 and non–insulin-treated type 2 diabetes. *The Journal of Clinical Endocrinology & Metabolism, 105*(3), e245–e254.

Jan, A., Saeed, M., Afridi, M. H., Khuda, F., Shabbir, M., Khan, H., Ali, S., Hassan, M., Samiullah, A., & Rani, Z. (2021). Association of HLA-B gene polymorphisms with type 2 diabetes in Pashtun ethnic population of Khyber Pakhtunkhwa, Pakistan. *Journal of Diabetes Research*, 10. https://doi.org/10.1155/2021/6669731

Kahanovitz, L., Sluss, P. M., & Russell, S. J. (2017). Type 1 diabetes—A clinical perspective. *Point of Care: The Journal of Near-Patient Testing & Technology, 16*(1), 37–40. https://doi.org/10.1097/POC.0000000000000125

King, H., Aubert, R. E., & Herman, W. H. (September 1, 1998). Global burden of diabetes, 1995–2025: Prevalence, numerical estimates, and projections. *Diabetes Care, 21*(9), 1414–1431. https://doi.org/10.2337/diacare.21.9.1414

Koning, F., Thomas, R., Rossjohn, J., et al. (2015). Coeliac disease and rheumatoid arthritis: Similar mechanisms, different antigens. *Nature Reviews Rheumatology, 11*, 450–461. https://doi.org/10.1038/nrrheum.2015.59

Lawrence, S. E., Chandran, M. M., Park, J. M., Sweiss, H., Jensen, T., Choksi, P., & Crowther, B. (2023). Sweet and simple as syrup: A review and guidance for use of novel antihyperglycemic agents for post-transplant diabetes mellitus and type 2 diabetes mellitus after kidney transplantation. *Clinical Transplantation, 37*(3), Article e14922. https://doi.org/10.1111/ctr.14922

Lee, C. H., & Lam, K. S. (2019). Obesity-induced insulin resistance and macrophage infiltration of the adipose tissue: A vicious cycle. *Journal of Diabetes Investigation, 10*, 29–31. https://doi.org/10.1111/jdi.12918

Li, X. G., Qi, M. Y., Li, X., & Ping, F. (2025). Exogenous insulin-associated autoimmunity and the emergence of double diabetes in type 2 diabetes. *World Journal of Diabetes, 16*(9), 109130.

Liane Ong, K., Stafford, L. K., McLaughlin, S. A., et al. (2023). Global, regional, and national burden of diabetes from 1990 to 2021, with projections of prevalence to 2050: A systematic analysis for the global burden of disease study 2021. *The Lancet, 402*(10397), 203–234. https://doi.org/10.1016/S0140-6736(23)01301-6

Ma, Z.-J., Sun, P., Guo, G., Zhang, R., & Chen, L.-M. (2013). Association of the *HLA-DQA1* and *HLA-DQB1* alleles in type 2 diabetes mellitus and diabetic nephropathy in the Han ethnicity of China. *Journal of Diabetes Research.* , Article 452537. https://doi.org/10.1155/2013/452537

Magliano, D. J., Boyko, E. J., & IDF Diabetes Atlas 10th edition scientific committee. (2021). *IDF diabetes Atlas* (10th ed.). Brussels: International Diabetes Federation. Table 3.4, Top 10 countries or territories for number of adults (20–79 years) with diabetes in 2021 and 2045 https://www.ncbi.nlm.nih.gov/books/NBK581940/table/ch3.t4/.

Manolio, T., Collins, F., Cox, N., et al. (2009). Finding the missing heritability of complex diseases. *Nature, 461*, 747–753. https://doi.org/10.1038/nature08494

McLaughlin, K. A., Gulati, K., Richardson, C. C., Morgan, D., Jonathan Bodansky, H., Feltbower, R. G., & Christie, M. R. (2014). HLA-DR4–Associated T and B cell responses to specific determinants on the IA-2 autoantigen in type 1 diabetes. *The Journal of Immunology, 193*(9), 4448–4456. https://doi.org/10.4049/jimmunol.1301902

Medhasi, S., & Chantratita, N. (2022). Human leukocyte antigen (HLA) system: Genetics and association with bacterial and viral infections. *Journal of Immunology Research, 2022*, 1–15. https://doi.org/10.1155/2022/9710376

Młynarska, E., Czarnik, W., Dzieża, N., Jędraszak, W., Majchrowicz, G., Prusinowski, F., Stabrawa, M., Rysz, J., & Franczyk, B. (2025). Type 2 diabetes mellitus: New pathogenetic mechanisms, treatment and the most important complications. *International Journal of Molecular Sciences, 26*(3), 1094.

Naito, T., Suzuki, K., Hirata, J., et al. (2021). A deep learning method for HLA imputation and trans-ethnic MHC fine-mapping of type 1 diabetes. *Nature Communications, 12*, 1639. https://doi.org/10.1038/s41467-021-21975-x

Nguyen, C., Varney, M. D., Harrison, L. C., & Morahan, G. (2013). Definition of high-risk type 1 diabetes HLA-DR and HLA-DQ types using only three single nucleotide polymorphisms. *Diabetes, 62*(6), 2135–2140. https://doi.org/10.2337/db12-1398

Nielsen, S. M., & Cummings, S. (2016). Genetic counseling: The role of genetic counselors on healthcare provider and endocrinology teams. In *Genetic diagnosis of endocrine disorders* (pp. 397–408). Elsevier. https://doi.org/10.1016/B978-0-12-800892-8.00028-2

Popoviciu, M. S., Kaka, N., Sethi, Y., Patel, N., Chopra, H., & Cavalu, S. (2023). Type 1 diabetes mellitus and autoimmune diseases: A critical review of the association and the application of personalized medicine. *Journal of Personalized Medicine, 13*(3), 422. https://doi.org/10.3390/jpm13030422

Prasad, R. B., & Groop, L. (2015). Genetics of type 2 diabetes—pitfalls and possibilities. *Genes, 6*(1), 87–123. https://doi.org/10.3390/genes6010087

Pugliese, A. (August 1, 2017). Autoreactive T cells in type 1 diabetes. *Journal of Clinical Investigation, 127* (8), 2881–2891. https://doi.org/10.1172/JCI94549

Quirant-Sánchez, B., Plans-Galván, O., Lucas, E., Argudo, E., Martinez-Cáceres, E. M., & Arméstar, F. (2023). HLA-DR expression on monocytes and Sepsis index are useful in predicting sepsis. *Biomedicines, 11*(7), 1836. https://doi.org/10.3390/biomedicines11071836

Rachana, R., & Sharma, K. (2024). *Novel nanotherapeutics for the management of diabetes*. Nanotrends-A Journal of Nano Technology & Its Applications. https://doi.org/10.37591/NTs.v26i01.160176

Rich, S. S., Erlich, H., & Concannon, P. (August 2018). Genetics of type 1 diabetes. In C. C. Cowie, S. S. Casagrande, A. Menke, M. A. Cissell, M. S. Eberhardt, J. B. Meigs, E. W. Gregg, W. C. Knowler, E. Barrett-Connor, D. J. Becker, F. L. Brancati, E. J. Boyko, W. H. Herman, B. V. Howard, K. M. V. Narayan, M. Rewers, & J. E. Fradkin (Eds.), *Diabetes in America* (3rd ed.). Bethesda (MD): National Institute of Diabetes and Digestive and Kidney Diseases (US).

Safiri, S., Nahid, K., Kaufman, J. S., Wilder, B. A., Aria, N. S., Sullman, M. J. M., Maziar, M.-L., Gary, C., & Ali-Asghar, K. (2022). Prevalence, deaths and disability-adjusted-life-years (DALYs) due to type 2 diabetes and its attributable risk factors in 204 countries and territories". *Frontiers in Endocrinology, 13*. https://doi.org/10.3389/fendo.2022.838027

Saxena, R., Elbers, C. C., Guo, Y., Peter, I., Gaunt, T. R., Mega, J. L., Lanktree, M. B., Tare, A., Castillo, B. A., Li, Y. R., Johnson, T., Bruinenberg, M., Gilbert-Diamond, D., Rajagopalan, R., Voight, B. F., Balasubramanyam, A., Barnard, J., Bauer, F., Baumert, J., … Keating, B. J. (2012). Large-scale gene-centric meta-analysis across 39 studies identifies type 2 diabetes loci. *The American Journal of Human Genetics, 90*(3), 410–425. https://doi.org/10.1016/j.ajhg.2011.12.022

Scott, R. A., Scott, L. J., Mägi, R., Marullo, L., Gaulton, K. J., Kaakinen, M., Pervjakova, N., Pers, T. H., Johnson, A. D., Eicher, J. D., Jackson, A. U., Ferreira, T., Lee, Y., Ma, C., Steinthorsdottir, V., Thorleifsson, G., Qi, L., Van Zuydam, N. R., Mahajan, A., , … Prokopenko, I., & the DIAbetes Genetics Replication And Meta-analysis (DIAGRAM) Consortium. (2017). An expanded genome-wide association study of type 2 diabetes in Europeans. *Diabetes, 66*(11), 2888–2902. https://doi.org/10.2337/db16-1253

Soltani, S., Mostafaei, S., Aslani, S., et al. (2020). Association of *KIR* gene polymorphisms with type 1 diabetes: A meta-analysis. *Journal of Diabetes and Metabolic Disorders, 19*, 1777–1786. https://doi.org/10.1007/s40200-020-00569-2

Sun, H., Saeedi, P., Karuranga, S., Pinkepank, M., Ogurtsova, K., Duncan, B. B., Stein, C., Basit, A., Chan, J. C. N., Mbanya, J. C., Pavkov, M. E., Ramachandran, A., Wild, S. H., James, S., Herman, W. H., Zhang, P., Bommer, C., Kuo, S., Boyko, E. J., & Magliano, D. J. (January 2022). IDF diabetes Atlas: Global, regional and country-level diabetes prevalence estimates for 2021 and projections for 2045. *Diabetes Research and Clinical Practice, 183*, Article 109119. https://doi.org/10.1016/j.diabres.2021.109119

Tandon, N., Anjana, R. M., Mohan, V., et al. (2018). The increasing burden of diabetes and variations among the states of India: The global burden of disease study 1990–2016. *Lancet Global Health, 6*(12), e1352–e1362. https://doi.org/10.1016/S2214-109X(18)30387-5

Valenzuela, N. M., & Reed, E. F. (2013). Antibodies in transplantation: The effects of HLA and non-HLA antibody binding and mechanisms of injury. In A. Zachary, & M. Leffell (Eds.), *Transplantation immunology, 1034* (pp. 41–70). Humana Press. https://doi.org/10.1007/978-1-62703-493-7_2

Valtierra-Alvarado, M. A., Castañeda-Delgado, J. E., Lugo-Villarino, G., Dueñas-Arteaga, F., Rivas-Santiago, B., Enciso-Moreno, J. A., & Serrano, C. J. (2022). Increased frequency of CD14+HLA-DR-/low cells in type 2 diabetes patients with poor glycemic control. *Human Immunology, 83*(11), 789–795. https://doi.org/10.1016/j.humimm.2022.08.011

Weiskopf, D., Angelo, M. A., Grifoni, A., O'Rourke, P. H., Sidney, J., Paul, S., De Silva, A. D., Phillips, E., Mallal, S., Premawansa, S., Premawansa, G., Wijewickrama, A., Peters, B., & Sette, A. (2016). HLA-DRB1 alleles are associated with different magnitudes of dengue virus–specific CD4+ T-cell responses. *The Journal of Infectious Diseases, 214*(7), 1117–1124. https://doi.org/10.1093/infdis/jiw309

Williams, R. C., Muller, Y. L., Hanson, R. L., Knowler, W. C., Mason, C. C., Bian, L., Ossowski, V., Wiedrich, K., Chen, Y. F., Marcovina, S., Hahnke, J., Nelson, R. G., Baier, L. J., & Bogardus, C. (2011). *HLA-DRB1* reduces the risk of type 2 diabetes mellitus by increased insulin secretion. *Diabetologia, 54,* 1684–1692. https://doi.org/10.1007/s00125-011-2122-8

World Health Organization. (2024). *Diabetes*. Retrieved [November 14, 2024], from https://www.who.int/news-room/fact-sheets/detail/diabetes.

Yeo, L., Pujol-Autonell, I., Baptista, R., Eichmann, M., Kronenberg-Versteeg, D., Heck, S., Dolton, G., Sewell, A. K., Härkönen, T., Mikk, M. L., Toppari, J., Veijola, R., Knip, M., Ilonen, J., & Peakman, M. (2020). Circulating β cell-specific CD8+ T cells restricted by high-risk HLA class I molecules show antigen experience in children with and at risk of type 1 diabetes. *Clinical and Experimental Immunology, 199*(3), 263–277. https://doi.org/10.1111/cei.13391

Further reading

Brooks-Worrell, B. M., Tjaden, A. H., Edelstein, S. L., Palomino, B., Utzschneider, K. M., Arslanian, S., Mather, K. J., Buchanan, T. A., Nadeau, K. J., Atkinson, K., Barengolts, E., Kahn, S. E., Palmer, J. P., & the RISE Consortium. (2021). Islet autoimmunity in adults with impaired glucose tolerance and recently diagnosed, treatment naïve type 2 diabetes in the restoring insulin SEcretion (RISE) study. *Frontiers in Immunology, 12,* Article 640251. https://doi.org/10.3389/fimmu.2021.640251

Gomez-Lopera, N., Alfaro, J. M., Rodriguez, A. M., et al. (November 2020). A non-coding RNASEH1 gene variant associated with type 1 diabetes and interacts with HLA tagSNPs in families from Colombia. *Pediatric Diabetes, 21*(7), 1183–1192. https://doi.org/10.1111/pedi.13057

Rodríguez-Ventura, A. L., Yamamoto-Furusho, J. K., Coyote, N., Dorantes, L. M., Ruiz-Morales, J. A., Vargas-Alarcón, G., & Granados, J. (2007). HLA-DRB1*08 allele may help to distinguish between type 1 diabetes mellitus and type 2 diabetes mellitus in Mexican children. *Pediatric Diabetes, 8,* 5–10. https://doi.org/10.1111/j.1399-5448.2006.00221.x

Zhao, L., Guo, S., Li, J., Liu, F., Chen, Y., Ge, Y., … Wang, N. (2016). Association of HLA-DQB1 polymorphisms with type 1 diabetes mellitus: A meta-analysis. *Scientific Reports, 6,* Article 35005. https://doi.org/10.1038/srep35005

Zhao, Y., & Zhao, B. (2021). The role of immune cells in the pathogenesis of type 1 diabetes. *Nature Reviews Disease Primers, 7*(1), 87. https://doi.org/10.1038/s41572-021-00287-3

9

Immune-mediated complications in type 2 diabetes mellitus (T2DM)

Taief Ahmad Dar[1] and Roaf Ahmad Rather[2]

[1]DEPARTMENT OF BIOCHEMISTRY, GOVERNMENT DEGREE COLLEGE KULGAM, KULGAM JAMMU & KASHMIR, INDIA; [2]DEPARTMENT OF AGRICULTURAL TECHNOLOGY, GOVERNMENT DEGREE COLLEGE KULGAM, KULGAM JAMMU & KASHMIR, INDIA

1. Introduction

Type 2 diabetes mellitus (T2DM) develops when the body becomes resistant to the action of insulin, and eventually the pancreas runs out of insulin to keep normal blood glucose levels within the body. This condition is called "insulin resistance" (Pickup & Crook, 1998). The hallmark of type 2 diabetes is insulin resistance, which happens when muscle, adipose, and liver cells lose their sensitivity to insulin, requiring greater doses to accomplish glucose absorption (De Luca & Olefsky, 2008; Leutholtz & Ripoll, 2011). This is also the major problem that arises in the early stages of type 2 diabetes. It is the most prevalent kind of diabetes, which manifests much later in life than type 1 diabetes, because it is primarily managed with tablets rather than only insulin, it is also known as noninsulin-dependent diabetes mellitus (Vijan, 2015). T2DM typically occurs due to a combined effect of genetic predisposition and lifestyle variables such as obesity, poor dietary habits and physical inactivity (Donath & Shoelson, 2011). This condition affects millions of people worldwide which poses significant challenges to healthcare systems globally and has shown an increase over time, which is expected to rise to 700 million cases in 2045 (Donath & Shoelson, 2011; Saeedi et al., 2019). It is a major global cause of illness and mortality, with immune dysregulation emerging as a significant contributor to its pathophysiology and complications.

Type 2 diabetes mellitus complications can be classified as either acute complications or chronic complications (Farmaki et al., 2021), the acute complications of type 2 diabetes mellitus incudes diabetic ketoacidosis and diabetic coma, hypoglycemia and hyperglycemia. One risky consequence of diabetes is diabetic ketoacidosis. The patient must be taken to the hospital right away because it is deemed an urgent event. Dehydration, acetone aspiration, and Kussmaul breath are all the signs present in the patient. One of the main side effects of treating diabetes is hypoglycemia, which happens when blood sugar is extremely low. The condition known as hyperglycemia occurs when

Type 2 Diabetes Mellitus. https://doi.org/10.1016/B978-0-443-33590-7.00006-X

blood sugar levels are excessively elevated. Diabetes-related chronic complications can be broadly divided into two main categories: Large artery damage, which is frequently referred to as macrovascular complications since it might result in issues of heart, brain, and legs. On the other hand, microvascular problems, also known as retinopathy, nephropathy, and neuropathy, impact the tiny blood arteries of eyes, kidneys, and nerves respectively (Fasanmade et al., 2008; Saeedi et al., 2020). Traditionally considered a metabolic disorder, T2DM involves a chronic, low-grade inflammatory state that affects multiple organ systems. Persistent immune activation contributes to insulin resistance, endothelial dysfunction, and progressive tissue damage, ultimately leading to severe complications such as cardiovascular disease (CVD), nephropathy, neuropathy, and retinopathy. One of the main causes of morbidity and mortality for people with type 2 diabetes is CVD (Ding et al., 2011; Mansour et al., 2023). Insulin resistance and hyperglycemia raise the risk of peripheral arterial disease, coronary artery disease, and stroke by promoting endothelial dysfunction, inflammation, and atherogenesis. Another frequent consequence of diabetes is diabetic nephropathy, which results in proteinuria and chronic kidney disease (CKD) due to damage to the kidneys' filtering units. The risk of end-stage renal disease (ESRD), which necessitates dialysis or a kidney transplant, is greatly increased by this illness. The peripheral and autonomic nerve systems are impacted by diabetic neuropathy, which can result in symptoms ranging from cardiovascular and gastrointestinal problems to pain and numbness in the extremities. Advanced glycation end products (AGEs), oxidative stress, and microvascular damage are some of the underlying causes. Similarly, damage to the retinal blood vessels causes hemorrhages, microaneurysms, and neovascularization in diabetic retinopathy, are one of the main causes of blindness (Giri et al., 2018; Guan et al., 2024; Li et al., 2023). This chapter delves into the role of immune mechanisms in mediating complications associated with T2DM, highlighting key cellular and molecular pathways involved.

2. Immunological basis of T2DM

2.1 Chronic inflammation and insulin resistance

T2DM complications are not limited to oxidative stress, metabolic disorders, and immune inflammation, and so on. Among these, inflammation plays an essential role in the pathogenesis of diabetes complications (Dror et al., 2017). Chronic low-grade inflammation brought on by excess adipose tissue in metabolically unhealthy obesity results in insulin resistance and beta-cell malfunction (Tsai et al., 2018). Proinflammatory cytokines such as TNF-α, IL-6, and MCP-1 are released by visceral fat, causing systemic inflammation that interferes with insulin signalling by promoting serine phosphorylation of insulin receptor substrate-1 (IRS-1), leading to reduced insulin sensitivity in skeletal muscle, liver, and adipose tissue. Tumor necrosis factor-α (TNF-α) disrupts insulin receptor substrate (IRS) signaling, decreasing glucose uptake, while increased free fatty acids in obesity worsen inflammation and further reduce insulin sensitivity (Solinas

& Karin, 2010). This on-going inflammation harms pancreatic beta cells, with inflammatory cytokines causing apoptosis thereby decreasing insulin production. Immune cell infiltration, particularly macrophages in the islets, increases proinflammatory cytokine levels, exacerbates beta-cell dysfunction, and contributes to insulin resistance and hyperglycemia (Berbudi et al., 2020).

Inflammation is a biomarker used to predict diabetes complications such as dilated cardiomyopathy (DCM), diabetic neuropathy (DPN), diabetic retinopathy (DR), and diabetic nephropathy (DN). Biomarkers could include inflammatory cytokines such as tumor necrosis factor-α (TNF-α), transforming growth factor-β (TGF-β), interleukins (ILs), adhesion molecules, and macrophage genes. Because of the numerous roles that inflammation plays in the occurrence and development of diabetes problems, its link has yet to be fully understood. Diabetic patients have higher levels of key inflammatory markers, including tumor necrosis factor-alpha (TNF-α), interleukin-6 (IL-6), and C-reactive protein (CRP) (Hotamisligil et al., 1995; Hotamisligil & Spiegelman, 1994; Roytblat et al., 2000; Sartipy & Loskutoff, 2003; Straczkowski et al., 2002; Visser et al., 1999).

2.2 Role of innate and adaptive immunity

T2DM pathogenesis is thought to be related to both innate and adaptive immunological mechanisms, which are recognized as significant etiological components in the development of insulin resistance (Goldberg, 2009). It has been suggested that T cells play important roles in the progression of T2DM. It demonstrated that T2DM was linked to overactivated T cells and the activation of inflammatory pathways (Shirakawa et al., 2016). During the long-term effect of high blood sugar levels, immune cells get activated, which triggers a series of responses. For instance, when macrophages are activated, they shift from an antiinflammatory M2 phenotype to a proinflammatory M1 phenotype, secreting inflammatory cytokines (Ieronymaki et al., 2019). Effector T cell differentiation is closely tied to the regulation process that impacts the generation of distinct sets of effector cytokines (Inácio et al., 2018). The TNF-α, IL-1β, IL-6, or other inflammatory factors being released will activate various inflammatory signaling pathways, such as nuclear factor kappa-B (NF-κB), signal transducer, activator of transcription 3 (STAT3), and so on, which exacerbate insulin resistance, resulting in organ damage (Kwak et al., 2016; Maris et al., 2012; Swaroop et al., 2012; Zheng et al., 2016).

$CD8^+$ T cells secrete cytokines like IFN-γ and TNF-α, which aid the adaptive immune response to infections. It has been well known that $CD8^+$ T lymphocytes may produce and express the proinflammatory cytokine IL-17, which is abundant in inflammatory tissues in numerous human inflammatory disorders (Srenathan et al., 2016). $CD8^+$ T cells contribute to inflammation by promoting macrophage activation, while $CD4^+$ T helper cells (Th1 and Th17 subsets) secrete proinflammatory cytokines that further impair insulin signaling. Th1 cells are developed $CD4^+$ T cells that produce proinflammatory interferon-γ (IFN-γ). Th2 cells differentiate from activated $CD4^+$ T cells, which stimulate the production of critical Th2 cell lineage-defining cytokines such as interleukin-4 (IL-4), IL-5, and IL-13. When $CD4^+$ T cells are exposed to IL-6 and TGF-β, they develop into Th17 cells, which can cause inflammatory diseases (Ansel et al., 2006; Raphael et al., 2015; Wilson et al., 2009; Zhu et al., 2010). B cells have been demonstrated to play a major role in the development of insulin resistance by producing IgG antibodies and activating T cells and macrophages, perpetuating the immune response in T2DM (Winer et al., 2011; Winer et al., 2009).

3. Immune-mediated complications of T2DM

Diabetes has several consequences, the most significant of which are vascular complications, which can be classified into microvascular problems and macrovascular complications based on different pathological mechanisms. Microvascular complications include diabetic neuropathy, nephropathy with glomerular damage and retinopathy, while the macrovascular complications include coronary heart disease (CHD), heart failure, arrhythmias, and sudden cardiac death. Patients with type 2 diabetes mellitus (T2DM) may develop cerebrovascular disease and peripheral artery disease, both of which are types of CVD. Complications associated with both forms of diabetes significantly increase morbidity and mortality rates (Fowler, 2011). CVD is the leading cause of death in individuals with type 2 diabetes. Long-term hyperglycemia activates a variety of inflammatory signal pathways and inflammatory mediators, which results in aggravating the development of diabetes complications, finally leading to the damage of various organs (Berbudi et al., 2020, p. 2). The most common immune-mediated complications of T2DM are CVD, nephropathy, retinopathy, and neuropathy (Fig. 9.1), which are discussed below.

3.1 Cardiovascular disease

Prolonged exposure to high glucose levels can cause arterial damage, leading to CVD such as coronary heart disease, atherosclerosis (AS), and dilated cardiomyopathy (Katakami, 2018) (Fig. 9.1). Subjects with T2DM are substantially more likely to develop these cardiovascular problems than those without diabetes mellitus (Henning, 2018).

Chronic inflammation in T2DM accelerates atherosclerosis through vascular endothelial injury that leads to cholesterol and platelet deposition in the walls of blood vessels, forming plaques, which finally results in vascular obstruction or stenosis (Gusev & Sarapultsev, 2023). High glucose levels can promote inflammation and malfunction of arterial endothelial cells, leading to adhesion between white blood cells and tiny blood capillaries over time. Meanwhile, the increased permeability of the vascular endothelial, causes low-density lipoprotein (LDL) to accumulate and oxidize to influence the monocytes (Clyne, 2021). Oxidized LDL induces macrophages to start expressing scavenger CD36, causing self-antigen presentation to diminish, which gets then transformed into foam cells. When the accumulation of foam cells and other inflammatory cells

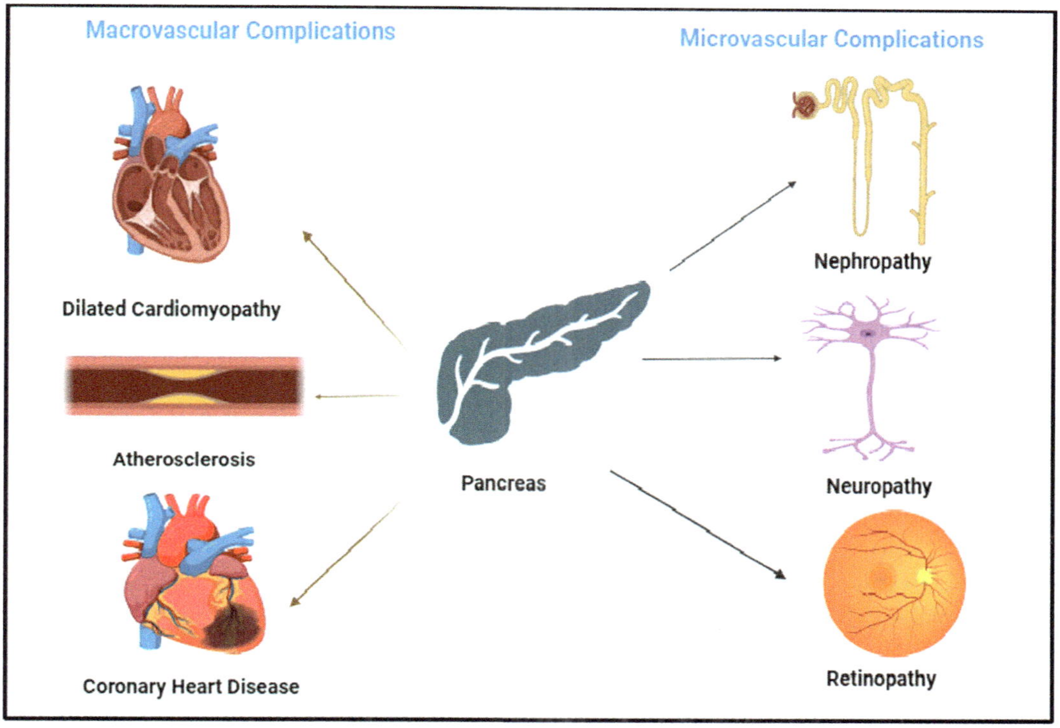

FIGURE 9.1 Macrovascular complications causes cardiovascular diseases (dilated cardiomyopathy, atherosclerosis and coronary heart disease) while microvascular damage affects nephron (nephropathy), neuron (neuropathy) and eyes (retinopathy).

occurs, it results in the formation of AS plaques. Moreover, when the inflammatory response persists, it induces the expression of various inflammatory cytokines, stimulating the activation of macrophages, which triggers a number of cascade reactions, finally accelerating AS (Ganesan et al., 2018). Thus, AS is intimately associated with macrophage activation and the release of inflammatory cytokines or adhesion molecules, as one of the most common causes of DM and AS. Dynamic variations in inflammation levels are strongly linked to the incidence of AS in T2DM subjects. The occurrence of AS in subjects with T2DM could be delayed by the Intervention of inflammatory levels (Zhao et al., 2024).

3.2 Diabetic nephropathy

Immune-mediated mechanisms contribute significantly to diabetic nephropathy. Diabetic nephropathy is renal injury caused by diabetic microangiopathy and is characterized by chronic proteinuria (Chen et al., 2022). Diabetic nephropathy is the most common CKD today, affecting more than half of all DM subjects (Martínez-Castelao et al., 2015). Inflammation has a role in several pathological processes associated with diabetic nephropathy, including renal tubular fibrosis, extracellular matrix buildup, inflammatory cell infiltration, podocyte autophagy, and so on. The aggravation of inflammation during the pathological process of diabetic nephropathy damages the kidney structure; as a result, the condition worsens (Kanasaki et al., 2013). During the early stages of diabetic nephropathy, inflammatory cytokines and immune cells cause tubular damage, glomerular hypertrophy, and glomerular basement membrane thickening. Glomerulosclerosis, tubulointerstitial fibrosis, and other symptoms emerge in the late stages of DN. Endothelial cells, the glomerular basement membrane, and podocytes make up the glomerular filtration membrane, which extends from inside to outside. TNF-α and IL-6 reduce the capillary space between endothelial cells, leading to decreased vasodilation (Dwivedi & Sikarwar, 2025). At the same time, inflammation enhances leukocyte adherence to endothelial cells, encouraging red blood cell folding, which inhibits nitric oxide (NO) generation, promotes EMT, and eventually leads to renal fibrosis (Black et al., 2019). During a high glucose environment, which is accompanied by thickening of the glomerular basement membrane, podocytes exhibit hypertrophy, EMT, apoptosis, and exfoliation, which disrupts the normal structure and function of glomeruli, eventually leading to abnormal glomerular filtration and proteinuria (Zhang et al., 2020). A large number of inflammatory actions affects structure and function of the kidney (Komada & Muruve, 2019). TNF-α damages podocytes and influences physiological indicators such albuminuria, plasma creatinine, and renal macrophage recruitment (Wang et al., 2022). IL-18 increases glomerular damage, while IL-6 causes podocyte death and growth inhibition at high glucose concentrations (Yaribeygi et al., 2019). IL-6 promotes podocyte hypertrophy in response to high glucose levels via the JAK2/STAT3 pathway (Jo et al., 2016). IL-17A regulates CD40 and TGF-β1 expression, contributing to podocyte damage and renal interstitial fibrosis. TGF-β1 transforms renal tubular epithelial cells into myofibroblasts, causing renal fibrosis by EMT (Sun et al., 2018). NLRP3 silencing enhances podocyte autophagy, which reduces podocyte damage and hence prevents renal fibrosis. TXNIP/NLRP3 pathway suppression prevents apoptosis (An et al., 2020). CXCR4 causes renal tubular epithelial cell death, while CXCL9 contributes to podocyte damage (Siddiqi et al., 2015). Inhibiting the NF-κB pathway decreases inflammation and improves renal fibrosis (Ren et al., 2024). The APMK/Sirt1/NF-κB route influences inflammation in DN, while the NF-κB/TNF-α pathway causes podocyte injury in DM rats (Rezaee et al., 2024). The absence of the TLR4 gene or inhibition of TLR4 expression improves urine protein, glomerular hypertrophy, and kidney tubular damage. TLR activation at high glucose levels triggers NF-κB, leading to inflammation and fibrosis (Garibotto et al., 2017). JNK inhibitor reduces the activity of NF-κB, expression of adhesion molecules, and the infiltration of inflammatory cells in diabetic nephropathy mice. The stimulation of the P38/JNK signaling pathway enhances podocyte death and worsens renal damage in diabetic nephropathy mice (Grynberg et al., 2017). JAK/STAT3 contributes to podocyte injury, renal interstitial fibrosis, and podocyte hypertrophy. The PI3K/AKT signal was implicated in renal tubulointerstitial fibrosis, tubulointerstitial cell damage, and glomerulosclerosis. Thus, inflammatory reactions will activate the damage to renal cells in diabetic nephropathy subjects and finally lead to renal dysfunction (Zhang et al., 2021).

3.3 Diabetic neuropathy

Chronic inflammation and immune activation are implicated in the pathogenesis of diabetic neuropathy, which affects both the central and peripheral nerve systems (Baum et al., 2021). Diabetic neuropathy is the most common type of diabetic complication, with symptoms including symmetrical pain and sensory abnormalities caused by peripheral nerve damage. Inflammation in DM patients modulates this situation (Sai Lakshmi and Prabhakar, 2021).

Inflammatory cytokines, immune cells, and the inflammasome all contribute to the control of nerve conduction velocity, neuronal death, nerve regeneration function, neurovascular function, and hyperalgesia. TNF-α decreases nerve conduction and destroys lamellar and axonal structures. Diabetic neuropathy causes damage to myelin axons and ultrastructure through IL-1β and its receptors. TGF-β promotes neuronal death by causing inflammation (Nashtahosseini et al., 2025). NLRP3 triggers excessive ROS, which causes Schwann cell pyroptosis. In diabetic neuropathy, adhesion molecules impede the conduction velocity of motor nerves. Related inflammatory signal pathways influenced nerve tissue shape and function. Activating NF-κB can target miR-146 genes, leading to inflammation, peripheral tissue blood perfusion, and thrombosis in diabetic neuropathy (Li et al., 2022). Ciliary neurotrophic factor activates NF-κB, protecting the peripheral nerve and promoting axon regrowth. TLRs promote cytokine and chemokine release, impacting sensory neuropathy early on through immunomodulation, and regulating axonal development and death in dorsal root ganglion neurons during hyperglycemia (Morel et al., 2020). The TLR4/MyD88/NF-κB signalling pathway promotes neuroprotection, while the JNK, JAK/STAT3, and PI3K/AKT/mTOR pathways regulate apoptosis, autophagy, and proliferation of Schwann cells (Zhao et al., 2024). Thus, inflammation can damage nerve tissues via signaling pathways, accelerating the progression of diabetic neuropathy (Cheng et al., 2024).

3.4 Diabetic retinopathy

Immune dysregulation contributes to microvascular retinal damage in T2DM. Diabetic retinopathy is a chronic disease in which eyesight is lost and, in severe cases, can lead to blindness. The mechanism which causes diabetic retinopathy is not completely understood, findings of research suggest a strong relationship with inflammation, caused by long-term hyperglycemia. The effect of Inflammation causes structural changes in the retina (Semeraro et al., 2015). Vascular permeability, capillary occlusion, and angiogenesis caused by excessive inflammatory action, which finally leads to damage to the blood–retinal barrier and retinal fibrosis (Capitão & Soares, 2016). Diabetic retinopathy is classified as nonproliferative or proliferative depending on how the disease progresses

(Danis & Davis, 2008). The first pathological change of DR is the loss of pericytes in capillaries. Nonfunctional blood vessels arise in the retina, creating an ischemic and anoxic environment that encourages neovascularization and eventually progresses to proliferative diabetic retinopathy due to pericyte loss and endothelial cell migration (Yang et al., 2020). During hyperglycemia, IL-1β promotes apoptosis of pericyte cells and, with the help of NF-κBsignaling pathway, causes increased vascular permeability, which stimulates TLR4 through AGE to increase expression within macrophages and microglia of angiogenic factor Galectin-1 (Yun, 2021). In diabetic retinopathy mice, TNF-α compromises the blood-retinal barrier through the regulatory action of IL-6. IL-17A affects retinal microvessels, Müller cells, and ganglion cells. The vascular remodeling and role in endothelial cell interaction are exerted by TGF-β1 (Homme et al., 2018). The vascular integrity mediated by macrophages is maintained by Ninjurin1, an adhesion molecule. Pathological neovascularization during the later stage of diabetic retinopathy and immune response of the retina occurs through NLRP3 (Raman & Matsubara, 2022). The pyrolysis mediated by NLRP3-caspase-1-GSDMD, causes partial loss of retinal pericytes by hyperglycemia. CXCL1 alters the blood-optic retina barrier in DR by recruiting neutrophils (Zhao et al., 2024). Activation of the NF-κB/STAT3 signaling pathway leads to an increase in IL-1β, IL-6, and TNF-α production, as well as polarization of M1 phenotypic microglia/macrophages, which demolish retinal structure. The damage to the retina and apoptosis by the inhibition of JNK improves DR. The PI3K/AKT/STAT3/NF-κB signalling pathway is crucial for maintaining the blood-retinal barrier and inhibiting microglia activity (Li et al., 2024). Thus, structural alterations in the retina involve a number of inflammatory cytokines, chemokines, the inflammasome, and other inflammatory signaling pathways (Kaur & Singh, 2021).

4. Conclusion

The role of immune mechanisms in the pathogenesis and complications of T2DM is increasingly recognized. Chronic inflammation, autoimmunity, and immune cell dysfunction contribute to diabetic complications, including CVD , nephropathy, neuropathy, and retinopathy. Understanding these immune-mediated pathways offers potential therapeutic targets for reducing morbidity and improving patient outcomes.

References

An, X., Zhang, Y., Cao, Y., Chen, J., Qin, H., & Yang, L. (2020). Punicalagin protects diabetic nephropathy by inhibiting pyroptosis based on TXNIP/NLRP3 pathway. *Nutrients, 12*(5), 1516. https://doi.org/10.3390/nu12051516

Ansel, K. M., Djuretic, I., Tanasa, B., & Rao, A. (2006). Regulation of TH2 differentiation and *Il4* Locus accessibility. *Annual Review of Immunology, 24*(1), 607–656. https://doi.org/10.1146/annurev.immunol.23.021704.115821

Baum, P., Toyka, K. V., Blüher, M., Kosacka, J., & Nowicki, M. (2021). Inflammatory mechanisms in the pathophysiology of diabetic peripheral neuropathy (DN)—New aspects. *International Journal of Molecular Sciences, 22*(19), Article 10835. https://doi.org/10.3390/ijms221910835

Berbudi, A., Rahmadika, N., Tjahjadi, A. I., & Ruslami, R. (2020). Type 2 diabetes and its impact on the immune system. *Current Diabetes Reviews, 16*(5), 442–449. https://doi.org/10.2174/1573399815666191024085838

Black, L. M., Lever, J. M., & Agarwal, A. (2019). Renal inflammation and fibrosis: A double-edged sword. *Journal of Histochemistry and Cytochemistry, 67*(9), 663–681. https://doi.org/10.1369/0022155419852932

Capitão, M., & Soares, R. (2016). Angiogenesis and inflammation crosstalk in diabetic retinopathy. *Journal of Cellular Biochemistry, 117*(11), 2443–2453. https://doi.org/10.1002/jcb.25575

Chen, J., Liu, Q., He, J., & Li, Y. (2022). Immune responses in diabetic nephropathy: Pathogenic mechanisms and therapeutic target. *Frontiers in Immunology, 13*, Article 958790. https://doi.org/10.3389/fimmu.2022.958790

Cheng, Y., Chen, Y., Li, K., Liu, S., Pang, C., Gao, L., Xie, J., Wenjing, L. V., Yu, H., & Deng, B. (2024). How inflammation dictates diabetic peripheral neuropathy: An enlightening review. *CNS Neuroscience and Therapeutics, 30*(4), Article e14477. https://doi.org/10.1111/cns.14477

Clyne, A. M. (2021). Endothelial response to glucose: Dysfunction, metabolism, and transport. *Biochemical Society Transactions, 49*(1), 313–325. https://doi.org/10.1042/BST20200611

Danis, R. P., & Davis, M. D. (2008). Proliferative diabetic retinopathy. In E. J. Duh (Ed.), *Diabetic retinopathy* (pp. 29–65). Humana Press. https://doi.org/10.1007/978-1-59745-563-3_2

De Luca, C., & Olefsky, J. M. (2008). Inflammation and insulin resistance. *FEBS Letters, 582*(1), 97–105. https://doi.org/10.1016/j.febslet.2007.11.057

Ding, J., Strachan, M. W. J., Fowkes, F. G. R., Wong, T. Y., MacGillivray, T. J., Patton, N., Gardiner, T. A., Deary, I. J., & Price, J. F. (2011). Association of retinal arteriolar dilatation with lower verbal memory: The Edinburgh type 2 diabetes study. *Diabetologia, 54*(7), 1653–1662. https://doi.org/10.1007/s00125-011-2129-1

Donath, M. Y., & Shoelson, S. E. (2011). Type 2 diabetes as an inflammatory disease. *Nature Reviews Immunology, 11*(2), 98–107. https://doi.org/10.1038/nri2925

Dror, E., Dalmas, E., Meier, D. T., Wueest, S., Thévenet, J., Thienel, C., Timper, K., Nordmann, T. M., Traub, S., Schulze, F., Item, F., Vallois, D., Pattou, F., Kerr-Conte, J., Lavallard, V., Berney, T., Thorens, B., Konrad, D., Böni-Schnetzler, M., & Donath, M. Y. (2017). Postprandial macrophage-derived IL-1β stimulates insulin, and both synergistically promote glucose disposal and inflammation. *Nature Immunology, 18*(3), 283–292. https://doi.org/10.1038/ni.3659

Dwivedi, S., & Sikarwar, M. S. (2025). Diabetic nephropathy: Pathogenesis, mechanisms, and therapeutic strategies. *Hormone and Metabolic Research, 57*(01), 7–17. https://doi.org/10.1055/a-2435-8264

Farmaki, P., Damaskos, C., Garmpis, N., Garmpi, A., Savvanis, S., & Diamantis, E. (2021). Complications of the type 2 diabetes mellitus. *Current Cardiology Reviews, 16*(4), 249–251. https://doi.org/10.2174/1573403X1604201229115531

Fasanmade, O. A., Odeniyi, I. A., & Ogbera, A. O. (2008). Diabetic ketoacidosis: Diagnosis and management. *African Journal of Medicine & Medical Sciences, 37*(2), 99–105.

Fowler, M. J. (2011). Microvascular and macrovascular complications of diabetes. *Clinical Diabetes, 29*(3).

Ganesan, R., Henkels, K. M., Wrenshall, L. E., Kanaho, Y., Di Paolo, G., Frohman, M. A., & Gomez-Cambronero, J. (2018). Oxidized LDL phagocytosis during foam cell formation in atherosclerotic plaques relies on a PLD2–CD36 functional interdependence. *Journal of Leukocyte Biology, 103*(5), 867–883. https://doi.org/10.1002/JLB.2A1017-407RR

Garibotto, G., Carta, A., Picciotto, D., Viazzi, F., & Verzola, D. (2017). Toll-like receptor-4 signaling mediates inflammation and tissue injury in diabetic nephropathy. *Journal of Nephrology, 30*(6), 719–727. https://doi.org/10.1007/s40620-017-0432-8

Giri, B., Dey, S., Das, T., Sarkar, M., Banerjee, J., & Dash, S. K. (2018). Chronic hyperglycemia mediated physiological alteration and metabolic distortion leads to organ dysfunction, infection, cancer progression and other pathophysiological consequences: An update on glucose toxicity. *Biomedicine & Pharmacotherapy, 107*, 306–328. https://doi.org/10.1016/j.biopha.2018.07.157

Goldberg, R. B. (2009). Cytokine and cytokine-like inflammation markers, endothelial dysfunction, and imbalanced coagulation in development of diabetes and its complications. *The Journal of Clinical Endocrinology & Metabolism, 94*(9), 3171–3182. https://doi.org/10.1210/jc.2008-2534

Grynberg, K., Ma, F. Y., & Nikolic-Paterson, D. J. (2017). The JNK signaling pathway in renal fibrosis. *Frontiers in Physiology, 8*, 829. https://doi.org/10.3389/fphys.2017.00829

Guan, H., Tian, J., Wang, Y., Niu, P., Zhang, Y., Zhang, Y., Fang, X., Miao, R., Yin, R., & Tong, X. (2024). Advances in secondary prevention mechanisms of macrovascular complications in type 2 diabetes mellitus patients: A comprehensive review. *European Journal of Medical Research, 29*(1), 152. https://doi.org/10.1186/s40001-024-01739-1

Gusev, E., & Sarapultsev, A. (2023). Atherosclerosis and inflammation: Insights from the theory of general pathological processes. *International Journal of Molecular Sciences, 24*(9), 7910. https://doi.org/10.3390/ijms24097910

Henning, R. J. (2018). Type-2 diabetes mellitus and cardiovascular disease. *Future Cardiology, 14*(6), 491–509. https://doi.org/10.2217/fca-2018-0045

Homme, R. P., Singh, M., Majumder, A., George, A. K., Nair, K., Sandhu, H. S., Tyagi, N., Lominadze, D., & Tyagi, S. C. (2018). Remodeling of retinal architecture in diabetic retinopathy: Disruption of ocular physiology and visual functions by inflammatory gene products and pyroptosis. *Frontiers in Physiology, 9*, 1268. https://doi.org/10.3389/fphys.2018.01268

Hotamisligil, G. S., Arner, P., Caro, J. F., Atkinson, R. L., & Spiegelman, B. M. (1995). Increased adipose tissue expression of tumor necrosis factor-alpha in human obesity and insulin resistance. *The Journal of Clinical Investigation, 95*(5), 2409–2415. https://doi.org/10.1172/JCI117936

Hotamisligil, G. S., & Spiegelman, B. M. (1994). Tumor necrosis factor alpha: A key component of the obesity-diabetes link. *Diabetes, 43*(11), 1271–1278. https://doi.org/10.2337/diab.43.11.1271

Ieronymaki, E., Theodorakis, E. M., Lyroni, K., Vergadi, E., Lagoudaki, E., Al-Qahtani, A., Aznaourova, M., Neofotistou-Themeli, E., Eliopoulos, A. G., Vaporidi, K., & Tsatsanis, C. (2019). Insulin resistance in macrophages alters their metabolism and promotes an M2-Like phenotype. *The Journal of Immunology, 202*(6), 1786–1797. https://doi.org/10.4049/jimmunol.1800065

Inácio, D. P., Amado, T., Silva-Santos, B., & Gomes, A. Q. (2018). Control of T cell effector functions by miRNAs. *Cancer Letters, 427*, 63–73. https://doi.org/10.1016/j.canlet.2018.04.011

Jo, H. A., Kim, J.-Y., Yang, S. H., Han, S. S., Joo, K. W., Kim, Y. S., & Kim, D. K. (2016). The role of local IL6/JAK2/STAT3 signaling in high glucose–induced podocyte hypertrophy. *Kidney Research and Clinical Practice, 35*(4), 212–218. https://doi.org/10.1016/j.krcp.2016.09.003

Kanasaki, K., Taduri, G., & Koya, D. (2013). Diabetic nephropathy: The role of inflammation in fibroblast activation and kidney fibrosis. *Frontiers in Endocrinology, 4*. https://doi.org/10.3389/fendo.2013.00007

Katakami, N. (2018). Mechanism of development of atherosclerosis and cardiovascular disease in diabetes mellitus. *Journal of Atherosclerosis and Thrombosis, 25*(1), 27–39. https://doi.org/10.5551/jat.RV17014

Kaur, G., & Singh, N. K. (2021). The role of inflammation in retinal neurodegeneration and degenerative diseases. *International Journal of Molecular Sciences, 23*(1), 386. https://doi.org/10.3390/ijms23010386

Komada, T., & Muruve, D. A. (2019). The role of inflammasomes in kidney disease. *Nature Reviews Nephrology, 15*(8), 501–520. https://doi.org/10.1038/s41581-019-0158-z

Kwak, S.-J., Kim, C.-S., Choi, M.-S., Park, T., Sung, M.-K., Yun, J. W., Yoo, H., Mine, Y., & Yu, R. (2016). The soy peptide Phe–Leu–Val reduces TNFα-Induced inflammatory response and insulin resistance in adipocytes. *Journal of Medicinal Food, 19*(7), 678–685. https://doi.org/10.1089/jmf.2016.3685

Leutholtz, B. C., & Ripoll, I. (2011). *Exercise and disease management* (0 ed.). CRC Press. https://doi.org/10.1201/b10856

Li, H., Li, B., & Zheng, Y. (2024). Role of microglia/macrophage polarisation in intraocular diseases (review). *International Journal of Molecular Medicine, 53*(5), 45. https://doi.org/10.3892/ijmm.2024.5369

Li, W., Liang, J., Li, S., Wang, L., Xu, S., Jiang, S., Song, M., Meng, H., Zhai, D., Tang, L., Yang, Y., Zhang, L., & Zhang, B. (2022). Research progress of targeting NLRP3 inflammasome in peripheral nerve injury and pain. *International Immunopharmacology, 110*, Article 109026. https://doi.org/10.1016/j.intimp.2022.109026

Li, Y., Liu, Y., Liu, S., Gao, M., Wang, W., Chen, K., Huang, L., & Liu, Y. (2023). Diabetic vascular diseases: Molecular mechanisms and therapeutic strategies. *Signal Transduction and Targeted Therapy, 8*(1), 152. https://doi.org/10.1038/s41392-023-01400-z

Mansour, A., Mousa, M., Abdelmannan, D., Tay, G., Hassoun, A., & Alsafar, H. (2023). Microvascular and macrovascular complications of type 2 diabetes mellitus: Exome wide association analyses. *Frontiers in Endocrinology, 14*, Article 1143067. https://doi.org/10.3389/fendo.2023.1143067

Maris, M., Overbergh, L., Gysemans, C., Waget, A., Cardozo, A. K., Verdrengh, E., Cunha, J. P. M., Gotoh, T., Cnop, M., Eizirik, D. L., Burcelin, R., & Mathieu, C. (2012). Deletion of C/EBP homologous protein (chop) in C57Bl/6 mice dissociates obesity from insulin resistance. *Diabetologia, 55*(4), 1167–1178. https://doi.org/10.1007/s00125-011-2427-7

Martínez-Castelao, A., Navarro-González, J., Górriz, J., & De Alvaro, F. (2015). The concept and the epidemiology of diabetic nephropathy have changed in recent years. *Journal of Clinical Medicine, 4*(6), 1207–1216. https://doi.org/10.3390/jcm4061207

Morel, L., Domingues, O., Zimmer, J., & Michel, T. (2020). Revisiting the role of neurotrophic factors in inflammation. *Cells, 9*(4), 865. https://doi.org/10.3390/cells9040865

Nashtahosseini, Z., Eslami, M., Paraandavaji, E., Haraj, A., Dowlat, B. F., Hosseinzadeh, E., Oksenych, V., & Naderian, R. (2025). Cytokine signaling in diabetic neuropathy: A key player in peripheral nerve damage. *Biomedicines, 13*(3), 589. https://doi.org/10.3390/biomedicines13030589

Pickup, J. C., & Crook, M. A. (1998). Is type II diabetes mellitus a disease of the innate immune system? *Diabetologia, 41*(10), 1241–1248. https://doi.org/10.1007/s001250051058

Raman, K. S., & Matsubara, J. A. (2022). Dysregulation of the NLRP3 inflammasome in diabetic retinopathy and potential therapeutic targets. *Ocular Immunology and Inflammation, 30*(2), 470–478. https://doi.org/10.1080/09273948.2020.1811350

Raphael, I., Nalawade, S., Eagar, T. N., & Forsthuber, T. G. (2015). T cell subsets and their signature cytokines in autoimmune and inflammatory diseases. *Cytokine, 74*(1), 5–17. https://doi.org/10.1016/j.cyto.2014.09.011

Ren, N., Wang, W.-F., Zou, L., Zhao, Y.-L., Miao, H., & Zhao, Y.-Y. (2024). The nuclear factor kappa B signaling pathway is a master regulator of renal fibrosis. *Frontiers in Pharmacology, 14*, Article 1335094. https://doi.org/10.3389/fphar.2023.1335094

Rezaee, A., Rahmanian, P., Nemati, A., Sohrabifard, F., Karimi, F., Elahinia, A., Ranjbarpazuki, A., Lashkarbolouki, R., Dezfulian, S., Zandieh, M. A., Salimimoghadam, S., Nabavi, N., Rashidi, M., Taheriazam, A., Hashemi, M., & Hushmandi, K. (2024). NF-κB axis in diabetic neuropathy, cardiomyopathy and nephropathy: A roadmap from molecular intervention to therapeutic strategies. *Heliyon, 10*(9), Article e29871. https://doi.org/10.1016/j.heliyon.2024.e29871

Roytblat, L., Rachinsky, M., Fisher, A., Greemberg, L., Shapira, Y., Douvdevani, A., & Gelman, S. (2000). Raised interleukin-6 levels in obese patients. *Obesity Research, 8*(9), 673–675. https://doi.org/10.1038/oby.2000.86

Saeedi, P., Petersohn, I., Salpea, P., Malanda, B., Karuranga, S., Unwin, N., Colagiuri, S., Guariguata, L., Motala, A. A., Ogurtsova, K., Shaw, J. E., Bright, D., & Williams, R. (2019). Global and regional diabetes prevalence estimates for 2019 and projections for 2030 and 2045: Results from the international diabetes Federation diabetes atlas, 9th edition. *Diabetes Research and Clinical Practice, 157*, Article 107843. https://doi.org/10.1016/j.diabres.2019.107843

Saeedi, P., Salpea, P., Karuranga, S., Petersohn, I., Malanda, B., Gregg, E. W., Unwin, N., Wild, S. H., & Williams, R. (2020). Mortality attributable to diabetes in 20–79 years old adults, 2019 estimates: Results from the international diabetes Federation diabetes Atlas, 9th edition. *Diabetes Research and Clinical Practice, 162*, Article 108086. https://doi.org/10.1016/j.diabres.2020.108086

Sai Lakshmi, M., & Prabhakar, O. (2021). Inflammatory biomarkers as a part of diagnosis in diabetic peripheral neuropathy. *Journal of Diabetes and Metabolic Disorders, 20*(1), 869–882. https://doi.org/10.1007/s40200-021-00734-1

Sartipy, P., & Loskutoff, D. J. (2003). Monocyte chemoattractant protein 1 in obesity and insulin resistance. *Proceedings of the National Academy of Sciences of the United States of America, 100*(12), 7265–7270. https://doi.org/10.1073/pnas.1133870100

Semeraro, F., Cancarini, A., dell'Omo, R., Rezzola, S., Romano, M. R., & Costagliola, C. (2015). Diabetic retinopathy: Vascular and inflammatory disease. *Journal of Diabetes Research, 2015*, 1–16. https://doi.org/10.1155/2015/582060

Shirakawa, K., Yan, X., Shinmura, K., Endo, J., Kataoka, M., Katsumata, Y., Yamamoto, T., Anzai, A., Isobe, S., Yoshida, N., Itoh, H., Manabe, I., Sekai, M., Hamazaki, Y., Fukuda, K., Minato, N., & Sano, M. (2016). Obesity accelerates T cell senescence in murine visceral adipose tissue. *Journal of Clinical Investigation, 126*(12), 4626–4639. https://doi.org/10.1172/JCI88606

Siddiqi, F. S., Chen, L.-H., Advani, S. L., Thai, K., Batchu, S. N., Alghamdi, T. A., White, K. E., Sood, M. M., Gibson, I. W., Connelly, K. A., Marsden, P. A., & Advani, A. (2015). CXCR4 promotes renal tubular cell survival in Male diabetic rats: Implications for ligand inactivation in the human kidney. *Endocrinology, 156*(3), 1121–1132. https://doi.org/10.1210/en.2014-1650

Solinas, G., & Karin, M. (2010). JNK1 and IKKβ: Molecular links between obesity and metabolic dysfunction. *The FASEB Journal, 24*(8), 2596–2611. https://doi.org/10.1096/fj.09-151340

Srenathan, U., Steel, K., & Taams, L. S. (2016). IL-17+ CD8+ T cells: Differentiation, phenotype and role in inflammatory disease. *Immunology Letters, 178*, 20–26. https://doi.org/10.1016/j.imlet.2016.05.001

Straczkowski, M., Dzienis-Straczkowska, S., Stêpieñ, A., Kowalska, I., Szelachowska, M., & Kinalska, I. (2002). Plasma interleukin-8 concentrations are increased in obese subjects and related to fat mass and tumor necrosis factor-alpha system. *The Journal of Clinical Endocrinology and Metabolism, 87*(10), 4602–4606. https://doi.org/10.1210/jc.2002-020135

Sun, B., Wang, H., Zhang, L., Yang, X., Zhang, M., Zhu, X., Ji, X., & Wang, H. (2018). Role of interleukin 17 in TGF-β signaling-mediated renal interstitial fibrosis. *Cytokine, 106*, 80–88. https://doi.org/10.1016/j.cyto.2017.10.015

Swaroop, J. J., Rajarajeswari, D., & Naidu, J. N. (2012). Association of TNF-α with insulin resistance in type 2 diabetes mellitus. *Indian Journal of Medical Research, 135*(1), 127–130. https://doi.org/10.4103/0971-5916.93435

Tsai, S., Clemente-Casares, X., Zhou, A. C., Lei, H., Ahn, J. J., Chan, Y. T., Choi, O., Luck, H., Woo, M., Dunn, S. E., Engleman, E. G., Watts, T. H., Winer, S., & Winer, D. A. (2018). Insulin receptor-mediated stimulation boosts T cell immunity during inflammation and infection. *Cell Metabolism, 28*(6), 922–934.e4. https://doi.org/10.1016/j.cmet.2018.08.003

Vijan, S. (2015). Type 2 diabetes. *Annals of Internal Medicine, 162*(5), ITC1–ITC16. https://doi.org/10.7326/AITC201503030

Visser, M., Bouter, L. M., McQuillan, G. M., Wener, M. H., & Harris, T. B. (1999). Elevated C-reactive protein levels in overweight and obese adults. *JAMA, 282*(22), 2131–2135. https://doi.org/10.1001/jama.282.22.2131

Wang, J., Feng, Y., Zhang, Y., Liu, J., Gong, L., Zhang, X., & Liao, H. (2022). TNF-α and IL-1β promote renal podocyte injury in T2DM rats by decreasing glomerular VEGF/eNOS expression levels and altering hemodynamic parameters. *Journal of Inflammation Research, 15,* 6657–6673. https://doi.org/10.2147/JIR.S391473

Wilson, C. B., Rowell, E., & Sekimata, M. (2009). Epigenetic control of T-helper-cell differentiation. *Nature Reviews Immunology, 9*(2), 91–105. https://doi.org/10.1038/nri2487

Winer, S., Chan, Y., Paltser, G., Truong, D., Tsui, H., Bahrami, J., Dorfman, R., Wang, Y., Zielenski, J., Mastronardi, F., Maezawa, Y., Drucker, D. J., Engleman, E., Winer, D., & Dosch, H.-M. (2009). Normalization of obesity-associated insulin resistance through immunotherapy. *Nature Medicine, 15*(8), 921–929. https://doi.org/10.1038/nm.2001

Winer, D. A., Winer, S., Shen, L., Wadia, P. P., Yantha, J., Paltser, G., Tsui, H., Wu, P., Davidson, M. G., Alonso, M. N., Leong, H. X., Glassford, A., Caimol, M., Kenkel, J. A., Tedder, T. F., McLaughlin, T., Miklos, D. B., Dosch, H.-M., & Engleman, E. G. (2011). B cells promote insulin resistance through modulation of T cells and production of pathogenic IgG antibodies. *Nature Medicine, 17*(5), 610–617. https://doi.org/10.1038/nm.2353

Yang, S., Zhang, J., & Chen, L. (2020). The cells involved in the pathological process of diabetic retinopathy. *Biomedicine & Pharmacotherapy, 132,* Article 110818. https://doi.org/10.1016/j.biopha.2020.110818

Yaribeygi, H., Atkin, S. L., & Sahebkar, A. (2019). Interleukin-18 and diabetic nephropathy: A review. *Journal of Cellular Physiology, 234*(5), 5674–5682. https://doi.org/10.1002/jcp.27427

Yun, J.-H. (2021). Interleukin-1β induces pericyte apoptosis via the NF-κB pathway in diabetic retinopathy. *Biochemical and Biophysical Research Communications, 546,* 46–53. https://doi.org/10.1016/j.bbrc.2021.01.108

Zhang, Y., Jin, D., Kang, X., Zhou, R., Sun, Y., Lian, F., & Tong, X. (2021). Signaling pathways involved in diabetic renal fibrosis. *Frontiers in Cell and Developmental Biology, 9,* Article 696542. https://doi.org/10.3389/fcell.2021.696542

Zhang, L., Wen, Z., Han, L., Zheng, Y., Wei, Y., Wang, X., Wang, Q., Fang, X., Zhao, L., & Tong, X. (2020). Research progress on the pathological mechanisms of podocytes in diabetic nephropathy. *Journal of Diabetes Research, 2020,* 1–15. https://doi.org/10.1155/2020/7504798

Zhao, L., Hu, H., Zhang, L., Liu, Z., Huang, Y., Liu, Q., Jin, L., Zhu, M., & Zhang, L. (2024). Inflammation in diabetes complications: Molecular mechanisms and therapeutic interventions. *MedComm, 5*(4), Article e516. https://doi.org/10.1002/mco2.516

Zheng, X., Ke, Y., Feng, A., Yuan, P., Zhou, J., Yu, Y., Wang, X., & Feng, W. (2016). The mechanism by which amentoflavone improves insulin resistance in HepG2 cells. *Molecules, 21*(5), 624. https://doi.org/10.3390/molecules21050624

Zhu, J., Yamane, H., & Paul, W. E. (2010). Differentiation of effector CD4 T cell populations. *Annual Review of Immunology, 28*(1), 445–489. https://doi.org/10.1146/annurev-immunol-030409-101212

10

Targeting immune pathways for T2DM treatment

Puja Kumari[1], Dhanusmita Barman[2] and Kripamoy Aguan[1]

[1]DEPARTMENT OF BIOTECHNOLOGY AND BIOINFORMATICS, NORTH EASTERN HILL UNIVERSITY, SHILLONG, MEGHALAYA, INDIA; [2]DEPARTMENT OF ZOOLOGY, AUXILIUM COLLEGE, UDALGURI, ASSAM, INDIA

1. Introduction

In 2023, the International Diabetes Federation (IDF) reported 540 million live cases of diabetes worldwide. It is anticipated that both developed and developing nations will see an increase in this number. It is projected that 629 million people worldwide will have diabetes by 2045 if current management controls are not addressed. Type 2 Diabetes Mellitus (T2DM) is a condition due to inadequate functioning of insulin, either due to insulin resistance or reduced insulin synthesis by β-islet cells of the pancreas. About 90% of all cases of diabetes are T2DM, where the blood glucose levels are elevated because of this illness. To compensate for insulin resistance, the pancreatic islets try to produce more insulin. However, when this attempt falls short of compensating for insulin resistance, T2DM develops. T2DM is a long-term chronic insulin resistance disorder that raises a number of concerns, including microvascular problems like nephropathy, neuropathy, retinopathy and macrovascular problems like atherosclerosis (Berbudi et al., 2020). Underlying T2DM is a complex interplay of genetic and epigenetic factors that includes metabolic, lifestyle and environmental parameters, all of which contribute to its widespread occurrence. Risk factors such as ethnicity and genetic predisposition (including family history) are nonmodifiable and play a significant role, as epidemiological studies indicate that a majority of diabetic cases can be prevented by addressing modifiable aspects. These include managing obesity, increasing physical activity, and adopting a healthier diet (Galicia-Garcia et al., 2020).

2. Molecular landscape involved in insulin resistance

At the molecular level, several inflammatory pathways are associated with insulin function inhibition, linking inflammation to insulin resistance. Among those, key pathways include JNK, IKK/NF-κB, JAK/STAT, etc., which contribute to chronic

Type 2 Diabetes Mellitus. https://doi.org/10.1016/B978-0-443-33590-7.00015-0

inflammation. Endogenous factors such as saturated fatty acids (SFAs) and heat shock proteins activate the pattern recognition receptors (PRRs), leading to the activation of inflammatory processes even without external pathogens. Inflammation results in cellular stress, tissue damage and inflammation and activates another class of molecules called -Associated Molecular Patterns (DAMP). Among PRRs the major ones are Toll like receptors (TLRs), RIG-I like RNA helicases (RLHs), NOD like receptors (NLRs) and AIM2-like receptors (ALRs). These molecules in particular detect pathogen-associated molecular patterns (PAMP) from pathogens and biological allergens such as bacterial DNA, lipopolysaccharides (LPS), and peptidoglycans. Recent studies have indicated that the proinflammatory molecule, such as leukotriene B4 (LTB4), also promotes insulin resistance via the JNK pathway. LTB4, a neutrophil chemotactic agent, is generated through arachidonic acid metabolism. It is produced by immune cells, including macrophages, eosinophils and by primary tissue cells such as adipocytes, hepatocytes, myocytes and endothelial cells. Elevated LTB4 levels significantly contribute to insulin resistance via the G protein-coupled receptor BLT-1, which is mostly present on immune and primary metabolic cells. Furthermore, LTB4 synthesis activates macrophage chemotaxis and migration, resulting in a positive feedback loop between macrophage LTB4 secretion and chronic tissue inflammation.

LTB4 administration has been reported to enhance JNK activity and increase the IRS-1 serine phosphorylation, thereby compromising insulin sensitivity in target cells. In vitro LTB4 treatment of adipocytes and hepatocytes also reported an induction of insulin resistance, while in obese mice, BLT-1 knockout improved the inflammation and insulin sensitivity. Insulin resistance is also linked to NF-κB activation through the action of TNF-α, a crucial inflammation-related transcription factor. IκB sequesters NF-κB, and IKK phosphorylation releases NF-κB, which helps in promoting inflammatory gene transactivation, exacerbating insulin resistance. IKK2 is vital for activating NF-κB in inflammatory responses, as demonstrated by improved glucose homeostasis in IKK2 heterozygous-deletion mice. Additionally, diet plays an important role, where the high-fat diet enhanced NF-κB activation and IKKε levels, while IKKε knockout mice show resistance to inflammation. The monocyte and macrophage-derived IL-1β also contributes to insulin resistance via the NF-κB pathway. Elevated IL-1β correlates with hyperglycaemia and increased T2DM risk. IL-1β binds to IL-1R1, activating JAK kinases and promoting NF-κB translocation to the nucleus, thereby enhancing inflammatory gene expression. IL-1β diminishes insulin signaling in tissues. Monocytes and macrophages express high levels of PPAR-γ, a nuclear receptor influencing inflammation, differentiation and metabolism. The natural ligands of PPAR-γ include lipids and prostaglandins, which, when elevated during inflammation, correlate positively with insulin resistance. Conversely, synthetic PPAR-γ agonists alleviate insulin resistance and are helpful in diabetes treatment. PPAR-γ inhibits NF-κB activity and inflammation by promoting p65 degradation and enhancing IRS protein levels, thereby mitigating obesity-induced insulin resistance. PPAR-γ knockout in macrophages results in impaired glucose tolerance and heightened insulin resistance, along with increased inflammatory markers. IL6 is essential for metabolism and immunity regulation. Its elevation in obese individuals negatively impacts metabolic homeostasis. The JAK2/STAT3 pathway is triggered by IL6 binding to its receptor, which results in the transcription of target genes such as SOCS-3. SOCS-3 inhibits IL6 signaling and adversely affects insulin signaling at the IRS protein level. The SOCS-3 induced by IL-6 results in the deterioration of IRS-1. Research on IL6's influence on insulin sensitivity has yielded inconsistent findings. Implementing a very-low-calorie diet significantly reduces IL6 levels and enhances insulin sensitivity. Acute IL6 injection in mice induces insulin resistance independent of obesity. Conversely, IL6 knockout mice exhibit insulin resistance as soon as they mature. Another investigation indicated IL6 deficient 4 months old mice experience glucose intolerance and increased adiposity (Li et al., 2022). Through these studies, it has been evident that inflammation and markers of inflammation play an essential role in establishing insulin resistance via dysregulation of immune and metabolic pathways. In the subsequent sections, we have comprehensively discussed the role of inflammation, immune cells and pathways with a distinct context on the potential therapeutic strategies that have been or can be explored against the upcoming diabetic pandemic.

3. Role of inflammation

In the development and progression of T2DM, chronic low-grade inflammation plays a fundamental role, particularly by contributing to insulin resistance and metabolic dysfunction. This inflammation is often exacerbated by lifestyle factors such as obesity, leading to a cascade of metabolic disturbances. Chronic inflammation has been reported in the gastrointestinal (GI) tract, pancreatic islets, muscle, liver, adipose tissue and central nervous system, showing the intricate, multiorgan crosstalk network involved in T2DM. The studies from the last 20 years significantly contributed to the underlying understanding of physiological and molecular mechanisms by which inflammation is linked to the development of insulin resistance and glucose intolerance (Lee & Olefsky, 2021). For instance, the involvement of TNFα in contributing to hyperglycemic conditions was reported to be involved through a seminal investigation done in the rodent model (Feingold et al., 1989). Similarly, other studies demonstrated to confers resistance against insulin, the uplift of the levels of TNFα in the adipose tissue of obese murine models for further neutralization of TNFα (Hotamisligil et al., 1994). In addition to TNFα, other studies have identified other molecules in the inflammatory signaling pathway that can block insulin signaling, such as JNK, IKK,β and other cytokines. Various studies have elucidated a mechanistic nexus between chronic inflammation and insulin resistance through the application of diverse genetic gain and loss of function methodologies in rodent models (Lee et al., 2018). For instance, genetically modified mice exhibiting global depletion of IKKβ, JNK, CCR2, and CCL2/MCP-1 demonstrated enhanced insulin sensitivity (Arkan et al., 2005; Weisberg et al., 2006). Moreover, knockout models targeting JNK, HIF-1α, NEMO, and TLR4 in either adipocytes or hepatocytes also resulted in improved insulin sensitivity (Jia et al., 2014). Conversely, the adipocyte-specific overexpression of CCL2 or HIF-1α was shown to precipitate insulin resistance and glucose intolerance even when subjected to a standard chow diet (Desai et al., 2017; Halberg et al., 2009). Notably, an extensive array of macrophage or hematopoietic cell-specific knockout studies involving inflammatory molecules has been reported, all indicating a protective effect against insulin resistance and glucose intolerance (Desai et al., 2017). Nevertheless, despite an abundance of studies conducted on human adipose tissue (Hill et al., 2018), hepatic tissue (Ghazarian et al., 2017), primary adipocytes (Liu et al., 1998), skeletal muscle (Austin et al., 2008), and pancreatic islets (Maedler et al., 2002) that substantiate this immunometabolism framework, the hypothesis positing that chronic inflammation induces insulin resistance and β-cell dysfunction remains to be conclusively validated in human populations. Recently, exosomes derived from macrophages have been reported to be involved in modulating the various aspects of inflammation-mediated insulin resistance (Lee & Olefsky, 2021). It has been found that the exosomes encapsulate a diverse array of bioactive molecules that facilitate inflammatory responses and can potentially interfere with insulin signaling pathways. Importantly, macrophages in adipose tissue secrete microRNAs, such as miR-210-3p, which hinder glucose uptake by downregulating GLUT4, thereby exacerbating the state of insulin resistance (Patra et al., 2024). Exosomes have been found to promote paracrine signaling, thereby influencing adjacent cells and contributing to the overarching phenomenon of systemic insulin resistance. Because of the disruption of glucose-lipid metabolism caused by the resulting β-cell malfunction eventually develop diabetes and their allied disorder. The understanding of exosomes' importance highlights their potential as effective therapeutic targets (Ghoshal, 2024).

Moreover, the presence of chronic low-grade inflammation serves as a crucial component in the progression of T2DM, affecting diverse organ systems (Wang et al., 2023). Low-grade systemic inflammation, characterized by elevated cytokines such as IL-6 and C-reactive protein (CRP), is increasingly recognized as a precursor to T2DM, particularly in individuals with obesity (Stanimirovic et al., 2022). Furthermore, when exposed to lifestyle-induced inflammation, genetic and epigenetic factors can impair the body's counter-regulatory responses to inflammation, making individuals more susceptible to T2DM. Genetic susceptibility, as evidenced by genetic risk scores (GRS), is linked with an elevated occurrence of diabetes, particularly when coupled with an elevated Lifestyle Inflammation Score (LIS) (Lee et al., 2024). Epigenetic alterations, including DNA methylation and histone modifications, modify immune cell functionality, thereby contributing to persistent inflammation and insulin resistance, which are integral to the pathogenesis of T2DM (Ding et al., 2022). Furthermore, dysregulated epigenetic changes can intensify inflammatory reactions, resulting in β-cell impairment. Lifestyle-related inflammatory variables interact strongly with genetic and epigenetic predispositions to increase susceptibility to T2DM. Genetic predispositions, such as particular single-nucleotide polymorphisms (SNPs), might amplify the impact of lifestyle factors like obesity, eating choices, and physical inactivity, resulting in an increased risk of diabetes. Furthermore, epigenetic changes influenced by the environment are crucial to immune cell function and inflammatory processes, both of which have a role in the development of T2DM. Genetic and Lifestyle Interactions Genetic Risk Scores (GRS) are connected with T2DM, with higher scores indicating an increased risk when combined with poor lifestyle choices. Certain lifestyle factors, such as tobacco use and food habits, interact with genetic susceptibilities to increase T2DM risk. Epigenetic changes caused by inflammation can affect immune cell activity, leading to insulin resistance and β-cell damage (Ding et al., 2022). It indicates the existence of a complicated crosstalk of genetic, environmental, and lifestyle parameters that warrants further investigation (Nunemaker, 2016).

4. Role of inflammatory markers

The development of insulin resistance in T2DM is certain, where chronic inflammation provides the platform. The connection between inflammation and insulin resistance primarily involves proinflammatory mediators like NF-Kβ, IKK-β, TNF-α, IL-6, IL-1β, and CRP. These mediators interfere with insulin signaling pathways, reducing the effectiveness of the body to respond to insulin, eventually leading to elevated blood glucose levels (Alzamil, 2020).

5. Tumor necrosis factor-α

Insulin resistance is a pivotal step for the onset and progression of T2DM, where tumor necrosis factor-α (TNF-α) is a major factor. Because it can affect various cell types, it is a pleiotropic cytokine (33). It is a material that immune cells and adipocytes make. It binds specifically to cell receptors and initiates specific pathways, such as the NF-κB and JNK pathways. They function similarly to switches, activating inflammatory processes inside the cells. These pathways alter IRS-1 (Insulin Receptor Substrate-1), a crucial protein implicated in insulin signaling, when they are triggered. Normally, IRS-1 permits glucose to enter cells, assisting cells in responding to insulin. However, TNF-α disrupts the normal function of IRS-1 by causing a phosphorylation change at serine 307. This modification acts as a negative modulator as IRS-1 cannot effectively transmit insulin signals inside the cells. This hampers the cells ability to uptake glucose properly, leading to increased blood sugar levels, which is a hallmark of T2DM. According to recent research, higher levels of TNF-α in the blood are assumed to be directly proportional to severe insulin resistance. Further supporting the idea that TNF-α is a key factor in developing insulin resistance and T2DM (Rehman & Akash, 2016).

6. Interleukin-1 beta (IL-1β)

IL-1β serves as a principal proinflammatory mediator, exerting a critical influence on the regulation of the expression of a multitude of other proinflammatory cytokines, adipokines, and chemokines. It initiates inflammatory processes through its interaction with interleukin-1 receptor type I (IL-1RI) and attenuates the expression of insulin receptor substrate-1 (IRS-1) at both ERK-dependent transcriptional and ERK-independent post-transcriptional levels. The synthesis of IL-1β is predominantly modulated by diet-induced metabolic stress. Investigative experimental studies have been conducted utilizing various animal models to explore the manifestations of inflammatory responses within the β-cells of pancreatic islets and peripheral tissues, which collectively suggest that IL-β functions as a primary proinflammatory mediator that significantly activates numerous other pro-inflammatory cytokines and chemokines through the engagement of various transcriptionally mediated pathways. Once inflammation is elicited, it precipitates detrimental effects on the β-cells of pancreatic islets, leading to compromised insulin secretion within these cells. Similarly, IL-β also assumes a critical role in instigating inflammation in peripheral tissues, consequently diminishing the capacity of these tissues to effectively utilize insulin in response to glucose, ultimately culminating in the development of insulin resistance in peripheral tissues (Rehman & Akash, 2016).

7. Interleukin-6 (IL-6)

Aging is linked to elevated plasma concentrations of interleukin-6 (IL-6), which can subsequently exhibit a positive correlation with insulin resistance. Furthermore, IL-6 activates suppressor of cytokine signaling (SOCS) proteins, which may impede the activation of transcription factors involved in the cytokine-mediated signaling pathway of the insulin receptor. Signal transducer and activator of transcription 5B (STAT5B) constitutes a member of the STAT family of transcription factors. STAT5B functions as both a signal transducer and a transcriptional regulator of the insulin receptor. In response to cytokine signaling, STAT5B undergoes phosphorylation mediated by kinases associated with the receptor. STAT5B plays a crucial role in the activation of insulin. Overnutrition increases blood glucose and free fatty acid (FFA) levels, leading to metabolic stress in pancreatic islet β-cells and insulin-sensitive tissues, including adipocytes. The metabolic stress in these tissues promotes the release of proinflammatory cytokines, including IL-1β and other cytokines and chemokines that rely on IL-1β. As a result, immune cells are attracted, which exacerbates tissue-specific inflammation. The generation of IL-1β causes inflammation in pancreatic islet β-cells. Prolonged exposure to FFAs and glucose activates IL-1β from pancreatic islet β-cells via transcriptional pathways including as TXNIP, MYD88, NF-κB, TLRs, caspases, and inflammasomes. Once activated, IL-1β recruits an array of additional proinflammatory mediators by binding to its receptor IL-1RI and through the involvement of MYD88 and NF-κB. Initially, the elevated levels of glucose and FFAs promote the expression and release of IL-1β from the β-cells of pancreatic islets. Chronic exposure to glucose and FFAs may result in the activation of IL-1β by triggering NF-κB and an auto-stimulatory amplification process. Upon activation and production, IL-1β act as the mediator to recruit various other proinflammatory cytokines, chemokines, and macrophages, which ultimately induce apoptosis, amyloidosis, and fibrosis in the pancreatic islet β-cells, leading to impaired insulin secretion, while in peripheral tissues, systemic inflammation fosters the development of insulin resistance. The transcription factor is activated by enhancing the activity of tyrosine kinase through binding to phosphor-tyrosine 960 of the insulin receptor. The activation of the insulin transcription factor is inhibited by SOCS proteins, which suppress the activity of tyrosine kinase through significant competition with STAT5B. SOCS proteins exert negative regulatory effects on insulin action, whereas IL-6 can activate these SOCS proteins. Hence, IL-6 is recognized as a significant biomarker for the manifestation of insulin resistance. The production of IL-6 is modulated by IL-1β via the activation of IL-1RI. The inhibition of IL-1RI activity using appropriate antiinflammatory agents, such as IL-1Ra, counteracts the agonistic effects of IL-1β, ultimately leading to a reduction in IL-6 production. AntiIL-6 receptor antibodies and soluble IL-6 receptors (sIL-6R) have demonstrated efficacy in diminishing the incidence of insulin resistance; however, this therapeutic strategy may not yield substantial effectiveness due to the dependency of IL-6 production on IL-1β activation, and the role of IL-1β in the progression of insulin resistance must not be overlooked (Makki et al., 2013).

8. C-reactive protein

In the context of type 2 diabetes, the modulation of diabetic inflammation is greatly aided by the regulation of C-reactive protein (CRP) expression. Chronic inflammation, which is linked to elevated CRP levels, is a major cause of insulin resistance and metabolic dysfunction in diabetes. T2DM patients have higher levels of inflammatory cytokines such TNF-α and IL-6, which are the main cause of CRP. Increased CRP levels exacerbate the consequences of diabetes by being correlated with vascular disease and endothelial dysfunction. The inflammatory environment in diabetes can be exacerbated by genetic variations in enhancer regions that affect immune responses and CRP production. Studies show that CRP levels are much greater in people with uncontrolled diabetes than in people with controlled diabetes, suggesting that it may be a useful bioindicator for inflammation in diabetics. Due to its active role in the inflammation network it might be considered as a therapeutic avenue to discard negative impact which is caused by type 2 diabetes (Stanimirovic et al., 2022).

9. IKKβ/NF-κB

IKKβ/NF-κB are the key players of the proinflammatory signaling pathway which serves as a critical regulatory mechanism and a pivotal point for antiinflammatory therapeutic interventions across a variety of pathological conditions. The IKKβ/NF-κB signaling cascade within the hypothalamus is integral to the understanding of pathophysiology of metabolic disorders, which encompass conditions such as hypertension, obesity, and resistance to leptin and insulin. In the absence of stimulation, NF-κB remains in an inactive form within the cytoplasm, where it associates with its inhibitory protein, IκB. The phosphorylation of IKKβ initiates downstream events such as phosphorylation of IκBα which ultimately culminates in the liberation of activated NF-κB., To facilitate the transcription of target genes, NF-κB translocases to the nucleus (Chen et al., 2020).

10. Innate and adaptive immune responses in T2DM

The onset and progression of obesity and type 2 diabetes are significantly influenced by adaptive immune cells, including T and B cells. One of the main causes of the beginning of these disorders is their activation and metabolic reprogramming. While dysregulated B cell activity leads to the overproduction of proinflammatory cytokines, which can worsen chronic inflammation, dysregulated T cells frequently produce changed amounts of cytokines, which can worsen inflammation. Immune dysfunction is linked to metabolic diseases by both conditions' additional impairment of insulin signaling pathways (25). Innate immune responses are dysregulated in type 2 diabetes mellitus (T2DM), which leads to metabolic dysfunction and persistent inflammation. The pathophysiology of insulin resistance, β-cell malfunction, and the related consequences observed in type 2 diabetes is largely attributed to this imbalance. Both innate and adaptive immunological factors, which are identified as significant etiological components in the development of insulin resistance, are associated with the pathogenesis of T2DM. Patients with T2DM have their immune systems activated due to obesity, which is linked to low-grade inflammation. Metabolic dysregulation can be brought on by an increase in fat mass in obese people. Additionally, it has been established that insulin resistance in obese people is closely related to adipose tissue inflammation. Table 10.1 provides the impact of different immune cells on the T2DM with the potential mechanisms involved.

Table 10.1 Mechanism and involvement of different immune cells in T2DM.

Immune cells	Effect of T2DM on cell recruitment	Potential mechanisms	References
Monocyte/ Macrophage	Enhanced macrophage presence in the retinas of diabetic rats induced by STZ	Mediated through the CCL2-CCR2 signaling pathway	Rangasamy et al. (2014)
	Increased macrophage recruitment in kidneys of diabetic mice treated with STZ	Linked to the CCL2-CCR2 axis	Tarabra et al. (2009)
	Higher monocyte adhesion to adipocytes in subcutaneous adipose tissue in T2DM patients	Elevated CX3CL1 levels in adipose tissue	R. Shah et al. (2011)
	Enhanced macrophage infiltration in white adipose tissue of obese mice on a high-fat diet	Increased CCR5 expression in white adipose tissue	Kitade et al. (2012)
	Elevated F4/80 and CD11c mRNA levels in adipose tissue of mice fed a high-fat diet	Upregulation of ICAM-1, VCAM-1, CCL2, and CXCL14	Kawanishi et al. (2010)
	Higher expression of F4/80 in adipose tissue of high-fat diet mice	Elevated ICAM-1 mRNA levels in adipose tissue	Brake et al. (2006)

Table 10.1 Mechanism and involvement of different immune cells in T2DM.—cont'd

Immune cells	Effect of T2DM on cell recruitment	Potential mechanisms	References
	Reduced RPMs and a shift to M2 polarization in db/db mice	Chronic inflammation in the peritoneal cavity	Liu et al. (2012)
	Reduced adhesion and phagocytic activity of RPMs in db/db mice (in vitro)	Altered microenvironment in diabetic mice	
	Lower monocyte/macrophage levels in lung tissue of diabetic DPP4H/M mice infected with MERS-CoV	Reduced Ccl2 and Cxcl10 expression in lung tissue	Kulcsar et al. (2019)
Dendritic cells	Increased CD11c high F4/80 low DCs in visceral adipose tissue of obese mice	Mechanisms not specified	Bertola et al. (2012)
	Higher CD11c + CD1c + cDCs in subcutaneous adipose tissue of obese humans	–	
	Elevated CD11c + cDCs numbers in adipose tissue of mice fed a high-fat diet	–	Chen et al. (2014)
Neutrophils	Increased neutrophil infiltration in visceral adipose tissue of mice after 3 days on a high-fat diet	Higher CD11b expression on neutrophils	Elgazar-Carmon et al. (2008)
	Sustained neutrophil infiltration in adipose tissue of mice on a high-fat diet for up to 90 days	Increased neutrophil elastase activity in adipose tissue	Talukdar et al. (2012)
$CD8^+$ T-cells	Enhanced infiltration of effector $CD8^+$ T-cells in visceral adipose tissue of high-fat diet mice	Activated by local endogenous stimuli	Nishimura et al. (2009)
	Fewer $CD8^+$ T-cells in the brains of db/db mice infected with West Nile virus	Decreased E-selectin and ICAM-1 expression in the brain	Kumar et al. (2014)
$CD4^+$ T-cells	Reduced $CD4^+$ T-cells in lung tissue of diabetic DPP4H/M mice infected with MERS-CoV	Lower expression of Ccl2 and Cxcl10	Kulcsar et al. (2019)
Tregs	Decreased regulatory T-cells in visceral adipose tissue of obese mice on a high-fat diet	Mechanisms not described	Nishimura et al. (2009)
	Reduced $CD4^+$ Tregs in high-fat diet mice	Lower adiponectin levels in fat tissue	Ilan et al. (2010)
B-cells	Elevated B-cell numbers in the bone marrow of high-fat diet mice	Mechanisms not specified	Trottier et al. (2012)
	Reduced B-cell count in the bone marrow of obese mice on a high-fat diet	Lower Pax5 expression in bone marrow	Chan et al. (2012)
Granulocytes	Decreased granulocyte levels in alveolar airspace of diabetic mice infected with Klebsiella pneumonia	Reduced levels of CXCL1, CXCL2, IL-1β, and TNF-α in lung tissue	Martinez et al. (2016)

11. Major immune pathways contributing to insulin resistance

Several immune pathways are involved in the pathophysiology of insulin resistance. The mechanism is majorly through the development and progression of chronic low-grade inflammation. Some key immune mechanisms that contribute to insulin resistance are.

12. Inflammatory cytokines-mediated insulin resistance

In adipose tissue, adipocytes and macrophages primarily secrete TNF-α promotes insulin resistance. TNF-α impairs insulin signaling by activating serine kinases that phosphorylate insulin receptor substrate (IRS), inhibiting downstream pathways like PI3K-Akt. TNF-α is predominantly synthesized within adipocytes and peripheral tissues which results in resulting in tissue-specific inflammation and insulin resistance and it is mediated through the production of reactive oxygen species (ROS) and the activation of various transcriptionally regulated pathways based on the mitogen-activated protein kinase (MAPK) signaling cascade. c-Jun N-terminal kinase (JNK), extracellular signal-regulated kinase (ERK), and p38 are the components of MAPK signaling cascade. Activator protein 1 (AP-1) is that transcription factor which governs the regulation of proinflammatory cytokine. The activation of AP-1 frequently occurs as a direct consequence of MAPK pathway modulation, particularly via the phosphorylation of c-Jun by JNK and the expression of c-Fos mediated by ERK1/2. The IKappaB kinase (IKK) complex is activated through the stimulation of TNF-α, leading to the phosphorylation and ubiquitination of IκBα. Subsequently, the nuclear factor kappa-light-chain-enhancer of activated B cells (NF-κB) transcription factor translocate from the cytoplasm to the nucleus after activation, thereby initiating the transcription of a variety of chemokines and cytokines, including IL-6, IL-1β, and MCP-1 as their target genes. TNF-α modulates the MAPK and NF-κB pathways, leading to inflammation and insulin resistance (Park & Han, 2024).

Chronic IL-6 levels, in addition to TNF-α, are connected to insulin resistance via increasing hepatic gluconeogenesis and compromising insulin signaling. Biazi et al. (2023) found that this cytokine promotes gluconeogenesis in the liver by increasing glucose synthesis from precursors such as alanine and glutamine. It also reduces insulin's suppressive effects on glycogenolysis, following similar pathways to TNF-α. Activated macrophages create IL-1β, which promotes inflammation and contributes to insulin resistance. Elevated glucose levels cause macrophages to produce IL-1β which in turn promotes insulin secretion. This creates a feedback loop that exacerbates insulin resistance (Holmes, 2017).

13. Toll-like receptors-mediated mechanisms

Toll-like receptors (TLRs)4 plays a significant role in recognizing pathogen-associated molecular patterns (PAMPs) and damage-associated molecular patterns (DAMPs) which include saturated fatty acids. Activation of TLR4 triggers the NF-κB pathway that leads to increased production of proinflammatory cytokines like TNF-α and IL-1β that can impair insulin signaling and contribute to insulin resistance. TLR2 is also implicated in inflammation-driven insulin resistance, especially in adipose tissue macrophages and skeletal muscle. TLR4 which is the most characterized TLR. TLR4 binds to LPS of gram-negative bacterial cell walls and consequently triggers the recruitment of MyD88 to the Toll/IL-1 receptor domain. This interaction triggers a downstream signaling cascade, activating the NF-κB pathway (Shi et al., 2006).

14. NOD-, LRR- and pyrin domain-containing protein 3 (NLRP3) inflammasome activation mechanism

The NLRP3 inflammasome is an immune sensor that detects various dangerous compounds which function as a metabolic danger signal. It is activated during endogenous danger signals including nucleic acids and lipo-oligosaccharides. Proinflammatory triglycerides such as palmitate and adipocyte-derived lyophosphatidylcholine stimulate the NLRP3 inflammasome that helps in initiating insulin resistance. Palmitate regulates inflammasome and IL-1β secretion by inhibiting AMP-activated protein kinase, suppressing autophagy, and increasing the generation of reactive oxygen species (ROS). Changes in ion concentration, primarily K^+ efflux, Ca^{2+} signal, and Cl^- efflux, are significant but not necessary during NLRP3 activation changes. Regulation of purinergic P2X7 receptors through enhanced ATP production with nigericin results in an intracellular decrease in K^+ ions, initiating inflammasome stimulation. Mitochondrial impairment and release of ROS initiate NLRP3 activation (Sehgal et al., 2021).

15. JNK pathway (c-Jun N-terminal kinase)

Chronic inflammation can activate JNK to phosphorylate insulin receptor substrates (IRS) 1 and 2 at Ser/Thr residues and dephosphorylate IRS-1 Tyr residues, preventing IRS from activating downstream PI3K and its upstream insulin receptor interaction. This leads to decreased sensitivity of target cells to insulin that helps in stimulating the body to continuously produce insulin to eliminate excess glucose in the blood. However, compensatory insulin synthesis in islet β cells forms hyperinsulinemia that adds the burden of islet β-cell secretion which leads to hyperproliferation and apoptosis that further results in insulin resistance. Studies have shown that JNK gene silencing decreases IRS-1 Ser 307 phosphorylation and increases Tyr phosphorylation that enhances insulin signaling and increases cell sensitivity to insulin (Feng et al., 2020).

16. Macrophage (M1 vs. M2) polarization

M1 macrophages are proinflammatory macrophages that secrete cytokines like TNF-α, IL-6 and IL-1β. The number of M1 macrophages in adipose tissue increases, promoting

Table 10.2 Factors that affect polarization of macrophages.

Proteins/Genes	Normal function	Impact on polarization
Lipopolysaccharides	Act as immune system stimulators	Promote M1 polarization
IL-12 and IL-23	Cytokines involved in immune regulation	Drive M1 polarization
IR-α	Facilitates immune modulation and antiviral responses	Encourages M1 polarization
TLR	Mediates nonspecific innate immune responses	Supports M2 polarization
IL-10	Antiinflammatory cytokine	Promotes M2 polarization
TGF-β	Cytokine regulating immune tolerance and repair	Drives M2 polarization

inflammation and insulin resistance whereas M2 macrophages are antiinflammatory macrophages and predominates in adipose tissue in lean individuals, maintaining insulin sensitivity through antiinflammatory cytokines like IL-10. M1 macrophages are glycolytic whereas M2 macrophages are involved in TCA cycling and mitochondrial oxidative phosphorylation and produce lactic acid and ATP which further downregulates tissue repair and inflammation. A shift from M2 to M1 macrophages in adipose tissue is a hallmark of insulin resistance. Table 10.2 highlights the major factors that can affect the macrophage polarization (Luo et al., 2024).

17. Involvement of NF-κB pathway

NF-κB is a crucial molecule in T2DM pathogenesis, activated by genotoxic, oxidative, and inflammatory stress. It regulates cytokine expression, cell-cycle progression, and inflammation. NF-κB activation causes insulin resistance and glucose metabolism. Upregulation in hepatocytes leads to T2DM, involving innate immune activation and inflammatory response. NF-κB activation in various tissues, such as adipose tissue, pancreas, and liver, contributes to the disease development (Matsumori, 2022).

18. Role of chemokines

It is integral to insulin resistance and diabetes complications. Circulating MCP-1 levels are elevated in type 2 diabetes. As an adipokine, MCP-1's heightened expression from adipose tissue promotes insulin resistance and macrophage infiltration. Insulin resistance poses a risk for type 2 diabetes, driving inflammation through MCP-1 production, leading to monocyte recruitment and macrophage activation. MCP-1 is linked to renal tubular damage and is exacerbated by heavy proteinuria, which facilitates diabetic nephropathy progression. In diabetic nephropathy patients, elevated serum MCP-1 acts as a potential biomarker. Urinary MCP-1 level rises as renal impairment progresses in T2DM patients. Retinal neurons produce MCP-1, activating retinal microglia and connecting it to diabetes pathogenesis. In a diabetic retinopathy rodent model, MCP-1 upregulation occurs early and intensifies with disease progression. Retinal resident cells are implicated in inflammatory responses in diabetic retinopathy via MCP-1 production. MCP-1 has been shown to aid diabetic wound healing by restoring macrophage response (Singh et al., 2021).

19. Targeting specific immune pathways in T2DM

Role of Interleukin-1 Beta (IL-1β) Pathway in Beta-Cell Dysfunction- Proinflammatory cytokines are one of the factors that affect beta-cell activity in both humans and animals. Those with T2DM have increased amounts of circulating proinflammatory cytokines and immune cell infiltration in the pancreatic islets. Local inflammation is made worse by cytokines and chemokines produced by the pancreatic islets and invading immune cells. Specifically, beta cell insulin secretion, survival and dedifferentiation are decreased by the proinflammatory cytokine interleukin-1β (IL-1β). In case of T2DM patients, blocking of the IL-1β receptor improves hyperglycemia and beta cell function and additionally it lowers inflammatory markers which indicate a role for IL-1β in T2DM. Significant alterations in gene expression occur in beta cells when they are exposed to IL-1β, which includes decreased expression of genes governing beta cell activity and increased expression of genes implicated in inflammatory processes. The expression of the gene Nos2 that codes for the enzyme-inducible nitric oxide synthase (iNOS) and other chemokines such as C-X-C motif ligand 1 (Cxcl1) that attracts and activates specific immune cells are among the genes that are induced by IL-1β. In beta cell lines of rodents and human islets, iNOS generates nitric oxide (NO), which, in high concentrations, suppresses glucose-stimulated insulin production. For e.g. the deactivation of mitochondrial aconitase lowers oxidative metabolism and depletion of ATP (Corbett et al., 1992). CASK is the membrane-associated guanylate kinase (MAGUK) family of proteins. CASK contributes to IL-1β-induced insulin secretion abnormalities, which may be primarily caused by activation of DNA methyltransferase via Inos (Wang, Liu, et al., 2020). NO is also a significant mediator of IL-1β-induced beta cell failure, causing DNA damage and controlling the production and activity of many proteins (Burke et al., 2014). IL-1β-induced gene expression is mediated by the activation of transcription factors, which are primarily nuclear factor-κB (Burke et al., 2015). P50 and/or p65 homodimers or heterodimers make up the dimeric transcription factor NF-κB, and they are attached to cytoplasmic IκB inhibitory proteins when not in use. The IκB kinase phosphorylates IκB in response to cytokine stimuli like IL-1β, which causes IκB to be degraded by proteasomes mediated by ubiquitin. This permits NF-κB to go into the nucleus, where it binds certain DNA fragments and then assembles the transcriptional machinery to start transcription. Since there are several levels at which NF-κB activity is regulated, finding activation inhibitors may be a useful strategy to stop IL-1β-induced beta cell failure. CASK is one of the family members of membrane-associated guanylate kinase (MAGUK) protein. CASK forms a part of IL-1β–inducing insulin secretion defects, which could be mainly exerted through activation of DNA methyltransferase via Inos (Wang, Liu, et al., 2020). Moreover, NO induces DNA-damage and regulates the expression and activity of several proteins, thus being a major mediator of IL-1β-induced beta cell failure (Burke et al., 2014). The activation of transcription factors, mainly nuclear factor-κB (NF-κB), mediates IL-1β-induced gene expression (Bhatt & Ghosh, 2014). NF-κB is a dimeric transcription factor consisting of homodimers or heterodimers of p50 and/or p65. In their inactive states, NF-κB is bound to IκB inhibitory proteins in the cytoplasm. Upon stimulation by cytokines (such as IL-1β) the IκB kinase phosphorylates IκB, which in turn induces ubiquitin-mediated proteasomal degradation. This allows nuclear translocation of NF-κB that binds specific DNA elements and subsequent assembly of the transcriptional machinery, which initiates transcription (Wang, Liu, et al., 2020). Regulation of NF-κB activity occurs at multiple levels and thus, identifying inhibitors of the activation has the potential to be an effective approach to prevent IL-1β-induced beta cell dysfunction.

20. Therapeutic significance of IL-1β inhibitors

The findings of clinical research on IL-1β inhibitors in T2DM have been encouraging, yet inconsistent. Canakinumab, a monoclonal antibody that targets IL-1β, and Anakinra, an IL-1 receptor antagonist, have shown promise in increasing pancreatic β-cell activity and glycemic management in many trials. It has been observed that both drugs are able to lower glycated hemoglobin (HbA1c) levels and boost insulin secretion. Although anakinra reduced inflammatory indicators, including CRP and IL-6, and enhanced β-cell function. It did not significantly increase insulin sensitivity in nondiabetic patients with metabolic syndrome. Larsen et al. conducted a follow-up study after an initial 13-week anakinra treatment period and observed sustained improvements in the proinsulin-to-insulin ratio, as well as persistent reductions in CRP and IL-6 levels for up to 39 weeks posttreatment, though HbA1c levels showed no further change. In a study of T2DM patients, gevokizumab, a monoclonal antiIL-1β antibody, was used, which markedly reduced HbA1c levels after 3 months, which was associated with better β-cell activity. According to these results, IL-1β inhibition may help T2DM patients achieve better glycemic control and less systemic inflammation, albeit the degree of the benefit may vary depending on the patient's features and stage of the disease (Guan et al., 2024).

21. Significance of protein kinase CK2 in the regulation of pancreatic beta-cells

Impairment of insulin secretion along with β-cell dysfunction are hallmarks of type 2 diabetes, and it is associated with the dysregulation of CK2 activity. CK2 activity increases due to the chronic elevation of glucose and fatty acids, which in turn suppresses insulin secretion. These two reasons are the critical elements of β-cell apoptosis (Dalle, 2024). The serine/threonine kinase protein CK2 (also known as CSNK2 or CK2) is important for controlling the physiology of pancreatic β-cells and insulin signaling pathways. Its impact on β-cell activity is complex, encompassing interactions with important signaling networks, transcriptional regulation, and insulin secretion modulation. CK2α (44 kDa) and CK2α' (36 kDa) are the catalytic subunit and two small noncatalytic CK2β subunits (25 kDa) make up its composition. The human enzyme CK2α is encoded by the CSNK2A1 gene. To control the metabolism of carbohydrates, CK2 also plays a crucial role. CK2 works by adding phosphate groups to its specific substrates, such as transcription factors and signaling molecules. In pancreatic β-cells, the transcription factor called pancreatic and duodenal homeobox-1 (PDX-1) is one of the promising targets. At serine 232 and threonine 231 of PDX-1 are phosphorylated by CK2, which suppresses the transcriptional activity of the protein. Increased PDX-1 stability and activity as a result of CK2 inhibition promote the transcription of insulin and other β-cell-specific genes (Klein et al., 2016). For appropriate insulin production and secretion in response to glucose levels, this regulatory system is essential. Additionally, CK2, which affects insulin secretion at various levels, functions as a molecular repressor of insulin production. Modulation of insulin receptor signaling is a function of CK2. The ability of CK2 to phosphorylate elements of the insulin signaling cascade, such as Akt, which is essential for the translocation of glucose transporter type 4 (GLUT4) to the cell membrane, has been demonstrated. Increased Akt activity from CK2 inhibition encourages GLUT4 translocation and boosts β-cell glucose absorption (Borgo et al., 2021). According to this, CK2 functions as a negative regulator of insulin signaling, and by inhibiting it, insulin sensitivity and glucose homeostasis can be improved. CK2 not only regulates transcription but also controls the release of insulin from β-cells. A negative regulator of receptor-mediated insulin release has been found to be CK2. For example, muscarinic M3 receptors (M3Rs) are phosphorylated by CK2 and so cannot induce insulin secretion (Doliba et al., 2017). By blocking the signaling cascade that causes calcium influx and subsequent insulin exocytosis. This phosphorylation emphasizes the function of CK2 in regulating the insulin release mechanism. For insulin production, calcium signaling pathways are also influenced by CK2. According to Scheuer et al. (2020) research shows that CK2 controls CaV2.1-dependent calcium currents in β-cells, which is necessary for the insulin granule exocytosis. CK2's control of these calcium channels can alter the total insulin secretion response to glucose as well as the intensity and duration of calcium signals that drive insulin release. Significant physiological ramifications result from CK2's regulatory functions in pancreatic β-cells, especially when diabetes mellitus is present. Therefore, targeting CK2 with specific inhibitors presents a potential therapeutic strategy to enhance β-cell function and improve glycemic control in diabetic patients.

22. Impact on cytokine-induced beta-cell damage

A key role for CK2 has been found in the regulation of pancreatic β-cell survival, especially when cytokine-induced damage is present. Influence of various cytokines such as IL-1β and tumor necrosis factor-alpha (TNF-α). Interleukin (IL)-1β, TNF-α, and IFN-γ are the major causes of inflammation. This inflammation led to the apoptosis of β-cells of the islet of Langerhans, which ultimately led to type 2 diabetes. The proapoptotic NFκB pathway is triggered as a result, which causes the mass of β-cells to drastically decrease. The NFκB component p65 is phosphorylated by CK2 on serine 529. The loss of this phosphorylation results in decreased transcriptional activity and, thus, protects against cytokine-induced apoptosis. The inhibition of CK2 by DRB and DMAT reduces the resynthesis of IκBα, which in turn inhibits the phosphorylation of p65 in β-cells. Inhibiting CK2 reduces IFN-α-stimulated phosphorylation of STAT1. Inhibiting CK2 can reduce inflammatory signaling pathways, potentially protecting β-cells from cytokine-induced cell death. Combining CK2 inhibitors with additional therapeutic drugs such as CSNK2 may give a dual approach to reduce β-cell loss caused by inflammatory cytokines. Moreover, understanding the precise mechanisms in β-cells where NF-κB and p53 pathways are modulated by CK2 and it could lead to the development of novel strategies to face chronic inflammation for the enhancement of β-cell survival (Rossi et al., 2015).

23. Role of G protein-coupled receptors (GPCRs) in modulation of insulin secretion

The role of G protein-coupled receptors (GPCRs) are essential for modulating insulin resistance, particularly in the setting of T2DM. These receptors have an impact on insulin secretion, glucose homeostasis and the body's general metabolic status through their participation in a number of signaling cascades. GPCR signaling and insulin resistance have a complex interaction that has attracted a lot of attention lately. A number of studies have found that targeting these receptors could be an effective therapy method. One of the primary ways GPCRs affect insulin resistance is by their role in controlling the release of insulin from pancreatic beta cells. GPCRs such as the glucose-dependent insulinotropic polypeptide receptor (GIPR) and the glucagon-like peptide-1 receptor (GLP-1R) have been shown to stimulate insulin production in response to glucose (Zheng et al., 2024). Moreover, the activation GPR119 receptor has been identified as a target because of its ability to boost insulin release and improvize glycemic control. By interacting with different metabolic pathways, GPCRs have a function in insulin production but are also linked to the development of insulin resistance. One way that specific GPCR activation may contribute to insulin resistance is by desensitizing insulin signaling pathways. According to studies, adipocytes interact, which in turn affects the inflammatory response linked to insulin resistance (Shah & Kowalski, 2010). There is evidence that a naturally occurring variation of the GIP receptor experiences greater desensitization, hence compromising its capacity to control adipose insulin sensitivity. The participation of certain G protein signaling pathways highlights the relevance of GPCRs in insulin resistance. Gαi and Gαq signaling pathways, for example, have been demonstrated to regulate β-cell activity and insulin secretion; modifications in these pathways are associated with reduced insulin release and glucose intolerance. Further evidence that the balance of GPCR signaling can have a substantial impact on metabolic outcomes comes from the identification of the regulatory G protein complex Gβ5-R7 as a positive modulator of insulin production (Wang, Henry, et al., 2020).

The problems of GPCR-targeted therapeutics for T2DM include receptor desensitization, off-target effects because GPCRs are widely expressed in tissues, and the inability to achieve signaling bias to preferentially activate favorable pathways.

Improved understanding of GPCR structure led to the development of selective drugs. The technique, such as cryo-electron microscopy, play a crucial role in the advancement of therapeutic management of type 2 diabetes. Along with various agonists and allosteric modulators act as promising techniques to improve efficacy while reducing side effects. To improve therapeutic accuracy, nanoparticle-based delivery approaches are being studied to target areas critical for glucose management. These developments have the potential to improve GPCR-targeted treatments for the treatment of T2DM and overcome current obstacles (Wootten et al., 2018).

24. Involvement of TLRs in inflammatory responses

The inflammatory response mediated by TLRs prominently involves TLR2, which typically forms heterodimers with either TLR1 or TLR6 to execute its functions. TLR2 activation activates downstream signaling cascades, including the NF-κB pathway, resulting in the release of proinflammatory cytokines such as TNF-α, IL-1β and IL-6. This mechanism is primarily driven by MyD88-dependent signaling. TLR2 and TLR4 both play important roles in sensing dietary lipids and influencing metabolic responses, especially in high-fat diet (HFD) circumstances. TLR2 signaling pathways play a crucial role in balancing β-cell quiescence and proliferation as indicated in the studies done in mice and humans. Under HFD conditions, models with TLR2 and TLR4 knockout mice show increased β-cell proliferation. TLR4 is activated by elevated levels of glucose, lipopolysaccharides (LPS), free fatty acids (FFAs), and damage-associated molecular patterns (DAMPs) such as degraded hyaluronic acid and oxidized phospholipids, which lead to the amplification of inflammatory responses. Activation of TLR4 induces the upregulation of caspase-3 and PARP along with an altered Bcl-2/BAX ratio, which culminates in excessive reactive oxygen species (ROS) production. ROS also activates the NLRP3 inflammasome and caspase-1, facilitating the maturation and release of IL-1β. Elevated IL-1β levels stimulate the secretion of additional proinflammatory cytokines and chemokines, including TNF and MCP-1, which promote macrophage infiltration into pancreatic islets. The inflammatory microenvironment further promotes a phenotypic shift of macrophages from the antiinflammatory M2 state to the proinflammatory M1 state. These M1 macrophages exacerbate β-cell dysfunction and apoptosis through the amplification of TLR4-mediated inflammatory signaling pathways, contributing to progressive β-cell failure (Wang, Ni, et al., 2020; Yehualashet, 2020).

25. Therapeutic potentials of TLR4 inhibitors

The reduction in TLR4 expression was associated with a substantial increase in insulin secretion in isolated pancreatic islets from rats, indicating that suppressing TLR4 expression may protect islet cells from damage caused by TLR4 ligands. In human monocytes and monocyte-derived dendritic cells (DCs), FP7, a small-molecule synthetic TLR4 antagonist, inhibited TLR4-mediated activation, reducing inflammatory signaling; in mice infected with the influenza virus, FP7 prevented excessive TLR4 activation, thereby controlling inflammation without suppressing the overall immune response. The therapeutic potential of a TLR4 antagonist was demonstrated in diabetic apolipoprotein E (ApoE)−/− mice, highlighting the antagonist's broader metabolic benefits. FP7 effectively blocks LPS-induced TLR4 signaling, reducing off-target effects, which are concerned with immunosuppressive therapies (Wang, Ni, et al., 2020).

26. Clinical trials of IL-1β inhibitors in T2DM

Canakinumab decreased blood levels of IL-6 and hs-CRP in patients with T2DM who had clinical IL-1β suppression. Prior research has documented comparable decreases in inflammatory indices in individuals with type 2 diabetes. Anakinra's antagonism of interleukin-1 signaling has been shown to improve glycemic control in T2DM patients, most likely by improving beta-cell secretory function. In fact, better measurements of beta-cell secretory capacity were associated with better glycemia in patients treated with anakinra.

Investigations on skeletal muscle, which are based on measurement of the oral glucose tolerance test as well as insulin-regulated gene expression, muscle, and serum adipokine levels, showed no change in insulin sensitivity (85). The CANTOS (Canakinumab AntiInflammatory Thrombosis Outcomes Study) found that targeting IL-1β can significantly reduce cardiovascular events without lowering blood pressure or cholesterol. In CANTOS, the degree of reduction in the downstream clinical biomarker CRP and the major signaling cytokine IL-6 was linked to the extent of the effect of this cytokine-targeted strategy on atherosclerosis treatment (Ridker, 2019).

27. Experimental therapies targeting CK2

Treatment of mouse pancreatic islets with CK2 inhibitor like CX4945, has been reported to cause a reduced phosphorylation of β-cell M3Rs caused by agonists. This, in turn, enhanced M3R-driven insulin secretion in both mouse and human islets (Rossi et al., 2015). The positive effect of CK2 inhibition might also be linked to its direct influence on the β-granule transport protein, kinesin heavy chain (KHC), which is essential for moving β-granules along microtubules in pancreatic β-cells (Doliba et al., 2017). Furthermore, kinase profiling demonstrated that KD025 effectively blocks the catalytic subunits of CK2, which is an always-active serine/threonine kinase. Experimental results confirmed that targeting the CK2A1 subunit (but not CK2A2) with KD025 improved β-cell survival under glucolipotoxic conditions. These findings suggest that KD025 protects β-cells from damage by inhibiting CK2 activity (Devkota et al., 2024).

28. GPCR-targeted drugs in preclinical studies

Table 10.3 provides the summary of the preclinical studies that have tested GPCR-targeting drugs with their possible mode of action (Su et al., 2024).

Table 10.3 GPCR-targeted drugs in preclinical studies in T2DM.

Intervention/Treatment	Mode of delivery	Mechanism of action
GLP-1 analogs	Subcutaneous injection	Stimulates GLP-1 receptors, leading to increased cAMP production and enhanced insulin release.
DPP4 inhibitors	Oral	Boosts GLP-1 receptor activity, raising cAMP levels and promoting insulin secretion.
Bromocriptine	Oral	Activates central D2 receptors, adjusts dopamine circadian rhythms, and improves insulin sensitivity.
Pramlintide	Subcutaneous injection	Engages the RAMP complex and reduces glucagon secretion to regulate glucose levels.

29. Drug development and translational challenges

Due to the disease's complexity and heterogeneity, the development of therapies for T2DM faces significant challenges. The identification of universal drug targets itself is a complex process due to the existence of variation in pathophysiology, genetic makeup, metabolic cause, and the environment. Most commonly, GPCR modulators, IL-1β inhibitors, and CK2 inhibitors are elaborated under promising therapeutic strategies to encounter unique obstacles of T2DM. To consider the GPCR-targeted treatments, maintenance of specificity and selectivity is essential to prevent desensitization and off-target effects. Due to the kinase's wide substrate profile, CK2 inhibitors struggle to achieve specificity, whereas IL-1β inhibitors carry the danger of infection and immunological suppression. Even to identify the dynamics of human-specific diseases in the preclinical models, it frequently falls short; as a result, translational gaps continue to exist. Furthermore, as T2DM is a chronic condition which sometimes comprises allied disorder so, ensuring long-term safety and efficacy are must, as a result, it raises the demands on clinical trials and regulations. Financial issues like expensive development expenses and other accessibility is further hampered (Donath & Shoelson, 2011; Hauser et al., 2017).

30. Potential side effects and safety concerns

T2DM therapies raise several safety issues that need to be resolved to guarantee effectiveness and reduce risk. Because GPCRs are widely distributed throughout tissues, off-target effects are a problem for GPCR-targeted medications, which are frequently employed in the treatment of T2D. Unintentional neurological, gastric, or cardiovascular problems may result from this. The long-term efficacy of the medication may be diminished by receptor desensitization brought on by prolonged use. IL-1β inhibitors, which target inflammation in relation to insulin resistance, have the potential to weaken the immune system and make people more vulnerable to infections like skin or respiratory infections. Over time, immune suppression may also impair the body's ability to respond to injuries or infections, and some evidence suggests a potential link to increased cancer risk (Donath & Shoelson, 2011).

31. Future research on immune modulation in T2DM

To manage T2DM, immunomodulation is a promising tool which is based on its complex inflammation network. Future studies should concentrate on the following important areas.

32. Therapies based on exosomes

Exosome-based treatments as drug delivery systems and targeted therapies may be investigated in future studies; they may also be used as biomarkers for illness monitoring and diagnosis. For instance, it has been demonstrated that adipocytes release exosomes containing the sonic hedgehog protein, which causes monocytes to become proinflammatory and ultimately results in insulin resistance (77).

33. Mesenchymal stromal cells

Mesenchymal stromal cells (MSCs) have shown potent immunomodulatory potential. They can ameliorate insulin resistance by targeting various pathways, such as activation of IRS-1/PI3K along with transition of macrophage from M1 to M2, suggesting MSCs as a promising avenue for T2DM therapy (Chen et al., 2021).

34. $CD4^+$ T cells and inflammatory pathways

$CD4^+$ T cells have been found to be important mediators of inflammation in type 2 diabetes, mainly via the TNF-a/STAT-3 signaling pathway. Inhibitors that target these pathways may be a useful treatment approach to reduce meta-inflammation in individuals with type 2 diabetes. For the treatment of type 2 diabetes nutrition and exercise are two lifestyle changes that have demonstrated immunomodulatory and antiinflammatory benefits for the treatment of type 2 diabetes. Micronutrients, phytoceuticals and diets such as the Mediterranean diet can modify immune responses and enhance glycemic management (Srividya et al., 2024).

35. Genetic and molecular biomarkers

Early diagnosis and management of type 2 diabetes can benefit from the identification of mRNA profiles associated with immunometabolism and inflammation. Research on the cGAS/STING and NOD-like receptor pathways may yield new biomarkers for tracking the progression of type 2 diabetes (94). To fully examine the function of metabolic pathways and translational machinery, research and treatment development must employ a variety of approaches. Understanding these interactions will be necessary to improve immune modulation strategies for type 2 diabetes in the future.

36. Conclusion

T2DM presents a huge burden on the global populations impacting around 10% of the population, with management costs of billions of dollars. Considering such an impact that is rapidly rising, Venkat Narayan, a Center for Drug Control epidemiologist, introduced the term "diabetes pandemic" for T2DM. T2DM can be classified as inflammation caused immunometabolism disorder that involves dysregulation and disruption of numerous signaling mechanisms contributing to insulin resistance and associated metabolic syndromes. Through this book chapter, we have comprehensively updated our understanding of the underlying molecular mechanisms, potential therapeutic targets that can be targeted or are currently explored with a particular consideration on the future of the T2DM therapeutics. Apart from certain genetic predispositions associated with T2DM, it is basically a metabolic disease where lifestyle choices, diet, and environment play a significant role that particularly contribute to the epigenetic regulation of the disease. Considering all the genetic, epigenetic and associated-molecular mechanisms in collaboration with the modern advancements in drug design and development, it has become quite possible to tackle the disease from its early stages to its complete elimination.

References

Alzamil, H. (2020). Elevated serum TNF-α is related to obesity in type 2 diabetes mellitus and is associated with glycemic control and insulin resistance. *Journal of Obesity, 2020*, Article 5076858. https://doi.org/10.1155/2020/5076858

Arkan, M. C., Hevener, A. L., Greten, F. R., Maeda, S., Li, Z.-W., Long, J. M., Wynshaw-Boris, A., Poli, G., Olefsky, J., & Karin, M. (2005). IKK-beta links inflammation to obesity-induced insulin resistance. *Nature Medicine, 11*(2), 191–198. https://doi.org/10.1038/nm1185

Austin, R. L., Rune, A., Bouzakri, K., Zierath, J. R., & Krook, A. (2008). siRNA-mediated reduction of inhibitor of nuclear factor-kappaB kinase prevents tumor necrosis factor-alpha-induced insulin resistance in human skeletal muscle. *Diabetes, 57*(8), 2066–2073. https://doi.org/10.2337/db07-0763

Berbudi, A., Rahmadika, N., Tjahjadi, A. I., & Ruslami, R. (2020). Type 2 diabetes and its impact on the immune system. *Current Diabetes Reviews, 16*(5), 442–449. https://doi.org/10.2174/1573399815666191024085838

Bertola, A., Ciucci, T., Rousseau, D., Bourlier, V., Duffaut, C., Bonnafous, S., Blin-Wakkach, C., Anty, R., Iannelli, A., Gugenheim, J., Tran, A., Bouloumié, A., Gual, P., & Wakkach, A. (2012). Identification of adipose tissue dendritic cells correlated with obesity-associated insulin-resistance and inducing Th17 responses in mice and patients. *Diabetes, 61*(9), 2238–2247. https://doi.org/10.2337/db11-1274

Bhatt, D., & Ghosh, S. (2014). Regulation of the NF-κB-Mediated transcription of inflammatory genes. *Frontiers in Immunology, 5*, 71. https://doi.org/10.3389/fimmu.2014.00071

Biazi, G. R., Uemura, I. G. F., Miksza, D. R., Ferraz, L. S., Diaz, B. F., Bertolini, G. L., & de Souza, H. M. (2023). Interleukin 6 acutely increases gluconeogenesis and decreases the suppressive effect of insulin on cAMP-stimulated glycogenolysis in rat liver. *Cell Biochemistry and Function, 41*(5), 609–618. https://doi.org/10.1002/cbf.3817

Borgo, C., D'Amore, C., Sarno, S., Salvi, M., & Ruzzene, M. (2021). Protein kinase CK2: A potential therapeutic target for diverse human diseases. *Signal Transduction and Targeted Therapy, 6*(1), 183. https://doi.org/10.1038/s41392-021-00567-7

Brake, D. K., Smith, E. O., Mersmann, H., Smith, C. W., & Robker, R. L. (2006). ICAM-1 expression in adipose tissue: Effects of diet-induced obesity in mice. *American Journal of Physiology. Cell Physiology, 291*(6), C1232–C1239. https://doi.org/10.1152/ajpcell.00008.2006

Burke, S. J., Lu, D., Sparer, T. E., Masi, T., Goff, M. R., Karlstad, M. D., & Collier, J. J. (2014). NF-κB and STAT1 control CXCL1 and CXCL2 gene transcription. *American Journal of Physiology. Endocrinology and Metabolism, 306*(2), E131–E149. https://doi.org/10.1152/ajpendo.00347.2013

Burke, S. J., Stadler, K., Lu, D., Gleason, E., Han, A., Donohoe, D. R., Rogers, R. C., Hermann, G. E., Karlstad, M. D., & Collier, J. J. (2015). IL-1β reciprocally regulates chemokine and insulin secretion in pancreatic β-cells via NF-κB. *American Journal of Physiology. Endocrinology and Metabolism, 309*(8), E715–E726. https://doi.org/10.1152/ajpendo.00153.2015

Chan, M. E., Adler, B. J., Green, D. E., & Rubin, C. T. (2012). Bone structure and B-cell populations, crippled by obesity, are partially rescued by brief daily exposure to low-magnitude mechanical signals. *The FASEB Journal, 26*(12), 4855–4863. https://doi.org/10.1096/fj.12-209841

Chen, Y., Tian, J., Tian, X., Tang, X., Rui, K., Tong, J., Lu, L., Xu, H., & Wang, S. (2014). Adipose tissue dendritic cells enhances inflammation by prompting the generation of Th17 cells. *PLoS One, 9*(3), Article e92450. https://doi.org/10.1371/journal.pone.0092450

Chen, Y.-M., Yu, X.-J., Liu, K.-L., Gao, H.-L., Li, Y., Sun, T.-Z., Shi, X.-L., Li, H.-B., Zhu, G.-Q., Qi, J., & Kang, Y.-M. (2020). Inhibition of hypothalamic inhibitor κB Kinase β/Nuclear transcription factor κB pathway attenuates metabolism and cardiac dysfunction in type 2 diabetic rats. *Neuroendocrinology, 110*(11–12), 899–913. https://doi.org/10.1159/000504444

Chen, J., Zheng, C.-X., Jin, Y., & Hu, C.-H. (2021). Mesenchymal stromal cell-mediated immune regulation: A promising remedy in the therapy of type 2 diabetes mellitus. *Stem Cells, 39*(7), 838–852. https://doi.org/10.1002/stem.3357

Corbett, J. A., Wang, J. L., Sweetland, M. A., Lancaster, J. R., & McDaniel, M. L. (1992). Interleukin 1 beta induces the formation of nitric oxide by beta-cells purified from rodent islets of Langerhans. Evidence for the beta-cell as a source and site of action of nitric oxide. *The Journal of Clinical Investigation, 90*(6), 2384–2391. https://doi.org/10.1172/JCI116129

Dalle, S. (2024). Targeting protein kinases to protect beta-cell function and survival in diabetes. *International Journal of Molecular Sciences, 25*(12). https://doi.org/10.3390/ijms25126425

Desai, H. R., Sivasubramaniyam, T., Revelo, X. S., Schroer, S. A., Luk, C. T., Rikkala, P. R., Metherel, A. H., Dodington, D. W., Park, Y. J., Kim, M. J., Rapps, J. A., Besla, R., Robbins, C. S., Wagner, K.-U., Bazinet, R. P., Winer, D. A., & Woo, M. (2017). Macrophage JAK2 deficiency protects against high-fat diet-induced inflammation. *Scientific Reports, 7*(1), 7653. https://doi.org/10.1038/s41598-017-07923-0

Devkota, R., Small, J. C., Carbone, K., Glass, M. A., Vetere, A., & Wagner, B. K. (2024). KD025 is a casein kinase 2 inhibitor that protects against glucolipotoxicity in β-Cells. *Diabetes, 73*(4), 585–591. https://doi.org/10.2337/db23-0506

Ding, Q., Gao, Z., Chen, K., Zhang, Q., Hu, S., & Zhao, L. (2022). Inflammation-related epigenetic modification: The bridge between immune and metabolism in type 2 diabetes. *Frontiers in Immunology, 13,* Article 883410. https://doi.org/10.3389/fimmu.2022.883410

Doliba, N. M., Liu, Q., Li, C., Chen, P., Liu, C., Naji, A., & Matschinsky, F. M. (2017). Inhibition of cholinergic potentiation of insulin secretion from pancreatic islets by chronic elevation of glucose and fatty acids: Protection by casein kinase 2 inhibitor. *Molecular Metabolism, 6*(10), 1240–1253. https://doi.org/10.1016/j.molmet.2017.07.017

Donath, M. Y., & Shoelson, S. E. (2011). Type 2 diabetes as an inflammatory disease. *Nature Reviews Immunology, 11*(2), 98–107. https://doi.org/10.1038/nri2925

Elgazar-Carmon, V., Rudich, A., Hadad, N., & Levy, R. (2008). Neutrophils transiently infiltrate intra-abdominal fat early in the course of high-fat feeding. *Journal of Lipid Research, 49*(9), 1894–1903. https://doi.org/10.1194/jlr.M800132-JLR200

Feingold, K. R., Serio, M. K., Adi, S., Moser, A. H., & Grunfeld, C. (1989). Tumor necrosis factor stimulates hepatic lipid synthesis and secretion. *Endocrinology, 124*(5), 2336–2342. https://doi.org/10.1210/endo-124-5-2336

Feng, J., Lu, S., Ou, B., Liu, Q., Dai, J., Ji, C., Zhou, H., Huang, H., & Ma, Y. (2020). The role of JNk signaling pathway in obesity-driven insulin resistance. *Diabetes, Metabolic Syndrome and Obesity: Targets and Therapy, 13,* 1399–1406. https://doi.org/10.2147/DMSO.S236127

Galicia-Garcia, U., Benito-Vicente, A., Jebari, S., Larrea-Sebal, A., Siddiqi, H., Uribe, K. B., Ostolaza, H., & Martín, C. (2020). Pathophysiology of type 2 diabetes mellitus. *International Journal of Molecular Sciences, 21*(17). https://doi.org/10.3390/ijms21176275

Ghazarian, M., Revelo, X. S., Nøhr, M. K., Luck, H., Zeng, K., Lei, H., Tsai, S., Schroer, S. A., Park, Y. J., Chng, M. H. Y., Shen, L., D'Angelo, J. A., Horton, P., Chapman, W. C., Brockmeier, D., Woo, M., Engleman, E. G., Adeyi, O., Hirano, N., … Winer, D. A. (2017). Type I interferon responses drive intrahepatic T cells to promote metabolic syndrome. *Science Immunology, 2*(10). https://doi.org/10.1126/sciimmunol.aai7616

Ghoshal, K. (2024). Exosomal RNA in type 2 diabetes mellitus and other metabolic diseases. In *Exosomal RNA* (pp. 135–165). Elsevier. https://doi.org/10.1016/B978-0-443-14008-2.00009-7

Guan, J., Abudouaini, H., Lin, K., & Yang, K. (2024). Emerging insights into the role of IL-1 inhibitors and colchicine for inflammation control in type 2 diabetes. *Diabetology & Metabolic Syndrome, 16*(1), 140. https://doi.org/10.1186/s13098-024-01369-x

Halberg, N., Khan, T., Trujillo, M. E., Wernstedt-Asterholm, I., Attie, A. D., Sherwani, S., Wang, Z. V., Landskroner-Eiger, S., Dineen, S., Magalang, U. J., Brekken, R. A., & Scherer, P. E. (2009). Hypoxia-inducible factor 1alpha induces fibrosis and insulin resistance in white adipose tissue. *Molecular and Cellular Biology, 29*(16), 4467–4483. https://doi.org/10.1128/MCB.00192-09

Hauser, A. S., Attwood, M. M., Rask-Andersen, M., Schiöth, H. B., & Gloriam, D. E. (2017). Trends in GPCR drug discovery: New agents, targets and indications. *Nature Reviews Drug Discovery, 16*(12), 829–842. https://doi.org/10.1038/nrd.2017.178

Hill, D. A., Lim, H.-W., Kim, Y. H., Ho, W. Y., Foong, Y. H., Nelson, V. L., Nguyen, H. C. B., Chegireddy, K., Kim, J., Habertheuer, A., Vallabhajosyula, P., Kambayashi, T., Won, K.-J., & Lazar, M. A. (2018). Distinct macrophage populations direct inflammatory versus physiological changes in adipose tissue. *Proceedings of the National Academy of Sciences of the United States of America, 115*(22), E5096–E5105. https://doi.org/10.1073/pnas.1802611115

Holmes, D. (2017). Immunometabolism: Physiologic role of IL-1β in glucose homeostasis. *Nature Reviews Endocrinology, 13*(3), 128. https://doi.org/10.1038/nrendo.2017.11

Hotamisligil, G. S., Murray, D. L., Choy, L. N., & Spiegelman, B. M. (1994). Tumor necrosis factor alpha inhibits signaling from the insulin receptor. *Proceedings of the National Academy of Sciences of the United States of America, 91*(11), 4854–4858. https://doi.org/10.1073/pnas.91.11.4854

Ilan, Y., Maron, R., Tukpah, A.-M., Maioli, T. U., Murugaiyan, G., Yang, K., Wu, H. Y., & Weiner, H. L. (2010). Induction of regulatory T cells decreases adipose inflammation and alleviates insulin resistance in ob/ob mice. *Proceedings of the National Academy of Sciences of the United States of America, 107*(21), 9765–9770. https://doi.org/10.1073/pnas.0908771107

Jia, L., Vianna, C. R., Fukuda, M., Berglund, E. D., Liu, C., Tao, C., Sun, K., Liu, T., Harper, M. J., Lee, C. E., Lee, S., Scherer, P. E., & Elmquist, J. K. (2014). Hepatocyte Toll-like receptor 4 regulates obesity-induced inflammation and insulin resistance. *Nature Communications, 5*, 3878. https://doi.org/10.1038/ncomms4878

Kawanishi, N., Yano, H., Yokogawa, Y., & Suzuki, K. (2010). Exercise training inhibits inflammation in adipose tissue via both suppression of macrophage infiltration and acceleration of phenotypic switching from M1 to M2 macrophages in high-fat-diet-induced obese mice. *Exercise Immunology Review, 16*, 105–118.

Kitade, H., Sawamoto, K., Nagashimada, M., Inoue, H., Yamamoto, Y., Sai, Y., Takamura, T., Yamamoto, H., Miyamoto, K., Ginsberg, H. N., Mukaida, N., Kaneko, S., & Ota, T. (2012). CCR5 plays a critical role in obesity-induced adipose tissue inflammation and insulin resistance by regulating both macrophage recruitment and M1/M2 status. *Diabetes, 61*(7), 1680–1690. https://doi.org/10.2337/db11-1506

Klein, S., Meng, R., Montenarh, M., & Götz, C. (2016). The phosphorylation of PDX-1 by protein kinase CK2 is crucial for its stability. *Pharmaceuticals, 10*(1). https://doi.org/10.3390/ph10010002

Kulcsar, K. A., Coleman, C. M., Beck, S. E., & Frieman, M. B. (2019). Comorbid diabetes results in immune dysregulation and enhanced disease severity following MERS-CoV infection. *Journal of Clinical Investigation Insight, 4*(20). https://doi.org/10.1172/jci.insight.131774

Kumar, M., Roe, K., Nerurkar, P. V., Orillo, B., Thompson, K. S., Verma, S., & Nerurkar, V. R. (2014). Reduced immune cell infiltration and increased pro-inflammatory mediators in the brain of Type 2 diabetic mouse model infected with West Nile virus. *Journal of Neuroinflammation, 11*, 80. https://doi.org/10.1186/1742-2094-11-80

Lee, Y. S., & Olefsky, J. (2021). Chronic tissue inflammation and metabolic disease. *Genes & Development, 35*(5–6), 307–328. https://doi.org/10.1101/gad.346312.120

Lee, H. A., Park, H., & Park, B. (2024). Genetic predisposition, lifestyle inflammation score, food-based dietary inflammatory index, and the risk for incident diabetes: Findings from the KoGES data. *Nutrition, Metabolism, and Cardiovascular Diseases, 34*(3), 642–650. https://doi.org/10.1016/j.numecd.2023.10.028

Lee, Y. S., Wollam, J., & Olefsky, J. M. (2018). An integrated view of immunometabolism. *Cell, 172*(1–2), 22–40. https://doi.org/10.1016/j.cell.2017.12.025

Li, H., Meng, Y., He, S., Tan, X., Zhang, Y., Zhang, X., Wang, L., & Zheng, W. (2022). Macrophages, chronic inflammation, and insulin resistance. *Cells, 11*(19). https://doi.org/10.3390/cells11193001

Liu, L. S., Spelleken, M., Röhrig, K., Hauner, H., & Eckel, J. (1998). Tumor necrosis factor-alpha acutely inhibits insulin signaling in human adipocytes: Implication of the p80 tumor necrosis factor receptor. *Diabetes, 47*(4), 515–522. https://doi.org/10.2337/diabetes.47.4.515

Liu, H.-F., Zhang, H.-J., Hu, Q.-X., Liu, X.-Y., Wang, Z.-Q., Fan, J.-Y., Zhan, M., & Chen, F.-L. (2012). Altered polarization, morphology, and impaired innate immunity germane to resident peritoneal macrophages in mice with long-term type 2 diabetes. *Journal of Biomedicine and Biotechnology, 2012*, Article 867023. https://doi.org/10.1155/2012/867023

Luo, M., Zhao, F., Cheng, H., Su, M., & Wang, Y. (2024). Macrophage polarization: An important role in inflammatory diseases. *Frontiers in Immunology, 15*, Article 1352946. https://doi.org/10.3389/fimmu.2024.1352946

Maedler, K., Sergeev, P., Ris, F., Oberholzer, J., Joller-Jemelka, H. I., Spinas, G. A., Kaiser, N., Halban, P. A., & Donath, M. Y. (2002). Glucose-induced beta cell production of IL-1beta contributes to glucotoxicity in human pancreatic islets. *The Journal of Clinical Investigation, 110*(6), 851–860. https://doi.org/10.1172/JCI15318

Makki, K., Froguel, P., & Wolowczuk, I. (2013). Adipose tissue in obesity-related inflammation and insulin resistance: Cells, cytokines, and chemokines. *ISRN Inflammation, 2013*, Article 139239. https://doi.org/10.1155/2013/139239

Martinez, N., Ketheesan, N., Martens, G. W., West, K., Lien, E., & Kornfeld, H. (2016). Defects in early cell recruitment contribute to the increased susceptibility to respiratory Klebsiella pneumoniae infection in diabetic mice. *Microbes and Infection, 18*(10), 649–655. https://doi.org/10.1016/j.micinf.2016.05.007

Matsumori, A. (2022). Novel biomarkers of inflammation for the management of diabetes: Immunoglobulin-free light chains. *Biomedicines, 10*(3). https://doi.org/10.3390/biomedicines10030666

Nishimura, S., Manabe, I., Nagasaki, M., Eto, K., Yamashita, H., Ohsugi, M., Otsu, M., Hara, K., Ueki, K., Sugiura, S., Yoshimura, K., Kadowaki, T., & Nagai, R. (2009). CD8+ effector T cells contribute to macrophage recruitment and adipose tissue inflammation in obesity. *Nature Medicine, 15*(8), 914–920. https://doi.org/10.1038/nm.1964

Nunemaker, C. S. (2016). Considerations for defining cytokine dose, duration, and milieu that are appropriate for modeling chronic low-grade inflammation in type 2 diabetes. *Journal of Diabetes Research, 2016*, Article 2846570. https://doi.org/10.1155/2016/2846570

Park, J.-E., & Han, J.-S. (2024). Improving the effect of ferulic acid on inflammation and insulin resistance by regulating the JNK/ERK and NF-κB pathways in TNF-α-Treated 3T3-L1 adipocytes. *Nutrients, 16*(2). https://doi.org/10.3390/nu16020294

Patra, D., Ramprasad, P., Sharma, S., Dey, U., Kumar, V., Singh, S., Dasgupta, S., Kumar, A., Tikoo, K., & Pal, D. (2024). Adipose tissue macrophage-derived microRNA-210-3p disrupts systemic insulin sensitivity by silencing GLUT4 in obesity. *Journal of Biological Chemistry, 300*(6), Article 107328. https://doi.org/10.1016/j.jbc.2024.107328

Rangasamy, S., McGuire, P. G., Franco Nitta, C., Monickaraj, F., Oruganti, S. R., & Das, A. (2014). Chemokine mediated monocyte trafficking into the retina: Role of inflammation in alteration of the blood-retinal barrier in diabetic retinopathy. *PLoS One, 9*(10), Article e108508. https://doi.org/10.1371/journal.pone.0108508

Rehman, K., & Akash, M. S. H. (2016). Mechanisms of inflammatory responses and development of insulin resistance: How are they interlinked? *Journal of Biomedical Science, 23*(1), 87. https://doi.org/10.1186/s12929-016-0303-y

Ridker, P. M. (2019). Anticytokine agents: Targeting interleukin signaling pathways for the treatment of atherothrombosis. *Circulation Research, 124*(3), 437–450. https://doi.org/10.1161/CIRCRESAHA.118.313129

Rossi, M., Ruiz de Azua, I., Barella, L. F., Sakamoto, W., Zhu, L., Cui, Y., Lu, H., Rebholz, H., Matschinsky, F. M., Doliba, N. M., Butcher, A. J., Tobin, A. B., & Wess, J. (2015). CK2 acts as a potent negative regulator of receptor-mediated insulin release in vitro and in vivo. *Proceedings of the National Academy of Sciences of the United States of America, 112*(49), E6818–E6824. https://doi.org/10.1073/pnas.1519430112

Scheuer, R., Philipp, S. E., Becker, A., Nalbach, L., Ampofo, E., Montenarh, M., & Götz, C. (2020). Protein kinase CK2 controls CaV2.1-Dependent calcium currents and insulin release in pancreatic β-Cells. *International Journal of Molecular Sciences, 21*(13). https://doi.org/10.3390/ijms21134668

Sehgal, A., Behl, T., Kaur, I., Singh, S., Sharma, N., & Aleya, L. (2021). Targeting NLRP3 inflammasome as a chief instigator of obesity, contributing to local adipose tissue inflammation and insulin resistance. *Environmental Science and Pollution Research International, 28*(32), 43102–43113. https://doi.org/10.1007/s11356-021-14904-4

Shah, R., Hinkle, C. C., Ferguson, J. F., Mehta, N. N., Li, M., Qu, L., Lu, Y., Putt, M. E., Ahima, R. S., & Reilly, M. P. (2011). Fractalkine is a novel human adipochemokine associated with type 2 diabetes. *Diabetes, 60*(5), 1512–1518. https://doi.org/10.2337/db10-0956

Shah, U., & Kowalski, T. J. (2010). GPR119 agonists for the potential treatment of type 2 diabetes and related metabolic disorders. *Vitamins and Hormones, 84*, 415–448. https://doi.org/10.1016/B978-0-12-381517-0.00016-3

Shi, H., Kokoeva, M. V., Inouye, K., Tzameli, I., Yin, H., & Flier, J. S. (2006). TLR4 links innate immunity and fatty acid-induced insulin resistance. *The Journal of Clinical Investigation, 116*(11), 3015–3025. https://doi.org/10.1172/JCI28898

Singh, S., Anshita, D., & Ravichandiran, V. (2021). MCP-1: Function, regulation, and involvement in disease. *International Immunopharmacology, 101*(Pt B), Article 107598. https://doi.org/10.1016/j.intimp.2021.107598

Srividya, N., Haldipur, A. C., & Yerra, H. (2024). Lifestyle modifications and nutritional modulation of immune system for prevention and management of diabetes mellitus: Current perspectives. In *Biochemical immunology of diabetes and associated complications* (pp. 313–330). Elsevier. https://doi.org/10.1016/B978-0-443-13195-0.00016-8

Stanimirovic, J., Radovanovic, J., Banjac, K., Obradovic, M., Essack, M., Zafirovic, S., Gluvic, Z., Gojobori, T., & Isenovic, E. R. (2022). Role of C-Reactive protein in diabetic inflammation. *Mediators of Inflammation, 2022*, Article 3706508. https://doi.org/10.1155/2022/3706508

Su, J., Xu, J., Hu, S., Ye, H., Xie, L., & Ouyang, S. (2024). Advances in small-molecule insulin secretagogues for diabetes treatment. *Biomedicine & Pharmacotherapy, 178*, Article 117179. https://doi.org/10.1016/j.biopha.2024.117179

Talukdar, S., Oh, D. Y., Bandyopadhyay, G., Li, D., Xu, J., McNelis, J., Lu, M., Li, P., Yan, Q., Zhu, Y., Ofrecio, J., Lin, M., Brenner, M. B., & Olefsky, J. M. (2012). Neutrophils mediate insulin resistance in mice fed a high-fat diet through secreted elastase. *Nature Medicine, 18*(9), 1407–1412. https://doi.org/10.1038/nm.2885

Tarabra, E., Giunti, S., Barutta, F., Salvidio, G., Burt, D., Deferrari, G., Gambino, R., Vergola, D., Pinach, S., Perin, P. C., Camussi, G., & Gruden, G. (2009). Effect of the monocyte chemoattractant protein-1/CC chemokine receptor 2 system on nephrin expression in streptozotocin-treated mice and human cultured podocytes. *Diabetes, 58*(9), 2109–2118. https://doi.org/10.2337/db08-0895

Trottier, M. D., Naaz, A., Li, Y., & Fraker, P. J. (2012). Enhancement of hematopoiesis and lymphopoiesis in diet-induced obese mice. *Proceedings of the National Academy of Sciences of the United States of America, 109*(20), 7622–7629. https://doi.org/10.1073/pnas.1205129109

Wang, Q., Henry, T. A. N., Pronin, A. N., Jang, G.-F., Lubaczeuski, C., Crabb, J. W., Bernal-Mizrachi, E., & Slepak, V. Z. (2020). The regulatory G protein signaling complex, Gβ5-R7, promotes glucose- and extracellular signal-stimulated insulin secretion. *Journal of Biological Chemistry, 295*(21), 7213–7223. https://doi.org/10.1074/jbc.RA119.011534

Wang, T.-Y., Liu, X.-J., Xie, J.-Y., Yuan, Q.-Z., & Wang, Y. (2020). Cask methylation involved in the injury of insulin secretion function caused by interleukin1-β. *Journal of Cellular and Molecular Medicine, 24* (24), 14247–14256. https://doi.org/10.1111/jcmm.16041

Wang, Z., Ni, X., Zhang, L., Sun, L., Zhu, X., Zhou, Q., Yang, Z., & Yuan, H. (2020). Toll-like receptor 4 and inflammatory micro-environment of pancreatic islets in Type-2 diabetes mellitus: A therapeutic perspective. *Diabetes, Metabolic Syndrome and Obesity: Targets and Therapy, 13*, 4261–4272. https://doi.org/10.2147/DMSO.S279104

Wang, H.-W., Tang, J., Sun, L., Li, Z., Deng, M., & Dai, Z. (2023). Mechanism of immune attack in the progression of obesity-related type 2 diabetes. *World Journal of Diabetes, 14*(5), 494–511. https://doi.org/10.4239/wjd.v14.i5.494

Weisberg, S. P., Hunter, D., Huber, R., Lemieux, J., Slaymaker, S., Vaddi, K., Charo, I., Leibel, R. L., & Ferrante, A. W. (2006). CCR2 modulates inflammatory and metabolic effects of high-fat feeding. *The Journal of Clinical Investigation, 116*(1), 115–124. https://doi.org/10.1172/JCI24335

Wootten, D., Christopoulos, A., Marti-Solano, M., Babu, M. M., & Sexton, P. M. (2018). Mechanisms of signalling and biased agonism in G protein-coupled receptors. *Nature Reviews Molecular Cell Biology, 19*(10), 638–653. https://doi.org/10.1038/s41580-018-0049-3

Yehualashet, A. S. (2020). Toll-like receptors as a potential drug target for diabetes mellitus and diabetes-associated complications. *Diabetes, Metabolic Syndrome and Obesity: Targets and Therapy, 13*, 4763–4777. https://doi.org/10.2147/DMSO.S274844

Zheng, W., Ji, X., Yin, Q. Q., Wu, C., Xu, C., Pan, H., & Wu, C. (2024). Exosomes as emerging regulators of immune responses in type 2 diabetes mellitus. *Journal of Diabetes Research, 2024*, Article 3759339. https://doi.org/10.1155/2024/3759339

11

Personalized medicine approaches based on immunogenetic profiling

Ghulam Mehdi Dar[1] and Bhawna Mahajan[1, 2]

[1]CENTRAL MOLECULAR LAB, GOVIND BALLABH PANT INSTITUTE OF MEDICAL EDUCATION AND RESEARCH, DELHI, NEW DELHI, INDIA; [2]DEPARTMENT OF BIOCHEMISTRY, GOVIND BALLABH PANT INSTITUTE OF MEDICAL EDUCATION AND RESEARCH, DELHI, NEW DELHI, INDIA

1. Introduction

1.1 Overview, epidemiology, and risk factors

Diabetes mellitus is defined as a condition of high blood sugar due to defective insulin secretion, action, or both. According to the WHO, the diabetic burden has increased significantly between 1990 and 2022, with 630 million new cases and a total of up to 828 million adults approximately affected by diabetes globally, where India and China account for the largest share, driven by their increasing population (Zhou et al., 2024). The racial and socioeconomic inequality impacts a higher prevalence of diabetes in black and Asian groups than in the white population (Hill-Briggs & Fitzpatrick, 2023). Diabetes mellitus can be classified into type 1 and type 2, where type 1 diabetes results from the insulin deficiency due to autoimmune destruction of pancreatic islet cells (American Diabetes Association, 2014). Meanwhile, the diabetic cases are characterized by the inadequate production of insulin by pancreatic islet β-cells, subpar compensatory response to insulin secretion, and insulin resistance (IR) in tissues failing to maintain glucose homeostasis (Chatterjee et al., 2017). The affected organs from T2DM are pancreatic cells—α and β, liver, adipose tissue, kidneys, skeletal muscle, and brain (DeFronzo, 2009), while the risk factors are multifaceted to include the genetic, environmental, and metabolic factors. The predisposition based on ethnicity and genetic basis are non-modifiable risk factors for a population, but for a considerable number of cases, the development of T2DM can be controlled by modifying dietary habits, physical activity, and lifestyle changes (Schellenberg et al., 2013). Patients with T2DM are characterized by obesity and aging populations, mainly with a sedentary lifestyle and high caloric diet consumption. Diets, especially the high-carb and fat-rich, are responsible for raising the levels of blood glucose, triglyceride-rich lipoproteins, and generation of reactive oxygen species (ROS) that leads to oxidative stress and subsequent

Type 2 Diabetes Mellitus. https://doi.org/10.1016/B978-0-443-33590-7.00004-6

inflammatory responses. This further causes oxidative damage through mitochondrial dysfunction, NADPH oxidase activation, and endoplasmic reticulum stress, contributing to the pathogenesis of T2DM and IR via sustained ROS levels (Galicia-Garcia et al., 2020). The elevated free fatty acids are also responsible for causing mitochondrial dysfunction by disruption of the respiratory chain and electron leakage, and together, these mechanisms drive IR and T2DM (Graciano et al., 2011). With a higher body fat fraction, the prevalence of T2DM also increases as the inflammatory response in the adipose tissue results in insulin resistance through numerous mechanisms that primarily cause dysregulation of fatty acid secretion and adipokines (Galicia-Garcia et al., 2020). Historically, the treatment for diabetes was more uniform in the context of broad population-based approaches. However, the complexity and heterogeneity of T2DM emphasize the personalized medicine approach, also known as precision medicine, based on genetic and phenotypic data. The integrative approach of understanding the genetic, epigenetic, and associated lifestyle factors can tailor personalized devices to optimize therapeutic outcomes while reducing the side effects. Furthermore, the promise of immunogenetics in personalizing T2DM treatment explores the genetic basis of immune responses in pathogenesis and identifies patient subgroups that may benefit from specific therapies (Roep et al., 2019). The field of pharmacogenetics and pharmacogenomics deals with the influence of drug response on genetic variations and thus emphasizes the need for genetic screening in patients for polymorphisms and specific responses to antidiabetic drugs (for example, Metformin, Sulfonylureas) to enhance treatment outcomes (Heo & Choi, 2019). More elaborate research is required to identify the biomarkers using omics technologies to predict drug responses and to understand disease progression through the complex interaction of genetics and environmental factors. GWAS and other methods of genetic research can also facilitate the identification of disease-associated genetic variants and move toward precision medicine approaches in clinical routine, enhancing therapeutic efficacy and reducing the economic burden of diabetes management globally.

Current scientific understanding has highlighted the importance of the immune response in the pathophysiology of T2DM, where both adaptive and innate responses collaboratively contribute to the progression of the disease. In this chapter, we review the interplay of the immune system involved in T2DM and personalized therapy through immunogenetic profiling approaches (Fig. 11.1).

1.2 Immunogenetic factors in T2DM

1.2.1 The immune system and T2DM

The pathophysiology of T2DM includes the components from both the adaptive and innate immune systems contributing to insulin resistance via mechanisms like proliferation of macrophages, altered T cells, and impaired functions of β cells and NK cells (Zhou et al., 2018). Previous studies evidence the role of the immune system in the pathogenesis of T2DM, particularly through its involvement in low-grade inflammation

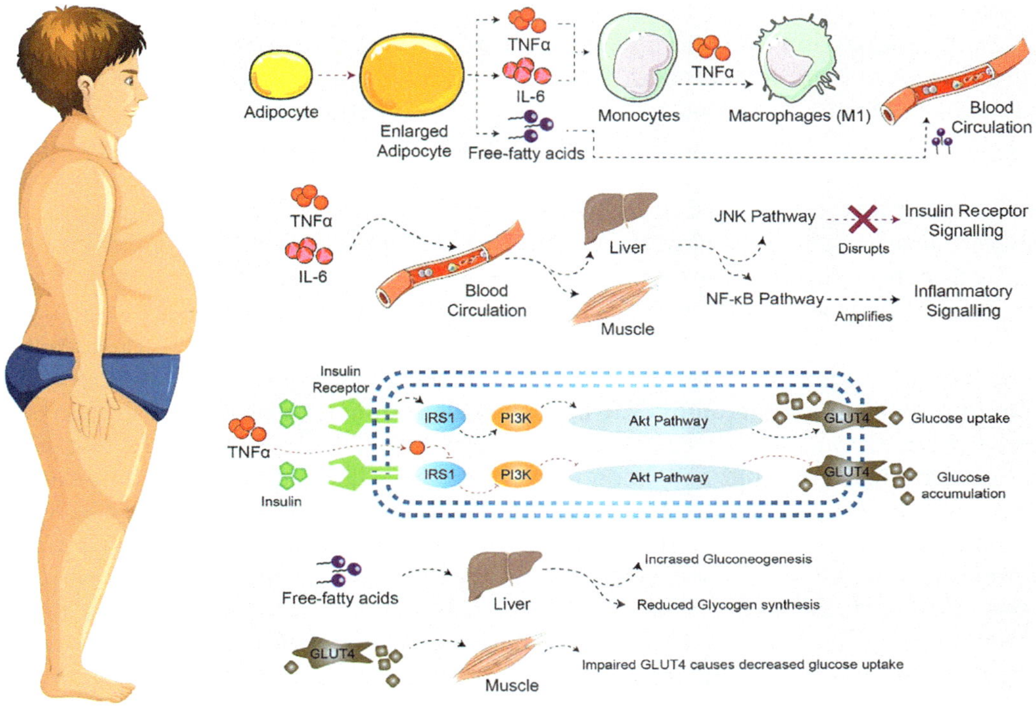

FIGURE 11.1 Mechanistic landscape of insulin resistance.

and metabolic dysregulation caused by environmental factors, including obesity. It is highlighted that NK-κβ activation is triggered by obesity factors and leads to expression of inflammatory genes, which in turn enhances monocyte-to-macrophage differentiation via binding of monocytes to smooth muscle cells and endothelial cells (Reddy & Natarajan, 2011). The activation of NK-κβ also elevates the expression levels of inflammatory cytokines that cause vascular inflammation and further generation of mediators like proteases and endothelial adhesion molecules (Guarner & Rubio-Ruiz, 2015). The inflammatory conditions arising from obesity are also mediated by Toll-like receptors that contribute to hypertension and insulin resistance (Reddy & Natarajan, 2011). Sedentary lifestyle and reduced physical activity also promote T2DM by increasing levels of proinflammatory molecules like IL-6, IL-1, CRP, and TNF-α, with IL-1, typically involved in impairing pancreatic β-cell function and promoting apoptosis. The inhibition of inflammasome, such as NLRP3, producing IL-1β and IL-18, has resulted in the prevention of T2DM by improving insulin sensitivity (Galicia-Garcia et al., 2020). Combating T2DM through boosting antiinflammatory components like IL-1 receptor antagonist and soluble TNF receptor and antioxidants like glutathione can be accomplished through regular physical activities in prediabetic and T2DM patients (Leeuwenburgh et al., 1994; Shamsuzzaman et al., 2004). As obesity is also linked with chronic inflammation in T2DM individuals, it leads to activation of the immune system. The polarization of macrophages toward proinflammatory M1 phenotype is typically marked in individuals with T2DM and obesity, which impairs insulin signaling and further immune activation to worsen the disease pathology (Ilan et al., 2010; Sell et al., 2012). As a component of the innate immune system, natural killer (NK) cells are also involved in dysfunction leading to T2DM. Impairment of their functions, as in the expression of NKG2D is found in individuals with T2DM, where a negative correlation of HbA1c levels is observed simultaneously, indicating the link with glycemic control. The dysfunction further leads to dysregulation of the overall immune system and complicates the disease management in T2DM (Sell et al., 2012). Understanding these mechanisms enhances the knowledge of the interaction between the immune system and T2DM and opens new avenues for targeted immunotherapeutic approaches that could improve patient outcomes. The immune cell populations and their functions are altered primarily in cases of T2DM. Patients with T2DM have been shown to exhibit abnormal proliferation and activation of immune cells like macrophages and T cells, which are found to contribute to chronic low-grade inflammation. The elevated levels of $CD45^+$ T cells mark the dysregulation of the immune system and evidence proinflammatory phenotype that escalates the metabolic disturbances associated with the disease (Sell et al., 2012; Sireesh et al., 2018). The imbalance between regulatory T cells and effector T cells, such as Th1 and Th17, is one of the critical aspects of immune dysregulation in T2DM. Regulatory T cells play an important role in the maintenance of immune homeostasis and the prevention of excessive inflammation. In patients with T2DM, their population is significantly reduced causing more inflammatory responses and insulin resistance. Conclusively, the altered scenario of T cells characterized by reduced regulatory T cells and increased proinflammatory Th cells contributes to the pathophysiology of T2DM (Zhang et al., 2014).

1.2.2 Role of HLA in T2DM progression

T2DM is found to be associated with the human leukocyte antigen (HLA) alleles and is involved in the regulation of the immune system (Chinniah et al., 2016). Though T2DM is primarily considered a metabolic disorder, studies suggested an overlap of genetic and immunological factors along with autoimmune conditions, where the specific HLA alleles, such as HLA-DRB1, HLA-DQA1, and HLA-DQB1, influence susceptibility to the disease (Zhao et al., 2024). Risk-associated alleles can facilitate presentation of abnormal peptides and self-antigens, leading to immune activation and prolonged inflammation, which can further damage pancreatic β-cells, impair insulin secretion, and exacerbate insulin resistance. In contrast, protective alleles enhance immune tolerance and reduce inflammatory activity. The genetic factors and environmental influences, such as dietary habits and physical activity, further influence the function of HLA alleles in disease development (Sheehy et al., 1989; Zhao et al., 2024). The HLA-DRB1 alleles are typically found to play a significant role in the development of T2DM. Research studies conducted on the South Indian population figured the variants of this allele, such as DRB103 and

DRB104, occur commonly among T2DM patients (Rathika et al., 2012). The association of these variants with the disease suggests its role in promoting immune dysregulation and metabolic dysfunction leading to the development of the disease (Groop et al., 1986; Tuomi, 2005). The study by Motala et al. (2005) shows that gender bias in predisposition of risk-associated allele DRB103, is more prevalent in women, indicating an interaction between genetic predisposition and sex-related factors like hormones that can influence immune system behavior (Motala et al., 2005).

The other two alleles: HLA-DQB1 and HLA-DQA1, are also major contributors to T2DM. For example, the allele DQB102, often in combination with DQA105:01, is found associated with increased disease susceptibility by forming heterodimer products that influence antigen presentation and can lead to immune activation along with chronic inflammation (Sheehy et al., 1989; Zhao et al., 2024). The genetic landscape of T2DM also extends into combining class I (HLA-A, HLA-B) and class II (HLA-DR, HLA-DQ) loci of HLA haplotypes. The A33-B40-DRB115-DQB106 haplotype is found to be strongly associated with T2DM risk (Chinniah et al., 2016). On the contrary, the DRB110 allele appears less frequently in individuals with T2DM, demonstrating a protective function that potentially mitigates inflammatory pathways related to the disease (Almawi et al., 2006). Similarly, the A01-B07-DRB110-DQB105 haplotype has shown protective effects (Chinniah et al., 2016). Other haplotypes like DQA103:03-DQB103:01, are also identified as protective and may assist in preventing the processes leading to T2DM.

This dual role of HLA alleles highlights the complex ways to modulate the immune environment and suggests that interactions between different HLA loci collectively determine the genetic predisposition to T2DM (Sheehy et al., 1989; Zhao et al., 2024). HLA polymorphisms also alter cytokine production and T-cell activity. Alleles linked to greater disease risk often correlate with higher production of proinflammatory cytokines, exacerbating chronic inflammation and metabolic disruption. Protective alleles, on the other hand, may increase regulatory T-cell activity, dampening immune responses and reducing the inflammatory environment. This dynamic highlight the dual roles of HLA alleles in promoting or mitigating the factors that drive T2DM progression (Zhao et al., 2024). The identification of specific HLA alleles and haplotypes associated with T2DM has significant implications for clinical practice and research. Screening for high-risk HLA profiles could enable earlier identification of individuals predisposed to T2DM, paving the way for targeted prevention strategies. Such individuals could benefit from personalized lifestyle modifications and pharmacological interventions to counteract their genetic risks. Moreover, understanding the interactions between HLA polymorphisms and environmental influences could lead to population-level strategies to reduce the incidence of T2DM. Incorporating HLA genotyping into clinical trials could also enhance patient selection, improving the evaluation and effectiveness of novel therapies. Lastly, targeted immunotherapies designed to neutralize the effects of high-risk alleles or enhance the functions of protective ones could revolutionize treatment approaches for T2DM (Chinniah et al., 2016; Zhao et al., 2024).

1.2.3 Cytokine genes involved in T2DM risk

Increasing evidence highlights the pivotal role of cytokines as antiinflammatory and proinflammatory factors involved in the pathogenesis of T2DM. The genetic variations in cytokine genes influence disease susceptibility and severity, and explore the potential of cytokine-targeted therapies in managing T2DM (Akash et al., 2018; Nadeem et al., 2015). Cytokine genes incorporate genetic polymorphism that plays a significant role in modulating resistance to insulin and inflammation. Among these, SNPs in the TNF-α gene have garnered particular attention. For instance, the G-308A polymorphism in the TNF-α promoter region enhances transcription factor binding, resulting in increased cytokine production, and is associated with heightened insulin resistance, particularly in obese populations, as it disrupts insulin signaling through phosphorylation of serine residue in insulin receptor substrate-1 (Nadeem et al., 2015). The IL-6 gene also exhibits SNPs that contribute to T2DM susceptibility. The -174G/C polymorphism affects promoter activity, altering IL-6 expression levels. Studies have shown that the combination of TNF-α -308A and IL-6 -174G polymorphisms significantly increases the risk of T2DM, highlighting the interplay between different cytokine gene variants. Gene-gene interactions amplify the impact of these SNPs, as seen in Indian populations where the combined presence of TNF-α and IL-6 variants elevates the risk of T2DM by several folds (Nadeem et al., 2015). Gene-environment interactions further modulate the effects of cytokine polymorphisms. Obesity, a critical risk factor for T2DM, exacerbates the influence of TNF-α and IL-6 polymorphisms by increasing cytokine production in adipose tissue. Environmental factors such as dietary habits and physical activity levels also interact with these polymorphisms, influencing serum cytokine levels and metabolic outcomes. This explains the ethnic variability observed in the association between cytokine SNPs and T2DM, as demographic and lifestyle differences shape the gene-environment interplay (Nadeem et al., 2015).

Variants in antiinflammatory cytokines, like interleukin-10 (IL-10), also impact T2DM pathogenesis. SNPs in the IL-10 promoter region alter transcriptional activity, influencing cytokine production and the ability to counteract proinflammatory mediators. These genetic variations have been linked to differences in T2DM susceptibility across populations, further emphasizing the role of antiinflammatory pathways in disease modulation (Nadeem et al., 2015). Proinflammatory cytokines such as IL-1β, TNF-α, and IL-6 are integral to the inflammatory cascade that underpins T2DM. TNF-α is produced predominantly by adipose tissue, impairs insulin signaling by activating NF-κβ, and induces IRS-1 serine phosphorylation. This disrupts downstream insulin receptor activity and glucose uptake, particularly in adipose tissue and skeletal muscle. Elevated TNF-α levels are consistently associated with increased insulin resistance, linking chronic inflammation to metabolic dysfunction (Akash et al., 2018). Meanwhile, IL-1β is another critical cytokine that is produced in response to hyperglycemia and lipotoxicity. It directly contributes to β-cell dysfunction by inducing apoptosis and reducing insulin secretion. IL-1β acts synergistically with TNF-α to amplify inflammation, creating a self-perpetuating cycle that accelerates β-cell failure and metabolic decline. Elevated IL-1β levels in patients with T2DM correlate with oxidative stress markers, further implicating it in disease progression (Li et al., 2023). IL-6 also plays a dual role in T2DM pathogenesis. While traditionally categorized as a proinflammatory cytokine, IL-6 exhibits context-dependent effects. Chronic elevation of IL-6 in adipose tissue contributes to systemic insulin resistance by promoting inflammatory signaling. However, IL-6 can also enhance glucose uptake during acute exercise, illustrating its complex involvement in metabolic regulation. The interplay between IL-6 and other cytokines underscores the intricate network of inflammatory mediators in T2DM (Akash et al., 2018). Antiinflammatory cytokines, including IL-10 and adiponectin, mitigate the harmful effects of proinflammatory mediators. IL-10 inhibits NF-κB signaling and suppresses the production of proinflammatory cytokines, thereby protecting against insulin resistance. Genetic variations in the IL-10 gene affect its expression and activity, influencing the balance between pro and antiinflammatory pathways in T2DM. These polymorphisms have been associated with variations in T2DM risk and progression across populations (Nadeem et al., 2015). Adiponectin is an antiinflammatory adipokine that enhances the sensitivity toward insulin by activating AMP-activated protein kinase and promoting lipid oxidation. SNPs in the ADIPOQ gene, such as -11377G/C, influence adiponectin levels and its protective effects on metabolic health. These genetic variations also interact with dietary factors, affecting the adiponectin-mediated regulation of glucose and lipid metabolism. Reduced adiponectin levels, often observed in obese individuals, exacerbate insulin resistance and highlight the critical role of antiinflammatory mediators in maintaining metabolic homeostasis (Nadeem et al., 2015). The identification of cytokines as key players in T2DM pathogenesis has spurred the development of targeted therapies. Antiinflammatory agents that are inhibitors to TNF-α (for example Etanercept, Infliximab) and IL-1 antagonists (e.g., anakinra, canakinumab) have demonstrated promising results in clinical trials. These therapies reduce systemic inflammation, improve sensitivity to insulin, and enhance β-cell function, addressing the inflammatory underpinnings of T2DM. Meta-analyses have shown that cytokine-targeted treatments significantly lower plasma glucose during fasting, C-reactive protein levels, and glycated hemoglobin (HbA1c), indicating their potential as effective interventions for T2DM (Li et al., 2023).

Combination therapies targeting multiple inflammatory pathways have shown enhanced efficacy. Diacerein, a dual inhibitor of TNF-α and IL-1β, outperforms monotherapies in reducing inflammatory markers and improving glycemic control. Such approaches leverage the synergistic effects of targeting interconnected cytokine networks, providing a comprehensive strategy to mitigate inflammation-driven metabolic dysfunction (Li et al., 2023) (Table 11.1).

Table 11.1 Role of immune cells in type 2 diabetes mellitus (T2DM).

Immune Cell(s) studied	Role in T2DM	Clinical significance	References
NK cells, B cells, T cells, macrophages	Abnormal differentiation and functional impairment contribute to T2DM progression.	Understanding immune dysregulation may support the development of immunotherapies for T2DM.	Zhou et al. (2018)
Adipose tissue-resident immune cells	Dysregulation promotes chronic inflammation and metabolic dysfunction	Targeting these immune populations may provide novel therapeutic avenues	Lu et al. (2019)
Macrophages	Promote insulin resistance and contribute to pancreatic β-cell damage	Insights into macrophage polarization can guide antiinflammatory therapeutic strategies	Odegaard and Chawla (2012)
T Cells	Drive chronic inflammation and exacerbates insulin resistance	Highlights T-cell–based immunomodulation as a potential treatment strategy	Xia et al. (2017)
$CD19^+$ $CD27^+$ B cells, monocytes, T cells	Higher circulating B-cell levels are associated with reduced T2DM risk	Suggests immune cell profiling as a biomarker for T2DM risk assessment	Olson et al. (2020)
Various immune cells	Inflammatory immune responses promote metabolic impairments	Emphasizes the importance of immunization and immune monitoring in T2DM patients	Daryabor et al. (2020)
Macrophages, immune mediators	Tissue infiltration and proinflammatory activity linked to insulin resistance	Identifies immune mediators as therapeutic targets for metabolic inflammation	Kolb and Mandrup-Poulsen (2005)
Innate immune mediators	Chronic inflammation impairs insulin secretion and insulin action	Highlights knowledge gaps and opportunities for antiinflammatory drug development	Donath et al. (2019)

2. Personalized medicine approaches based on immunogenetic profiling

2.1 Risk stratification

The initial steps in T2DM management are the screening of individuals at higher risk of developing the disease. This risk stratification is accomplished by using genetic risk scores (GRS) that account for the multi-factorial nature of T2DM and consider the interplay of genetic predisposition and environmental factors. The heritability of the disease is found to range from 40% to 70% (Scott et al., 2017; Zhao et al., 2017), with more than 500 identified loci (Mahajan et al., 2018) contributing to the susceptibility of T2DM. The application of GRS quantifies genetic risk and predicts the disease onset, enabling early management. Traditionally, single-trait models for GRS were used on the basis of associated individual genetic variants to predict the risk, but such models only reflected a fraction of the causal factors underlying T2DM. A more comprehensive approach is obtained by using multi-trait GRS that link genetic variation with correlated phenotypes such as body mass index and blood pressure. In the study conducted by Rohde et al. (2021), it was shown that the accuracy of prediction for T2DM risk is enhanced by using multi-trait GRS by 12.5%–94% in several datasets for validation. Particularly, the consideration of traits like BMI and medication use contributed significantly to the improved predictive ability of multi-trait GRS. These findings highlight the need for consideration of pleiotropic genetic effects and intricate interactions between metabolic conditions and T2DM (Evangelou et al., 2018; Locke et al., 2015). In addition to the application of multi-trait GRS, designing population-specific risk scores has further shown to improve the accuracy of disease prediction. A study conducted by Shitomi-Jones et al. (2023) with a focus on the Jat Sikh community - an endogamous North Indian population—having higher rates of T2DM prevalence, utilized weighted GRS based on the susceptible 10 validated loci. The results included two genetic variants KCNQ1 (rs2237892) and TCF7L2 (rs7903146), that are notorious contributors in pathogenesis and risk of T2DM. They also included clinical parameters such as lipid profiles and waist circumference in the GRS, which resulted in a good-performing predictive model with an area under the curve (AUC) of 0.844. This study, thus, underscores the importance of the incorporation of a greater number of clinical and genetic parameters along with improvising population specific development of GRS models due to the genetic or lifestyle variability found across different ethnic groups (Shitomi-Jones et al., 2023). With the advancement in machine learning methods, the predictive power of GRS has been boosted with the inclusion of multiple datasets that optimize the performance of the model. Wang et al. developed predictive T2DM risk models applying various advanced machine learning algorithms, including random forests (RF), artificial neural networks (ANN), and gradient boosting machines (Wang et al., 2021) that considered conventional risk factors such as age, plasma glucose levels during fasting, and BMI. They reported the greatest improvement in AUC up to 3.3% while including GRS. Further, it showed enhanced discriminatory ability of the model, as among all classifiers, the net reclassification index (NRI) was found to increase by 40% for the additional value of GRS. This shows the capability of machine learning prediction models in efficient intervention of T2DM patients (Friedman, 2001; Hastie, 2009).

2.2 Optimizing treatment strategies

To obtain better patient outcomes and reduced adverse effects, treatment strategies need to be optimized for a precision medicine approach. Pharmacogenetics is an emerging research area to explore and understand differences in drug responses and metabolism within different T2DM patients. Drugs like metformin and sulfonylureas are widely studied in combination with different genetic polymorphisms, providing insights into personalized treatment (Bozkurt et al., 2007; Maruthur et al., 2014; Phani et al., 2014). Sulfonylureas, which act on pancreatic cells to stimulate insulin secretion, are metabolized primarily by the enzyme CYP2C9. Variants such as CYP2C9*2 and CYP2C9*3 are linked to decreased enzymatic activity, leading to slower drug clearance and prolonged action. This pharmacokinetic variation results in an increased risk of hypoglycemia among carriers of these alleles. Bozkurt et al. (2007) reported that the CYP2C9*3 allele is associated with a 50% reduction in oral clearance of glyburide, emphasizing the need for tailored dosing regimens in patients with these genetic profiles (Bozkurt et al., 2007). Metformin, a widely used first-line therapy in T2DM, demonstrates pharmacogenetic interactions with the SLC30A8 gene, encoding the transporter molecule for zinc - ZnT8. This transporter plays a vital role in the secretion of insulin. The rs1326634 polymorphism within SLC30A8 has been associated with variable responses to metformin therapy. Specifically, individuals carrying the TT genotype of rs1326634 exhibit better glycemic control compared to other genotypes, suggesting a genotype-dependent mechanism for metformin action. Phani et al. (2014) demonstrated that the TT genotype correlates with improved therapeutic response, likely mediated by enhanced pancreatic beta-cell function (Phani et al., 2014). These pharmacogenetic interactions underscore the importance of genetic testing in diabetes management. Personalized medicine, guided by genetic information, enables clinicians to minimize adverse effects, optimize therapeutic outcomes, and provide patient-centered care. For sulfonylureas, this could involve genotype-guided dosing adjustments to reduce hypoglycemia risk. For metformin, genetic insights might help identify patients who would benefit most from the therapy or require alternative treatments (Bozkurt et al., 2007; Maruthur et al., 2014). Recent advances in immunotherapy highlight its transformative potential beyond oncology, with T2DM emerging as a novel domain of interest. Immune checkpoint pathways, originally explored in cancer immunotherapy, offer intriguing opportunities to modulate immune-mediated insulin resistance, a hallmark of T2DM pathophysiology (Moore et al., 2022; Orabona et al., 2018). PD-1 and CTLA-4 are checkpoint molecules that regulate immune cell activation and tolerance. Their inhibition has shown promise in resetting aberrant immune responses in malignancies, yet similar interventions in metabolic diseases remain nascent. PD-1 signaling, mediated through SHP2 phosphatase recruitment, inhibits inflammatory responses critical in autoimmunity and cancer (Orabona et al., 2018).

However, its dysregulation in T2DM contributes to chronic low-grade inflammation, aggravating insulin resistance. Utilizing immune checkpoint inhibitors (ICIs) could reprogram immune circuits to enhance insulin sensitivity, akin to mechanisms observed in Type 1 Diabetes Mellitus (T1DM) trials targeting PD-1 and CTLA-4 pathways (Moore et al., 2022). Moreover, enzymes such as indoleamine 2,3-dioxygenase (IDO1) influence immune tolerance through the kynurenine pathway. Deficient IDO1 activity correlates with exacerbated inflammatory states, suggesting that its therapeutic restoration might alleviate T2DM-induced metabolic dysregulation. Tocilizumab-mediated modulation of IDO1 activity in T1DM provides a conceptual framework for extending these strategies to T2DM (Orabona et al., 2018). Personalized interventions targeting IDO1 polymorphisms could refine therapeutic efficacy and minimize off-target effects (Moore et al., 2022; Orabona et al., 2018).

2.3 Drug response prediction

T2DM affects millions globally, presenting challenges in disease management due to interindividual variability in drug response and adverse effects. Personalized medicine, guided by pharmacogenomics, promises optimized therapeutic strategies by considering genetic influences on drug metabolism and response. Pharmacogenomic studies have found major links between genetic variants and the therapeutic efficacy of antidiabetic drugs. For metformin, polymorphisms in the SLC22A1 and SLC22A2 genes, which encode organic cation transporters (OCT1 and OCT2), critically influence drug pharmacokinetics and glycemic control. Variants such as rs12208357 and rs628031 modulate metformin transport and efficacy. Carriers of reduced-function alleles often exhibit suboptimal glycemic outcomes or increased risk of adverse effects, underscoring the potential of genotyping in therapeutic decision-making (Mannino et al., 2019; Reitman et al., 2007). Studies also highlight the influence of the rs8192675 SNP in SLC2A2 on metformin's glycemic response. This variant reduces GLUT2 expression, impairing metformin's efficacy. Despite these insights, inconsistencies across ethnic groups indicate that population-specific genetic data are critical for clinical translation (Mannino et al., 2019; Pollastro et al., 2015). Sulfonylureas, another mainstay of T2DM treatment, target ATP-sensitive potassium channels (KATP) to enhance insulin secretion. The genes ABCC8 and KCNJ11, encoding the sulfonylurea receptor 1 (SUR1) and the Kir6.2 channel, respectively, harbor variants associated with drug response variability. The rs5219 variant in KCNJ11, resulting in the K23E substitution, is linked to differential glycemic outcomes. Homozygous carriers of the risk allele exhibit higher glycemic reduction after sulfonylurea therapy, suggesting tailored dosing strategies based on genetic testing. Similarly, the A1369S variant (rs757110) in ABCC8 significantly impacts therapeutic efficacy and secondary failure rates. These findings emphasize the importance of incorporating genetic profiling in prescribing sulfonylureas, minimizing risks such as hypoglycemia and ensuring sustained efficacy (Mannino et al., 2019; Pollastro et al., 2015). Thiazolidinediones (TZDs), including pioglitazone and rosiglitazone, act as peroxisome proliferator-activated receptor-gamma (PPARγ) agonists to improve insulin sensitivity. Genetic variations in PPARG, such as the Pro12Ala polymorphism, are pivotal in modulating TZD response. Carriers of the Ala allele demonstrate improved insulin sensitivity and lipid profiles, highlighting this polymorphism's potential as a biomarker for TZD responsiveness. Furthermore, rare variants in CYP2C8, involved in TZD metabolism, also influence drug efficacy and adverse event risk. The CYP2C8*3 haplotype is associated with altered drug clearance, necessitating dose adjustments in affected individuals.

Comprehensive pharmacogenomic screening could preemptively identify patients at risk for adverse reactions, such as fluid retention and weight gain, commonly associated with TZDs (Mannino et al., 2019; Pollastro et al., 2015). The variability in drug response is not solely attributed to pharmacokinetics but also extends to pharmacodynamics. Variants in genes influencing downstream signaling pathways, such as TCF7L2 and IRS1, further compound interindividual differences in treatment outcomes. The rs7903146 polymorphism in TCF7L2, a transcription factor implicated in insulin secretion, is associated with reduced sulfonylurea efficacy. Likewise, the Gly972Arg variant in IRS1 impacts insulin signaling and contributes to secondary treatment failure. These genetic determinants reinforce the complexity of pharmacogenomic interactions in T2DM management (Mannino et al., 2019; Pollastro et al., 2015). Genetic profiling also holds promise for identifying individuals at risk for adverse drug reactions. For instance, polymorphisms in the SLC47A1 gene, encoding the multidrug and toxin extrusion protein 1 (MATE1), modulate metformin renal clearance. Variants such as rs2289669 are linked to altered drug accumulation, increasing the risk of lactic acidosis, a rare but severe complication. Similarly, genetic markers in CYP2C9, including the *2 and *3 alleles, influence sulfonylurea metabolism and hypoglycemia risk. Preemptive genotyping could mitigate these adverse events by guiding drug selection and dosage adjustments (Mannino et al., 2019; Pollastro et al., 2015; Reitman et al., 2007).

2.4 Immunotherapy for T2DM

Advances in immunogenetics have transformed the understanding and treatment of T2DM, emphasizing the role of immune dysfunction in its pathophysiology. Chronic low-grade inflammation mediated by immune cells, such as macrophages, T cells, and dendritic cells, plays a critical role in the progression of insulin resistance and β-cell dysfunction. Targeting these immune mechanisms using personalized medicine approaches, informed by immunogenetic profiling, offers novel therapeutic avenues (Dinarello, 2011; Esser et al., 2014; Kiyotani et al., 2021; Martin et al., 2015; Roth-Walter et al., 2021). Fig. 11.2 provides a comprehensive illustration of the role of major immune cells in the progression of T2DM.

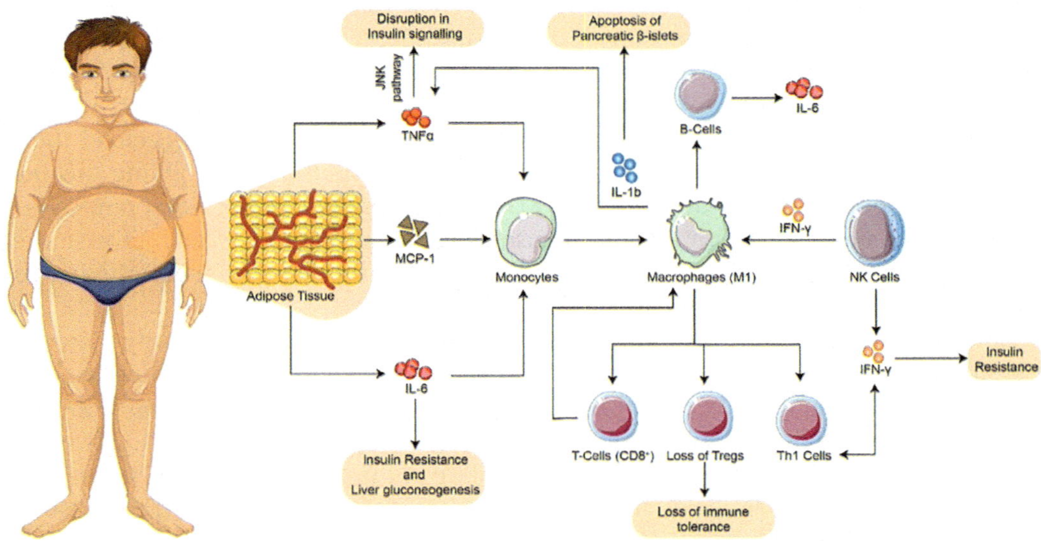

FIGURE 11.2 Role of different immune cells and cytokines in the progression of T2DM.

Macrophages, particularly their polarization states, are central to the inflammatory environment in T2DM. Proinflammatory M1 macrophages dominate in insulin-resistant tissues, releasing cytokines such as tumor necrosis factor-alpha (TNF-α) and interleukin-6 (IL-6), which impair insulin signaling and exacerbate systemic inflammation. Conversely, M2 macrophages exhibit antiinflammatory properties, promoting tissue repair and insulin sensitivity. Therapeutic strategies aimed at modulating macrophage polarization have shown potential in preclinical studies. For instance, nanoparticles delivering antiinflammatory agents or CD163 agonists have been reported to shift macrophage polarization toward the M2 phenotype, thereby alleviating insulin resistance (Esser et al., 2014; Martin et al., 2015; Roth-Walter et al., 2021). T cells also contribute significantly to the inflammatory milieu in T2DM. Studies have demonstrated an imbalance between proinflammatory T helper (Th1) and Th17 cells and regulatory T cells (Tregs), with a lower Treg-to-Th1 ratio observed in patients with T2DM. This imbalance promotes inflammation through the secretion of interferon-gamma (IFN-γ) and interleukin-17 (IL-17). Enhancing Treg function through low-dose interleukin-2 (IL-2) therapy or adoptive transfer of autologous Tregs has shown promise in animal models and early clinical trials, reducing inflammatory markers and improving glycemic control (Dinarello, 2011; Martin et al., 2015). Additionally, single-cell transcriptomics has enabled the identification of T cell subsets involved in diabetic inflammation, providing a basis for the development of targeted therapies (Kiyotani et al., 2021). Cytokines like TNF-α and IL-1β are critical drivers of inflammation in T2DM. IL-1β has been shown to impair insulin secretion and promote β-cell apoptosis. Clinical trials investigating IL-1 receptor antagonists, such as anakinra, have demonstrated significant improvements in glycemic control and reductions in systemic inflammation (Dinarello, 2011). Similarly, TNF-α inhibitors like etanercept, commonly used for autoimmune diseases, have shown potential in improving insulin sensitivity in obese patients with insulin resistance (Esser et al., 2014). These findings underscore the importance of targeting cytokine signaling pathways to mitigate inflammation and preserve β-cell function. The JAK-STAT signaling pathway is another potential target for T2DM therapy. Dysregulation of this pathway has been implicated in the chronic inflammatory state characteristic of T2DM. Selective JAK inhibitors, such as tofacitinib, which are already approved for autoimmune conditions, are now being evaluated for their ability to reduce inflammation and improve metabolic outcomes in T2DM patients (Roth-Walter et al., 2021). Immunogenetic profiling may help identify patients with hyperactivation of the JAK-STAT pathway, enabling precision-targeted interventions. Autologous stem cell transplantation (ASCT) has emerged as a transformative approach in the management of diabetes. By resetting immune homeostasis and promoting pancreatic β-cell regeneration, ASCT offers a dual mechanism for addressing T2DM pathophysiology. Mesenchymal stem cells (MSCs) are noted for their immunomodulatory properties, including the secretion of transforming growth factor-beta (TGF-β) and antiinflammatory cytokines such as IL-10. MSC-based therapies have shown efficient results in trials for type 1 diabetes, demonstrating the ability to reduce exogenous insulin requirements and preserve β-cell function. The extension of these approaches to T2DM patients with significant β-cell dysfunction could offer new therapeutic possibilities (Kiyotani et al., 2021). Chimeric antigen receptor (CAR)-T cell therapy represents another innovative immunotherapy approach for T2DM. CAR-T cells engineered to target proinflammatory immune cells, such as macrophages, or cytokine-producing T cells, have demonstrated efficacy in preclinical models of obesity-induced diabetes. This precision approach could offer a targeted method for reducing inflammation in diabetic tissues and improving insulin sensitivity (Roth-Walter et al., 2021).

Despite these advancements, several challenges hinder the clinical application of personalized immunotherapy in T2DM. The heterogeneity of the disease, influenced by genetic, environmental, and lifestyle factors, complicates the identification of universal therapeutic targets. Immunogenetic profiling is critical for stratifying patients based on their unique immune and metabolic profiles, enabling personalized interventions. However, high costs and limited accessibility of advanced diagnostic tools remain significant barriers to implementation (Esser et al., 2014). Long-term efficacy data are essential to evaluate the clinical utility of these therapies. For example, cytokine-targeting therapies may impair immune defense mechanisms, increasing susceptibility to infections and malignancies. Rigorous clinical trials with extended follow-up periods are necessary to address these concerns (Martin et al., 2015). Furthermore, combining immunotherapies with existing glucose-lowering agents, such as metformin or GLP-1 receptor agonists, may enhance outcomes by addressing both metabolic and inflammatory pathways (Dinarello, 2011).

3. Immunogenetic profiling techniques

Immunogenetic profiling involves the application of high-resolution methods to study the genetic and immune-related factors influencing the pathogenesis of T2DM and enhance understanding of disease progression.

3.1 HLA typing

HLA typing deciphers the specific HLA genes and cell surface protein markers present in an individual to understand the predisposing genetic factors and immune signaling leading to T2DM. Serological methods are conventional methods based on antibody-antigen interaction, used in the detection of HLA antigens on cell surfaces, but come along with the limitations of low resolution and indistinguishable alleles that are closely related. These drawbacks of typing result in discrepancies and failed detection of alleles, such as in the detection of HLA-C alleles, serological methods ensued significant undetectable antigen percentage (Bunce & Welsh, 1994; Feng et al., 2020). Therefore, serological approaches are found to provide erroneous diagnoses frequently as compared to molecular methods (Wu et al., 2004), like PCR-SSP, which presents high specificity for the detection of HLA alleles. This rapid and accurate molecular technique enables identification of both nonserologically and serologically defined alleles (Bunce et al., 1993, 1995).

PCR-SSP is used in typing HLA class I and II genes, overcoming the limitations of serological methods by providing higher specificity and resolution (Maruya et al., 1996). NGS revolutionized the resolution to the allele-level with accuracy and provides comprehensive profiling of HLA diversity. The rare and novel variants can also be identified using NGS technologies that provide an in-depth understanding of HLA alleles in T2DM progression. Large-scale clinical studies can be facilitated through this rapid and low-cost HLA sequencing (Kask et al., 2023). Single-cell sequencing is another technique to identify HLA expression, providing an understanding of antigen presentation dynamics in the immune cells at single-cell resolution. The heterogeneity of immune responses and function of specific HLA alleles in T2DM can be revealed through single cell approaches to delve deeper into immunological aspect of the disease (Kask et al., 2023).

3.2 Genome-wide association studies

Genome-wide association studies (GWAS) has immense contribution in exploring genetic variation across extensive cohorts suffering from T2DM. GWAS assists in the identification of specific loci associated with the disease, such as key loci - TCF7L2 and CDKN2A/B, which are consistently associated with T2DM risk across populations (Cirillo et al., 2018; Visscher et al., 2017). Identification of TCF7L2 association further revealed the mechanism of disease progression through the Wnt signaling pathway that regulates pancreatic β-cell development and its function. The variants in this locus are found to affect insulin secretion and thus are robustly found in multiple studies regarding T2DM. Similarly, the other locus—CDKN2A/B, which regulates the progression to cell cycle are responsible for replication and survival of β cells (Bailey et al., 2016; Cirillo et al., 2018; Visscher et al., 2017). GWAS have also pinpointed the role of immune-related genes in initiating inflammation and causing metabolic dysregulation in T2DM.

The polymorphisms in the IL-6R gene are observed to alter interleukin-6 receptor functionality and cause inflammation that ultimately leads to insulin resistance. Alongside, variants of TLR have been linked with altered immune responses and pathogenesis of T2DM. These association studies highlight the multifaceted aspects of immune dysregulation contributing to metabolic disturbances in T2DM (Bailey et al., 2016; Visscher et al., 2017). Among the major issues posed in GWAS is the interpretation of the functional implications for the identified variants, particularly those located in noncoding regions. The noncoding variants associated with the disease are mostly regulatory elements that modulate gene expression, as in the case of eQTL studies that demonstrated SNPs near TCF7L2 affect its expression levels in the islet cells of the pancreas and hinder insulin secretion, though the understanding of its mechanism is limited (Bailey et al., 2016). Further research is required to delve into the intricate mechanisms of regulation by noncoding variants. Another critical limitation is population diversity, where most research studies are based on the European population, leading to a biased genetic picture of T2DM. Genetic variants showed differential effects on different populations, for example, ABCA1 and LPL functions in lipid metabolism and glucose regulation in nonEuropean population which limits the generalization of risk prediction (Bailey et al., 2016; Visscher et al., 2017). To combat these drawbacks, GWAS data is complemented with additional secondary analyses like pathway analysis that associates SNPs with biological processes and provides insights about the disease mechanism. For instance, major GWAS dataset pathways revealed that PI3K-Akt signaling pathway, along with the Wnt signaling pathway, play important roles in insulin-mediated glucose uptake (Bailey et al., 2016; Mahajan et al., 2018; Visscher et al., 2017). Further, integration of GWAS findings with eQTL data has linked SNPs of both coding and noncoding regions to the changes in expression level of the genes, enhancing the functional aspect of GWAS variants. Tissue-specific analyses of eQTLs, as in liver, adipose tissue, and pancreatic islets, deciphered roles of noncoding SNPs. It was observed that SNPs in the FTO locus that are previously shown to be linked with obesity, influence expression of adipogenesis genes and indirectly pose T2DM risk (Bailey et al., 2016; Visscher et al., 2017). Gene-environmental interactions are also considered in GWAS where environmental and lifestyle factors were integrated, and it was observed that the effects of SNPs in TCF7L2 locus have been modulated by dietary habits, paving the way for a personalized strategy. The study also showed that the linkage of genetic variants associated with traits like insulin resistance is connected with lipid metabolism and adipose tissue function, while β-cell dysfunction is associated with pancreatic pathways (Bailey et al., 2016). The polygenic nature of T2DM was elucidated through GWAS variants, and therefore, polygenic risk scores (PRS) were taken into consideration that aggregate the combined effects of multiple variants in an individual to measure genetic predisposition. PRS is a potential measure for early intervention, though it is limited by the generalization of a diverse population with different genetic backgrounds (Bailey et al., 2016; Cirillo et al., 2018). GWAS also supports the discovery of novel therapeutic targets, such as the identification of the PPARG gene involved in adipogenesis and insulin sensitivity, which has assisted in the development of thiazolidinediones as a potential drug. Similarly, a potential drug target for SLC30A8 that encodes a zinc transporter in β cells was identified (Bailey et al., 2016; Cirillo et al., 2018; Visscher et al., 2017).

3.3 Next-generation sequencing

Next-generation sequencing (NGS) and Whole-Genome Sequencing (WGS) have emerged as pivotal methods to capture the genetic landscape, including rare mutations and structural variants influencing the development and progression of T2DM. Immunogenetic categorization has drastically changed the knowledge about T2DM due to the disclosure of the genetic risk and its relationship with the immune system. New approaches, particularly molecular profiling through NGS, enable researchers to map intricate and more precise genomic variations associated with T2DM. NGS allows for the detection of SNPs, structural variants, and epigenetic changes, showing how genetic and immune system players interact as related to the disease process and initiation (Bewicke-Copley et al., 2019; Cao et al., 2019). WGS, an extensive NGS application, enables the analysis of the entire genome with regard to genes and introns. This is especially important in T2DM because functionally important noncoding regions hold regulatory elements that control genes involved in insulin synthesis, inflammation, and metabolism. As WGS looks for rare mutations and structural variants, the genetic architecture of T2DM, represented as polygenic and multifactorial, can be fully appreciated. These insights allow identifying previously unknown regions within the GWAS genes, which influence susceptibility in individuals. Moreover, WGS contributes to the development of the new individualized approach to T2DM therapy. The inclusion of genotypes in clinical practice is useful in that risk-stratified populations can be identified, and therapies targeting the immune or metabolic cascade can be developed. This strategy minimizes therapeutic efficacy and augments potential adverse effects, which testifies to the novelty of genomic technologies in clinical practice (Bewicke-Copley et al., 2019; Cao et al., 2019).

3.4 Whole exome sequencing

WES has emerged as a central diagnostic test for the analysis of genetic susceptibility and molecular mechanisms of T2DM. Because most documented disease-associated mutations occur in protein-coding regions, WES offers an economical and practical substitute to WGS. This technique identifies both frequent and low-frequency SNPs and Indels associated with T2DM pathogenesis (Malhotra et al., 2023; Zhou et al., 2021). In T2DM analysis, WES has contributed positively to the identification of multiple genetic factors linked to insulin responsiveness and release. For example, there are case reports of familial mutation dealing with genes like the CAMKK2 and PNLIPRP1, which belong to the pathway of glucose metabolism and insulin signaling. These outcomes raise the possibility of using WES for identifying potential genes for subsequent functional characterization and therapeutic intervention (Feng et al., 2020; Malhotra et al., 2023). Further, WES gives perceptions about the polygenic nature of T2DM. The study of a huge population has revealed more than 75 regions associated with the disease, and many of the "risk" SNPs have moderate ORs. These outcomes suggest multiple genetic factors that play a role in the expression of diseases, together with the multiple environmental factors that contribute to the onset of diseases. Furthermore, WES can identify undetectable mutations by targeted panels and therefore advance a more comprehensive understanding of the genetic architecture involved in T2DM (Malhotra et al., 2023; Zhou et al., 2021). As a cost-effective and targeted strategy, WES can be employed both for detecting key genetic changes and for explaining the mechanisms of T2DM development. This has seen its application remain useful in enhancing precision medicine by offering a platform for genomic development of targeted interventions (Feng et al., 2020).

3.5 Targeted sequencing

Consequently, targeted sequencing methods, mostly NGS, offer a suitable framework for analyzing immunogenic DNA sequences and genes involved in immune recognition, signaling, and CPRs. These approaches allow a more detailed analysis of immunogenetic differences as well as immunity on an individual and population level (Chen et al., 2021; Kask et al., 2023; Minervina et al., 2019). Especially noteworthy, as polymorphic genes involved in the mechanism of antigen presentation, HLA loci are outstanding. The advancement of high-speed platforms like long-read nanopore sequencing makes HLA typing more precise within the regions of high polymorphism and with more depth. This advancement enables detailed immune phenotyping, which is essential in deciphering T-cell-mediated action in T2DM. Furthermore, these approaches decrease the time and cost, making them superior to traditional genotyping techniques for clinic and research purposes (Chen et al., 2021; Kask et al., 2023). Further, the methods for predicting HLA alleles and other immune gene variants from whole-genome or exome sequencing data have been greatly enhanced through computational methods. It needs to be understood that these tools yield 97% concordance in terms of HLA allele typing, making them useful clinically. When combined with specific algorithms applicable to sequence data, T2DM's immunogenetic pertinence can be unveiled with more detailed analysis on how each variant in immunologically related genes relates to disease risk (Chen et al., 2021). In addition, by targeting cytokines and pattern recognition receptors, immune repertoire sequencing shows differences in adaptive immunity, including T cell receptor and B cell receptor repertoires. Next-generation sequencing can be used to accurately measure the variables and immune signaling related to T2DM, allowing for the discovery of new biomarkers for disease progression. The combined approach of genetic and immune risk prediction thus forms a solid base for progressive development of individual-specific therapies in T2DM (Minervina et al., 2019).

4. Single-cell omics

4.1 Single-cell RNA-Seq (scRNA-Seq)

Single-cell RNA sequencing technique, also known as scRNA-Seq is revolutionizing the study of the development of T2DM. This technology makes it possible to delineate and determine various cell subpopulations and activation profiles, as well as the inflammatory markers that are cardinal in the development of T2DM. Among the key findings resulting from scRNA-Seq is the elucidation of the pathophysiology of pancreatic β-cell dysfunction in T2DM. Understanding redox signaling in relationship to β-cells has revealed that modifications in this aspect of the signaling pathway are implicated in β-cell dysfunction and, therefore, in the disease's onset (Marques et al., 2021). In addition, the help of scRNA-Seq to study such molecular changes in pancreatic islets shows the complexity of T2DM at the cellular level (Wang & Sander, 2021). The use of scRNA-Seq is not limited to pancreatic cells only. It has been applied to determine common features between T2DM and other diseases, including colorectal cancer, through molecular and immune features (Luo et al., 2024). This approach has shown that several genes, including EVPL and ENTPD3, are involved in T2DM and cancer and therefore can be targets for drug treatment. Also, in T2DM, scRNA-Seq has led to the discovery of new therapeutic targets and possible drugs. For instance, the CCR5 gene is a potential target, and demonstrative drugs may be able to bind the target well according to the scRNA-Seq data, suggesting the way forward for precise medication (Zhou et al., 2022). It underlines that scRNA-Seq contributes not only to the explication of diseases but also to the identification of new treatment targets.

4.2 Epigenomic profiling

Epigenomic profiling is a powerful tool for understanding the molecular mechanisms underlying T2DM. This approach involves analyzing DNA methylation, histone modifications, and chromatin accessibility to identify epigenetic changes that may contribute to the disease.

4.3 DNA methylation analysis

DNA methylation changes are crucial in regulating gene expression, particularly in immune-related genes such as cytokine genes. These changes can serve as markers for predicting T2DM risk. An epigenome-wide association study (EWAS) identified novel CpG sites associated with T2DM risk, i.e., alterations of methylation at specific CpG sites of genes like MIR1287 and EDN2-SCMH1 (Giri et al., 2023). Bisulfite sequencing and methylation-specific PCR, though demands high costs, are standard methods for profiling DNA methylation. An economical alternative is the DNA pooling technique, which allows for large-scale epigenetic investigations by generating precise quantitative assessments by taking the mean value of group DNA methylation, thus reducing the time and required DNA sample (Docherty et al., 2010).

4.4 High-throughput genotyping

High-throughput genotyping technologies such as microarray-based genotyping, MassARRAY technology, and digital droplet PCR (ddPCR) are trend-setting technologies as they embark on achieving these goals. These techniques make it possible to perform the examination of single-nucleotide polymorphisms and to determine rare genetic variants and differences that disclose the molecular pathogenesis of T2DM (Bortolin et al., 2004; Iwasaki et al., 2002; Pastinen et al., 2000). Microarray-based genotyping enables large-scale screening of SNPs by using allele-specific primers immobilized on arrays, where hybridization distinguishes genetic variations. This method's efficacy lies in its ability to process thousands of genetic loci simultaneously, with high specificity and accuracy. Pastinen et al. demonstrated its utility in identifying SNPs linked to multifactorial diseases, including metabolic disorders like T2DM, by achieving a success rate nearing 100% across diverse genetic variants (Pastinen et al., 2000). Moreover, advancements in enzyme-assisted primer extension have enhanced the sensitivity of microarray platforms, ensuring the robust detection of even minor allele frequencies

(Pastinen et al., 2000). MassARRAY technology combines mass spectrometry with multiplex PCR, offering precise SNP genotyping with exceptional accuracy and scalability. Its high-throughput capabilities make it particularly advantageous for investigating immune-related genetic variants in T2DM. By leveraging the precision of mass spectrometry, this technique minimizes errors associated with traditional genotyping approaches, thus providing a reliable method for profiling disease-associated SNPs (Bortolin et al., 2004). Furthermore, MassARRAY technology provides an additional layer of precision by integrating mass spectrometry. This approach is particularly suited for fine mapping immune-related genes in T2DM, where identifying functional variants is critical. The multiplex nature of MassARRAY enables the analysis of numerous SNPs in a single reaction, reducing time and reagent costs. Its robustness in detecting both common and rare variants makes it a valuable tool for genome-wide association studies (GWAS) targeting immune pathways in T2DM (Bortolin et al., 2004). Moreover, its ability to resolve ambiguous genotypes through mass spectrometric analysis of nucleotide mass adds an extra dimension of reliability. Digital droplet PCR (ddPCR) represents a breakthrough in detecting low-frequency variants, including rare immune gene mutations implicated in T2DM. Its partition-based approach allows for the absolute quantification of DNA molecules, ensuring unparalleled sensitivity and specificity. Iwasaki et al. validated the ddPCR technique's potential in analyzing SNPs across various genomic regions, highlighting its suitability for rare variant detection in complex diseases like T2DM (Iwasaki et al., 2002). The advent of digital droplet PCR (ddPCR) has revolutionized rare variant detection. Unlike traditional PCR, ddPCR partitions the DNA sample into thousands of droplets, allowing independent amplification events. This partitioning minimizes background noise and increases the detection sensitivity for low-abundance alleles. In the context of T2DM, where rare immune gene mutations may play a pivotal role, ddPCR provides a powerful means to detect these variants with high specificity. For instance, studies leveraging ddPCR have uncovered low-frequency SNPs in immune regulatory genes, providing new avenues for understanding their contributions to T2DM pathogenesis (Iwasaki et al., 2002). Microarray-based genotyping also addresses challenges in studying large population cohorts. By employing oligonucleotide probes for allele-specific hybridization, this technique achieves high accuracy in distinguishing between homozygous and heterozygous genotypes. Iwasaki et al. reported that microarray platforms demonstrated a genotyping accuracy of 99.9% when compared with single-base extension and direct sequencing methods (Iwasaki et al., 2002). The integration of fluorescent probes and multiplex PCR amplification further enhances this platform's utility, enabling simultaneous analysis of multiple genetic loci in a high-throughput manner. The combination of these high-throughput genotyping methods has significantly enhanced our ability to identify genetic variants associated with T2DM. For instance, microarray-based genotyping has been employed in studies to map SNPs in inflammatory cytokine genes, revealing their associations with insulin resistance and beta-cell dysfunction. Similarly, MassARRAY technology has been instrumental in fine mapping the HLA region, identifying alleles that confer susceptibility to T2DM through immune modulation. ddPCR, with its unparalleled sensitivity, has uncovered previously undetectable rare variants in immune signaling pathways, shedding light on novel mechanisms of disease progression (Bortolin et al., 2004; Iwasaki et al., 2002; Pastinen et al., 2000). These technologies are also instrumental in identifying gene-environment interactions in T2DM. By enabling the simultaneous analysis of genetic variants and their epigenetic modifications, high-throughput genotyping methods provide a holistic view of the molecular landscape driving T2DM. For example, studies using microarrays have revealed methylation patterns in immune gene promoters that correlate with T2DM risk. MassARRAY's precision has been used to validate these findings, providing quantitative insights into the extent of epigenetic changes. ddPCR, with its high resolution, has further corroborated these results by quantifying allele-specific expression patterns, linking immune gene variants to altered metabolic outcomes (Bortolin et al., 2004; Iwasaki et al., 2002). The clinical implications of these findings are profound. By pinpointing immune gene variants associated with T2DM, researchers can develop targeted therapeutic strategies aimed at modulating immune responses. For instance, inhibitors targeting proinflammatory cytokines identified through microarray studies are currently under investigation for their potential to improve insulin sensitivity. MassARRAY's contributions to pharmacogenomics have identified SNPs influencing drug metabolism, paving the way for personalized medicine approaches in T2DM management. ddPCR's role in rare variant detection has opened new avenues for gene-editing therapies aimed at correcting pathogenic mutations (Bortolin et al., 2004; Pastinen et al., 2000).

5. Proteomic and metabolomic profiling

5.1 Mass spectrometry-based proteomics

Protein mass spectrometry is now a central tool for analyzing immune signaling proteins, cytokines, and HLA-bound peptides, especially in relation to T2DM. This strategy provides a broad survey of the inherent proteome, as well as allowing for the prioritization of several proteins and their involvement in immune signaling and disease development. Protein identification and quantification can be achieved in high throughput through the application of mass spectrometry, also known as MS. It is especially applied in proteomics due to its capability for the separation of protein complexes and the detection of modified peptides. Technology has evolved over time to increase sensitivity, quantitative precision, and sample turnaround, making it an essential tool in current proteomics analysis (Cox & Mann, 2008; Deutsch et al., 2023; Navarrete-Perea et al., 2018). The immune-signaling proteins have been identified using proteomics employing MS in several cellular systems. These proteins have important functions in the regulation of immune reactions and are associated with the pathogenesis of autoimmune diseases and T2DM. For example, the Trans-Proteomic Pipeline (TPP) is equipped with unparalleled spectrum processing and protein inference capabilities that are critical in the discovery of immune signaling proteins from heavily alienated biological mixtures (Deutsch et al., 2023). Cytokines are essential in cell communication and signaling, and their misregulation is linked with inflammation, T2DM, and other allied disorders. Cytokines are well characterized as signaling molecules, and their quantities and effects can be elucidated by MS-based proteomics. However, integrating proteomics with other techniques like mass cytometry to dissect cytokine signaling networks and drive immune cell function remains to be profound (Wang et al., 2023). The analysis of bound HLA-peptides is relevant to the assessment of antigen presentation and immune recognition. As a result, algorithms derived from MS have been designed to provide a precise identification of complexes of HLA molecules with the ligands, which form a part of the so-called HLA peptidome (Navarrete-Perea et al., 2018).

5.2 Metabolomics

Metabolomics for T2DM concerns the analysis of metabolites, especially those associated with immune cells, including inflammatory lipid mediators. This field employs such analytical strategies as Nuclear Magnetic Resonance (NMR) spectroscopy and Liquid Chromatography-Mass Spectrometry (LC-MS) to understand the metabolic perturbation linked with T2DM (Kopriva et al., 2020). One of the applications of NMR spectroscopy is in quantitative analysis of body fluids, including urine samples and blood plasma, because of its ability to handle large numbers of samples. However, the fact that 1H NMR operates at a relatively low frequency means that the resolution of the signal is poor, and often signals can be masked in complex mixtures — a typical problem in metabolomics. To overcome this, a strategy known as nonnegative least squares (NNLS) has been introduced in the quantification of overlapping metabolites in 1H NMR spectra. This method involves using a database of pure component spectra by which the complex mixture spectra are resolved into a series of metabolite concentrations. Inas much as applying this approach in T2DM, the aim has been to pinpoint metabolites that differentiate T2DM patients from control subjects. More than all, 63 of them were identified as having significant differences between the T2DM group and the healthy control group, and 46 metabolites exhibited significantly different levels between the controls and T2DM patients. These results are cross-verified using other analytical tools and are consistent with the literature supplemented by NMR-based metabolomics for the discovery of biomarkers for T2DM (Kopriva et al., 2020).

Another important approach mentioned in metabolomics is LC-MS, which provides an additional view on the intracellular metabolism, or more specifically, immune cells. Immunometabolism is an essential subject in elucidating T2DM, as it is established that metabolism in immune cells is abnormal in this disease. Recent research used LC-MS in a project related to the identification of changes in the human monocytes' metabolic profile in response to lipopolysaccharide (LPS) stimulation, an immune activation model. This work used methanol-based extraction and raw HILIC for the comprehensive sampling of monocyte metabolites. The study showed that metabolism in monocytes was affected beginning 4 hours after LPS stimulation for the following: amino acids and Krebs cycle metabolites were increasing; aspartate and β-alanine were decreasing. These alterations are paralleled by enhanced cytokine release, indicating that metabolic modifications are possibly tightly connected with activating the immune defense system. The overall metabolite profiling approach identified 154 significantly altered metabolites, while pathway analysis revealed alterations in inositol metabolism, glycolysis, and the pentose phosphate pathway. Consequently, these studies demonstrate the potency of LC-MS in characterizing the metabolic basis for immune cell activation in T2DM (Leacy et al., 2023). The use of NMR and coupled LC-MS offers a systematic approach toward understanding the metabolomics of T2DM. The ratio of L/B to NMR is relatively high, providing quantitative information about biofluids, whereas LC-MS gives metabolomic and immune cell metabolic information. Combined, these approaches help establish metabolic biomarkers and the associations between T2DM and altered metabolic pathways that may be targeted for treatment. The selectivity in identifying targeted immune cell metabolite levels is especially useful since immune cells and inflammation are essential in T2DM development and progression (Kopriva et al., 2020; Leacy et al., 2023).

6. Cytometric techniques

6.1 Flow cytometry

Flow cytometry remains a valuable approach to the analysis of immune cell populations and their activation status, especially in T2DM. This technique enables sample scientists to dissect T cell and β cell subpopulations that are important in the study of the immune pathology present in T2DM. It is highly utilized to evaluate the immunophenotyping of T cells and serves to study T cell receptor clonality and MRD in different diseases that are characterized by neoplasia. The technique is known as T-cell receptor (TCR) νβ repertoire analysis, which is specific in identifying T-cell clonality. These techniques have been employed to identify T cell neoplasia and estimate MRD in clinical practice (Tembhare et al., 2011). The assessment of T-cell clonality by flow cytometry is often difficult because of complex techniques and suboptimal sensitivity, particularly when used to determine low disease burden. Therefore, there are new trends in the methodology that have enhanced the detection of T-cell receptor clonality, such as the use of TRBC1 expression analysis (Berg et al., 2020). In T2DM, the immune system disease, and the key subsets of T cells and B cells are directly involved in the development of the disease. Flow cytometry helps in the identification of various immune cell populations at once, and besides T and B cells, other cells can also be identified through multicolor labeling. This capability is particularly important for dissecting the immune-related factors in T2DM patients (Horan et al., 1986). Flow cytometry can be used to perform a detailed phenotyping of the T cells, where T cell subsets like the $CD4^+$ and the $CD8^+$ T cells, as well as their effector memory, can be determined. These results provide insight into the functional specialization of T cells and their potential ability to either maintain immunological self-tolerance or participate in autoimmunity, which is considered in T2DM (Mousset et al., 2019). Subsequently, the development of more advanced flow cytometry panels, including 43 color panels, further refined the differentiation of immune cell populations. These panels allow for the dissection of both traditional and atypical T cells, B cells, NK cells, monocytes, dendritic cells, and ILCs. Such comprehensive panels are useful specifically when the number of specimens is low, as they provide a more complete understanding of the immune system in T2DM patients (Mousset et al., 2019). These include spectral flow cytometry, which employs conjugated fluorochromes with overlapping emission profiles, thus enhancing the analytical capability of the equipment. This advancement enables the utilization of spectrally similar fluorochrome pairs in a single panel, which enables the detailed depiction of immune cells in T2DM (Mousset et al., 2019).

6.2 Mass cytometry

Mass cytometry, also known as Cytometry by Time-of-Flight (CyTOF), is a transformative technology that enables high-dimensional immune profiling by simultaneously measuring dozens of markers at the single-cell level. This capability is particularly valuable in the context of T2DM, where understanding the immune landscape can provide insights into disease mechanisms and potential therapeutic targets. CyTOF technology utilizes metal-tagged antibodies to achieve high-dimensional single-cell analysis, allowing researchers to profile complex biological samples with unprecedented detail. This is particularly useful for monitoring systemic immune changes, such as those that may occur in T2DM or during cancer immunotherapy (Saederup et al., 2022). The technology's ability to resolve over 40 markers in a single panel without the need for compensation makes it ideal for routine immunophenotyping and comprehensive immune profiling (Selvanantham et al., 2022). The vast amount of data generated by CyTOF poses significant analytical challenges. Traditional methods like manual gating are labor-intensive and can introduce bias.

To address these challenges, new computational tools and frameworks have been developed. For instance, ImmCellTyper is a novel toolkit designed for CyTOF data analysis, incorporating a semisupervised clustering tool called BinaryClust. This tool automatically identifies main cell types and outperforms existing clustering tools in accuracy and speed, providing a comprehensive solution for CyTOF data analysis (Sun et al., 2024a; 2024b). In the context of T2DM, CyTOF can be used to explore the immune cell populations involved in the disease. The technology's ability to provide a high-resolution multiparametric landscape of single cells allows for the identification of novel cellular subsets and the characterization of immune cell phenotypes. This is crucial for understanding the immune dysregulation associated with T2DM and for identifying potential biomarkers for disease progression and treatment response (Mujib et al., 2021). Recent innovations in CyTOF technology have further expanded its capabilities. For example, the development of new mass tags based on nanometal organic frameworks (NMOFs) has improved the sensitivity and multiplexing detection ability of CyTOF. These NMOF-based mass tags provide significant signal amplification and are compatible with existing mass tag systems, enhancing the technology's utility for high-dimensional single-cell immune profiling (Dang et al., 2021). CyTOF is often integrated with other technologies and analytical platforms to enhance its utility. For instance, automated analysis platforms like Astrolabe can streamline data processing and analysis, making it easier to track batch variability and ensure data quality. Additionally, the use of continuous metrics and trajectory inference methods can provide deeper insights into the dynamics of immune cell states, which is particularly useful in translational research and clinical trials (Sidiropoulos et al., 2022).

6.3 Functional genomics

Recent advancements in functional genomics have provided new insights into the pathogenesis of T2DM, particularly through the usage of state-of-the-art technologies like CRISPR/Cas9 screens and RNA interference (RNAi) techniques. CRISPR/Cas9 technology enables precise gene editing and allows researchers to systematically knock out genes in immune cells to identify the critical ones involved in T2DM pathogenesis. When this technology is combined with genome-scale guide RNA libraries, it provides unbiased phenotypic screening of genetic elements. This technique is thus crucial in the discovery and annotation of genes involved in immune responses to cause T2DM (Shalem et al., 2015). One such innovative application popularly used is the CHimeric IMmune Editing (CHIME) system that bypasses ex vivo manipulation and enables in vivo screening of both innate and adaptive immune cells. By using a bone marrow delivery system, this technique allows efficient gene deletion in immune lineages without hindering their development and function. The CHIME system has been used to identify genes like Ptpn2-a negative regulator of $CD8^+$ T cell-mediated responses- and therefore can also be implemented in dissecting immune responses in T2DM by knocking out specific genes to study cell behavior and identify potential therapeutic targets (LaFleur et al., 2019). RNA interference (RNAi) is another powerful tool used in functional genomics to study the role of specific genes in inflammation and insulin resistance, both of which are key components of T2DM. RNAi works by silencing specific genes, allowing researchers to investigate their function and contribution to disease processes. This technique is particularly useful for studying immune genes involved in T2DM, as it can help elucidate the molecular mechanisms underlying inflammation and insulin resistance (LaFleur et al., 2019). In comparison to CRISPR/Cas9, RNAi opts for a different approach to gene silencing. While the former technique permanently knocks out genes, RNAi temporarily reduces gene expression, providing a reversible method to study gene function. This can be advantageous in cases where permanent gene knockout may lead to compensatory mechanisms or is found to be lethal, which could obscure the gene's role in disease (Shalem et al., 2015). RNAi has been used extensively to study the role of immune genes in T2DM. By silencing genes involved in inflammatory pathways, researchers can assess their impact on insulin signaling and glucose metabolism. This approach has led to the identification of several key genes that contribute to insulin resistance, providing insights into potential therapeutic targets for T2DM. The integration of CRISPR/Cas9 and RNAi technologies offers a comprehensive approach to studying the genetic basis of T2DM. While CRISPR/Cas9 provides a robust method for gene knockout and functional annotation, RNAi offers a complementary approach for gene silencing and functional analysis. Together, these technologies enable a deeper understanding of the complex interactions between immune genes and T2DM pathogenesis (LaFleur et al., 2019).

6.4 Multi-omics integration

Owing to the complexity of T2DM, integration of various data derived from genomics, transcriptomics, proteomics, and epigenomics potentially provides a broad landscape of immune regulation associated with the disorder. Multi-omics data are integrated through advanced machine learning and network analysis approaches that enhance understanding of underlying mechanisms and identification of novel biomarkers and therapeutic targets. Machine learning models handle high-dimensional multi-omics data to discover complex patterns and interactions that are often overlooked through a single approach (Ivanisevic & Sewduth, 2023). The effective combination of different omics layers offers novel insights into biological systems through various integration methods like early, mixed, intermediate, late, and hierarchical integration strategies (Picard et al., 2021). Machine learning methods assist powerful prediction and interpretation through enabling omics data transformation into illustrations and facilitating downstream analysis (Hu et al., 2023). Similarly, network analysis is an effective technique to map interactions between immune-associated pathways in T2DM progression. The regulatory nodes and pathways involved in the disease are highlighted through complex mapping among genes, proteins, and metabolites (Sanches et al., 2024). Analyses and visualization of the interaction webs of regulatory nodes provide insights into potential therapeutic targets. The interplay between different omics layers and simultaneous effects of T2DM is better understood using network-based methods such as interactome and coexpression analysis that further enhances our understanding of disease pathology and potential therapeutic targets (Nicora et al., 2020).

7. Emerging techniques

7.1 Spatial transcriptomics

Spatial transcriptomics is an innovative technology that provides a high-resolution map of gene expression within the spatial context of tissues. This technology has significant implications for understanding the pathophysiology of T2DM, particularly in linking gene expression to specific tissue microenvironments such as inflamed adipose tissue or pancreatic islets (Kim & Lee, 2023). Spatial transcriptomics allows researchers to map gene expression patterns in specific tissues affected by T2DM, such as visceral adipose tissue, liver, skeletal muscle, and pancreas. This mapping is crucial for identifying tissue-specific expression quantitative trait loci (eQTL) that influence gene expression in these tissues (Kim & Lee, 2023). By understanding these patterns, researchers can identify genes and pathways that are dysregulated in T2DM, providing insights into the disease's molecular mechanisms. The integration of spatial transcriptomics with genome-wide association studies (GWAS) has led to the identification of spatial eGenes that are colocalized with T2DM GWAS signals. These eGenes are enriched in various biological pathways, with a notable emphasis on the lysosomal pathway in pancreatic tissue (Kim & Lee, 2023). They suggest that the lysosomal pathway plays a critical role in the autophagic processes associated with T2DM, highlighting a potential area for therapeutic intervention (Kim & Lee, 2023). Recent advancements in spatial transcriptomics technologies have enabled the development of highly multiplexed methods and single-cell resolution techniques. These advancements allow for a more detailed analysis of gene expression patterns within their native spatial context, providing a deeper understanding of tissue architecture and cellular interactions (Robles-Remacho et al., 2023). The ability to analyze gene expression at such a high resolution is particularly beneficial for studying complex diseases like T2DM, where multiple tissues and cell types are involved.

8. Challenges and future directions

T2DM is thus a complex disorder that poses significant challenges for its clinical management. With advancing research, several clinical, technical, and ethical issues are addressed while developing precision medicine against this disorder. Privacy concerns rise from the vast amount of data generated, owned, and shared, necessitating robust data security measures to protect patient information. The integration of genetic technologies and genome-wide testing also holds the potential for stigma as personalized medicine becomes prevalent (Ormond & Cho, 2014). Hence, the ethical medical practice of informed consent should be mandated during genetic testing for T2DM. Genetic counseling, including the information about implications of genetic testing and potential risks/benefits, should be provided to the patients to help them make informed decisions benefiting them as well as research studies. The major challenge in developing countries is that access to precision medicine is limited by socioeconomic factors and low-resource settings. The cost of personalized genetic testing is found to be high, and even access to these modern technologies is required to carry out significant disease management (Ormond & Cho, 2014; Thomas et al., 2016). The technical challenges surrounding T2DM are the complexity of the disorder. The issue is to pinpoint a specific marker while the nature of the disease is polygenic and requires a comprehensive study of genomic and epigenetic interactions. To develop effective personalized medicine, these complex interactions need to be explored and targeted simultaneously for the treatment of T2DM (Venkatachalapathy et al., 2021). The understanding of immune mechanisms in the development of T2DM is limited, and further research is required to elucidate these complex mechanisms for the development of targeted therapy (Chen et al., 2012). The reduced interest in clinical trials in the case of T2DM is due to disease heterogeneity, where incorporating genetic, environmental, and socioeconomic factors poses major challenges. Robust trial designs to include all these variabilities are therefore crucial to advance personalized medicine approaches. Overall, the integrated usage of multi-omics and advances in pharmacogenomics has enhanced our understanding and paved the way for individualized therapies based on genetic and genomic information in healthcare. The identification of biomarkers has revolutionized the treatment of T2DM through better prediction and response, improving patient outcomes and reducing diabetic burden (Philipson, 2019).

References

Akash, M. S. H., Rehman, K., & Liaqat, A. (2018). Tumor necrosis factor-alpha: Role in development of insulin resistance and pathogenesis of type 2 diabetes mellitus. *Journal of Cellular Biochemistry, 119* (1), 105–110.

Almawi, W. Y., Wakim-Ghorayeb, S. F., Arekat, M. R., Najm, P., Keleshian, S. H., Al-Sayed, N., Blanchon, B., Samaha, H. R., & Irani-Hakime, N. (2006). Association of selective HLA class II susceptibility-conferring and protective haplotypes with type 2 diabetes in patients from Bahrain and Lebanon. *Clinical and Vaccine Immunology, 13*(11), 1296–1298.

American Diabetes Association. (2014). Diagnosis and classification of diabetes mellitus. *Diabetes Care, 37*(Suppl. 1), S81–S90.

Bailey, J. N. C., Loomis, S. J., Kang, J. H., Allingham, R. R., Gharahkhani, P., Khor, C. C., Burdon, K. P., Aschard, H., Chasman, D. I., Igo Jr, R. P., et al. (2016). Genome-wide association analysis identifies TXNRD2, ATXN2 and FOXC1 as susceptibility loci for primary open-angle glaucoma. *Nature Genetics, 48*(2), 189–194.

Berg, H., Otteson, G. E., Corley, H., Shi, M., Horna, P., Jevremovic, D., & Olteanu, H. (2020). Flow cytometric evaluation of TRBC1 expression in tissue specimens and body fluids is a novel and specific method for assessment of T-cell clonality and diagnosis of T-cell neoplasms. *Cytometry Part B: Clinical Cytometry, 100*, 361–369. https://doi.org/10.1002/cyto.b.21881

Bewicke-Copley, F., Kumar, E. A., Palladino, G., Korfi, K., & Wang, J. (2019). Applications and analysis of targeted genomic sequencing in cancer studies. *Computational and Structural Biotechnology Journal, 17*, 1348–1359.

Bortolin, S., Black, M., Modi, H., Boszko, I., Kobler, D., Fieldhouse, D., Lopes, E., Lacroix, J.-M., Grimwood, R., Wells, P., et al. (2004). Analytical validation of the Tag-It high-throughput microsphere-based universal array genotyping platform: Application to the multiplex detection of a panel of thrombophilia-associated single-nucleotide polymorphisms. *Clinical Chemistry, 50*(11), 2028–2036.

Bozkurt, O., De Boer, A., Grobbee, D. E., Heerdink, E. R., Burger, H., & Klungel, O. H. (2007). Pharmacogenetics of glucose-lowering drug treatment: A systematic review. *Molecular Diagnosis and Therapy, 11*, 291–302.

Bunce, M., Fanning, G., & Welsh, K. I. (1995). Comprehensive, serologically equivalent DNA typing for HLA-B by PCR using sequence-specific primers (PCR-SSP). *Tissue Antigens, 45*(2), 81–90.

Bunce, M., Taylor, C., & Welsh, K. (1993). Rapid HLA-DQB typing by eight polymerase chain reaction amplifications with sequence-specific primers (PCR-SSP). *Human Immunology, 37*(4), 201–206.

Bunce, M., & Welsh, K. (1994). Rapid DNA typing for HLA-C using sequence-specific primers (PCR-SSP): Identification of serological and non-serologically defined HLA-C alleles including several new alleles. *Tissue Antigens, 43*(1), 7–17.

Cao, J., Chen, L., Li, H., Chen, H., Yao, J., Mu, S., Liu, W., Zhang, P., Cheng, Y., Liu, B., et al. (2019). An accurate and comprehensive clinical sequencing assay for cancer targeted and immunotherapies. *The Oncologist, 24*(12), e1294–e1302.

Chatterjee, S., Khunti, K., & Davies, M. J. (2017). Type 2 diabetes. *The Lancet, 389*(10085), 2239–2251.

Chen, J., Madireddi, S., Nagarkar, D., Migdal, M., Vander Heiden, J., Chang, D., Mukhyala, K., Selvaraj, S., Kadel III, E. E., Brauer, M. J., et al. (2021). In silico tools for accurate HLA and KIR inference from clinical sequencing data empower immunogenetics on individual-patient and population scales. *Briefings in Bioinformatics, 22*(3), Article bbaa223.

Chen, L., Magliano, D., & Zimmet, P. (2012). The worldwide epidemiology of type 2 diabetes mellitus—present and future perspectives. *Nature Reviews Endocrinology, 8*, 228–236. https://doi.org/10.1038/nrendo.2011.183

Chinniah, R., Vijayan, M., Sivanadham, R., Ravi, P. M., Panneerselvam, D., & Karuppiah, B. (2016). Association of HLA-A, B, DRB1* and DQB1* alleles and haplotypes in south Indian T2DM patients. *Gene, 592*(1), 200–208.

Cirillo, E., Kutmon, M., Gonzalez Hernandez, M., Hooimeijer, T., Adriaens, M. E., Eijssen, L. M., Parnell, L. D., Coort, S. L., & Evelo, C. T. (2018). From SNPs to pathways: Biological interpretation of type 2 diabetes (T2DM) genome wide association study (GWAS) results. *PLoS One, 13*(4), Article e0193515.

Cox, J., & Mann, M. (2008). MaxQuant enables high peptide identification rates, individualized p.p.b.-range mass accuracies and proteome-wide protein quantification. *Nature Biotechnology, 26*, 1367–1372. https://doi.org/10.1038/nbt.1511

Dang, J., Li, H., Zhang, L., Li, S., Zhang, T., Huang, S., Li, Y., Huang, C., Ke, Y., Shen, G., Zhi, X., & Ding, X. (2021). New structure mass tag based on Zr-NMOF for multiparameter and sensitive single-cell interrogating in mass cytometry. *Advanced Materials, 33*. https://doi.org/10.1002/adma.202008297

Daryabor, G., Atashzar, M. R., Kabelitz, D., Meri, S., & Kalantar, K. (2020). The effects of type 2 diabetes mellitus on organ metabolism and the immune system. *Frontiers in Immunology, 11*, 1582.

DeFronzo, R. A. (2009). From the triumvirate to the ominous octet: A new paradigm for the treatment of type 2 diabetes mellitus. *Diabetes, 58*(4), 773–795.

Deutsch, E., Mendoza, L., Shteynberg, D. D., Hoopmann, M., Sun, Z., Eng, J., & Moritz, R. (2023). Trans-proteomic pipeline: Robust mass spectrometry-based proteomics data analysis suite. *Journal of Proteome Research*. https://doi.org/10.1021/acs.jproteome.2c00624

Dinarello, C. A. (2011). Interleukin-1 in the pathogenesis and treatment of inflammatory diseases. *Blood, 117*(14), 3720–3732.

Docherty, S. J., Davis, O. S., Haworth, C. M., Plomin, R., & Mill, J. (2010). DNA methylation profiling using bisulfite-based epityping of pooled genomic DNA. *Methods, 52*(3), 255–258.

Donath, M. Y., Dinarello, C. A., & Mandrup-Poulsen, T. (2019). Targeting innate immune mediators in type 1 and type 2 diabetes. *Nature Reviews Immunology, 19*(12), 734–746.

Esser, N., Legrand-Poels, S., Piette, J., Scheen, A. J., & Paquot, N. (2014). Inflammation as a link between obesity, metabolic syndrome and type 2 diabetes. *Diabetes Research and Clinical Practice, 105*(2), 141–150.

Evangelou, E., Warren, H. R., Mosen-Ansorena, D., Mifsud, B., Pazoki, R., Gao, H., Ntritsos, G., Dimou, N., Cabrera, C. P., Karaman, I., et al. (2018). Genetic analysis of over 1 million people identifies 535 new loci associated with blood pressure traits. *Nature Genetics, 50*(10), 1412–1425.

Feng, Z., Scheuenpflug, J., Tan, M., & Wang, D. (2020). *Whole-exome sequencing based immunogenomic profiling with potential clinical applicability in circulating cell-free DNA and tissue from advanced stage colorectal cancer patients.*

Friedman, J. H. (2001). Greedy function approximation: A gradient boosting machine. *Annals of Statistics*, 1189–1232.

Galicia-Garcia, U., Benito-Vicente, A., Jebari, S., Larrea-Sebal, A., Siddiqi, H., Uribe, K. B., Ostolaza, H., & Martín, C. (2020). Pathophysiology of type 2 diabetes mellitus. *International Journal of Molecular Sciences, 21*(17), 6275.

Giri, A. K., Prasad, G., Parekatt, V., Rajashekar, D., Tandon, N., & Bharadwaj, D. (2023). Epigenome-wide methylation study identified two novel CpGs associated with T2DM risk and a network of co-methylated CpGs capable of patient classification. *Human Molecular Genetics, 32*(16), 2576–2586.

Graciano, M. F., Valle, M., Kowluru, A., Curi, R., & Carpinelli, A. (2011). Regulation of insulin secretion and reactive oxygen species production by free fatty acids in pancreatic islets. *Islets, 3*(5), 213–223.

Groop, L. C., Bottazzo, G. F., & Doniach, D. (1986). Islet cell antibodies identify latent type I diabetes in patients aged 35–75 years at diagnosis. *Diabetes, 35*(2), 237–241.

Guarner, V., & Rubio-Ruiz, M. E. (2015). Low-grade systemic inflammation connects aging, metabolic syndrome and cardiovascular disease. *Aging and Health—A Systems Biology Perspective, 40*, 99–106.

Hastie, T. (2009). *The elements of statistical learning: Data mining, inference, and prediction.*

Heo, C. U., & Choi, C.-I. (2019). Current progress in pharmacogenetics of second-line antidiabetic medications: Towards precision medicine for type 2 diabetes. *Journal of Clinical Medicine, 8*. https://doi.org/10.3390/jcm8030393

Hill-Briggs, F., & Fitzpatrick, S. L. (2023). Overview of social determinants of health in the development of diabetes. *Diabetes Care, 46*(9), 1590–1598.

Horan, P., Slezak, S. E., & Poste, G. (1986). Improved flow cytometric analysis of leukocyte subsets: Simultaneous identification of five cell subsets using two-color immunofluorescence. *Proceedings of the National Academy of Sciences USA, 83*(21), 8361–8365.

Hu, M., Zhu, J., Peng, G., Lu, W., Wang, H., & Xie, Z. (2023). IMOVNN: Incomplete multi-omics data integration variational neural networks for gut microbiome disease prediction and biomarker identification. *Briefings in Bioinformatics, 24*(6). https://doi.org/10.1093/bib/bbad394

Ilan, Y., Maron, R., Tukpah, A.-M., Maioli, T. U., Murugaiyan, G., Yang, K., Wu, H. Y., & Weiner, H. L. (2010). Induction of regulatory T cells decreases adipose inflammation and alleviates insulin resistance in ob/ob mice. *Proceedings of the National Academy of Sciences, 107*(21), 9765–9770.

Ivanisevic, T., & Sewduth, R. (2023). Multi-omics integration for the design of novel therapies and the identification of novel biomarkers. *Proteomes, 11*. https://doi.org/10.3390/proteomes11040034

Iwasaki, H., Ezura, Y., Ishida, R., Kajita, M., Kodaira, M., Knight, J., Daniel, S., Shi, M., & Emi, M. (2002). Accuracy of genotyping for single nucleotide polymorphisms by a microarray-based single nucleotide polymorphism typing method involving hybridization of short allele-specific oligonucleotides. *DNA Research, 9*(2), 59–62.

Kask, O., Knappenberger, M., Lee, H., Stone, A. V., & Anderson, K. S. (2023). HLA-popseq: High throughput, multiplexed six-locus human leukocyte antigen typing for population-scale T cell immune profiling using rapid long-read nanopore sequencing. *The Journal of Immunology, 210*(Suppl. 1), 250–310.

Kim, Y., & Lee, C. (2023). Enrichment of spatial eGenes colocalized with type 2 diabetes mellitus genome-wide association study signals in the lysosomal pathway. *Applied Sciences.* https://doi.org/10.3390/app131810447

Kiyotani, K., Toyoshima, Y., & Nakamura, Y. (2021). Personalized immunotherapy in cancer precision medicine. *Cancer Biology and Medicine, 18*(4), 955.

Kolb, H., & Mandrup-Poulsen, T. (2005). An immune origin of type 2 diabetes? *Diabetologia, 48,* 1038–1050.

Kopriva, I., Jeric, I., Hadžija, M., Hadzija, M., & Lovrenčić, M. (2020). Non-negative least squares approach to quantification of 1H nuclear magnetic resonance spectra of human urine. *Analytical Chemistry.* https://doi.org/10.1021/acs.analchem.0c02837

LaFleur, M., Nguyen, T. H., Coxe, M. A., Yates, K. B., Trombley, J. D., Weiss, S. A., Brown, F. D., Gillis, J. E., Coxe, D. J., Doench, J. G., Haining, W., & Sharpe, A. (2019). A CRISPR-Cas9 delivery system for in vivo screening of genes in the immune system. *Nature Communications, 10.* https://doi.org/10.1038/s41467-019-09656-2

Leacy, E., Batten, I., Sanelli, L., McElheron, M., Brady, G., Little, M., & Khouri, H. (2023). Optimal LC-MS metabolomic profiling reveals emergent changes to monocyte metabolism in response to lipopolysaccharide. *Frontiers in Immunology, 14.* https://doi.org/10.3389/fimmu.2023.1116760

Leeuwenburgh, C., Fiebig, R., Chandwaney, R., & Ji, L. L. (1994). Aging and exercise training in skeletal muscle: Responses of glutathione and antioxidant enzyme systems. *American Journal of Physiology, 267*(2), R439–R445.

Li, D., Zhong, J., Zhang, Q., & Zhang, J. (2023). Effects of anti-inflammatory therapies on glycemic control in type 2 diabetes mellitus. *Frontiers in Immunology, 14,* Article 1125116.

Locke, A. E., Kahali, B., Berndt, S. I., Justice, A. E., Pers, T. H., Day, F. R., Powell, C., Vedantam, S., Buchkovich, M. L., Yang, J., et al. (2015). Genetic studies of body mass index yield new insights for obesity biology. *Nature, 518*(7538), 197–206.

Lu, J., Zhao, J., Meng, H., & Zhang, X. (2019). Adipose tissue-resident immune cells in obesity and type 2 diabetes. *Frontiers in Immunology, 10,* 1173.

Luo, Y., Yang, L., Wu, H., Xu, H., Peng, J., Wang, Y., & Zhou, F. (2024). Exploring the molecular mechanism of comorbidity of type 2 diabetes mellitus and colorectal cancer: Insights from bulk omics and single-cell sequencing validation. *Biomolecules, 14.* https://doi.org/10.3390/biom14060693

Mahajan, A., Taliun, D., Thurner, M., Robertson, N. R., Torres, J. M., Rayner, N. W., Payne, A. J., Steinthorsdottir, V., Scott, R. A., Grarup, N., et al. (2018). Fine-mapping type 2 diabetes loci to single-variant resolution using high-density imputation and islet-specific epigenome maps. *Nature Genetics, 50*(11), 1505–1513.

Malhotra, R., Javle, V., Tanwar, N., Gowda, P., Varghese, L., Madhusudhan, N., Jaiswal, N., Bhargavi, K. S., Chatterjee, M., Prabhash, K., et al. (2023). An absolute approach to using whole exome DNA and RNA workflow for cancer biomarker testing. *Frontiers in Oncology, 13,* Article 1002792.

Mannino, G. C., Andreozzi, F., & Sesti, G. (2019). Pharmacogenetics of type 2 diabetes mellitus, the route toward tailored medicine. *Diabetes, 35*(3), Article e3109.

Marques, E., Formato, E., Liang, W., Leonard, E. R., & Timme-Laragy, A. (2021). Relationships between type 2 diabetes, cell dysfunction, and redox signaling: A meta-analysis of single-cell gene expression of human pancreatic β-cells. *Journal of Diabetes, 14,* 34–51. https://doi.org/10.1111/1753-0407.13236

Martin, S., Coukos, G., Holt, R., & Nelson, B. (2015). Targeting the undruggable: Immunotherapy meets personalized oncology in the genomic era. *Annals of Oncology, 26*(12), 2367–2374.

Maruthur, N. M., Gribble, M. O., Bennett, W. L., Bolen, S., Wilson, L. M., Balakrishnan, P., Sahu, A., Bass, E., Kao, W. L., & Clark, J. M. (2014). The pharmacogenetics of type 2 diabetes: A systematic review. *Diabetes Care, 37*(3), 876–886.

Maruya, E., Saji, H., & Yokoyama, S. (1996). PCR-LIS-SSCP (low ionic strength single-stranded conformation polymorphism)—a simple method for high-resolution allele typing of HLA-DRB1, -DQB1, and -DPB1. *Genome Research, 6*(1), 51–57. https://doi.org/10.1101/gr.6.1.51

Minervina, A., Pogorelyy, M., & Mamedov, I. (2019). T-cell receptor and B-cell receptor repertoire profiling in adaptive immunity. *Transplant International, 32*(11), 1111–1123.

Moore, E. K., Strazza, M., & Mor, A. (2022). Combination approaches to target PD-1 signaling in cancer. *Frontiers in Immunology, 13*, Article 927265.

Motala, A. A., Busson, M., Al-Harbi, E. M., Khuzam, M. A., Al-Omari, E. M., Arekat, M. R., & Almawi, W. Y. (2005). Susceptible and protective human leukocyte antigen class II alleles and haplotypes in Bahraini type 2 (non-insulin-dependent) diabetes mellitus patients. *Clinical and Vaccine Immunology, 12*(1), 213–217.

Mousset, C. M., Hobo, W., Woestenenk, R., Preijers, F., Dolstra, H., & van der Waart, A. B. (2019). Comprehensive phenotyping of T cells using flow cytometry. *Cytometry, Part A, 95*. https://doi.org/10.1002/cyto.a.23724

Mujib, S., Li, S., Zabinyakov, N., & Loh, C. (2021). A single-tube, 44-marker CyTOF assay to assess antigen-specific immunity in whole blood human samples with data analysis solution. *The Journal of Immunology*. https://doi.org/10.4049/jimmunol.206.supp.27.09

Nadeem, A., Mumtaz, S., Naveed, A. K., Aslam, M., Siddiqui, A., Lodhi, G. M., & Ahmad, T. (2015). Gene-gene, gene-environment, gene-nutrient interactions and single nucleotide polymorphisms of inflammatory cytokines. *World Journal of Diabetes, 6*(4), 642.

Navarrete-Perea, J., Yu, Q., Gygi, S., & Paulo, J. (2018). Streamlined tandem mass tag (SL-TMT) protocol: An efficient strategy for quantitative (phospho)proteome profiling using tandem mass tag-synchronous precursor selection-MS3. *Journal of Proteome Research, 17*(6), 2226–2236. https://doi.org/10.1021/acs.jproteome.8b00217

Nicora, G., Vitali, F., Dagliati, A., Geifman, N., & Bellazzi, R. (2020). Integrated multi-omics analyses in oncology: A review of machine learning methods and tools. *Frontiers in Oncology, 10*. https://doi.org/10.3389/fonc.2020.01030

Odegaard, J. I., & Chawla, A. (2012). Connecting type 1 and type 2 diabetes through innate immunity. *Cold Spring Harbor Perspectives in Medicine, 2*(3), Article a007724.

Olson, N. C., Doyle, M. F., Sitlani, C. M., De Boer, I. H., Rich, S. S., Huber, S. A., Landay, A. L., Tracy, R. P., Psaty, B. M., & Delaney, J. A. (2020). Associations of innate and adaptive immune cell subsets with incident type 2 diabetes risk: The MESA study. *Journal of Clinical Endocrinology and Metabolism, 105*(3), e848–e857.

Orabona, C., Mondanelli, G., Puccetti, P., & Grohmann, U. (2018). Immune checkpoint molecules, personalized immunotherapy, and autoimmune diabetes. *Trends in Molecular Medicine, 24*(11), 931–941.

Ormond, K., & Cho, M. (2014). Translating personalized medicine using new genetic technologies in clinical practice: The ethical issues. *Personalized Medicine, 112*, 211–222. https://doi.org/10.2217/pme.13.104

Pastinen, T., Raitio, M., Lindroos, K., Tainola, P., Peltonen, L., & Syvänen, A.-C. (2000). A system for specific, high-throughput genotyping by allele-specific primer extension on microarrays. *Genome Research, 10*(7), 1031–1042.

Phani, N., Rai, P., Adhikari, P., Nagri, S., D'Souza, S., Gopinath, M., & Satyamoorthy, K. (2014). Impact of KCNJ11, TCF7L2, SLC30A8, IGF2BP2, PPARG, SLC47A1, STK11, HHEX, KCNQ1, CDKAL1, FTO, CYP2C9, ADIPOQ, CAPN10 gene polymorphisms on risk of type 2 diabetes and therapeutic response to sulfonylurea and metformin therapy. *Molecular Cytogenetics, 7*, 1–2.

Philipson, L. (2019). Harnessing heterogeneity in type 2 diabetes mellitus. *Nature Reviews Endocrinology, 16*, 79–80. https://doi.org/10.1038/s41574-019-0308-1

Picard, M., Scott-Boyer, M.-P., Bodein, A., Périn, O., & Droit, A. (2021). Integration strategies of multi-omics data for machine learning analysis. *Computational and Structural Biotechnology Journal, 19*, 3735–3746. https://doi.org/10.1016/j.csbj.2021.06.030

Pollastro, C., Ziviello, C., Costa, V., & Ciccodicola, A. (2015). Pharmacogenomics of drug response in type 2 diabetes: Toward the definition of tailored therapies? *PPAR Research, 2015*(1), Article 415149.

Rathika, C., Balakrishnan, K., Manikandan, T., Raja, N., Palani Kumaran, V., & Prasad, N. (2012). Involvement of HLA-DR/DQ, APOE and ACE I/D gene polymorphisms in development of secondary complication in South Indian T2DM patients. *International Journal of Human Genetics, 12*(1), 21–32.

Reddy, M. A., & Natarajan, R. (2011). Epigenetic mechanisms in diabetic vascular complications. *Cardiovascular Research, 90*(3), 421–429.

Reitman, M. L., Schadt, E. E., et al. (2007). Pharmacogenetics of metformin response: A step in the path toward personalized medicine. *The Journal of Clinical Investigation, 117*(5), 1226–1229.

Robles-Remacho, A., Sanchez-Martin, R. M., & Díaz-Mochón, J. (2023). Spatial transcriptomics: Emerging technologies in tissue gene expression profiling. *Analytical Chemistry, 95*, 15450–15460. https://doi.org/10.1021/acs.analchem.3c02029

Roep, B., Wheeler, D. C. S., & Peakman, M. (2019). Antigen-based immune modulation therapy for type 1 diabetes: The era of precision medicine. *Lancet Diabetes and Endocrinology, 7*(1), 65–74. https://doi.org/10.1016/S2213-8587(18)30109-8

Rohde, P. D., Nyegaard, M., Kjolby, M., & Sørensen, P. (2021). Multi-trait genomic risk stratification for type 2 diabetes. *Frontiers of Medicine, 8*, Article 711208.

Roth-Walter, F., Adcock, I. M., Benito-Villalvilla, C., Bianchini, R., Bjermer, L., Boyman, O., Caramori, G., Cari, L., Fan Chung, K., Diamant, Z., et al. (2021). Immune modulation via T regulatory cell enhancement: Disease-modifying therapies for autoimmunity and their potential for chronic allergic and inflammatory diseases—an EAACI position paper of the task force on immunopharmacology (TIPCO). *Allergy, 76*(1), 90–113.

Saederup, N., Yao, H., Cohen, M. J., & Fung, L. (2022). Abstract 1977: Extending the capabilities of a high-parameter immunophenotyping assay with cytoplasmic staining applications for mass cytometry. *Cancer Research*. https://doi.org/10.1158/1538-7445.am2022-1977

Sanches, P., de Melo, N. C., Porcari, A., & de Carvalho, L. M. (2024). Integrating molecular perspectives: Strategies for comprehensive multi-omics integrative data analysis and machine learning applications in transcriptomics, proteomics, and metabolomics. *Biology*. https://doi.org/10.3390/biology13110848

Schellenberg, E. S., Dryden, D. M., Vandermeer, B., Ha, C., & Korownyk, C. (2013). Lifestyle interventions for patients with and at risk for type 2 diabetes: A systematic review and meta-analysis. *Annals of Internal Medicine, 159*(8), 543–551.

Scott, R. A., Scott, L. J., Mägi, R., Marullo, L., Gaulton, K. J., Kaakinen, M., Pervjakova, N., Pers, T. H., Johnson, A. D., Eicher, J. D., et al. (2017). An expanded genome-wide association study of type 2 diabetes in Europeans. *Diabetes, 66*(11), 2888–2902.

Sell, H., Habich, C., & Eckel, J. (2012). Adaptive immunity in obesity and insulin resistance. *Nature Reviews Endocrinology, 8*(12), 709–716.

Selvanantham, T., Li, S. K. H., Zabinyakov, N., Bouzekri, A., Jong, R., Sullivan, M., Laboda, A., Majonis, D., & Loh, C. (2022). Abstract 3908: A streamlined and automated approach to high-content cytometric immunophenotyping with CyTOF XT. *Cancer Research*. https://doi.org/10.1158/1538-7445.am2022-3908

Shalem, O., Sanjana, N. E., & Zhang, F. (2015). High-throughput functional genomics using CRISPR–Cas9. *Nature Reviews Genetics, 16*, 299–311. https://doi.org/10.1038/nrg3899

Shamsuzzaman, A. S., Winnicki, M., Wolk, R., Svatikova, A., Phillips, B. G., Davison, D. E., Berger, P. B., & Somers, V. K. (2004). Independent association between plasma leptin and C-reactive protein in healthy humans. *Circulation, 109*(18), 2181–2185.

Sheehy, M., Scharf, S., Rowe, J., DeGimenez, M. N., Meske, L., Erlich, H., Nepom, B., et al. (1989). A diabetes-susceptible HLA haplotype is best defined by a combination of HLA-DR and -DQ alleles. *The Journal of Clinical Investigation, 83*(3), 830–835.

Shitomi-Jones, L. M., Akam, L., Hunter, D., Singh, P., & Mastana, S. (2023). Genetic risk scores for the determination of type 2 diabetes mellitus (T2DM) in North India. *International Journal of Environmental Research and Public Health, 20*(4), 3729.

Sidiropoulos, D. N., Stein-O'Brien, G., Danilova, L. V., Gross, N. E., Charmsaz, S., Xavier, S., Leatherman, J., Wang, H., Yarchoan, M., Jaffee, E., Fertig, E., & Ho, W. J. (2022). Integrated T cell cytometry metrics for immune-monitoring applications in immunotherapy clinical trials. *JCI Insight, 7.* https://doi.org/10.1172/jci.insight.160398

Sireesh, D., Dhamodharan, U., Ezhilarasi, K., Vijay, V., & Ramkumar, K. M. (2018). Association of NF-E2-related factor 2 (NRF2) and inflammatory cytokines in recent onset type 2 diabetes mellitus. *Scientific Reports, 8*(1), 5126.

Sun, J., Choy, D., Sompairac, N., Jamshidi, S., Mishto, M., & Kordasti, S. (2024a). ImmCellTyper facilitates systematic mass cytometry data analysis for deep immune profiling. *eLife, 13.* https://doi.org/10.7554/eLife.95494

Sun, J., Choy, D., Sompairac, N., Jamshidi, S., Mishto, M., & Kordasti, S. (2024b). ImmCellTyper: An integrated computational pipeline for systematic mining of mass cytometry data to assist deep immune profiling. bioRxiv. https://doi.org/10.1101/2024.01.15.575790.

Tembhare, P., Yuan, C., Xi, L., Morris, J., Liewehr, D., Venzon, D., Janik, J., Raffeld, M., & Stetler-Stevenson, M. (2011). Flow cytometric immunophenotypic assessment of T-cell clonality by V repertoire analysis: Detection of T-cell clonality at diagnosis and monitoring of minimal residual disease following therapy. *American Journal of Clinical Pathology, 135*(6), 890–900. https://doi.org/10.1309/AJCPV2D1DDSGJDBW

Thomas, P., Alshehri, S., van Kranen, H. V., & Ambrosino, E. (2016). The impact of personalized medicine of type 2 diabetes mellitus in the global health context. *Personalized Medicine, 13*(4), 381–393. https://doi.org/10.2217/pme-2016-0029

Tuomi, T. (2005). Type 1 and type 2 diabetes: What do they have in common? *Diabetes, 54*(Suppl. 2), S40–S45.

Venkatachalapathy, P., Padhilahouse, S., Sellappan, M., Subramanian, T., Kurian, S. J., Miraj, S. S., Rao, M., Raut, A., Kanwar, R., Singh, J. N., Khadanga, S., Mondithoka, S., & Munisamy, M. (2021). Pharmacogenomics and personalized medicine in type 2 diabetes mellitus: Potential implications for clinical practice. *Pharmacogenomics and Personalized Medicine, 14*, 1441–1455. https://doi.org/10.2147/PGPM.S329787

Visscher, P. M., Wray, N. R., Zhang, Q., Sklar, P., McCarthy, M. I., Brown, M. A., & Yang, J. (2017). 10 years of GWAS discovery: Biology, function, and translation. *The American Journal of Human Genetics, 101*(1), 5–22.

Wang, H., Luo, F., Shao, X., Gao, Y., Jiang, N., Jia, C., Li, H., & Chen, R. (2023). Integrated proteomics and single-cell mass cytometry analysis dissects the immune landscape of ankylosing spondylitis. *Analytical Chemistry.* https://doi.org/10.1021/acs.analchem.3c00809

Wang, G., & Sander, M. (2021). A multi-omics roadmap of β-cell failure in type 2 diabetes mellitus. *Nature Reviews Endocrinology, 17*, 641–642. https://doi.org/10.1038/s41574-021-00556-4

Wang, Y., Zhang, L., Niu, M., Li, R., Tu, R., Liu, X., Hou, J., Mao, Z., Wang, Z., & Wang, C. (2021). Genetic risk score increased discriminant efficiency of predictive models for type 2 diabetes mellitus using machine learning: Cohort study. *Frontiers in Public Health, 9*. https://doi.org/10.3389/fpubh.2021.606711

Wu, D.-L., Ling, H.-X., & Tang, H. (2004). [Comparative studies of serological typing and HLA-A, B antigen genotyping with PCR using sequence-specific primers]. *Di1 Jun Yi Da Xue Xue Bao = Academic Journal of the First Medical College of PLA, 24*(11), 1267–1270.

Xia, C., Rao, X., & Zhong, J. (2017). Role of T lymphocytes in type 2 diabetes and diabetes-associated inflammation. *Journal of Diabetes Research, 2017*(1), Article 6494795.

Zhang, C., Xiao, C., Wang, P., Xu, W., Zhang, A., Li, Q., & Xu, X. (2014). The alteration of Th1/Th2/Th17/Treg paradigm in patients with type 2 diabetes mellitus: Relationship with diabetic nephropathy. *Human Immunology, 75*(4), 289–296.

Zhao, L. P., Papadopoulos, G. K., Skyler, J. S., Pugliese, A., Parikh, H. M., Kwok, W. W., Lybrand, T. P., Bondinas, G. P., Moustakas, A. K., Wang, R., et al. (2024). HLA class II (DR, DQ, DP) genes were separately associated with the progression from seroconversion to onset of type 1 diabetes among participants in two diabetes prevention trials (DPT-1 and TN07). *Diabetes Care, 47*(5), 826–834.

Zhao, W., Rasheed, A., Tikkanen, E., Lee, J.-J., Butterworth, A. S., Howson, J. M., Assimes, T. L., Chowdhury, R., Orho-Melander, M., Damrauer, S., et al. (2017). Identification of new susceptibility loci for type 2 diabetes and shared etiological pathways with coronary heart disease. *Nature Genetics, 49*(10), 1450–1457.

Zhou, X., Guo, W., Yin, H., Chen, J., Ma, L., Yang, Q., Zhao, Y., Li, S., Liu, W., & Li, H. (2021). Whole exome sequencing study in a family with type 2 diabetes mellitus. *International Journal of General Medicine*, 8217–8229.

Zhou, T., Hu, Z., Yang, S., Sun, L., Yu, Z., & Wang, G. (2018). Role of adaptive and innate immunity in type 2 diabetes mellitus. *Journal of Diabetes Research, 2018*(1), Article 7457269.

Zhou, W., Liu, Q., Wang, W., Yuan, X., Xiao, C., & Ye, S. (2022). Comprehensive network analysis reveals the targets and potential multitarget drugs of type 2 diabetes mellitus. *Oxidative Medicine and Cellular Longevity, 2022*. https://doi.org/10.1155/2022/8255550

Zhou, B., Rayner, A. W., Gregg, E. W., Sheffer, K. E., Carrillo-Larco, R. M., Bennett, J. E., Shaw, J. E., Paciorek, C. J., Singleton, R. K., Pires, A. B., et al. (2024). Worldwide trends in diabetes prevalence and treatment from 1990 to 2022: A pooled analysis of 1108 population-representative studies with 141 million participants. *The Lancet, 404*(10467), 2077–2093.

Further reading

Abelin, J. G., Keskin, D., Sarkizova, S., Hartigan, C. R., Zhang, W., Sidney, J., Stevens, J., Lane, W., Zhang, G., Eisenhaure, T., Clauser, K., Hacohen, N., Rooney, M. S., Carr, S., & Wu, C. J. (2017). Mass spectrometry profiling of HLA-associated peptidomes in mono-allelic cells enables more accurate epitope prediction. *Immunity, 46*, 315–326. https://doi.org/10.1016/j.immuni.2017.02.007

Acharya, D., & Mukhopadhyay, A. (2024). A comprehensive review of machine learning techniques for multi-omics data integration: Challenges and applications in precision oncology. *Briefings in Functional Genomics*. https://doi.org/10.1093/bfgp/elae013

Ammar, R., Paton, T., Torti, D., Shlien, A., & Bader, G. D. (2015). Long read nanopore sequencing for detection of HLA and CYP2D6 variants and haplotypes. *F1000Research, 4*. https://doi.org/10.12688/f1000research.6037.2

Becker, J. P., & Riemer, A. (2022). The importance of being presented: Target validation by immunopeptidomics for epitope-specific immunotherapies. *Frontiers in Immunology, 13*. https://doi.org/10.3389/fimmu.2022.883989

Cantor, E., & Koschmann, C. (2019). Multiplatform molecular profiling: A precision medicine victory built on cytotoxic chemotherapy. *The Cancer Journal, 25*(2), 80.

Gide, T. N., Mao, Y., Scolyer, R. A., Long, G. V., & Wilmott, J. S. (2024). Tissue-based profiling techniques to achieve precision medicine in cancer: Opportunities and challenges in melanoma. *Clinical Cancer Research, 30*(23), 5270–5280.

Grbesa, I., Tannenbaum, M., Sarusi-Portuguez, A., Schwartz, M., & Hakim, O. (2017). Mapping genome-wide accessible chromatin in primary human T lymphocytes by ATAC-seq. *Journal of Visualized Experiments, 129.* https://doi.org/10.3791/56313

Guan, H., Zhao, S., Li, J., Wang, Y., Niu, P., Zhang, Y., Zhang, Y., Fang, X., Miao, R., & Tian, J. (2024). Exploring the design of clinical research studies on the efficacy mechanisms in type 2 diabetes mellitus. *Frontiers in Endocrinology, 15.* https://doi.org/10.3389/fendo.2024.1363877

He, J., Shen, J., Luo, W., Han, Z., Xie, F., Pang, T., Liao, L., Guo, Z., Li, J., Li, Y., & Chen, H. (2022). Research progress on application of single-cell TCR/BCR sequencing technology to the tumor immune microenvironment, autoimmune diseases, and infectious diseases. *Frontiers in Immunology, 13.* https://doi.org/10.3389/fimmu.2022.969808

Jamieson, N. B., & Maker, A. V. (2017). Gene-expression profiling to predict responsiveness to immunotherapy. *Cancer Gene Therapy, 24*(3), 134–140.

Koelzer, V. H., Sirinukunwattana, K., Rittscher, J., & Mertz, K. D. (2019). Precision immunoprofiling by image analysis and artificial intelligence. *Virchows Archiv, 474*(4), 511–522.

Kupai, K., Várkonyi, T., Török, S., Gáti, V., Czimmerer, Z., Puskás, L., & Szebeni, G. (2022). Recent progress in the diagnosis and management of type 2 diabetes mellitus in the era of COVID-19 and single-cell multi-omics technologies. *Life, 12.* https://doi.org/10.3390/life12081205

Kwarta, K., Campbell, T., Northcutt, A., & Schwarz, S. (2023). Precise spatial multiplexing of protein biomarkers for immune profiling in tissue samples with chip cytometry. *Cancer Research, 83*(Suppl. 7), 6769.

Lang, J. (2023). Nano2NGS: A framework for converting nanopore sequencing data to NGS-like sequencing data for data analysis. *Cancer Research.* https://doi.org/10.1158/1538-7445.am2023-2081

Lee, D., Cook, S., Jung, Y., Lim, M., Lee, J. E., Im, H.-J., Lee, D., & Choi, H. (2024). Automated tumor microenvironment analysis for multiple samples by image-based spatial transcriptomics on tissue microarray. *Cancer Research.* https://doi.org/10.1158/1538-7445.am2024-4948

Li, M., Zeng, T., Liu, R., & Chen, L. (2014). Detecting tissue-specific early warning signals for complex diseases based on dynamical network biomarkers: Study of type 2 diabetes by cross-tissue analysis. *Briefings in Bioinformatics, 15*(2), 229–243.

Liang, Y., Wang, C., Liang, Z., Zhang, L., & Zhang, Y. (2022). C18-functionalized amine-bridged hybrid monoliths for mass spectrometry-friendly peptide separation and highly sensitive proteomic analysis. *Analytical Chemistry.* https://doi.org/10.1021/acs.analchem.1c04405

Liu, C. (2020). A long read to rapid high-resolution HLA typing: The nanopore perspective. *Human Immunology.* https://doi.org/10.1016/j.humimm.2020.04.009

Malone, E. R., Oliva, M., Sabatini, P. J., Stockley, T. L., & Siu, L. L. (2020). Molecular profiling for precision cancer therapies. *Genome Medicine, 12,* 1–19.

Matern, B., Olieslagers, T., Groeneweg, M., Duygu, B., Wieten, L., Tilanus, M., & Voorter, C. (2020). Long-read nanopore sequencing validated for HLA-class I typing in routine diagnostics. *Journal of Molecular Diagnostics.* https://doi.org/10.1016/j.jmoldx.2020.04.001

Mohd Rizal, M. F., Abdul Maulud, K. N., Ganasegeran, K., Abdul Manaf, M. R., Safian, N., Mustapha, F. I., & Waller, L. A. (2024). A scoping review of supervised machine learning techniques in predicting the prevalence of type 2 diabetes mellitus. *Medicine and Health, 19*(2), 380–399. https://doi.org/10.17576/MH.2024.1902.03

Mosbruger, T., Dinou, A., Duke, J., Ferriola, D., Mehler, H., Pagkrati, I., Damianos, G., Mbunwe, E., Sarmady, M., Lyratzakis, I., Tishkoff, S., Dinh, A., & Monos, D. (2020). Utilizing nanopore sequencing technology for the rapid and comprehensive characterization of eleven HLA loci; addressing the need for deceased donor expedited HLA typing. *Human Immunology, 81*, 413–422. https://doi.org/10.1016/j.humimm.2020.06.004

Mukherjee, S. (2019). Genomics-guided immunotherapy for precision medicine in cancer. *Cancer Biotherapy and Radiopharmaceuticals, 34*(8), 487–497.

Nelde, A., Schuster, H., Bilich, T., Bauer, J., Roerden, M., Schroeder, S., Heitmann, J., Rucker-Braun, E., Rammensee, H., Salih, H., & Walz, J. (2022). Abstract 3168: Immunopeptidome-defined acute myeloid leukemia progenitor cell-associated antigens are targeted in vivo by AML patients' T cells. *Cancer Research*. https://doi.org/10.1158/1538-7445.am2022-3168

Payet, M., Dargai, F., Gasque, P., & Guillot, X. (2021). Epigenetic regulation (including microRNAs, DNA methylation and histone modifications) of rheumatoid arthritis: A systematic review. *International Journal of Molecular Sciences, 22*(22), Article 12170.

Rai, V., Quang, D. X., Erdos, M. R., Cusanovich, D. A., Daza, R. M., Narisu, N., Zou, L. S., Didion, J. P., Guan, Y., Shendure, J., et al. (2020). Single-cell ATAC-seq in human pancreatic islets and deep learning upscaling of rare cells reveals cell-specific type 2 diabetes regulatory signatures. *Molecular Metabolism, 32*, 109–121.

Ramarathinam, S. H., & Purcell, A. W. (2021). *Proteomics special issue: Precision immunology and oncology*.

Reel, P., Reel, S., Pearson, E., Trucco, E., & Jefferson, E. (2021). Using machine learning approaches for multi-omics data analysis: A review. *Biotechnology Advances*. Article 107739. https://doi.org/10.1016/j.biotechadv.2021.107739

Solleder, M., Guillaume, P., Racle, J., Michaux, J., Pak, H., Müller, M., Coukos, G., Bassani-Sternberg, M., & Gfeller, D. (2020). Mass spectrometry-based immunopeptidomics leads to robust predictions of phosphorylated HLA class I ligands. *Molecular and Cellular Proteomics, 19*(2), 390–404. https://doi.org/10.1074/mcp.TIR119.001641

Thibodeau, A., Khetan, S., Eroglu, A., Tewhey, R., Stitzel, M., & Ucar, D. (2020). CoRE-ATAC: A deep learning model for the functional classification of regulatory elements from single cell and bulk ATAC-seq data. *PLoS Computational Biology, 17*. https://doi.org/10.1371/journal.pcbi.1009670

Weisbrod, L., Capriotti, L., Hofmann, M., Spieler, V., Dersch, H., Voedisch, B., Schmidt, P., & Knake, S. (2024). FastMap—a flexible and scalable immunopeptidomics pipeline for HLA- and antigen-specific T-cell epitope mapping based on artificial antigen-presenting cells. *Frontiers in Immunology, 15*. https://doi.org/10.3389/fimmu.2024.1386160

Xu, C., Yang, J., Kosters, A., Babcock, B. R., Qiu, P., & Ghosn, E. (2021). Comprehensive multi-omics single-cell data integration reveals greater heterogeneity in the human immune system. *iScience, 25*. https://doi.org/10.1016/j.isci.2022.105123

12

Emerging trends in immunogenetic research in type 2 diabetes mellitus (T2DM)

Jai Vardhan[1], Shriram Sisodia[1], Prem Shankar Mishra[1], Aryan Kumar[1], Mohd Rizwan Jameel[2] and Abid Ali Sheikh[3]

[1]*FACULTY OF PHARMACY, VIDYA UNIVERSITY, MEERUT, UTTAR PRADESH, INDIA;* [2]*CENTRE FOR INTERDISCIPLINARY RESEARCH IN BASIC SCIENCE, JAMIA MILIA ISLAMIA, DELHI, NEW DELHI, INDIA;* [3]*NATIONAL INSTITUTE OF BIOLOGICALS, NOIDA, UTTAR PRADESH, INDIA*

1. Introduction

Diabetes mellitus is a group of metabolic diseases involving carbohydrate, lipid, and protein metabolism. It is characterized by persistent hyperglycemia, as a result of defects in insulin secretion, insulin action or a combination of both, defective secretion and incorrect action. There are two main types of diabetes mellitus: Type 1 (insulin-dependent), and type 2 (non-insulin-dependent, Karamanou, 2016). According to estimates from the Global Burden of Diseases, Injuries, and Risk Factors Study (GBD) 2019, diabetes was the eighth leading cause of death and disability combined in the world, with nearly 460 million people across every country and age group living with the disease in 2019.6 Diabetes represents a substantial burden to health-care systems, 2,7–9 with estimates by the International Diabetes Federation (IDF) indicating that 537 million people worldwide had diabetes in 2021, resulting in health expenditures of US$966 billion globally, forecast to reach more than $1054 billion by 2045 (Ong et al., 2023). Type 2 diabetes affects more than 400 million people worldwide. It's a chronic disease, and both genes and your environment play a role. At its core, the problem is insulin resistance and when the β-cells in your pancreas stop working as they should. What causes that? Things like β-cells losing their identity, mitochondria getting sluggish, and too much oxidative stress all come into play (White et al., 2016). Treatment should be based on nonpharmacological therapy. Strategies such as increased physical activity, dietary

Type 2 Diabetes Mellitus. https://doi.org/10.1016/B978-0-443-33590-7.00007-1

modifications, cognitive-behavioral therapy are important in maintaining normal glycemia (Bizimana, 2024). These treatments are supported and strengthened with the help of Advanced therapies, among which SGLT2 inhibitors and GLP-1 receptor agonists can be singled out, which provide a solid glycemic control, weight control, and cardiovascular risk reduction. Inflammatory complications of Type 2 diabetes mellitus (T2DM), like diabetic kidney disease, retinopathy, and neuropathy, call for early diagnosis and thorough management that would lead to better patient outcomes and quality of life (Młynarska et al., 2025). T2DM isn't just about metabolism—there's a big immune system story here too. People now see it as a condition marked by ongoing, low-level inflammation and a messed-up immune response. Blood cells such as T cells and monocytes are the main culprits that lead to the inflammation (Li et al., 2024). The issues of the immune system are the core of the main cause of T2DM. Inflammatory and immune reactions that are disordered, most of the time, are the reason for insulin resistance and the malfunction of beta cells. Furthermore, alterations in the expression of immune-related genes may also serve as crucial determinants in the development of diabetes. Therefore, a complete understanding of the involvement of these immune genes in the cognitive impairment of individuals with T2DM is imperative (Gao et al., 2024). The CTLA-4 gene is an important regulator of T-cell activation involved in the downregulation of immune response & CTLA-4 has been linked to susceptibility to several autoimmune diseases, including Type 1 diabetes mellitus and T2DM (Qi et al., 2014). Only a few common variants in PPARG, KCNJ11, and TCF7L2 were shown to be associated with type 2 diabetes. With the advent of GWA studies, there are at least 20 loci identified today that are associated with the risk of type 2 diabetes. The first GWA study in the French population revealed SLC30A8 and HHEX as new loci for type 2 diabetes in addition to replicating the strong association with TCF7L2 (Chauhan et al., 2010). Epigenetics plays an important role in the transmission of T2DM from one generation to another. Epigenetic changes are also implicated in the two basic pathogenic components of T2DM, namely insulin resistance and impaired insulin secretion. Hyperglycaemia induced permanent epigenetic modifications of the expression of DNA are responsible for the phenomenon of metabolic memory. Epigenetics influences the development of micro and macrovascular complications of T2DM (Mannar et al., 2023). Multi-omics aided the dramatic discovery that diabetes was associated with the intestinal flora. The altered microbiota observed in genetically obese mice or people is sufficient to promote increased adiposity in lean mice that receive a microbiota transplant. Germ-free mice, which lack a microbiota, have reduced adiposity and improved tolerance to glucose and insulin when compared to their counter parts. They are also free from diet-induced obesity when fed a Western-style diet. Taken together, the correlation between intestinal flora, obesity, and diabetes demonstrates that the microbiota contributes to the regulation of adiposity and T2DM. However, the precise mechanism is still not clear (Wang et al., 2021). Diabetes is a complex disease that involves multiple molecular mechanisms. Recent advances in multi-omics sequencing techniques have significantly enhanced the understanding of the pathogenesis of diabetes (Cai et al., 2025). The interaction of T-cells with monocytes in T2DM is essential and, as a result, it significantly changes the immune regulation, inflammation, and autoimmunity processes, which are the main factors not only of the disease's progression but also of its management. Knowing these communications helps one figure out the mechanisms of immune dysregulation that result in chronic inflammation and insulin resistance in T2DM (Li et al., 2024).

2. The immune system and T2DM: A paradigm shift

Type 2 diabetes, which is frequently abbreviated as T2D, is, in essence, insulin resistance combined with the gradual loss of pancreatic beta cells. A scenario like this generally leads to chronic hyperglycemia. Macrophages are the main impactful cells that initiate and prolong insulin resistance. Basically, they constitute a significant part of the innate immune system, and they are very reactive to inflammation. In turn, they themselves alter their metabolism. These aspects are very important because they are directly linked with the core repertoires of T2D macrophages, which have great plasticity and can shift their polarization toward not only inflammatory but also antiinflammatory ones. In the case of T2D, the ones that are proinflammatory and use glycolysis worsen insulin resistance. They along with proinflammatory cytokines also release high amounts of nitric oxide. Moreover, proresolutive macrophages, which are able to restore glucose homeostasis switch their metabolism toward fatty acid oxidation. For instance, proinflammatory macrophages trigger meta-inflammation, whereby the latter term denotes chronic, low-grade, inflammation, which significantly contributes to the development of T2D, thus forming an environment that is very favorable for metabolic dysfunctions. This review paper is an attempt to explain the role of macrophages in the progression of type 2 diabetes. It gives some details about their inflammatory responses and the metabolic changes they undergo. These features are the main contributors to insulin resistance and, thus, the major problems at the core of the disease. Furthermore, the paper strives to shed more light on the molecular and metabolic pathways that underlie these phenomena. Very early on, it leads to a better understanding of the impact of the disease on the way of life of millions of people all over the world (Witcoski Junior et al., 2024).

T2DM is one of the major chronic ailments that has become very common. It is responsible for over 90% of the diabetes cases globally. The main feature of the condition is the resistance of the cells to insulin, accompanied by hyperglycemia that lasts for a long time (Ahmad et al., 2022). T2DM does not stop at metabolic issues only. It is associated with significant changes in the immune system. Cells such as macrophages, neutrophils, and natural killer cells become dysfunctional. The immune dysfunction in diabetic patients contributes to their increased susceptibility to infections. The condition also causes more inflammation and is involved in the diabetics' complications (Vaibhav et al., 2024). Long-term high blood sugar causes the body to start an inflammatory reaction, which then prevents the body's natural immune defense and so makes the management of diseases even more difficult. This chapter delves into the complex interplay between T2DM and the immune system, pointing out that the impairment of immune cells is one of the factors that aggravate insulin resistance. In addition, the chapter discusses the influence of proinflammatory markers and cellular responses in the development and progression of diabetes. The chronically flooded glucose milieu results in many physiological and pathophysiological alterations. There are a number of mechanisms through which hyperglycemia can aggravate its toxic effects on the cells, tissues, and organ systems. Hyperglycemia causes oxidative stress, increases the activity of the polyol pathway, activates protein kinase C (PKC), increases the hexosamine biosynthetic pathway (HBP), facilitates the formation of advanced glycation end-products (AGEs), and in the end, gene expression is modified (Giri et al., 2018). Prolonged hyperglycemic condition leads to severe diabetic conditions by damaging the pancreatic β-cell and inducing insulin resistance (Kim et al., 2005). Hyperglycemia activates protein kinase C, and this inhibits neutrophil migration, phagocytosis, superoxide production and microbial killing (Jafar et al., 2016). High glucose concentrations decrease the formation of neutrophil extracellular traps. Hyperglycemia can also induce Toll like receptor expression and inhibit neutrophil function and apoptosis. High glucose concentrations decrease vascular dilation and increase permeability during the initial inflammatory responses, possibly through protein kinase C activation (Jafar et al., 2016). Hyperglycemia can cause direct glycosylation of proteins and alter the tertiary structure of complement; these changes inhibit immunoglobulin-mediated opsonization of bacteria and complement fixation to bacteria and decrease phagocytosis. Hyperglycemia also stimulates the production and release of cytokines. Several trials have demonstrated that better glycemic control reduces nosocomial infections in critically ill patients and surgical site infections. Fig. 12.1 demonstrates the inhibition of insulin, causing hyperglycemia.

3. Genetic susceptibility and immune-related genes

Type 2 diabetes (T2D) is the result of an interaction between environmental factors and a strong hereditary component. Very few T2D risk genes were identified using candidate

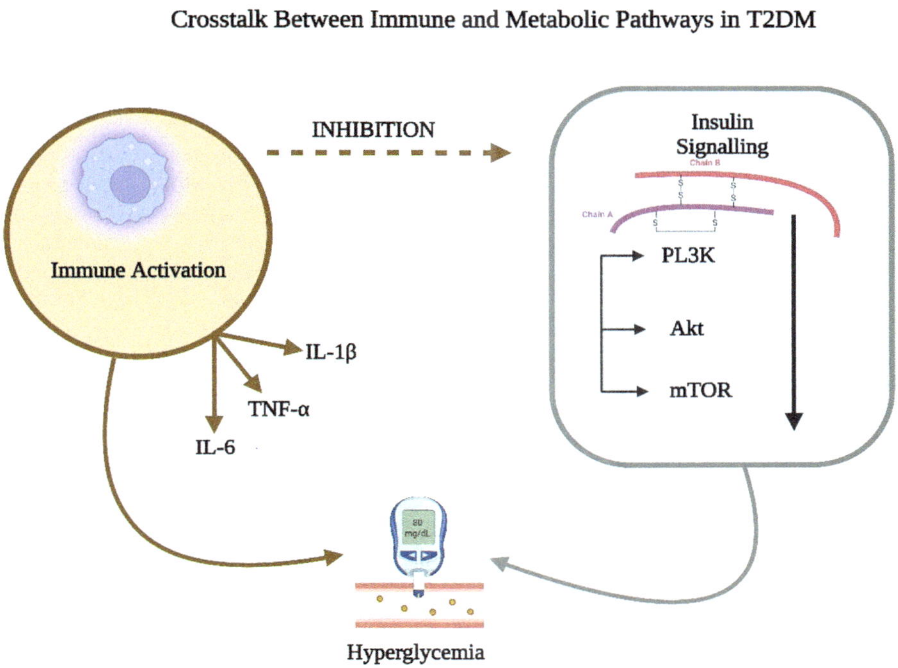

FIGURE 12.1 Crosstalk between immune and metabolic pathways in Type 2 Diabetes Mellitus (T2DM).

gene and linkage-based studies, but the advent of genome-wide association studies has led to the identification of multiple genes, including several that were not previously known to play any role in T2D. Highly replicated genes, for example, TCF7L2, KCNQ1 and KCNJ11(23), **TCF7L2 is** the most potent locus known for T2D risk. The TCF7L2 gene is a downstream effector of the canonical Wnt/b-catenin signaling pathway, which permits TCF7L2 to control a great variety of functions by virtue of the complexity of its expression with numerous mRNA isoforms. This gene has been associated with several fundamental processes, including adipogenesis, natural selection, and alternative splicing, and various and diverse diseases, including different types of cancer. Continued efforts are underway to understand the genomic variation associated with T2D and its functional implications. Future interinstitutional collaborations are needed to guarantee that the clinical translation of this knowledge leads to improved patient care (Del Bosque-Plata et al., 2021). Table 12.1 summarizes major susceptibility genes identified in T2DM, including their specific polymorphisms/single-nucleotide polymorphism (SNPs), functional consequences, associated disease risks, ethnic variability in prevalence, and

Table 12.1 Clinical applications of immunogenetics and personalized medicine in T2DM.

Gene	Polymorphism/ SNP	Key findings	Associated risks	Ethnic variation	Function
TCF7L2	N/A	Most potent locus for T2DM risk. Involved in the Wnt/b-catenin signaling pathway, affecting adipogenesis, alternative splicing, and cancer development.	Strong association with T2DM susceptibility.	Found in multiple populations with consistent results, particularly in European and Asian populations.	Affects adipogenesis, gene expression, and signaling pathways, influencing insulin resistance and beta-cell function.
KCNQ1	rs2237892	SNP is highly associated with T2DM risk. Significant association with susceptibility to T2DM, particularly in East Asian populations.	Higher risk of developing T2DM, especially with the C allele.	Strong effect in East Asian populations; inconsistent findings in other populations (e.g., European).	Involved in regulating insulin secretion and glucose metabolism.
KCNJ11	rs5219 (E23K), rs5215, rs5210	SNPs associated with T2DM risk. The rs5219 (E23K) variant is the strongest.	Significant association with T2DM risk, particularly in East Asian and European populations.	Ethnic differences in effect: stronger association in East Asian and European populations.	Influences insulin secretion by regulating potassium channels in pancreatic beta cells.
SLC30A8	rs13266634 (Trp325Arg)	Decreases insulin levels and increases proinsulin ratio, which enhances T2DM risk. Mouse model studies show ZNT8 deletion reduces islet zinc, causing abnormal insulin granules.	Increased risk of T2DM due to disrupted zinc homeostasis and abnormal insulin secretion.	No significant ethnic bias in the association.	Zinc transporter crucial for insulin crystallisation and beta-cell function. Rare mutations in this gene can protect against T2DM.
PTPN22	rs2476601 (CT), rs33996649 (GA)	SNPs linked to T2DM and tuberculosis interaction. rs2476601-CT reduces pulmonary tuberculosis risk, while rs33996649-GA increases the risk of T2DM and PTB.	T2DM risk is higher for those with rs33996649-GA, especially when combined with metabolic conditions like T2DM.	Significant findings in the Chinese Uyghur population, particularly with metabolic diseases like T2DM and tuberculosis.	Affects immune cell signaling and inflammatory response, potentially influencing both autoimmune diseases and metabolic disorders like T2DM.

their mechanistic roles in insulin secretion, β-cell function, and immune-metabolic regulation.

KCNQ1 T2DM is a multifactorial trait in which both environmental and genetic factors contribute to its pathogenesis. The most common SNP of the potassium voltage-gated channel subfamily Q member 1 (KCNQ1) gene, rs2237892, is highly associated with the risk of T2DM. The KCNQ1 has been identified as a susceptibility gene of T2DM by several GWASs performed in different ethnicities, such as European and Asian populations, but various studies show conflicting results. Some GWAS consistently showed that KCNQ1 is a strong susceptibility gene for T2DM, especially in the East Asian population, but studies on population showed there is no significant difference found between the rs2237892 variant and T2DM (Erfani et al., 2020). Studies show that the findings indicated that although the rs2237895 KCNQ1 gene polymorphism was not linked to type 2 diabetes, its presence considerably reduced the risk of renal problems (Afshardoost et al., 2019). The KCNQ1 gene rs2237895 was significantly associated with susceptibility to T2DM in an Asian population. Carriers of the C allele had a higher risk of T2DM. The KCNQ1 gene rs2237895 was significantly associated with susceptibility to T2DM in an Asian population. Carriers of the C allele had a higher risk of T2DM. This association was not significant in nonAsian populations

kcnj11 Meta analysis studies study was performed to evaluate the relation between kcnj11 gene polymorphism and type 2 diabetes risk. In this study, mainly rs5219(e23k), rs5215 and rs5210 variants are analyze. Result demonstrated that these variants have a significant association with the T2dm, and among them, rs5219 is to be found strongest variant The study also showed there is ethnics difference present, in which there is an east Asian and European populations showed more strong effect. Overall conclusion is this kcnj11 is an important susceptible gene for t2dm, further functional studies are required to clarify its exact role (Moazzam-Jazi et al., 2022).

SLC30a8 genes encode ZNT8 Zinc transporter, and they play an important role in maintaining zinc homeostasis within the beta cell of the pancreas and maintaining insulin crystallization. Its common variant rs13266634(Trp325Arg) decreases the insulin level and increases the proinsulin ratio, as a result, chance of type it enhances the risk of type 2 dm. Mouse model study demonstrated that deletion of znt8 causes a decrease in islet zinc, and insulin granules become abnormal. But glucose tolerance and secretion depend on the environment and genetic background. Other than this one important mechanism demonstrated through recent studies, low zinc secretion increases hepatic insulin clearance because the circulating insulin level becomes lower. One other interesting finding is this from recent studies: rare loss-of-function mutation protects from T2DM means partial loss of ZnT8 is harmful, but complete loss may be protective

4. PTPN22

The study conducted on the Chinese Uygur population evaluated the interaction of ptpn22 gene polymorphism and T2DM with tuberculosis. The result revealed that the rs2476601-CT genotype of PTP, N22 reduce the risk of pulmonary tuberculosis, while **rs33996649-GA** genotype increases the risk of PTB. The most important aspect of this study is who have T2DM with rs33996649-GA variant have a very high risk of ptb development.t So it is clear with this PTPN22 genetic variants themselves affect the disease susceptibility, but it shows a synergistic effect when combined with metabolic conditions like T2DM (Wang et al., 2017). Fig. 12.2 explains the immunogenetic and epigenetic mechanisms for type 2 diabetes.

5. Epigenetic and transcriptomic advances

T2DM pathogenesis is not a result of only genetic mutation but rather environmental factors and epigenetic modification like DNA methylation play a major role in it (Nadiger

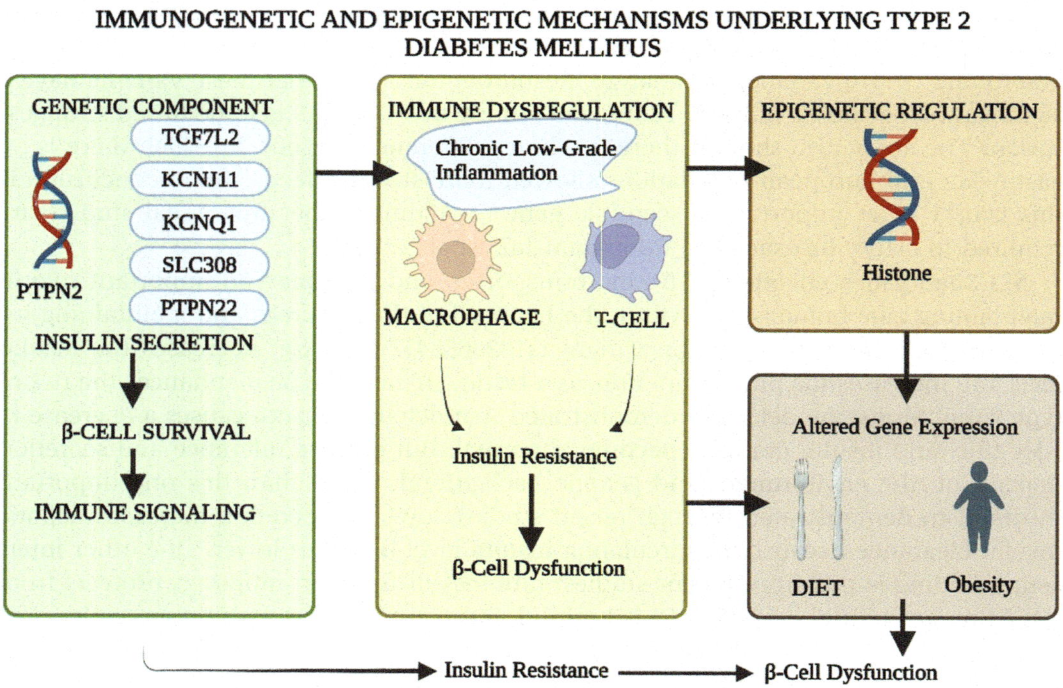

FIGURE 12.2 Immunogenetic and epigenetic mechanisms underlying type 2 diabetes mellitus.

et al., 2024). DNA methylation is a relatively stable epigenetic modification that can regulate and stabilize gene expression patterns and hence establish cell identity. Because metabolic intermediates are key factors of DNA methylation and demethylation, perturbations in metabolic homeostasis can trigger alterations in cell-specific patterns of DNA methylation and contribute to disease development, including type 2 diabetes (Kim, 2019). Studies on monozygotic twins revealed that environmental factor has modulate gene expression at the epigenetic level, and this important pathway of glucose is also disturbed. In the adipose tissue of t2dm patient amount of mitochondrial DNA found to be comparatively lower, and glycan metabolism, immune response and inflammation pathways upregulated, but their oxidative phosphorylation and lipid/ carbohydrate metabolism pathway is downregulated (Das, 2014). The integration of DNAmethylation and gene expression can lead to the development of new targets and therapeutic approaches. Wang et al. (2023) evaluated T2dm patients in the Tibetan and Han population and found that clinical and disease difference is majorly due to transcriptomic and epigenetic variation. Recent studies have integrated the data with epigenomic and revealed that, genetic and epigenetic factors play an important role in the pathogenesis of T2DM. DNA methylation and gene expression patterns show that some gene dysregulated in the metabolic, inflammatory and insulin signaling pathways (Wu et al., 2023). This integrative approach identifies multiple novel candidate genes and molecular mechanism which involve in the progression and development of T2DM. Other than DNA methylation, histone marks, chromatin accessibility, noncoding RNAs play an important role in epigenetic regulation.

6. Multi-omics and systems biology approach

Since the concept of genomes and genomics was introduced, "omics" research has profoundly affected systems biology discoveries. Multi-omics research enables researchers to identify the differences in genes, proteins, and metabolites that lead to understanding overall functional disturbances in diseases, including T2DM. Multi-omic studies have provided breakthroughs and directions to guide traditional molecular biology research. The expansion of "omics" data and the continuous advancement of bioinformatics analysis technology will surely continue the advancement of our knowledge on the mechanisms of T2DM, especially on intestinal flora perturbation and dyslipidemia (Wang et al., 2021). Traditional methodologies often fall short in addressing the complexity of biological systems. In this regard, systems biology omics have brought invaluable tools for conducting comprehensive analysis. Current sequencing capabilities have revolutionized genetics and genomics studies, as well as the characterization of transcriptional profiling and dynamics of several species and sample types. Biological systems experience complex biochemical processes involving thousands of molecules. These processes occur at different levels that can be studied using mass spectrometry-based (MS-based) analysis, enabling high-throughput proteomics, glycoproteomic, glycomics, metabolomics, and lipidomics analysis. Here, we present the most up-to-date techniques utilized in the completion of omics analysis. Additionally, we include some interesting examples of the applicability of multi-omics to a variety of biological systems (Reyes et al., 2024). Certain impacts of chronic hyperglycemia on gastric metabolism and protein synthesis in mice have been observed, based on the findings of a transcriptome, proteomics, and metabolomics study. The mechanism of action of diabetic gastrointestinal lesions may be closely related to the digestion and absorption of vitamins, glycerophospholipid metabolism, and the arachidonic acid metabolism pathway by applying the BKS-db/db spontaneous diabetic mouse model (Zhang et al., 2024). The endoplasmic reticulum (ER) is a membranous organelle involved in calcium storage, lipid biosynthesis, protein folding and processing. Many pathophysiological conditions and pharmacological agents are known to perturb normal ER function and can lead to ER stress, which severely compromises protein folding mechanisms and hence poses a high risk of proteotoxicity. Upon sensing ER stress, the different stress signaling pathways interconnect with each other and work together to preserve cellular homeostasis. ER stress response is a part of the integrative stress response (ISR) and might play an important role in the pathogenesis of chronic neurodegenerative diseases, where misfolded protein accumulation and cell death are common. The initiation, manifestation and progression of ER stress-mediated unfolded protein response (UPR) is a complex procedure involving multiple proteins, pathways and cellular organelles. To understand the cause and consequences of such complex processes, the implementation of an integrative, holistic approach is required to identify novel players and regulators of ER stress. As multi-omics data-based systems analyses have shown potential to unravel the underlying molecular mechanism of complex biological systems, it is important to emphasize the utility of this approach in understanding the ER stress biology. In this review, we first discuss the ER stress signaling pathways and regulatory players, along with their interconnectivity. We next highlight the importance of systems and network biology approaches using multi-omics data in understanding ER stress-mediated cellular responses. This report would help advance our current understanding of the multivariate spatial interconnectivity and temporal dynamicity of ER stress (Mallick et al., 2022). These state-of-the-art models can serve as a scaffold for integrating multi-omics data, thereby enabling the identification of signatures of dysregulated metabolism by systems approaches. For example, increased plasma mannose levels due to decreased uptake in the liver have been identified as a potential biomarker of early insulin resistance by multiomics approaches (Son et al., 2020).The developments in the multi-omics area, which consist of genomics, transcriptomics, proteomics, microbiomics, and metabolomics, have created a connection between genetic differences and regulatory components to the disease properties viewed from the systems level. The single-cell technologies also play a major role in this perspective by pinpointing the specific cell type drivers for B-cell failure, the dysregulation of hepatic glucose, and inflammation in adipose tissue. hitherto, AI-driven analysis and machine learning have worked together to combine these high-dimensional datasets, revealing the molecular and regulatory networks that are engaged in insulin signaling, lipid metabolism, mitochondrial function, and immune-metabolic crosstalk. This article collects current proof concerning the molecular structure of T2D, drawing attention to important pathways like PI3K-Akt, AMPK, mTOR, JNK, and sirtuins (Qi & Zalloua, 2025).

7. Immunogenetics and personalized medicine in T2DM

A paradigm shift that personalized medicine approach will have in managing patients with T2DM (Gloyn & Drucker, 2018), targeting to customize the treatment and prevention methods according to the patient's genomic profile, living habits, and surroundings. In T2DM, the interaction of heredity and the environment determines when, how fast, and which treatments will be given to patients' reactions (Fitipaldi et al., 2018). The rapid advancement of genomic technologies has resulted in the identification of more than 100 genetic loci as contributors to the risk of T2DM, thus shedding light on the genetic mechanisms involved in the disease. The information has also greatly increased the power of predicting an individual's T2DM predisposition and customizing treatments based on that, leading to care that is more accurate and effective (Dennis, 2020).

One important aspect of an individualized-medicine approach to type 2 diabetes is the utilization of genetic information to identify individuals at risk, even before clinical symptoms are exhibited (Kleinberger & Pollin, 2015). Consistently, genetic variants found in genes such as TCF7L2, KCNJ11 and PPARG, which affect insulin secretion, insulin sensitivity, and glucose metabolism, have been associated with a higher risk of developing T2DM. The integration of genetic testing into standard healthcare would enable doctors to make more accurate predictions regarding the patient's disease susceptibility, thus opting for an early intervention through the means of either lifestyle changes or the use of preventive treatments (Franks & Poveda, 2017). As an example, persons having certain genetic variations might receive help from targeted measures such as modifications in diet or drugs that directly affect the basic genetic pathways. Such a preventive method could possibly postpone the occurrence of T2DM and lessen the medical problems connected with it, like heart disease, kidney damage, and nerve damage.

Personalized medicine has already gone beyond risk prediction and is now expected to increase the effectiveness of treatment through a selection process whereby patients are coupled with the most suitable therapies based on their genetic profiles. A case in point is that certain genetic changes impact the response of patients to diabetes drugs like metformin, SGLT2 inhibitors, and GLP-1 receptor agonists (Tonin et al., 2025). The healthcare professionals will be able to optimize drug schedules by comprehensively getting these genetic interactions and that will allow them to lessen the negative effects and at the same time, prolong the positive outcomes. This method not only improves the standard of treatment but also cuts down the trial-and-error procedure that is usually a part of the treatment of long-lasting diseases like T2DM. Furthermore, the inclusion of genomics with other "omics" data (like proteomics, metabolomics, and microbiomics) opens the door to a more comprehensive understanding of the disease by enabling the incorporation of data related to the functioning of a patient's metabolic and immune systems at the molecular level (Awasthi, n.d.).

Moreover, immunogenetics is a new and promising area in the personalized treatment of T2DM. The role of inflammation and immune disorders in the T2DM development has become more and more evident. The major immune response genes, CTLA-4 and PTPN22, are among those affected by environmental factors that may lead to the development of diabetes (Sharma et al., 2021). Autoimmune diseases and T2DM have both been associated with this, indicating that the malfunctioning of the immune system is a major factor contributing to the insulin resistance and beta-cell failure. The genetic underpinnings of T2DM-related immune system defects being elucidated can lead to the discovery of novel strategies of treatment. One example is that directing the interventions toward certain immune pathways might, as a consequence, assist in controlling the inflammation and also in lessening the chronic low-level inflammatory state which is typical of T2DM (Donath et al., 2019). With the continual advancement of immunogenetics research, the likelihood of precision treatments that specifically address immune dysfunction is getting higher and higher, thus presenting a new frontier in the management of T2DM.

The incorporation of multi-omics technologies has a great impact on the personalized approach in diabetes mellitus type 2 by offering a comprehensive perspective of the disease (Saikia & Kalita, 2025; Srivastav et al., 2024). By merging genomics, transcriptomics, proteomics, metabolomics, and microbiomics data, the complex interactions between genes, proteins, metabolites, and the microbiota driving T2DM can be revealed. This comprehensive approach has the power to identify novel biomarkers, therapeutic targets, and predictive models of disease progression. Besides, machine learning and AI-driven analytical methodologies also contribute significantly to interpreting multi-omics data for proposing personalized treatment strategies with better efficacy in the management of the disease and prevention of complications (Ali, 2023). Eventually, this would translate into the fact that the integration of genomic data with clinical practice would mark the future of management in T2DM and ensure a more personalized, efficient, and effective approach toward diabetes care.

8. Clinical applications

The therapeutic uses of immunogenetics and personalized medicine are fundamentally transforming the management of T2DM (Venkatachalapathy et al., 2021). But as we begin to dig deeper and truly understand the genetic and immunological underpinnings of T2DM, clinicians are more prepared than ever to offer highly tailored patient-specific approaches, strategies not just to improve treatment outcomes but actually to help prevent the disease from starting in the first place. Traditional management of diabetes has, for a long time now, relied mostly on generalized approaches, such as simple lifestyle changes and standard drugs (Tiwari, 2015). The game has completely changed with the advent of genetic screening, pharmacogenomics, and epigenetic research. This opens massive new doors for precision medicine, where therapeutic strategies will be custom-designed to match the unique genetic, environmental, and immune characteristics of every single patient. The clinical applications are not confined to prescribing different drugs but now also extend to lifestyle interventions, early detection of disease, monitoring of disease, and modulation of immune response (Sorensen, 2024). Putting it all together, the integration of multi-omics technologies, genomics, transcriptomics, proteomics, and microbiomics further enhances our capacity to personalize care and provides a truly holistic approach to the management of T2DM. As these powerful innovations continue to evolve, they hold great potential to significantly improve not only the prevention but also the treatment of T2DM, thus reducing the huge global burden of this chronic metabolic disease. This section, therefore, appraises various clinical applications, with an emphasis on the increasing role of immunogenetics and personalized medicine in totally reimagining diabetes care.

9. Genetic screening for risk prediction and early detection of T2DM

Genetic screening is quickly becoming an essential tool for nailing down an individual's risk of developing T2DM (Lyssenko & Laakso, 2013). With over 100 genetic loci connected to the illness, this might identify high-risk people before they feel sick. That is enormous, enabling early lifestyle changes or pharmacological therapy to block or delay T2DM. Insulin resistance and glucose metabolism are linked to TCF7L2, KCNJ11, and PPARG variations (Piek, 2025). By integrating genetic screening into clinical practice, physicians will then be able to stratify patients depending on their inherited risk and offer them truly personalized care plans aimed at meeting their unique needs. Finding these risk alleles early is especially powerful for people with a strong family history of diabetes.

10. Pharmacogenomics in tailoring T2DM treatment

Let's now discuss the reason why managing type 2 diabetes used to be so unpredictable: trial and error. This is where pharmacogenomics comes into play, essentially resolving the issue down to prescribing a medication based on a patient's genetic data (Khan, n.d.). The problem is that depending on a person's genetic background, several popular diabetic medications—including GLP-1 receptor agonists, SGLT2 inhibitors, and metformin—work very differently. We now understand that certain gene variations, such as SLC30A8 or KCNJ11, are the primary determinants of a drug's ability to reach its intended target (Marin et al., 2024). By truly understanding those genetic factors at work that influence drug response, clinicians will be able to literally skip the frustrating guesswork. They can prescribe the right drug immediately, meaning way fewer side effects and dramatically greater efficacy. The whole approach completely eliminates that old, inefficient trial-and-error process and dramatically boosts patient outcomes.

11. Immune modulation therapy for T2DM management

Emerging research is strongly suggesting that immune system dysregulation is a huge factor in how T2DM develops (Brooks-Worrell et al., 2012). Inflammatory pathways and the immune response itself directly cause insulin resistance and beta-cell dysfunction. Therefore, for the final management of type 2 diabetes, the therapeutic application of immunogenetics is refocusing on determining how to effectively modulate these immunological pathways (Pilla et al., 2016). Focusing on these areas may be a great way to lessen the persistent low-grade inflammation that is characteristic of type 2 diabetes. Immune modulation therapies have the potential to greatly enhance glucose homeostasis and reduce the risk of catastrophic consequences, including nephropathy and cardiovascular disease. This method may be in its infancy, but it has great potential for the treatment of diabetes in the future.

12. Personalized lifestyle and behavioral interventions

Personalized lifestyle interventions, informed by genetic, epigenetic, and metabolic data, are emerging as a vital clinical application for the management of T2DM (Williams et al., 2022). Clinicians may finally stop giving patients the same old advice because of this smartly combining traditional genetic testing with extensive patient data (microbiome composition, metabolic profile, environmental exposures, etc.) allows them to develop individualized plans that include dietary restrictions, exercise programs, and behavioral therapies targeted at controlling blood sugar, decreasing obesity, and improving overall health (Alkhatib, 2020). For example, some variants in the PPARG gene may enable one patient to flourish on a particular diet, while their copatient requires an entirely different regimen. Even behavioral interventions can be personalized, matching an individual patient's distinctive psychological profile and facilitating the resolution of deep-seated emotional issues that may hinder the effective management of diabetes. Table 12.2 describes the precision medicine-based strategies originating from the genetic, immunological, and multi-omics discoveries in T2DM, based on their purpose, respective technologies or biomarkers, and potential benefit for early risk prediction, optimized treatment selection, immune modulation, and personalized lifestyle intervention.

Table 12.2 Clinical applications of immunogenetics and personalized medicine in T2DM.

Clinical application	Description	Key examples/ Technologies	Potential benefits
Genetic Screening for Risk Prediction and Early Detection	Utilizes genetic information to identify individuals at high risk of developing T2DM, even before clinical symptoms appear.	- TCF7L2, KCNJ11, and PPARG gene variants.	- Early identification of at-risk individuals. - Preemptive interventions to prevent T2DM onset.
Pharmacogenomics in Tailoring T2DM Treatment	Uses genetic profiles to predict how individuals will respond to various diabetes medications, enabling more precise and effective treatment.	- SGLT2 inhibitors, Metformin, GLP-1 receptor agonists.	- Optimized drug choice based on genetic makeup. - Reduced side effects and improved efficacy.
Immune Modulation Therapy for T2DM Management	Targets immune pathways involved in chronic inflammation, which contributes to insulin resistance and beta-cell dysfunction.	- Monoclonal antibodies targeting immune cells and cytokines.	- Reduction in chronic inflammation. - Improved insulin sensitivity and glucose metabolism.
Personalized Lifestyle and Behavioral Interventions	Tailor lifestyle interventions (diet, exercise, and behavioral therapies) based on genetic, epigenetic, and metabolic profiles.	- Diet adjustments for individuals with specific genetic variants. - Personalized exercise programs.	- More effective weight management. - Better control of blood glucose and overall metabolic health.
Targeting Epigenetic Modifications in T2DM Treatment	Focuses on altering epigenetic modifications (such as DNA methylation) that contribute to insulin resistance and beta-cell dysfunction in T2DM.	- Epigenetic modulators to influence gene expression. - CRISPR-based gene editing.	- Potential reversal of epigenetic changes contributing to T2DM. - Long-term improvements in glucose regulation.
Multi-Omics for Comprehensive Disease Management	Combines genomic, transcriptomic, proteomic, metabolomic, and microbiomics data to create a detailed, systems-level understanding of T2DM in individual patients.	- AI-driven analysis of multi-omics data. - Biomarker identification.	- Holistic approach to personalized treatment. - Identification of new biomarkers and treatment targets.
Immunogenetic-Based Biomarkers for Early Diagnosis and Monitoring	Uses immune-related genetic biomarkers to diagnose T2DM early and monitor disease progression, enabling more personalized monitoring strategies.	- Genetic variants in CTLA-4, PTPN22 for autoimmune involvement.	- Early diagnosis and intervention. - Improved monitoring of disease progression and complications.

13. Targeting epigenetic modifications in T2DM treatment

Now that we know that epigenetic modifications, such as changes in DNA methylation and histone modifications, play a significant role in the onset of type 2 diabetes, let's learn more about them. Indeed, the present state of knowledge centers on the mechanisms by which environmental and lifestyle variables may cause epigenetic changes, which in turn affect gene expression and advance the illness (Yang et al., 2022). These changes can directly influence insulin secretion, insulin resistance, and inflammation in T2DM. The amazing thing is that with an understanding of these epigenetic mechanisms, completely new therapeutic strategies have been developed aimed at either reversing or modulating the modifications. For instance, simple interventions that may influence DNA methylation patterns can effectively "reset" gene expression in such a way as to improve insulin sensitivity (Odimegwu et al., 2024). We may soon witness new medications or therapies developed to target these changes, providing an interesting new angle on treating type 2 diabetes, as this study progresses.

14. Multi-omics for comprehensive disease management

The integration of multi-omics technologies, including genomics, transcriptomics, proteomics, metabolomics, and microbiomics, is essential for achieving a comprehensive understanding of the complexities associated with T2DM (Hasin et al., 2017). Clinical applications for multi-omics allow us to understand at a systems level how all those different molecular pathways are interacting as the disease progresses. Think of combining genomic data together with proteomic and metabolomic information; this gives deep insight to the clinician into specific molecular changes occurring in every single patient, finally allowing truly personalized treatment strategies (Chen et al., 2023). For example, distinct variations in the composition of gut microbiota have been conclusively associated with insulin resistance and obesity. Multi-omics approaches are highly valued for uncovering biomarkers of early detection and progression, which directly enable the development of more targeted therapies (Xiao et al., 2022). Advanced biology tools are utilized to identify complex gene-environment interactions that influence disease outcome, resulting in refined and individualized care plans for patients with T2DM.

15. Immunogenetic-based biomarkers for early diagnosis and monitoring

Biomarkers are essential for the early diagnosis and continuous monitoring of T2DM (Ortiz-Martínez et al., 2022). Most promising, however, are biomarkers based on immunogenetics, which are directly derived from genetic and immune system information. They offer incredible diagnostic tools for flagging individuals with high risk and tracking the course of the disease. These biomarkers can give critical insight into the inflammatory process underlying T2DM and changes in immune cell function (Laakso, 2019). For example, specific genetic variants in immune-related genes such as *CTLA-4* and *PTPN22* could serve as indicators of autoimmune involvement in T2DM, helping us with both early detection and intervention (Nygård, 2021). Beyond that, the measurement of specific immune markers in the blood can indicate to doctors the extent of the disease's progression, the real effectiveness of the treatments being applied, and even enable the forecasting of possible complications. In the immediate future, these immunogenetic biomarkers will be used together with traditional diagnostics, including blood glucose and HbA1c, to provide a much more complete picture of health status.

16. Future directions in T2DM research and treatment

The future of T2DM management appears promising due to significant advancements in personalized medicine, immunogenetics, and multi-omics technologies (Kupai et al., 2022). The huge game-changer here is how AI and machine learning seamlessly blend to analyze genetic data, clinical data, and lifestyle data. This technology is poised to totally upend how we predict and handle T2DM, largely because it builds incredibly precise predictive models that fully take into account a patient's entire genetic and health profile. What does this mean in practical terms? By leveraging AI, researchers are identifying novel genetic variations, biomarkers, and extremely personalized treatment techniques that allow for earlier intervention and more effective care.

Gene therapy is one of the most promising and exciting research fields. Recent progress in CRISPR-Cas9 and other genome-editing techniques has enabled the correction of the specific genetic defects leading to insulin resistance and beta-cell dysfunction in T2DM (Golkar, 2020). Use is not restricted to managing the condition only; they open up the possibility of genetic curing of the disease, which makes this area of research very attractive to futurists. The researchers aim to normalize the production and action of insulin in patients by specifically altering and targeting the genes related to T2DM pathogenesis, thus giving them an actual long-term solution (Doudna, 2020).

The microbiome is the research frontier that is causing the most significant changes in T2DM. The gut microbiota studies have shown very clearly that it is not just a passive player; instead, it has a huge impact on controlling the activities of metabolism, the immune system, and insulin sensitivity, among others (Upadhyaya & Banerjee, 2015). The next generation of therapies, therefore, becomes really interesting: scientists are looking into ways of treating conditions by the gut and metabolic health, ranging from mere probiotics and prebiotics to advanced fecal microbiota transplants, which are done to actively change the gut. Besides, the possibility of metabolic surgery and other gut-related treatments is being investigated as new smart methods for modifying the microbiome to combat obesity and T2DM directly (Brunkwall & Orho-Melander, 2017). In the initial phases, this entire method has already opened up a very interesting and completely different path for treating patients with obesity-induced T2DM, particularly those who are resistant to current treatments.

The application of immunomodulatory therapies will totally take over the management of T2DM. The rationale is very plain: chronic inflammation is a primary contributor to T2DM, and an immune system disorder is a significant factor in insulin resistance. Consequently, as immunogenetics research proceeds, it will be easier to develop more precise immunotherapies by discovering the exact immune-related genes and pathways that regulate T2DM (Singh et al., 2024). The primary aim is to alter the immune reaction, efficiently minimize the persistent, chronic low-grade inflammation, and raise the insulin sensitivity. Just imagine the possibilities: monoclonal antibodies specifically designed to attack certain immune cells or inflammatory cytokines might provide a really new option for the treatment of patients suffering from both immune dysregulation and T2DM.

17. Challenges in T2DM research and clinical application

The immunogenetics and personalized medicine approaches are still facing significant challenges in their clinical applications despite the remarkable advances made in T2DM research (KN et al., 2025). Why? One of the main problems with T2DM is its drastic differences among patients. There are no two cases of the same type; instead, there are huge amounts of variations in resistance to insulin, beta-cell failure, and complications. Such remarkable diversity makes it completely impossible to come up with one-size-fits-all treatment plans. The truth is that patient-specific treatment, which takes into account each person's individual genetic make-up and disease symptoms, is absolutely indispensable (Sulashvili et al., 2025). The central problem we have to solve at present is coming up with the design of treatment plans that are stratified more effectively and, at the same time, nicely blend all the different genetic and environmental factors that are responsible for the advancement of the disease.

The incorporation of all the crucial multi-omics data, such as genomics, transcriptomics, proteomics, metabolomics, and microbiomics, into regular clinical practice is proving to be one of the most significant challenges (Mani et al., 2025). Indeed, the utilization of these technologies reflects tremendous insight into the molecular basis of T2DM; however, bringing all that individual information together into an integrated, patient-specific approach is highly complex (Buriani et al., 2017). Access is the big problem: the huge flow of data from high-dimensional sources requires modern computational models and bioinformatics tools for correct analysis; frankly speaking, such things are not very common and widely applicable in a usual hospital. Besides, there is a pronounced need for longitudinal studies that would follow the T2DM patients over several years in order to understand the long-term effects of genetic and epigenetic changes. The problem is that these studies require enormous resources and time, which in turn makes large-scale implementation really difficult.

Immunogenetics and personalized medicine also face serious ethical challenges. The use of genetic tests for predicting diseases and choosing appropriate therapy in some diseases raises significant problems concerning patient confidentiality, consent, and possible genetic discrimination (Santaló & Berdasco, 2022). What constitutes an ethical practice here is the complete and clear information that patients get and their understanding of the implications of genetic testing and data handling. Moreover, the new technologies of gene therapy and CRISPR-based technology for the treatment of T2DM raise questions about ethics in a very difficult way because of the genetic engineering of humans and the uncertain long-term effects of such powerful interventions (Salari & Larijani, 2017). Of course, the determinants of our regulatory frameworks need to change quickly to cope with these state-of-the-art issues and ensure that these revolutionary technologies are used in a safe and responsible way.

The access and affordability of personalized medicine for T2DM are major barriers to its broad application. Genetic testing, advanced treatments, and multi-omics technologies are expensive and hence beyond the reach of many patients (Hamza et al., 2025), especially those situated in low-resource conditions. The healthcare delivery systems are called to draw up planned and determined measures to fully support the inclusion of these powerful technologies in daily assistance and not unintentionally create differences in the participation of patients in the treatment. The problem of accessibility is further intensified by the requirement that medical staff continuously update their knowledge of the fast-paced genetic and personalized medicine practices (Fierz, 2004). Immediately, there is a growing requirement for specific educational and training programs that will allow healthcare personnel to gain the knowledge and acquire the tools for the effective integration of these crucial developments into daily clinical practice.

Eventually, we encounter unending obstacles related to getting regulatory approval and clinical validation of the latest therapies. While immunogenetic research is advancing, new treatments such as immunomodulatory therapies and gene-based interventions will have to undergo testing in patients who are extremely strict to ensure their safety and effectiveness (Amsaveni et al., 2025). The regulatory approval process for these kinds of treatments is quite complicated and lengthy by nature; thus, new therapies being available to patients gets delayed. Moreover, finding a way to turn fantastic research results into daily clinical applications requires a lot of interaction among the academic world, healthcare professionals, and drug companies in order to make sure that the new things are properly used (Grimshaw et al., 2012).

18. Conclusion

To sum up, the new directions in immunogenetics studies bring about a revolutionary way to deal with T2DM, with personalized treatment being the main highlight of the progress. With genetics and immune factors becoming more and more the focus as primary causes of T2DM, the prospect of risk prediction and the creation of treatment planning based on one's genetic makeup is a grand one. Combining genomic information with other "omics" technologies, such as proteomics and microbiomics, provides the full view of the disease at the molecular level that subsequently sustains the elaboration of highly effective and precise therapies. Immunomodulatory treatments targeted at the immune system's dysfunction and inflammation, together with the rapid development of gene therapy, constitute major changes in T2DM management. However, the personalization of T2DM treatment comes along with the problem of disease heterogeneity, complexity of multi-omics data integration, ethical issues related to genetic testing and therapies, as well as challenges concerning access and affordability, especially in low-resource settings. Nevertheless, the future management of T2DM is probably going to be more personal, highly effective, and sustainable, thus making treatment choices that can have a significant and positive impact on patient care and quality of life. Consequently, ongoing and interdisciplinary research and collaboration will be the way not only "to overcome these obstacles" but also "to ensure that T2DM patients everywhere can benefit from the world's innovations".

References

Afshardoost, S., Sarhangi, N., Afshari, M., Aghaei Meybodi, H. R., & Hasanzad, M. (2019). The influence of a genetic variant in the KCNQ1 gene on type 2 diabetes mellitus development. *Gene Reports, 17* (August), Article 100529. https://doi.org/10.1016/j.genrep.2019.100529

Ahmad, E., Lim, S., Lamptey, R., Webb, D. R., & Davies, M. J. (2022). Type 2 diabetes. *The Lancet, 400* (10365), 1803–1820. https://doi.org/10.1016/S0140-6736(22)01655-5

Ali, H. (2023). Artificial intelligence in multi-omics data integration: Advancing precision medicine, biomarker discovery and genomic-driven disease interventions. *International Journal of Science and Research Archive, 8*(1), 1012–1030.

Alkhatib, A. (2020). Personalising exercise and nutrition behaviours in diabetes lifestyle prevention. *European Medical Journal, 5*(1), 67–77.

Amsaveni, S., Radha, M., Chandrasekaran, V., Chanchal, D. K., Mathew, S., Sharma, M. C., Shiekmydeen, J., & Ali, S. S. (2025). Immune modulation strategies in gene therapy: Overcoming immune barriers and enhancing efficacy. *Current Gene Therapy, 25*(4), 374–393.

Awasthi, A. (n.d.). Understanding genomic, transcriptomic, proteomic, and metabolomics approaches. Molecular Plant Pathology, 38.

Bizimana, R. T. (2024). The impact of lifestyle modifications on type 2 diabetes prevention and management. *Idosr Journal of Biochemistry, Biotechnology and Allied Fields, 9*(3), 18–24. https://doi.org/10.59298/idosr/jbbaf/24/93.1824000

Brooks-Worrell, B., Narla, R., & Palmer, J. P. (2012). Biomarkers and immune-modulating therapies for type 2 diabetes. *Trends in Immunology, 33*(11), 546–553.

Brunkwall, L., & Orho-Melander, M. (2017). The gut microbiome as a target for prevention and treatment of hyperglycaemia in type 2 diabetes: From current human evidence to future possibilities. *Diabetologia, 60*(6), 943–951.

Buriani, A., Fortinguerra, S., & Carrara, M. (2017). Clinical perspectives in diagnostic-omics and personalized medicine approach to monitor effectiveness and toxicity of phytocomplexes. In *Toxicology of herbal products* (pp. 385–476). Springer.

Cai, F. Hong, Qian, Cui, F., Li, long, B., Li, dong, L., Liao, hong, B., Yu, min, Z., Fang, Q. li, Li, Y. yu, Dong, F. juan, Zhou, wei, L., Li, C., Wang, Q. yu, & Liu, J. hua (2025). DiabetesOmic: A comprehensive multi-omics diabetes database. *Computational and Structural Biotechnology Journal, 27*(May), 2147–2154. https://doi.org/10.1016/j.csbj.2025.05.008

Chauhan, G., Spurgeon, C. J., Tabassum, R., Bhaskar, S., Kulkarni, S. R., Mahajan, A., Chavali, S., Kumar, M. V. K., Prakash, S., Dwivedi, O. P., Ghosh, S., Yajnik, C. S., Tandon, N., Bharadwaj, D., & Chandak, G. R. (2010). The risk of type 2 diabetes in 5, 164 Indians. *Diabetes, 59*(August), 2068–2074. https://doi.org/10.2337/db09-1386.G.C

Chen, C., Wang, J., Pan, D., Wang, X., Xu, Y., Yan, J., Wang, L., Yang, X., Yang, M., & Liu, G. (2023). Applications of multi-omics analysis in human diseases. *MedComm, 4*(4), Article e315.

Das, S. K. (2014). Integrating transcriptome and epigenome: Putting together the pieces of the type 2 diabetes pathogenesis puzzle. *Diabetes, 63*(9), 2901–2903. https://doi.org/10.2337/db14-0757

Del Bosque-Plata, L., Martínez-Martínez, E., Espinoza-Camacho, M.Á., & Gragnoli, C. (2021). The role of TCF7L2 in type 2 diabetes. *Diabetes, 70*(6), 1220–1228. https://doi.org/10.2337/DB20-0573

Dennis, J. M. (2020). Precision medicine in type 2 diabetes: Using individualized prediction models to optimize selection of treatment. *Diabetes, 69*(10), 2075–2085.

Donath, M. Y., Dinarello, C. A., & Mandrup-Poulsen, T. (2019). Targeting innate immune mediators in type 1 and type 2 diabetes. *Nature Reviews Immunology, 19*(12), 734–746.

Doudna, J. A. (2020). The promise and challenge of therapeutic genome editing. *Nature, 578*(7794), 229–236.

Erfani, T., Sarhangi, N., Afshari, M., Abbasi, D., Meybodi, H. R. A., & Hasanzad, M. (2020). KCNQ1 common genetic variant and type 2 diabetes mellitus risk. *Journal of Diabetes and Metabolic Disorders, 19*(1), 47–51. https://doi.org/10.1007/s40200-019-00473-4

Fierz, W. (2004). Challenge of personalized health care: To what extent is medicine already individualized and what are the future trends. *Medical Science Monitor, 10*(5), 111–123.

Fitipaldi, H., McCarthy, M. I., Florez, J. C., & Franks, P. W. (2018). A global overview of precision medicine in type 2 diabetes. *Diabetes, 67*(10), 1911–1922.

Franks, P. W., & Poveda, A. (2017). Lifestyle and precision diabetes medicine: Will genomics help optimise the prediction, prevention and treatment of type 2 diabetes through lifestyle therapy? *Diabetologia, 60*(5), 784–792.

Gao, J., Zou, Y., Lv, X.-Y., Chen, L., & Hou, X.-G. (2024). Novel insights into immune-related genes associated with type 2 diabetes mellitus-related cognitive impairment. *World Journal of Diabetes, 15*(4), 735–757. https://doi.org/10.4239/wjd.v15.i4.735

Giri, B., Dey, S., Das, T., Sarkar, M., Banerjee, J., & Dash, S. K. (2018). Chronic hyperglycemia mediated physiological alteration and metabolic distortion leads to organ dysfunction, infection, cancer progression and other pathophysiological consequences: An update on glucose toxicity. *Biomedicine & Pharmacotherapy, 107*(July), 306–328. https://doi.org/10.1016/j.biopha.2018.07.157

Gloyn, A. L., & Drucker, D. J. (2018). Precision medicine in the management of type 2 diabetes. *Lancet Diabetes & Endocrinology, 6*(11), 891–900.

Golkar, Z. (2020). CRISPR: A journey of gene-editing based medicine. *Genes & Genomics, 42*(12), 1369–1380.

Grimshaw, J. M., Eccles, M. P., Lavis, J. N., Hill, S. J., & Squires, J. E. (2012). Knowledge translation of research findings. *Implementation Science, 7*(1), 50.

Hamza, N., Chen, L. L., Ahmed, N., & Zainaba, N. (2025). *Advancing diabetes care the role of personalized medicine in type 2 diabetes management.*

Hasin, Y., Seldin, M., & Lusis, A. (2017). Multi-omics approaches to disease. *Genome Biology, 18*(1), 83.

Jafar, N., Edriss, H., & Nugent, K. (2016). The effect of short-term hyperglycemia on the innate immune system. *The American Journal of the Medical Sciences, 351*(2), 201–211. https://doi.org/10.1016/j.amjms.2015.11.011

Karamanou, M. (2016). Milestones in the history of diabetes mellitus: The main contributors. *World Journal of Diabetes, 7*(1), 1. https://doi.org/10.4239/wjd.v7.i1.1

Khan, P. A. (n.d.). Personalized medicine: Optimizing treatment with the right drug, for the right patient, and at the right dose through pharmacogenomics.Pristyn Research Solutions.

Kim, M. (2019). DNA methylation: A cause and consequence of type 2 diabetes. *Genomics & Informatics, 17*(4), e38. https://doi.org/10.5808/gi.2019.17.4.e38

Kim, W. H., Lee, J. W., Suh, Y. H., Hong, S. H., Choi, J. S., Lim, J. H., Song, J. H., Gao, B., & Jung, M. H. (2005). Exposure to chronic high glucose induces β-cell apoptosis through decreased interaction of glucokinase with mitochondria: Downregulation of glucokinase in pancreatic β-cells. *Diabetes, 54*(9), 2602–2611. https://doi.org/10.2337/diabetes.54.9.2602

Kleinberger, J. W., & Pollin, T. I. (2015). Personalized medicine in diabetes mellitus: Current opportunities and future prospects. *Annals of the New York Academy of Sciences, 1346*(1), 45–56.

Kn, P., Dr, B., Ahmed, S. S., & Bm, J. (2025). Precision medicine in diabetes management: From theory to clinical practice. *International Journal of Pharmaceutical Investigation, 15*(2).

Kupai, K., Várkonyi, T., Török, S., Gáti, V., Czimmerer, Z., Puskás, L. G., & Szebeni, G. J. (2022). Recent progress in the diagnosis and management of type 2 diabetes mellitus in the era of COVID-19 and single cell multi-omics technologies. *Life, 12*(8), 1205.

Laakso, M. (2019). Biomarkers for type 2 diabetes. *Molecular Metabolism, 27*, S139–S146.

Li, H., Zou, L., Long, Z., & Zhan, J. (2024). Immunometabolic alterations in type 2 diabetes mellitus revealed by single-cell RNA sequencing: Insights into subtypes and therapeutic targets. *Frontiers in Immunology, 15*(January), 1–15. https://doi.org/10.3389/fimmu.2024.1537909

Lyssenko, V., & Laakso, M. (2013). Genetic screening for the risk of type 2 diabetes: Worthless or valuable? *Diabetes Care, 36*(Suppl. 2), Article S120.

Młynarska, E., Czarnik, W., Dzieża, N., Jędraszak, W., Majchrowicz, G., Prusinowski, F., Stabrawa, M., Rysz, J., & Franczyk, B. (2025). Cite 11. *International Journal of Molecular Sciences, 26*(3).

Mallick, P., Maity, S., Chakrabarti, O., & Chakrabarti, S. (2022). BBA - Molecular Cell Research Role of systems biology and multi-omics analyses in delineating spatial interconnectivity and temporal dynamicity of ER stress mediated cellular responses. *BBA - Molecular Cell Research, 1869*(4), Article 119210. https://doi.org/10.1016/j.bbamcr.2022.119210

Mani, S., Lalani, S. R., & Pammi, M. (2025). Genomics and multiomics in the age of precision medicine. *Pediatric Research*, 1–12.

Mannar, V., Boro, H., Patel, D., Agstam, S., Dalvi, M., & Bundela, V. (2023). Epigenetics of the pathogenesis and complications of type 2 diabetes mellitus. *TouchREVIEWS in Endocrinology, 19*(1), 46–53. https://doi.org/10.17925/EE.2023.19.1.46

Marin, J. J. G., Serrano, M. A., Herraez, E., Lozano, E., Ortiz-Rivero, S., Perez-Silva, L., Reviejo, M., & Briz, O. (2024). Impact of genetic variants in the solute carrier (SLC) genes encoding drug uptake transporters on the response to anticancer chemotherapy. *Cancer Drug Resistance, 7*, 27.

Moazzam-Jazi, M., Najd-Hassan-Bonab, L., Masjoudi, S., Tohidi, M., Hedayati, M., Azizi, F., & Daneshpour, M. S. (2022). Risk of type 2 diabetes and KCNJ11 gene polymorphisms: A nested case–control study and meta-analysis. *Scientific Reports, 12*(1), 1–13. https://doi.org/10.1038/s41598-022-24931-x

Nadiger, N., Veed, J. K., Chinya Nataraj, P., & Mukhopadhyay, A. (2024). DNA methylation and type 2 diabetes: A systematic review. *Clinical Epigenetics, 16*(1), 1–25. https://doi.org/10.1186/s13148-024-01670-6

Nygård, L. (2021). *Autoimmunity-associated polymorphisms and their effects on the immunophenotype: Cohort generation and subject immunophenotyping in the Finnish Diabetes Prediction and Prevention study*.

Odimegwu, C. L., Uwaezuoke, S. N., Chikani, U. N., Mbanefo, N. R., Adiele, K. D., Nwolisa, C. E., Eneh, C. I., Ndiokwelu, C. O., Okpala, S. C., & Ogbuka, F. N. (2024). Targeting the epigenetic marks in type 2 diabetes mellitus: Will epigenetic therapy be a valuable adjunct to pharmacotherapy? *Diabetes, Metabolic Syndrome and Obesity*, 3557–3576.

Ong, K. L., Stafford, L. K., McLaughlin, S. A., Boyko, E. J., Vollset, S. E., Smith, A. E., Dalton, B. E., Duprey, J., Cruz, J. A., Hagins, H., Lindstedt, P. A., Aali, A., Abate, Y. H., Abate, M. D., Abbasian, M., Abbasi-Kangevari, Z., Abbasi-Kangevari, M., ElHafeez, S. A., Abd-Rabu, R., … Vos, T. (2023). Global, regional, and national burden of diabetes from 1990 to 2021, with projections of prevalence to 2050: A systematic analysis for the Global Burden of Disease Study 2021. *The Lancet, 402*(10397), 203–234. https://doi.org/10.1016/S0140-6736(23)01301-6

Ortiz-Martínez, M., González-González, M., Martagón, A. J., Hlavinka, V., Willson, R. C., & Rito-Palomares, M. (2022). Recent developments in biomarkers for diagnosis and screening of type 2 diabetes mellitus. *Current Diabetes Reports, 22*(3), 95–115.

Piek, L. (2025). *Advances in genetic screening and their societal impact: Implications for diabetes mellitus*.

Pilla, S. J., Quan, A. Q., Germain-Lee, E. L., Hellmann, D. B., & Mathioudakis, N. N. (2016). Immune-modulating therapy for rheumatologic disease: Implications for patients with diabetes. *Current Diabetes Reports, 16*(10), 91.

Qi, X., Wang, J., Xu, Z., Sun, J., Keller, L., & Xu, W. (2014). Relationship of CTLA-4 gene to latent autoimmune diabetes in adults and type 2 diabetes: A population-based case–control study. *Diabetes Management, 4*(2), 131–139. https://doi.org/10.2217/dmt.13.70

Qi, L., & Zalloua, P. (2025). *From omics to AI — Mapping the pathogenic pathways in type 2 diabetes* (pp. 1–37). https://doi.org/10.1002/1873-3468.70115

Reyes, C. D. G., Alejo-jacuinde, G., Sanchez, B. P., Reyes, J. C., Onigbinde, S., Mogut, D., Hern, I., Calder, D., Quintanar, J. L., & Mechref, Y. (2024). *Multi omics applications in biological systems* (pp. 5777–5793).

Saikia, A. P., & Kalita, A. (2025). Artificial intelligence and multi-omics integration in obesity: A review of computational models for predicting metabolic comorbidities. *Clinical & Translational Metabolism, 23*(1), 7.

Salari, P., & Larijani, B. (2017). Ethical issues surrounding personalized medicine: A literature review. *Acta Medica Iranica*, 209–217.

Santaló, J., & Berdasco, M. (2022). Ethical implications of epigenetics in the era of personalized medicine. *Clinical Epigenetics, 14*(1), 44.

Sharma, C., Ali, R., B., Osman, W., Afandi, B., Aburawi, E. H., Beshyah, S. A., Al-Mahayri, Z., Al-Rifai, R. H., Al Yafei, Z., & ElGhazali, G. (2021). Association of variants in PTPN22, CTLA-4, IL2-RA, and INS genes with type 1 diabetes in Emiratis. *Annals of Human Genetics, 85*(2), 48–57.

Singh, K., Gupta, J. K., Chanchal, D. K., Varma, A., Shanno, K., Kumar, S., & Shamim. (2024). Deciphering the genetic landscape: Exploring the relationship between HLA-DQA1, HLA-DQB1, and HLA-DRB1 genes in diabetes mellitus. *Current Pharmacogenomics and Personalized Medicine, 21*(3), 125–135.

Son, J. W., Shoaie, S., & Lee, S. (2020). *Review article systems biology : A multi-omics integration approach to metabolism and the microbiome* (pp. 507–514).

Sorensen, J. (2024). The art and science of lifestyle medicine: A practical guide to transforming your health. *eBookIt. com*.

Srivastav, S., Lavanya, Avasthi, A., Kaur, N., Gaertner, W., Kesheri, M., Kanchan, S., & Sharda, S. (2024). Integromics: Tracking the multi-omic expanse in theragnostics. In *Microbial omics in environment and health* (pp. 135–173). Springer.

Sulashvili, N., Yaduvanshi, U., Yaduvanshi, N., Yadav, M., Abzianidze, E., Chichoyan, N., Gabunia, L., Gorgaslidze, N., Alavidze, N., & Abuladze, N. (2025). The scientific discourse of manifestation on key issue aspects of features, role and function of the family doctor in the 21 century in general. *Georgian Scientists, 7*(3), 485–521.

Tiwari, P. (2015). Recent trends in therapeutic approaches for diabetes management: A comprehensive update. *Journal of Diabetes Research, 2015*(1), Article 340838.

Tonin, G., Goričar, K., Blagus, T., Janež, A., Dolžan, V., & Klen, J. (2025). Genetic variability in sodium-glucose cotransporter 2 and glucagon-like peptide 1 receptor effect on glycemic and pressure control in type 2 diabetes patients treated with SGLT2 inhibitors and GLP-1RA in the everyday clinical practice. *Frontiers in Endocrinology, 16*, Article 1547920.

Upadhyaya, S., & Banerjee, G. (2015). Type 2 diabetes and gut microbiome: At the intersection of known and unknown. *Gut Microbes, 6*(2), 85–92.

Vaibhav, Nishad, S. S., Dongare, D., Tripathi, A. C. P., Tripathi, T., & Tripathi, P. (2024). Deciphering the intricacies of immune system dysfunction and its impact on diabetes mellitus: Revisiting the communication strategies to manage diabetes mellitus. *Health Sciences Review, 13*(September), Article 100201. https://doi.org/10.1016/j.hsr.2024.100201

Venkatachalapathy, P., Padhilahouse, S., Sellappan, M., Subramanian, T., Kurian, S. J., Miraj, S. S., Rao, M., Raut, A. A., Kanwar, R. K., & Singh, J. (2021). Pharmacogenomics and personalized medicine in type 2 diabetes mellitus: Potential implications for clinical practice. *Pharmacogenomics and Personalized Medicine*, 1441–1455.

Wang, X., Liu, J., Wang, Q., & Chen, Q. (2023). The transcriptomic and epigenetic alterations in type 2 diabetes mellitus patients of Chinese Tibetan and Han populations. *Frontiers in Endocrinology, 14* (February), 1–13. https://doi.org/10.3389/fendo.2023.1122047

Wang, X. H., Ma, A. G., Han, X. X., Chen, L., Liang, H., Aishan-Litifu, A.-A., & Xue, F. (2017). Protein tyrosine phosphatase nonreceptor type 22 (PTPN22) gene single nucleotide polymorphisms and its interaction with T2DM on pulmonary tuberculosis in Chinese Uygur population. *Oncotarget, 8*(39), 65601–65608. https://doi.org/10.18632/oncotarget.19274

Wang, S., Yong, H., & He, X.-D. (2021). Multi-omics: Opportunities for research on mechanism of type 2 diabetes mellitus. *World Journal of Diabetes, 12*(7), 1070–1080. https://doi.org/10.4239/wjd.v12.i7.1070

White, M. G., Shaw, J. A. M., & Taylor, R. (2016). Type 2 diabetes: The pathologic basis of reversible β-cell dysfunction. *Diabetes Care, 39*(11), 2080–2088. https://doi.org/10.2337/dc16-0619

Williams, D. M., Jones, H., & Stephens, J. W. (2022). Personalized type 2 diabetes management: An update on recent advances and recommendations. *Diabetes, Metabolic Syndrome and Obesity: Targets and Therapy*, 281–295.

Witcoski Junior, L., de Lima, J. D., Somensi, A. G., de Souza Santos, L. B., Paschoal, G. L., Uada, T. S., Bastos, T. S. B., de Paula, A. G. P., Dos Santos Luz, R. B., Czaikovski, A. P., Davanso, M. R., & Braga, T. T. (2024). Metabolic reprogramming of macrophages in the context of type 2 diabetes. *European Journal of Medical Research, 29*(1), 497. https://doi.org/10.1186/s40001-024-02069-y

Wu, Y. L., Lin, Z. J., Li, C. C., Lin, X., Shan, S. K., Guo, B., Zheng, M. H., Li, F., Yuan, L. Q., & Li, Z. hong (2023). Epigenetic regulation in metabolic diseases: Mechanisms and advances in clinical study. *Signal Transduction and Targeted Therapy, 8*(1). https://doi.org/10.1038/s41392-023-01333-7

Xiao, Y., Bi, M., Guo, H., & Li, M. (2022). Multi-omics approaches for biomarker discovery in early ovarian cancer diagnosis. *EBioMedicine, 79.*

Yang, Y., Luan, Y., Feng, Q., Chen, X., Qin, B., Ren, K.-D., & Luan, Y. (2022). Epigenetics and beyond: Targeting histone methylation to treat type 2 diabetes mellitus. *Frontiers in Pharmacology, 12*, Article 807413.

Zhang, Y., Zhang, Y., Yin, R., & Fang, X. (2024). *Multi-omics characterization of type 2 diabetes mellitus-induced gastroenteropathy in the db/db mouse model* (pp. 1–11). https://doi.org/10.3389/fcell.2024.1417255

13

Unresolved questions and challenges in immunogenetics

Rahul Kumar[1, 5], Prem Shankar Mishra[1], Abid Ali Sheikh[2], SK Abdul Rahman[4], Rakhi Mishra[3] and Sakshi Patel[1, 5]

[1]FACULTY OF PHARMACY, VIDYA UNIVERSITY, MEERUT, UTTAR PRADESH, INDIA; [2]NATIONAL INSTITUTE OF BIOLOGICALS, NOIDA, UTTAR PRADESH, INDIA; [3]NOIDA INSTITUTE OF ENGG. & TECHNOLOGY (PHARMACY INSTITUTE), NOIDA, UTTAR PRADESH, INDIA; [4]DEPARTMENT OF PHARMACEUTICAL SCIENCES, VIGNAN'S FOUNDATION FOR SCIENCE, TECHNOLOGY AND RESEARCH, GUNTUR, ANDHRA PRADESH, INDIA; [5]FACULTY OF PHARMACY, SWAMI VIVEKANAND SUBHARTI UNIVERSITY, MEERUT, UTTAR PRADESH, INDIA

1. Introduction

The study of the relationships between genetic variables and immunological phenotypes or immunity-related disorders is centered on the discipline of immunogenetics. The term immunogenetics, which combines the terms "immunization" and "genetics," refers to the study of immune system genetics. "Genetics" comes from the Greek term genesis, which means origin, and "immunity" from the Latin word immunis, which means "exempt." These days, one of the most difficult fields in immunogenetic biology is immunogenetics (Isaghazadeh and Rezaei, 2019). It has recently moved to the forefront of contemporary sciences with the introduction of cutting-edge methods like genetic modification and monoclonal antibodies. Immunology is the study of how the body fights against infectious diseases caused by bacteria, viruses, protozoa, fungi, and parasitic microorganisms like helminth worms (Boehncke & Brembilla, 2018).

The study of immunogenetics includes genetics, immunological system, hereditary immune reaction control, development, immunologically significant molecular arrangement, immunogenetics of reproductive biology, tissue separation, and susceptibility to illness. The fundamental elements of immunogenetics include sequences, nucleotides, genes, proteins, immunoglobins, or antibodies such as human leukocyte antigen (HLA) and major histocompatibility complex (MHC) receptors on T cells (Langerak, 2022a). The diagnosis, treatment, and engineering of autoimmune diseases, acquired immunodeficiency disorders, and infectious diseases (AIDS, etc.) can all benefit from immunogenetics.

Type 2 Diabetes Mellitus. https://doi.org/10.1016/B978-0-443-33590-7.00013-7

In order to identify, prevent, and cure a variety of infectious illnesses, this chapter will examine MHC and HLA immunogenetics and assess their therapeutic application potential. At the intersection of immunology and genetics, the intriguing field of immunogenetics investigates the genetic basis of immune system response and function. It simplifies autoimmune illnesses, highlights the intricate relationship between our genetic makeup and the body's defenses against infections, and provides focused therapy alternatives (Potts, 2002).

The importance, tenets, and uses of immunogenetics in deciphering the immune system will all be discussed in this article. Immunogenetics, at its core, studies the effects of genetic differences on the immune system's capacity to recognize, respond to, and retain infections. The body's immune system is a sophisticated network of tissues, materials, and cells that cooperate to defend the body against outside dangers and identify them from everyday ones. Genes that encode proteins essential to immune responses control this complex system (Lefranc, 2003). The investigation of the Major Histocompatibility Complex is one of the main areas of interest in immunogenetics (MHC). Human leukocyte antigens (HLAs), or MHC genes, are proteins that are expressed in humans. These molecules are essential in exposing foreign antigens to T cells, which triggers the immune system. Genetic differences in the MHC region can affect a person's vulnerability to autoimmune conditions, viral illnesses, and transplant rejection (Traherne, 2008). The hereditary tendency to autoimmune illnesses, in which the body's tissues are wrongly targeted by the immune system, has been clarified by immunogenetics. Using genome-wide association studies (GWAS) and linkage analysis, researchers have discovered many susceptibility loci linked to autoimmune diseases such as multiple sclerosis, type 1 diabetes, and rheumatoid arthritis. The genetic underpinnings of autoimmunity must be understood in order to develop personalized therapies and interventions (Lefranc, 2005). Immunogenetics is a key field in infectious disease research that helps us understand vaccination responses and host-pathogen interactions. Genetic differences in immune-related genes can affect a person's capacity to develop a successful immune response after vaccination, as well as their vulnerability to infections. Researchers can create vaccines specific to certain groups and enhance immunization efforts by clarifying these genetic characteristics (Giudicelli et al., 2005). Immunogenetics provides important findings that have ramifications for translational medicine. Within the field of immunogenetics, pharmacogenomics examines how genetic differences affect a person's reaction to drugs used to treat autoimmune diseases, cancer, and immunotherapy. Clinicians can avoid adverse responses and optimize medicine selection and administration by taking into account a patient's genetic profile. Immunogenetics is developing along with technology, opening up new fields of study and treatment options (Baum et al., 2004).

The fields of systems biology, CRISPR/Cas9 gene editing, and high-throughput sequencing are transforming our knowledge of immune-related genetic variants and their functional implications. Furthermore, combining immunogenetics with other omics fields like transcriptomics and proteomics could yield a thorough grasp of immune system control. By elucidating the genetic underpinnings of immune system function, autoimmunity, infectious illnesses, and therapeutic responses, immunogenetics is at the cutting edge of biomedical research. Immunogenetics holds the key to custom medicine, in which unique genetic profiles are used to inform treatment decisions by understanding the complex interactions between DNA and the immune system (Monod et al., 2004). Immunogenetics will keep fostering medical innovation as knowledge expands and technology develops, providing promise for better treatments and diagnostics as well as, eventually, better health outcomes for people all around the world.

2. Principles of immunogenomics

The core of immunogenetics theory is an understanding of how genetic variations impact immune system development and regulation. It includes research on how immune response-related chemicals are encoded by genes, how genetic differences impact immunological function, and how these variations influence vaccination responses, treatment results, and disease risk. This is a thorough overview of the immunogenetics' guiding concepts (Bach & Bach, 1972).

3. Immune system components genetic foundation

The body's defense mechanism against diseases and foreign substances is the immune system, which is composed of several cell, tissue, and molecular types. The proteins and receptors necessary for immunological function are encoded by genes. Genes, for instance, encode proteins linked to the immune system, major histocompatibility complex (MHC) components, B cell receptors (BCRs), T cell receptors (TCRs), and cytokines. polymorphisms in the structure, expression, and function of immune components can be caused by genetic polymorphisms within these genes, and this can impact the immune response's overall efficacy (Roederer et al., 2015).

3.1 Key histocompatibility complex (MHC) and presentation of antigens

Antigen presentation is a crucial initial step in initiating adaptive immune responses, and it is assisted by the human leukocyte antigen (HLA) system, which is sometimes referred to as the MHC.MHC gene-encoded cell surface proteins transmit antigenic peptides to T cells, which trigger immunological responses. In autoimmune illnesses, these peptides may come from the body's cells or from infections.Different MHC molecules are produced by genetic variations in MHC genes, which affect an individual's capacity to present a variety of antigens and assess immunological response (Fuggle & Taylor, 2012, pp. 55–75).

3.2 Immunogenetics of autoimmunity

When the immune system mistakenly assaults and targets body tissues, autoimmune diseases result. Research in immunogenetics has shown genetic variations linked to a higher risk of developing autoimmune diseases, including rheumatoid arthritis, type 1 diabetes, and systemic lupus erythematosus (Farid, 1990). These genetic variants may impact immune regulation, self-tolerance, or the recognition of self-antigens, which can lead to autoimmune disease.

3.3 Immunogenetics in infectious diseases

The vulnerability of an individual to infectious illnesses and their capacity to develop a successful immune response toward pathogens can be influenced by genetic variants within immune-related genes. Genetic variations in genes that encode cytokines, chemokines, and pattern recognition receptors (PRRs) can affect how infectious pathogens are recognized, signaled, and removed from the body. Furthermore, immunogenetic variables affect vaccination reactions, impacting the effectiveness and persistence of protective immunity after immunization (Alves et al., 2006).

3.4 Pharmacogenomics and immunogenetics

Pharmacogenomics is the study of how genetic differences affect a person's reaction to medications, such as immunomodulatory therapies for cancer, autoimmune illnesses, and organ transplants. The effectiveness, toxicity, and side effects of drugs can be impacted by genetic variations in genes related to drug metabolism, pharmacological targets, or immunological pathways (Poland et al.).

Generally speaking, immunogenetics emphasizes how genetic variations affect immunological responses, susceptibility to disease, and treatment outcomes. It also demonstrates the complex interplay between immunity and heredity. By making these ideas more understandable, immunogenetics contributes to personalized medicine by enabling treatments to be tailored to the genetic profile of each patient for improved safety and effectiveness (Qadir & Majid, 2022). The immune system is an intricate network of molecules and cells that defends the body against infections, foreign substances, and abnormal cells. The immune system's remarkable adaptability allows it to recognize and hold onto certain illnesses, allowing it to develop a stronger fight against them later on (Ali et al., 2022a).

Genomic science is the study of an organism's whole DNA sequence, which includes all of its genes and non-coding regions. Scientists can now identify genetic variations connected to certain traits, diseases, and treatment responses because of advancements in genomics. The goal of immunogenomics is to integrate these two domains to get a deeper comprehension of the immune system's genetic foundation and how genetic differences might impact immune response and disease propensity (Ali et al., 2022b). Researchers can find genes and pathways involved in immune activity and control by examining the transcriptome and genome of immune cells.

3.5 The range of immunological diseases and immunogenetics

The innate immune system serves as the primary defense against foreign antigens through interactions with pattern recognition receptors (PRRs) such as nucleotide-binding oligomerization domain-like receptors (NLRs) and Toll-like receptors (TLRs), as well as signal-transducing molecules such as interleukin-1 receptor-associated kinase 4 (IRAK4). An underactive system leads to an underdetection of exogenous chemicals, which increases an individual's susceptibility to infection.

Another undesirable function of this system is reacting to its own components, as seen in autoimmune illnesses. In any case, this prevents the immune system from working as it should (Hill, 2001). For example, genetic factors increase the body's susceptibility to viral and autoimmune illnesses. By focusing on autoimmune diseases and infections, immunogenetics attempts to address the HLA and non-HLA repercussions for each of the aforementioned categories, which stand for the two extremes of the spectrum of immune disorders (Lamont et al., 2022).

4. Autoimmune diseases

A robust immune system protects the body against illness and infection. However, when the immune system isn't working properly, it starts attacking healthy tissues, cells, and organs. referred described as an autoimmune illness.

4.1 Diabetes mellitus

One significant and ever more significant cardiovascular risk factor is diabetes mellitus (DM). Over 240 million individuals worldwide are estimated to have diabetes mellitus (DM), with 439 million predicted to have the illness by 2030. Cardiovascular disease is the main killer of diabetics. It has long been known that people with diabetes are more likely to die from cardiovascular disease and other conditions. In a similar vein, the primary cause of death for those with rheumatoid arthritis (RA) is cardiovascular disease. Furthermore, RA patients have a higher death rate from cardiovascular disease than one would anticipate in a healthy individual. It's unclear, though, if a higher-than-normal frequency of DM is related to RA. The relationship between DM risk and RA has been the subject of much research; however, These studies' results differed because of variations in study design, sample size, controls, and geographical areas (Morran et al., 2015). To date, no meta-analysis has focused on the association between RA and the risk of DM (Table 13.1).

4.1.1 Diabetes mellitus Type 1 (T1DM)

The pancreatic beta cells that create insulin are damaged in type 1 diabetes mellitus, also known as simply type 1 diabetes. It is a persistent autoimmune disease. A hormone called insulin helps cells absorb glucose from the circulation so they can use it to

Table 13.1 Representing the diseases caused by Diabetic Mellitus.

Immunogenetic diseases caused by Diabetic Mellitus	Diabetic mellitus Type 1 Diabetic mellitus Type 2 Psoriasis Rheumatoid arthritis (RA) Cardiovascular disease Diabetic Nephropathy Neurological diseases Multiple sclerosis (MS) Retinopathy Diabetes and Asthma Diabetes and lung disease Diabetic vascular disease

produce energy. When a person has type 1 diabetes, their immune system accidently kills these beta cells, which prevents them from making adequate insulin (Noble, 2015).

It is unclear what exactly triggers the autoimmune reaction that destroys beta cells, although it is thought to be a result of a complicated interaction between immunological dysregulation, viral infections, and genetic vulnerability. The symptoms may appear suddenly and be severe, and in certain cases, they proceed quickly to hyperglycemia (high blood sugar) and diabetic ketoacidosis (DKA). Dehydration, electrolyte abnormalities, metabolic acidosis, and elevated blood ketone levels are the hallmarks of DKA, a potentially fatal condition (Fernandes et al., 2005).

Glycated hemoglobin (HbA1c) readings, which indicate the average blood glucose levels over the two to 3 months before, are measured, fasting blood glucose levels are tested for, and clinical indications of type 1 diabetes are looked for. Autoantibodies such as islet cell antibodies (ICA), which are directed against pancreatic beta cells, insulin autoantibodies (IAA), antibodies against zinc transporter 8 (ZnT8), and glutamic acid decarboxylase (GADA) can be discovered to demonstrate that the disorder is autoimmune. Maintaining blood sugar levels within the prescribed range is the aim of treatment to avoid both immediate consequences (like hypoglycemia and diabetic ketoacidosis) and long-term effects (such as neuropathy, renal disease, cardiovascular disease, and retinopathy) (Mimura et al., 1990).

The constant management of diabetes by those with type 1 diabetes might have negative psychological repercussions. The difficulties in managing type 1 diabetes, the fear of adverse consequences, and the stigma associated with the condition can induce mental distress, worry, hopelessness, and suffering from diabetes. Comprehensive diabetes care must include emotional support, education, and counseling (Reece et al., 1991).

4.1.2 Type 2 diabetes T2DM

Approximately 90% of all instances of diabetes are T2DM mellitus. Insulin resistance is the term used to describe a person with type 2 diabetes who is less sensitive to insulin. Adults over 45 are most frequently diagnosed with type 2 diabetes. But because obesity, lack of exercise, and energy-dense diets are on the rise, it is becoming more common among kids, teens, and young adults. Immunogenetics influences type 2 diabetes mellitus (T2DM), however in a different way than it has historically been linked to autoimmune diseases like type 1 diabetes. The hallmarks of type 2 diabetes are insulin resistance, a condition in which the body's cells become less sensitive to insulin, and a relative insulin shortfall brought on by compromised beta-cell activity (Olokoba et al., 2012).

Although T2DM is commonly thought to be a metabolic disease, new research indicates that dysregulation of the immune system and mild inflammation may play a role in the disease's onset. There is evidence to suggest that some genetic variations raise the risk of type 2 diabetes. These variations may have an impact on beta-cell function, insulin signaling pathways, and immunological response. Numerous susceptibility loci have been found by genome-wide association studies (GWAS), some of which are linked to genes associated to the immune system, including those that control inflammation, cytokine signaling, and adaptive immunological responses. Type 2 diabetes, insulin resistance, and obesity are frequently associated with chronic low-grade inflammation, which is marked by high levels of inflammatory markers such as C-reactive protein (CRP), tumor necrosis factor-alpha (TNF-α), and interleukin-6 (IL-6).

There are several potential causes of this inflammation, such as metabolic stress, dysfunctional adipose tissue, and activation of innate immune pathways (Goyal et al., 2024). Specifically, visceral adipose tissue secretes pro-inflammatory cytokines termed adipokines and chemokines, acting as an active endocrine organ. Insulin resistance and systemic inflammation, two variables that contribute to obesity and type 2 diabetes, are made worse by adipose tissue inflammation, which is characterized by the invasion of immune cells such as T lymphocytes and macrophages.

Genetic variants affecting immune cell recruitment, inflammation of adipose tissue, and adipokine production may influence the susceptibility to type 2 diabetes. It has been discovered that the etiology of type 2 diabetes and insulin resistance involves the dysregulation of immune cell types such as T cells, dendritic cells, and macrophages. Variations in the ratio of pro-to-anti-inflammatory (M1) macrophage phenotypes to T cell subsets (Th1, Th2, Th17, Treg) may be involved in the development of chronic inflammation linked to type 2 diabetes, beta-cell dysfunction, and poor glucose homeostasis. Metabolic homeostasis and immune response regulation are significantly influenced by gut flora. Type 2 diabetes, insulin resistance, and obesity have all been connected to dysbiosis, or alterations in the make-up and activity of the microbial communities that reside in the gut (Ginter & Simko, 2013, pp. 42–50).

Gene expression patterns can be altered by epigenetic processes, including DNA methylation, histone modifications, and non-coding RNA regulation, in response to a variety of environmental stressors, including nutrition, exercise, and metabolic stress. Epigenetic changes that affect genes related to the immune system, metabolism, and insulin sensitivity may have an impact on the incidence and progression of type 2 diabetes. Although insulin resistance and beta-cell dysfunction are the primary causes of type 2 diabetes mellitus (T2DM), immunogenetic factors such as genetic predisposition, low-grade inflammation, adipose tissue dysfunction, immune cell dysregulation, gut microbiota composition, and epigenetic alterations also play important roles in the pathogenesis of the disease (Chen et al., 2012). Knowing how immunological and genetic variables interact in type 2 diabetes (T2DM) may help develop new treatment targets, provide light on the disease's causes, and direct individualized approaches to the prevention and treatment of the condition.

4.2 Diabetic nephropathy

One prevalent and potentially fatal side effect of diabetes mellitus, particularly type 1 diabetes (T1DM) and type 2 diabetes is diabetic nephropathy, also known as diabetic kidney disease (T2DM). The condition is typified by the increasing impairment of the glomerular filtration units (GLUTs) in the kidneys, culminating in the development of proteinuria, hypertension, end-stage renal disease (ESRD), and fading renal function. A person's hereditary risk factors account for most cases of diabetic nephropathy. A heritable component of diabetic kidney disease has been found through research on twins and family history, which may point to a potential genetic susceptibility. Genome-wide association studies (GWAS) have connected a number of genetic variants associated to immune-related genes, including those that cause inflammation and fibrosis, to an elevated risk of diabetic nephropathy and renal function. Chronic low-grade inflammation is linked to the development of diabetic nephropathy. Diabetes causes hyperglycemia and metabolic abnormalities, which lead to the production of pro-inflammatory cytokines, chemokines, and reactive oxygen species. These factors also cause endothelial dysfunction, glomerular hypertrophy, podocyte damage, and interstitial fibrosis (Asgarbeik et al., 2021). Immune cells that enter the kidneys and release inflammatory mediators, such as T cells, dendritic cells, and macrophages, worsen renal damage. Some Human Leukocyte Antigen (HLA) alleles in diabetics have been linked to an increased risk of diabetic nephropathy. For instance, some alleles of HLA-DRB1 and HLA-DQB1 have been connected to a higher risk of diabetic nephropathy in both T1DM and T2DM. These HLA correlations suggest that immune-mediated processes and underlying immune system dysfunction might play a role in the etiology of diabetic kidney disease. Although diabetic nephropathy is typically thought of as a non-immune-mediated consequence of diabetes, there is mounting evidence that suggests renal impairment may occasionally be caused by autoimmune processes. Diabetes-related nephropathy patients have been shown to have autoantibodies against renal antigens, including mesangial cells and extracellular matrix proteins (Mlynarski et al., 2005). This finding raises the possibility of immune complex deposition and immunological-mediated glomerular damage. The pathophysiology of diabetic nephropathy may involve genetic variables that affect autoantibody synthesis, immune complex formation, and renal tissue vulnerability to immunological-mediated injury.

All things considered, immunological dysregulation, inflammation, hereditary vulnerability, and anomalies in metabolism all play a role in the multifactorial condition known as diabetic nephropathy. Knowing the immunogenetic foundation of diabetic nephropathy may help to identify patients who are more likely to experience renal problems, provide light on the disease's causes, and guide the development of individualized treatment plans that include immunomodulatory medication.

4.3 Psoriasis

When psoriasis was first discovered, it was thought to be a condition caused by aberrant keratinocyte growth, which often manifested as persistent plaque and put sufferers at risk for joint, psychological, and cardiovascular problems. Long-term autoimmune skin condition psoriasis results in red, scaly, and inflammatory patches of skin. Although psoriasis mostly affects the skin, it is becoming more well acknowledged that it is a systemic inflammatory illness that may have consequences for a number of comorbidities, such as diabetes mellitus. Here is the immunogenetic relationship between psoriasis and diabetes, namely type 2 diabetic mellitus (T2DM) (Harden et al., 2015). Dysregulated immunological responses, typified by aberrant immune cell activation and persistent inflammation, are characteristics of psoriasis and type 2 diabetes. Immune cells such as T cells, dendritic cells, and macrophages can permeate the skin during psoriasis. These cells produce proliferating keratinocytes, which further aids in the formation of skin lesions, as well as inflammatory cytokines including interleukin-17 and tumor necrosis factor-alpha. Similarly, insulin resistance, beta-cell dysfunction, and systemic metabolic abnormalities are linked to chronic low-grade inflammation in type 2 diabetes (T2DM), which is defined by higher levels of pro-inflammatory cytokines, adipokines, and acute-phase reactants. Numerous comorbidities, such as metabolic syndrome, cardiovascular disease, and type 2 diabetes, are linked to an increased risk of psoriasis.

Epidemiological studies have demonstrated time and time again that the prevalence of type 2 diabetes is higher in psoriasis patients than in the general population (Schneeberger et al., 2015). The clustering of these illnesses may be explained by the existence of shared underlying processes, such as hereditary vulnerability, insulin resistance, and chronic inflammation. Psoriasis and type 2 diabetes have been related to environmental factors in its development. These variables include smoking, food, stress, physical inactivity, and obesity.

These substances may exacerbate immunological dysregulation, promote chronic inflammation, and contribute to the initiation or progression of both diseases. When common environmental variables are taken into account, there may be a stronger correlation between type 2 diabetes and psoriasis. Inflammation-targeting psoriasis therapies may improve metabolic parameters and lower the risk of type 2 diabetes, per a recent research. Nevertheless, it has been demonstrated that a variety of drugs used to treat type 2 diabetes, such as glucagon-like peptide-1 receptor agonists (GLP-1 RAs) and thiazolidinediones (TZDs), lessen the severity of psoriasis in those who co-occurring type 2 diabetes and psoriasis (Mak et al., 2009).

4.4 Multiple sclerosis (MS)

Both diabetes and multiple sclerosis (MS) are autoimmune illnesses, which means that the body's tissues are attacked by the immune system. Although MS affects the central nervous system and diabetes affects the pancreas and insulin control, there may be an immunogenetic connection between the two conditions despite their distinct organ effects. The study of how hereditary variables affect the immune system and how it reacts to illnesses is known as immunogenetics. It has been shown that there is a hereditary component to both diabetes and MS and that specific genetic abnormalities may raise the likelihood of getting these disorders (Hollenbach & Oksenberg, 2015).

Studies have indicated that there are certain genetic similarities between multiple sclerosis (MS) and type 1 diabetes, an autoimmune variant of the disease. Both illnesses have been linked to a number of genes that control inflammation and the immune system. For example, there is a connection between the HLA (human leukocyte antigen) genes, which are critical for the immune system, and an increased risk of MS and type 1 diabetes. Moreover, some studies have suggested that an individual with one autoimmune disease may be more vulnerable to another.

This phenomenon is called poly autoimmunity or autoimmune disease clustering. Due to a common underlying immune dysregulation, people who already have one autoimmune illness, such as MS or type 1 diabetes, may be more susceptible to developing another autoimmune ailment. But despite data pointing to possible genetic similarities and common pathways between diabetes and multiple sclerosis, there is still much to learn about the precise nature of these connections and the underlying processes (McDonald et al., 1984). To completely comprehend how these illnesses could interact at the immunogenetic level, more research is required.

4.5 Rheumatoid arthritis (RA)

A chronic inflammatory illness of the synovial joints, rheumatoid factor (RF) and anti-citrullinated protein antibody (ACPA) production, synovial hyperplasia, abnormalities of the bone, and systemic symptoms are the hallmarks of rheumatoid arthritis (RA). RA largely affects the joints, resulting in insulin insufficiency and hyperglycemia, whereas T1DM is primarily related to inflammation, discomfort, and eventually degeneration of the joints owing to the autoimmune death of insulin-producing beta cells in the pancreas (Messemaker et al., 2015). These conditions differ in their pathophysiological causes and clinical manifestations, but they are similar in that they are associated with autoimmune dysregulation and immunogenetics.There is a significant hereditary component to both T1DM and RA, as some genetic variations make people more susceptible to developing autoimmune diseases. Genome-wide association studies have identified a large number of susceptibility loci for T1DM and RA (GWAS). Numerous genes relevant to immunity, such as those encoding cytokines, signaling molecules involved in immune regulation, and human leukocyte antigens (HLAs), are associated with several of these loci.

There is substantial evidence linking specific HLA alleles to a higher risk of T1DM or RA development. For example, there is a strong correlation between the likelihood of developing RA and certain HLA-DRB1 alleles, such as those encoding the shared epitope (SE), particularly in seropositive individuals with rheumatoid factor (RF) or anti-citrullinated protein antibodies (ACPAs). Similarly, individuals with certain HLA class II alleles, such as HLA-DRB104:01 and HLA-DQB103:02, are more likely to develop type 1 diabetes because they are more vulnerable to the autoimmune destruction of their pancreatic beta cells.

Dysregulated immune responses leading to autoantibodies, inflammatory cytokines, and immune cell infiltration into target tissues are the hallmarks of both RA and T1DM (Walport et al., 1992). Because autoantibodies primarily target self-antigens in the joints, they specifically target synovial inflammation and joint degradation in RA patients with RF and ACPAs. Autoantibodies against pancreatic beta-cell antigens, including insulin, glutamic acid decarboxylase (GAD), and insulinoma-associated antigen 2 (IA-2), have been related with beta cell death and inadequate insulin production in patients with type 1 diabetes mellitus. Even while genetic factors significantly increase the risk of the illness, environmental triggers have a significant role in initiating and sustaining inflammatory responses in both RA and T1DM. Environmental factors such as infections, diet, smoking, and hormone changes can lead to immune dysregulation and autoimmunity in genetically susceptible individuals, thereby precipitating the onset or exacerbation of disease. An illustration of the interdependence of autoimmune illnesses and the complexity of their genetic and immunological underpinnings is provided by autoimmune polyendocrine syndrome type 3 (APS-3), which is defined by the presence of autoimmune thyroiditis, type 1 diabetes, and other autoimmune ailments (Onengut-Gumuscu & Concannon, 2006).

Generally, immunogenetic characteristics such as genetic predisposition, HLA linkages, autoimmune dysregulation, and environmental triggers are shared by both RA and T1DM, despite the fact that they are separate autoimmune illnesses that affect different target organs.

4.6 Cardiovascular disease

Diabetes mellitus (T2DM) and cardiovascular disease (CVD) have complex etiologies that involve the interaction of immunogenetic, inflammatory, and metabolic variables. Individuals who have diabetes have a much higher risk of cardiovascular problems compared to the general population. Diabetes's immunogenetic components raise the risk of cardiovascular disease in a number of ways. Genetics has a role in diabetes and cardiovascular disease; genome-wide association studies (GWAS) have found many risk loci for these conditions. Numerous genes linked to the immune system, inflammation, lipid metabolism, and cardiovascular risk factors are associated with these genetic variations.

Pro-inflammatory cytokines, chemokines, and acute-phase reactants are produced in diabetes due to hyperglycemia, insulin resistance, and metabolic abnormalities. These factors also cause endothelial dysfunction, vascular inflammation, atherosclerosis, and plaque instability (Candore et al., 2006). Immune cells that enter vascular tissues, such as dendritic cells, T cells, and macrophages, release inflammatory mediators that exacerbate vascular damage and promote atherogenesis. The genetic predisposition to thrombosis, platelet dysfunction, and coagulation pathways may increase the risk of cardiovascular problems in diabetics.

The majority of cardiovascular events are caused by atherosclerosis and plaque instability, which is increased in people with diabetes. These plaques are more likely to rupture and cause thrombosis when diabetes is present. Acute cardiovascular events are more likely to occur in diabetics due to genetic variables that affect the stability, composition, and susceptibility to rupture of plaque (Limas et al., 2002). Knowing the intricate interactions between inflammatory, metabolic, and genetic factors may help to clarify the mechanisms underlying diabetes-related cardiovascular complications and guide the development of focused prevention and management plans for this high-risk population.

4.7 Neurological diseases

The genesis of neurological illnesses, which can include complex interplay between genetic vulnerability and environmental variables, poses considerable challenges to public health. Understanding the etiology and course of different neurological illnesses has led to a major focus on immunogenetics, the study of genetic implications on immunological responses.

The intricate interactions that occur between the immune system and the central nervous system (CNS) in neuroinflammatory diseases, highlighting the role that hereditary factors play in controlling autoimmune reactions and neuroinflammation.

We also discuss about the challenges associated with studying immunogenetics in neurological disorders, including the need for lengthy cooperative research initiatives, the complexity of disease pathophysiology, and the range of patient populations. Notwithstanding these obstacles, developments in immunogenetics provide promise for precision medicine methods in neurology, providing chances for individualized prognosis, diagnosis, and therapeutic approaches (Ash & Roy, 2022). We stress the significance of transdisciplinary research projects, data-sharing programs, and multidisciplinary cooperation in order to overcome these obstacles and hasten the knowledge and treatment of neurological illnesses.

4.8 Retinopathy

Diabetic retinopathy, which is typified by ocular blood vessel destruction in the retina, is a common outcome of diabetes mellitus. The development and progression of diabetic retinopathy have been connected to many genes related to oxidative stress, inflammation, and vascular function. These genes may change the way the body responds to oxidative stress, blood vessel growth, inflammation, and other processes that may raise the risk of retinal damage in diabetics (Stewart et al., 1993).

Chronic low-grade inflammation is thought to play a major part in the development of diabetic retinopathy because it causes aberrant blood vessel formation and vascular damage in the retina. An individual's capacity to manage oxidative damage in the retina may be impacted by genetic differences in genes encoding antioxidant enzymes and other components of oxidative stress pathways, which may in turn impact the risk of diabetic retinopathy (Wang et al., 2023). Moreover, genes about vascular function, particularly those controlling the integrity and creation of blood vessels, are probably implicated in the onset of diabetic retinopathy. Variations in these genes may impact the integrity and functionality of retinal blood vessels, making diabetics more vulnerable to injury.

To fully understand the intricate interactions among vascular disease, immunological dysregulation, and genetic variables in diabetic retinopathy, more research is necessary. While the immunogenetics of this issue is still being studied, pinpointing certain genetic risk factors may help predict a person's likelihood of developing diabetic retinopathy and may result in the creation of tailored approaches to screening, prevention, and treatment.

4.9 Diabetes and asthma

Asthma is a long-term inflammatory respiratory disease that affects 1%–8% of the population. Diabetes increases a person's risk of asthma. According to epidemiologic research, type 1 diabetes incidence has been increasing globally at a rate of 3% per year, while the prevalence of type 2 diabetes and asthma has been steadily rising in industrialized countries (Cookson, 2004). According to a retrospective countrywide population-based cohort research, asthma attacks were far more common among type 2 diabetes patients than in the general population. This finding suggests that insufficient glycemic management in children may potentially increase their susceptibility to asthma. Asthma and diabetes have been linked to certain genetic variations. For example, these illnesses have been associated with several gene variants related to inflammation, immune system function, and insulin regulation (Howell, 1994). The Human Leukocyte Antigen (HLA) system, which encodes essential immune system proteins, has been connected to a higher risk of diabetes and asthma.

In a manner similar to this, the immune system attacks and destroys the pancreatic beta cells responsible for producing insulin in type 1 diabetes. Numerous immunological systems and cell types linked to asthma may be involved in the development of diabetes, especially type 1 diabetes, according to studies (Borish, 1999). Diabetes and asthma attacks can have an impact on the severity and onset of attacks depending on environmental factors such pollution, nutrition, and lifestyle decisions. For example, type 2 diabetes risk factors including obesity and insulin resistance can cause asthma. Knowing the immunogenetic causes of diabetes and asthma might lead to more specialized treatments and medications (Sandford et al., 1996). Finding shared immune systems or genetic pathways might result in the creation of innovative therapies that can treat both illnesses at once. Overall, it is evident that both diabetes and asthma have intricate genetic and immunological components, even if the precise immunogenetic interactions between the two conditions are still being worked out (Bragina et al., 2014).

4.10 Diabetes and lung disease

Diabetes suggests a long-term state of hyperglycemia, which causes nonenzymatic protein glycosylation, which is a significant cause of multi-organ dysfunction. The respiratory system has been targeted by diabetes in recent decades, in addition to the most frequent repercussions of diabetes, which include atherosclerosis, neuropathy, nephropathy, and retinopathy.

Most studies have focused on the damage to the pulmonary vascular bed and alveolar surface that causes pulmonary microangiopathy, pulmonary capillary basal laminae, and thickening of the alveolar epithelia based on autopsy data from diabetic patients (Krishna et al., 2024). One of the main causes of tissue damage in diabetics is the elevated production of reactive oxygen and nitrogen species brought on by hyperglycemia.

Actuality, it damages DNA among other biological constituents. Asthma and diabetes, particularly Type 1 diabetes, have common inflammatory pathways despite their differing symptoms. The hallmarks of asthma include inflammation of the airways, which causes bronchoconstriction and increased mucus production (Xin et al., 2023). Both disorders are impacted by signaling proteins known as cytokines, which affect the immune system. For instance, elevated levels of TNF-alpha and interleukin-6 (IL-6) have been linked to Type 2 diabetes and asthma, which may indicate a common immune activation route.

The goal of current research is to have a deeper understanding of the immunological and genetic links between asthma and diabetes (Khadhraoui et al., 2020). By comprehending this, medical professionals can develop more potent therapies that target the underlying immunological malfunction rather than just the symptoms. For instance, therapies that alter inflammatory pathways shared by the two illnesses may have two advantages.

Furthermore, by identifying these connections, individuals at risk for both diseases might benefit from improved screening and preventative measures. In conclusion, common inflammatory pathways, hereditary variables, and immune system dysfunctions are involved in the link between diabetes and asthma in the context of immunogenetics (Lu et al., 2024).

4.11 Diabetic vascular disease

Atherosclerosis and its consequence are caused by a predisposition to thrombosis in conjunction with abnormalities in the function of vascular smooth muscle cells and endothelium (DeGraba, 2004). In order to maintain vascular homeostasis, which prevents thrombosis and leukocyte diapedesis and ensures enough blood flow and nutrient supply, normal endothelium cells create and release biologically active substances. Endothelial NO synthase (eNOS) constitutively produces nitric oxide (NO), which is one of the major chemicals generated by the endothelial cell. It does this by oxidizing the guanidine-nitrogen terminal of L-arginine by five electrons.

An essential indicator of arterial health is the NO bioavailability (Kristensen, 1984). When NO stimulates guanylyl cyclase on adjacent vascular smooth muscle cells, vasodilation takes place. Additionally, NO mediates chemical signals that prevent platelets and leukocytes from interacting with the vascular wall, limiting the migration and proliferation of vascular smooth muscle cells and shielding the blood vessel from endogenous damage or atherosclerosis. On the other hand, a decrease in NO produced from the endothelium allows for increased activation of nuclear factor kappa B (NF-), which in turn stimulates the expression of leukocyte adhesion molecules and the synthesis of chemokines and cytokines.

These pathways facilitate the migration of monocytes and vascular smooth muscle cells into the intima, resulting in the formation of macrophage foam cells and the first anatomical abnormalities connected to atherosclerosis. Reduced endothelium-dependent, NO-mediated relaxation is a sign of endothelial dysfunction in cellular and experimental types of diabetes (Bossini-Castillo et al., 2015).

Consequently, diabetes may have an atherogenic predisposition since it reduces NO levels. The equilibrium between NO production by NOS and its degradation, especially by oxygen-derived free radicals, is reflected in the bioavailability of NO.Endothelial cell activity is abnormally affected by some metabolic disorders associated with diabetes, such as insulin resistance, hyperglycemia, and excessive release of free fatty acids, which all influence the production or breakdown of NO (Ünlü et al., 2022).

5. Infectious diseases

A substance that damages a person's health, frequently a form of bacterium, is the source of an infection.

5.1 Human immunodeficiency virus (HIV)

Reduced endothelium-dependent, NO-mediated relaxation in cellular and experimental forms of diabetes indicates endothelial dysfunction.Clinical studies have shown that most but not all cases of type 1 or type 2 diabetes are associated with abnormal endothelium-dependent vasodilation. Because diabetes lowers NO levels, it may consequently have an atherogenic propensity (Medhasi & Chantratita, 2022). The equilibrium between NO production by NOS and its degradation, especially by oxygen-derived free radicals, is reflected in the bioavailability of NO.Endothelial cell activity is abnormally affected by several metabolic illnesses associated with diabetes, such as insulin resistance, hyperglycemia, and excessive release of free fatty acids. These diseases also influence the production or breakdown of NO. The CCR5-Δ32 mutation confers resistance to HIV infection by shortening the CCR5 receptor, which stops the virus from infecting host cells (Lisanwork Arage et al., 2021). Changes in the genes that encode cytokines, chemokines, and other immune signaling molecules can impact the kind and intensity of the immune response to HIV, as well as the development of immunological activation and chronic inflammation, which are characteristics of HIV infection (Hajdarevic).

Furthermore, the rate at which HIV disease advances and the onset of AIDS-related complications may be influenced by host genetic characteristics. Genetic differences in genes associated to host-pathogen interactions, immunological modulation, and viral replication can affect the balance between immune control and replication.

This may affect how quickly the sickness advances and how likely it is to have opportunistic infections and other AIDS-related disorders (Arage et al.). Understanding the immunogenetic variables that determine HIV susceptibility, progression, and treatment results is critical for creating tailored approaches to HIV prevention, treatment, and care (Li et al., 2021). By discovering genetic markers linked to HIV susceptibility and disease development, researchers may better anticipate individual risk profiles and adapt therapies to match the unique requirements of infected people. Different people have different levels of immunity to HIV. HLA genes provide HIV resistance by interacting with $CD4^+$ helper T cells and $CD8^+$ cytotoxic T cells to facilitate the start of anti-HIV adaptive immunological responses (Basler & Groettrup, 2020). Increased vulnerability to infection, lowered viral load, accelerated or delayed disease progression, and infection prevention have all been linked to HLA genes. HIV resistance has also been linked to KIR genes (Pao et al., 2022). What's more fascinating is that HIV patients' distinct immunogenetic composition, at least in part, impacts the onset of tuberculosis (TB).

5.2 Viruses that cause hepatitis B (HBV) and hepatitis C (HCV) infection

Immunogenetics of Hepatitis B and HCV infections is the study of how genetic differences impact treatment results and susceptibility in individuals with Hepatitis B virus (HBV) and Hepatitis C virus (HCV), as well as how these variations affect the immune response to these viruses (Ding et al., 2024). Genetic variations in genes encoding elements of the immune system, including as human leukocyte antigens (HLAs), cytokines, chemokines, and other immune-related molecules, might affect an individual's susceptibility to HBV or HCV infection as well as the progression of the illness. A higher or lower incidence of HBV or HCV infection, the start of chronic hepatitis, the development of cirrhosis or hepatocellular carcinoma (HCC), and other conditions have all been associated with certain HLA alleles (Ashhab et al., 2020).

Genetic differences in genes associated with immune response pathways may impact the ability of the immune system to control an HBV or HCV infection. Changes in the genes encoding immunological signaling molecules such as cytokines, chemokines, and Toll-like receptors (TLRs) can affect the course of viral infection, the degree of immune response, and the development of chronic inflammation and liver damage (Al-Mayah, 2024).

The balance between viral replication and immunological control can be influenced by genetic variations in genes related to immune modulation, host-pathogen interactions, and viral replication. This can affect the severity of liver disease and the risk of developing cirrhosis, liver failure, or hepatocellular carcinoma (HCC) (Soleiman-Meigooni et al., 2024). Genetic variations in drug metabolic routes, transporters, and drug targets can all have an impact on the pharmacokinetics and pharmacodynamics of antiviral medicines, resulting in variances in treatment effectiveness, toxicity, and outcomes among HBV and HCV infected people (Tao et al., 2022). Researchers can more accurately predict individual risk profiles, customize interventions to the unique needs of affected individuals, and optimize treatment strategies to improve outcomes and lessen the burden of viral hepatitis by identifying genetic markers linked to viral susceptibility, disease progression, and treatment response.

People who have HBV or HCV infection are more prone to developing cirrhosis, hepatocellular carcinoma, and chronic liver disease due to the altered expression of intrahepatic genes (Su et al., 2020). Comprehending the kinetics of virus-specific T-cell responses can help with tracking clinical recovery as they are essential for the removal of infected hepatocytes. The formation of HBV-specific T cells in peripheral blood indicates that after a year, about 2% of individuals with chronic HBV infection will spontaneously eradicate their virus (Kemming et al., 2020). Using genome-wide association studies (GWASs), genes associated to both HLA and non-HLA groups have been linked to chronic HBV infection, disease progression, and the risk of developing HBV-related hepatocellular carcinoma. Again, both HLA and non-HLA genes have been associated with spontaneous clearance of HCV. Two genes are associated with HCV-related hepatocellular carcinoma: MICA and DEPDC5.

5.3 Tuberculosis (TB)

Tuberculosis (TB) and diabetic mellitus (DM) have a complex association, and immunogenetics play an important part in how these illnesses interact with one another.The immunological response to tuberculosis includes a variety of genetic variables that determine infection susceptibility, illness development, and treatment response (Ndong et al., 2023). An individual's capacity to react to tuberculosis (TB) may be impacted by variations in the genes that generate cytokines, chemokines, and other chemicals related to the immune system.

There is evidence linking variations in the genes encoding TNF-α, IFN-γ, and ILs to the severity and susceptibility to tuberculosis (TB). Chronic hyperglycemia is the outcome of insulin action, production, or both issues in diabetes mellitus, a metabolic condition (Kumar & Meena, 2020). Numerous genes contribute to the etiology of both diabetes type 1 and type 2, which include inherited components. The manufacture of insulin, sensitivity, and other metabolic processes are all impacted by these genes.

Variations in the genes encoding insulin (INS), insulin receptor (INSR), and other transcription factors linked to the function of pancreatic beta cells can raise the risk of diabetes (Varzari et al., 2024). Diabetes makes a person more susceptible to TB and makes their outcomes worse than those of non-diabetics. The immunosuppressive effects of hyperglycemia on the immune system, impaired macrophage function, and dysregulated cytokine production are thought to be the causes of this heightened sensitivity (Ridolfi et al., 2023).

Genetic variables that impact immunological function, such as those involved in the host response to tuberculosis, may also influence the risk and severity of tuberculosis in people with diabetes. Furthermore, several genetic variations associated with diabetes may alter susceptibility to tuberculosis or responsiveness to anti-TB therapy (Singh et al., 2021).

5.4 Immunogenetics and immunosenescence

Immunosenescence, the aging process that weakens the immune system, increases the risk of infection, linked diseases, and death in the elderly (Caruso et al., 2022). It is typified by a chronic low-grade inflammation caused by abnormal innate and adaptive immune responses. Numerous illnesses are linked to it, such as type 2 diabetes, atherosclerosis, cancer, neurological conditions, obesity, osteoporosis, and osteoarthritis (Lian et al., 2020). Over the past 40 years, immunosenescence has received a lot of attention from geneticists. But because different approaches were used, we are unable to apply the results to all senior people (Rehman et al.). The immunogenetic network that spans the human lifespan appears to be influenced by non-HLA genes linked to both innate and adaptive immunity in addition to HLA genes.

5.5 Immunogenetics of skin disorders

The three chronic illnesses that children are most commonly affected by are asthma, hay fever (allergic rhinitis), and eczema (atopic dermatitis). Given their close relationship, atopic dermatitis and asthma are both classified as forms of atopic disorders (Martin et al., 2020). The term “atopy” can be used to describe a range of illnesses, such as asthma, food allergies, urticaria, and allergic rhinitis. It is thought that Th2 cytokines drive IgE + memory B and plasma cells to synthesize IgE, which is how atopy is caused (Lee et al., 2022).

Genome scans show that 60% of atopic disorders are often heritable, suggesting that the MHC gene, located on the short arm of chromosome 6, may be shared by genes that cause atopy and other autoimmune diseases (Kanikowska et al., 2021). Since the airway epithelium in particular affects asthma, there is a good chance that common genes will result in asthma as well as other epithelial-based conditions like psoriasis and Crohn's disease.

Moreover, genes that code for cytokines and innate immune receptors, (Vaseghi-Shanjani et al., 2021) are part of the immunogenetic network linked to atopy and are necessary for the start and development of allergic reactions.

6. Adversomics and vaccomics: Immunogenetics and vaccination response

In general, immunogenetic data is used by vaccinomics and adversomics to anticipate vaccination effectiveness and safety, which promotes the creation of more potent vaccines. Vaccinomics' main goal is to target the genes that might account for a substantial amount of this diversity.

For instance, research indicates that the diversity in antibody response to the measles, mumps, rubella, and hepatitis B surface antigen (HBsAg) is 60%, 88%, 38%, and 45% hereditary, respectively (Kennedy et al., 2020). TLRs, cell surface receptors, and HLA and non-HLA-encoding genes generally impact immunological responses to vaccinations such as HBV, smallpox, MMR, and seasonal influenza (De la Fuente & Contreras, 2021). The goal of immunogenetics is to find and treat the genetically altered immune systems that cause functional defects in the immune system.

6.1 Diagnosis

Immunogenetics plays a major role in the autoimmune illness known as Type 1 diabetes mellitus (T1DM) (Black & Zorina, 2020). The immunogenetic elements of Type 2 diabetes (T2DM) are less prevalent but still very important, especially in understanding the inflammatory pathways that contribute to insulin resistance.

6.2 Type 1 diabetes mellitus (T1DM) and immunogenetics

Typically, hyperglycemia and one or more autoantibodies specific to diabetes are found to be the first signs of T1DM. Further information can be obtained by immunogenetic testing, particularly by identifying genetic markers associated with a higher chance of developing type 1 diabetes (Monar et al., 2022).

6.2.1 Test for autoantibodies

Look for antibodies that are commonly associated with type 1 diabetes.

Islet cell cytoplasmic autoantibodies (ICA) are a common kind of autoantibodies.

Autoantibodies to insulin (IAA).

Autoantibodies against glutamic acid decarboxylase (GADA).

Autoantibodies against tyrosine phosphatase IA-2 (IA-2A).

Autoantibodies against zinc transporter 8 (ZnT8A)

6.2.1.1 HLA typing

Identify genetic susceptibility to T1DM.

Examine for the alleles of the HLA-DR and HLA-DQ genes, which are closely linked to type 1 diabetes. T1DM risk is increased by the presence of certain HLA haplotypes (e.g., DR3-DQ2, DR4-DQ8) (Minniakhmetov et al., 2024).

6.2.1.2 Insulin therapy

Replace the insulin that your body cannot make. Use an insulin pump or inject insulin to regulate blood glucose levels. Think about customizing insulin dosages according to genetic factors affecting insulin sensitivity and metabolism.

6.2.1.3 Immunomodulatory therapies

To avoid pancreatic beta cell death, target the immune system. Use immunosuppressive medicines (e.g., corticosteroids, cyclosporine), immune modulators (e.g., anti-CD3 monoclonal antibodies), or biologics (e.g., anti-IL-1β agents) to manage the autoimmune response (Thomas et al., 2023). Genetic profiling may assist in identifying people who are more likely to benefit from certain immunomodulatory medications.

6.2.1.4 Islet cell transplantation

restore insulin production by transplanting pancreatic islet cells. Consider islet cell transplantation in selected patients, particularly those with frequent severe hypoglycemia or hypoglycemia unawareness. Genetic factors may influence the success and long-term outcomes of transplantation (Johnson et al., 2020).

6.2.1.5 Genetic counseling

Provide patients and families with information and assistance about the hereditary elements of type 1 diabetes (Zhang et al., 2021). Provide genetic counseling to assist patients in understanding genetic risk factors, inheritance patterns, and implications for family planning.

6.3 Immunogenetics in diabetes mellitus type 2 (T2DM)

Diagnosing type 2 diabetes usually involves measuring plasma glucose levels, such as A1C, 2-hour plasma glucose during a 75-gram oral glucose tolerance test, or fasting plasma glucose. Immunogenetic variables, however, could be important (Chinniah et al., 2021), notably in terms of inflammation and insulin resistance.

6.3.1 Genetic markers of inflammation

Identify genetic variations that alter the inflammatory pathways that contribute to insulin resistance.

Example: Variants in genes such as TNF-α and IL-6 can disrupt metabolic pathways and lead to insulin resistance.

6.3.2 *Polygenic risk scores*

Evaluate the cumulative effect of several modest genetic variants, each of which marginally raises the risk of T2DM (Borysewicz-Sańczyk et al., 2020). Using genetic data, generate a score that predicts the chance of getting T2DM depending on the existence of these variants.

6.4 Treatment

Diabetes mellitus therapy, particularly in the context of immunogenetics, entails controlling both the metabolic elements of the disease as well as immune system dysregulation, particularly in Type 1 diabetes (T1DM).

Lifestyle changes such as nutrition, exercise, and weight management can help to improve insulin sensitivity and glucose control.Encourage patients to adopt healthy lifestyle choices customized to their genetic predispositions and metabolic profiles.

6.4.1 *Pharmacological therapies*

Boost insulin secretion, decrease glucose production, or improve insulin sensitivity. Provide medication, such as metformin, sulfonylureas, SGLT-2 inhibitors, DPP-4 inhibitors, or GLP-1 receptor agonists, based on the specifics of each patient, taking into account hereditary factors that may impact drug response and metabolism (Zhao et al., 2024).

6.4.2 *Precision medicine approaches*

Personalize treatment plans based on genetic and immunological characteristics. Consider combining genetic testing and polygenic risk scores to identify people who can benefit from certain drugs or lifestyle modifications.

6.4.3 *Inflammatory modulation*

Address the chronic inflammation linked with type 2 diabetes and its consequences. Investigate medicines that target inflammatory pathways involved in insulin resistance and beta-cell malfunction (Osman et al., 2022), taking into consideration genetic variations linked with inflammation.

7. Challenges of immunogenomics

Though immunogenomics has the potential to improve healthcare, there are various problems involved with this topic, including (Figs. 13.1 and 13.2).

7.1 Complexity of the immune system

Immunogenetic research must traverse the immune system's enormous complexity, which includes many genes, their interconnections, and their varied expressions under diverse situations (Qadir & Majid, 2022). This intricacy makes it difficult to pinpoint

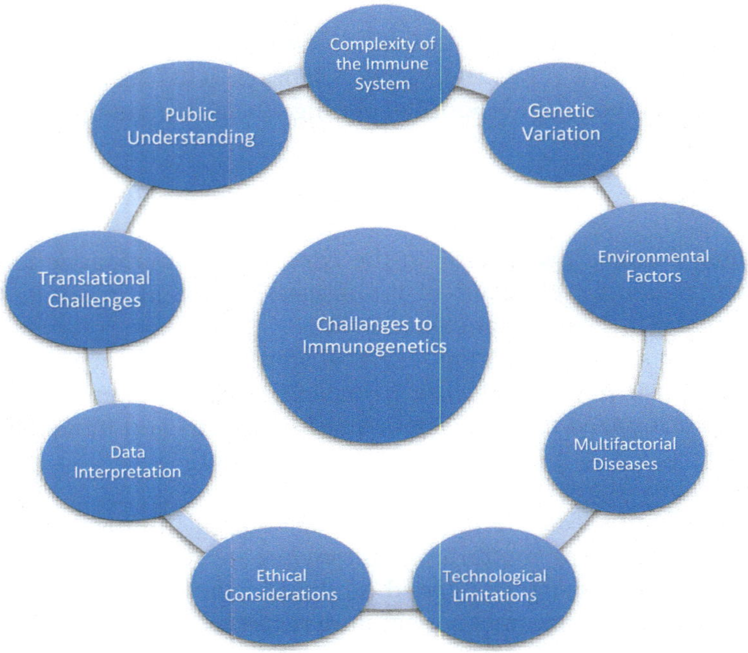

FIGURE 13.1 Representing the challenges of immunogenetics.

FIGURE 13.2 Representing strategies for improvement in immunogenetics.

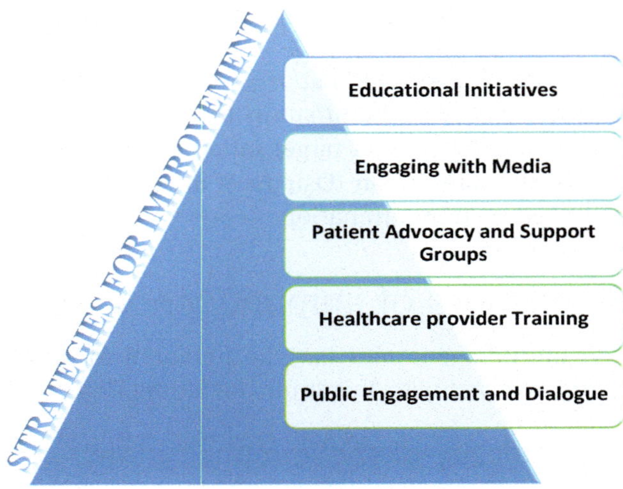

particular genetic components that are responsible for immunological responses, such as,

- Immune characteristics are inherited polygenically.
- Interactions between genes and the environment can affect immune-related geneexpression.
- Genetic variation makes it difficult to replicate results across groups.

Large-scale GWAS has identified polymorphic polygenic variations, which are the largest group and do not provide useful functional information on individual variants (Kiyotani et al., 2021). Conversely, these variances may be used to calculate an individual's total genetically based risks (PRS), which can then be used as the basis for suggestions for medical interventions or alterations in behavior to help reduce the risks (Addala et al., 2024). However, before any of these claims can be validated for practical use, in-depth population-by-population study will be required (Ros et al., 2019).

Currently, the challenge is to use limited genetic association studies to identify single-unit changes with significant functional effects. The best ways to do this are to 1) research rare mutations, which are usually chosen after thorough candidate evaluation, and 2) carefully choose phenotypes (Hollenbach et al., 2013), They are frequently the most extreme examples of a quantitative variable or traits with a high heritability. Therefore, rare variants with relatively large impacts will serve as the main foundation for identifying functional variations that are uniquely recognizable. These variations will help understand the molecular basis of complicated diseases and traits, which will ultimately lead to improved disease prevention and treatment (Mack et al., 2009).

7.2 Environmental effect

The environmental impact on immunogenetics is an important topic of research because it investigates how external variables influence genetic predispositions in the immune system (Siddique, 2023).The environmental influences on immunogenetics emphasize the need of taking into account both genetic predispositions and environmental interactions while examining immunological responses. This comprehensive approach is critical for designing more effective disease preventive measures, medicines, and public health interventions suited to specific surroundings and populations (Emam).

7.3 Infection exposure

The field of immunogenetics focuses on understanding healthy immune systems and identifying genetic variations that lead to immune system illnesses. This research aims to identify new treatment targets (Wolf & Samuels, 2018). The immune system, which is the body's primary defensive mechanism, responds differently to various pathogenic illnesses. Unlike other species, viruses replicate by using their host's resources. Genes that encode human leukocyte antigens (HLA), such as those of the human histocompatibility system, regulate the immune system (Petersdorf, 2006). Human HLA is regarded as the major polymorphic genetic system since it has a variety of alleles and hence numerous potential combinations. Because of this polymorphism, which is strongly linked to both species genetic diversity and variations in disease susceptibility across genetically varied populations, large-scale epidemics are consequently less likely to develop (Gonzalez-Galarza et al., 2021). HLA antigens are crucial for both disease susceptibility and resistance. The main elements influencing a person's susceptibility to infectious diseases include genetics. Different immune responses may be seen by infected individuals against the same infectious disease (Hill, 2001).

7.4 Genetic variations

In immunogenetics, the concept of genetic variation is essential to comprehend the diversity of immunological responses in individuals and groups (Kamatani & Nakamura, 2021). It affects immunity to infections, how the body reacts to vaccinations, and the reasons certain people are more susceptible to allergies or autoimmune diseases. Talk about the main types of genetic variations that affect immunogenetics and its implications here.

7.5 Single nucleotide polymorphisms (SNPs)

In the human genome, SNPs are the most common genetic variation. A single nucleotide alteration in a DNA sequence can affect the production of genes or the function of proteins, which can influence the immune system (Chen et al., 2021).SNPs in genes that encode cytokines or cytokine receptors can change immunological responses, resulting in differences in infection susceptibility, illness severity, and the outcome of inflammatory disorders. For example, specific SNPs in the IL-10 gene promoter might cause varying levels of IL-10 production (Kim & Jeong, 2020), influencing inflammatory and autoimmune illnesses.

7.6 Copy number variations (CNVs)

CNVs are duplications or deletions of larger regions of DNA, ranging in size from a 1000 to millions of base pairs (Marcon et al., 2020). These polymorphisms can alter the amount of gene copies, possibly influencing gene dosage and phenotypic results. The quantity of immunological receptors on cells, for example, is one immune system component that can be impacted by CNVs, which might impact the immune system's capacity to recognize and react to infections (Zhu et al., 2022). For example, CNVs in complement component genes might disrupt the effectiveness of the complement system, which is critical for innate immunity.

7.7 Gene rearrangements

The genes that code for the antigen receptors on B and T cells, notably the immunoglobulin (Ig) and T-cell receptor (TCR), are highly significant in immunogenetic research

(Vlachonikola et al., 2023a). These rearrangements are a type of somatic genetic diversity necessary for the development of a broad repertoire of antibodies and TCRs.

The huge number of potential rearrangements enables the identification of an equally vast number of antigens, which is required for successful adaptive immunity (Sinkora et al., 2022). Errors in these rearrangements can cause immunodeficiencies or malignancies like lymphomas.

7.8 Epigenetic modifications

Epigenetic modifications impact gene expression instead of the DNA sequence. Examples of modifications that are susceptible to both hereditary and environmental influences are histone acetylation and DNA methylation (Cao & Yan, 2020). Epigenetic alterations have the ability to regulate the expression of genes involved in immunological responses, hence influencing an individual's response to immunizations and infections. Numerous autoimmune diseases and allergies are associated with epigenetic instability (Looi et al., 2023).

7.9 Mitochondrial DNA variations

Though less typically mentioned in immunogenetics, differences in mitochondrial DNA (mtDNA) can have an impact on immune function since mitochondria are involved in energy generation, apoptosis, and immunological signaling pathways (Lo Faro et al., 2021). Variations in mtDNA can influence how immune cells operate, possibly impacting inflammation and susceptibility to viral illnesses.

8. Multifunctional disease

Immunogenetics researchers are particularly interested in multifunctional illnesses, which are complicated diseases that impact several body systems, including the immune system (Yang et al., 2022). Genetic predispositions, environmental factors, and immune responses often combine in these illnesses, leading to complicated disease processes and a variety of clinical manifestations. Examples include diabetes, heart disease, autoimmune diseases, and some cancers (Yang et al., 2022; Kung et al., 2022). These multifactorial disorders can have a significant influence on immunogenetics, making understanding this interplay critical for creating targeted medicines and interventions. Certain genetic predispositions in multifunctional disorders can have an impact on immune system function (Tam et al., 2020; Kiyotani et al., 2021; Addala et al., 2024).

8.1 Technological limitations

The field of immunogenetics, which studies the genetics of immune system behavior, relies heavily on technological advancements. However, limitations in technology limit our ability to fully understand and manipulate immunogenetic data, affecting research and clinical applications (Hussain & Shabir, 2022). Our grasp of sophisticated algorithms, such as natural language processing and data mining approaches, which uncover patterns, risk factors, and predictors of vaccination effectiveness and safety, has been drastically altered by the application of AI, which has led to substantial advancements in immunology and genetics (Agathangelidis et al., 2022).

Artificial neural network-based deep learning technologies have become powerful instruments for the analysis of massive genomic datasets. These algorithms have been utilized by researchers to find hidden connections and patterns that might otherwise be missed by employing more conventional techniques (Xu et al., 2021). Because it makes it easier to identify possible immunogenicity hazards and encourages the creation of safer and more effective treatment methods, this knowledge is crucial to the development of novel medications (Ansari et al., 2023). This makes it possible to study the intricate relationships that exist between genetic variations and immune responses, which has led to important discoveries into the mechanisms behind autoimmune diseases, cancer immunotherapy, and vaccine development (Klau et al., 2023).

These algorithms successfully cluster cells based on their gene expression patterns using unsupervised learning techniques, providing important insights into the diversity of immune cell populations and their function in maintaining health and the emergence of illness. These uses highlight AI's great potential to increase immunogenetics research and discovery, which will ultimately lead to better disease management and the development of customized medicines (Klau et al., 2023).

8.2 Data interpretation

The heterogeneity of immunological data gathered from many sources, including imaging, genomic, proteomic, and electronic health records, makes it difficult to integrate and harmonize various data types while preserving high data quality (Cotet et al., 2023). The development and functionality of AI models can be impacted by a number of problems, including inconsistent data, missing information, and unclear data formats. Moreover, facilitating interoperability across diverse data systems and platforms is crucial for fostering seamless data sharing and cooperation (Farzan, 2024).

8.3 Translational challenges

Over the last decade, there has been a considerable advancement in clinical immunology. In the United States, screening programs for additional inborn immune disorders, such as severe combined immunodeficiency, are being expanded internationally. Severe combined immunodeficiency screening for newborns is currently common (Garg, 2023).We learned more about important immune responses and found additional immune gene abnormalities during the COVID-19 pandemic (Malkan et al., 2023; Sen et al., 2021). Managing patients with immune dysregulated organ damage presents a unique major clinical challenge, with management often lacking standardization ranging from endocrine, rheumatologic, and neurologic complications to autoimmune cytopenias, enteropathy, and liver disease (Haznedaroglu, 2020).

8.4 Public awareness

The public's awareness of immunogenetics is critical for impacting views, attitudes, and actions regarding genetic research, customized treatment, and healthcare decisions. Effective communication and education are critical for bridging the gap between complicated scientific concepts and general awareness (Peng et al., 2021; Hao et al., 2022). Raising awareness of genetic testing's usefulness, limitations, and implications can assist individuals in making informed decisions about testing and translating results. Immunogenetics is a complicated discipline containing scientific ideas that the general public may find difficult to grasp (Shah et al., 2023; Wang et al., 2021). It is critical to ensure that immunogenetic information is accessible and culturally sensitive to varied people with varying educational backgrounds, languages, and belief systems.

8.5 Strategies for improvement

The field of diabetic immunogenetics investigates how the immune system and genetics interact to cause and progress type 1 diabetes (T1D), an autoimmune disease. Improving our understanding and efforts in this area may result in more accurate diabetes prediction, prevention, and treatment (Mahdi & Ni,).

Several techniques are now being investigated or might be used to improve the study and clinical treatment of diabetic immunogenetics.

8.6 Educational initiatives

Educational activities in immunogenetics are critical for increasing knowledge and skills in the area among students, healthcare professionals, and the general public (Liu et al., 2023).Creating educational programs, workshops, and materials customized to various audiences, such as schools, community organizations, and the general public, can improve knowledge and awareness of immunogenetics (Al-Rashed et al., 2020). Effective instruction in this sector involves a multidisciplinary approach that combines ideas from genetics immunology, bioinformatics, and patient care (Gao et al., 2020).

8.7 Engaging with media

Effective media engagement in immunogenetics is critical for promoting public awareness, disseminating new research findings, and altering public health policy (Lewis et al., 2022). Researchers can collaborate directly with journalists on feature pieces that highlight the complexities of immunogenetics and its influence on medicine (Maruthamuthu et al., 2022).

8.8 Patient advocacy and support groups

In the field of immunogenetics, patient advocacy and support organizations are essential, especially because genetic discoveries might have significant effects on individuals with linked disorders (Feldtkeller et al., 2000). Collaborating with patient advocacy and support organizations can help to address immunogenetics-related issues, offer trustworthy information, and promote peer-to-peer education. Provide clear, reliable information regarding genetic immune disorders to patients and their families (De Miranda & Scheeren, 2024).

8.9 Healthcare provider training

Immunogenetics education for healthcare professionals is crucial to incorporating the most recent genetic discoveries into clinical practice (Gragert). Particularly for disorders like autoimmune illnesses, malignancies, and infectious diseases that have a significant genetic component, this training can improve diagnosis, therapy, and customized medicine approaches (Niedeggen et al., 2019).

8.9.1 Public engagement and dialog

Improving public-scientific community awareness, trust, and support in immunogenetics requires public participation and discourse. The ethical, legal, and societal issues that may come up as a result of genetic research developments are also addressed by this interaction (Pichini et al., 2022). Fostering trust, transparency, and collaboration between academics, healthcare providers, politicians, and the community may be achieved via encouraging public involvement, participation in research debates, and open communication regarding immunogenetics. Encourage candid conversations on the advantages and moral implications of immunogenetics (Shahrier et al., 2023; Ozdemir et al., 2011).

9. Unresolved questions in immunogenetics

Combining genetics and immunology, immunogenetics is a fast-developing science that aims to explain how immune system diversity affects genetic variation. Many unanswered issues remain despite tremendous progress mostly because immune responses are complicated and have a variety of roles in both health and illness (Carton & Nappi, 2001). It is important to address these issues to create vaccinations and therapies that work better. These are a few of the major immunogenetics unanswered questions.

9.1 Basis of immune response variability

Individual differences in immune responses can occur even when immunizations or infections are the same. It is still difficult to fully understand the genetic, epigenetic, and environmental components that lead to this heterogeneity (Castrillo). Comprehending the genetic underpinnings of intricate, multifaceted illnesses is imperative in order to ascertain risk factors, evaluate the impact of gene-environment interactions, forecast individualized responses to particular medications, and explore novel avenues for drug discovery (Bastin et al., 1996).

The Major Histocompatibility Complex [MHC] is a useful marker system for assessing genes that predispose to sickness due to its high genetic diversity and "enbloc" transmission of its genes in the form of haplotypes. Such a polymorphism could also give a genetic basis for the observed variation in immunological reactivity among communities and individuals, as well as the ensuing profiles of vulnerability to and resistance from disease (Hadzidimitriou et al., 2011).

9.2 Genetics of autoimmune diseases

Various genetic factors increase a person's chance of developing an autoimmune disease.Such as HLA genes have been linked to an elevated risk of autoimmune illnesses. Heredity has a major role in the development of most autoimmune diseases (Lee et al., 2015). Despite the quick progress being made in genetic research, a significant portion of heritable risk still results from either the contribution of an unknown, encoded component of risk or the unidentified effects of known risk loci (Misra et al., 2018). The primary use of this knowledge would be in the logical development of innovative treatments that capitalize on the ways in which these significant pathways impact disease (Miller, 1995).

9.3 Role of epigenetics

Epigenetic modifications have a critical role in regulating gene expression in response to environmental stimuli. Our immune cell memory and function have the potential to completely transform the way we administer immunizations and treat disorders connected to the immune system (Zhou et al., 2014). The interactions between immune cells and malignancies depend on epigenetic processes such as DNA methylation, histone post-translational changes, and chromatin structural manipulation. Consequently, immunomodulatory medications with epigenetic targeting are appealing and will significantly influence immuno-oncology (Vinciguerra et al., 2020).

9.4 Genetic architecture of the immune system

It is an enormous task to identify every gene implicated in immune responses and to comprehend their roles and interactions. This involves the thorough mapping of poorly understood genes and non-coding areas that control the expression of immune genes (Pouget, 2018). It is essential to comprehend this genomic architecture in order to create therapy, preventative, and prediction techniques. Although T2DM's immune genetic architecture is less well understood than that of T1DM, inflammation is a key factor in the disease's etiology such as genes TNF-α, IL-6, and IL-1β are associated with insulin resistance and systemic inflammation.

9.5 Impact of microbial genomes

Immune responses are significantly influenced by the human microbiome, however, it is unclear what genetic foundation underlies these interactions (Qadri et al., 2022). The immune response is often triggered by a sequence of consecutive processes in which the complex antigen is taken up by T helper lymphocytes, and activating B cells, cytotoxic T cells, and suppressor subpopulations. Highly polymorphic genes that are a component of the major histocompatibility complex (MHC)/human leukocyte antigen (HLA) system control some aspects of human behavior (Lefranc et al., 2005).The relationship between several microbiological diseases (viral, bacterial, fungal, and parasitic) and the host's HLA system has been the subject of numerous investigations (Haralambieva et al., 2013).

9.6 Pathogen Co-evolution

Human immune systems and disease virulence factors engage in a genetic arms race as a result of coevolving human populations and pathogens (Le Pendu et al., 2014). Pathogen genetic diversity can provide selection pressure to the human immune system, causing immune genes to evolve. Research is ongoing to determine the dynamics of this connection and how it affects a person's vulnerability to certain illnesses (Rausell & Telenti, 2014).

9.6.1 Examples of Co-evolution

HLA System and Viral Infections: Human HLA (human leukocyte antigen) systems provide as an example of how immune responses are shaped via co-evolution. Depending on how well an HLA allele presents viral peptides to immune cells, it can either enhance or decrease vulnerability to illnesses like HIV (Antonides).

Red Queen Hypothesis: According to this evolutionary theory, organisms must continuously change, adapt, and multiply to live against other species that have evolved to counteract their adaptations not to get a reproductive advantage (Hirayasu et al., 2012).

9.7 Somatic hypermutation and immune repertoire

Somatic hypermutation in the variable (V) regions of immunoglobulin genes in B cells found in secondary lymphoid organs like the spleen and lymph nodes happens during the germinal center response (Karan-Djurasevic & Pavlovic, 2017). The wide variety of distinct antigen receptors found in the immune system, such as antibodies made by B cells and T-cell receptors expressed on T cells, is known as immune repertoire diversity. The V(D)J recombination process, which takes place during the formation of B and T cells in the bone marrow and thymus, respectively, broadens the immunological repertoire (Langerak et al., 2017).

9.8 Translational immunogenetics

How might immunogenetic knowledge be applied to develop successful treatments? The field of translational immunogenetics facilitates the creation of customized strategies for managing diseases by utilizing individual genetic profiles (Langerak, 2022b). For instance, HLA allele testing is used genetically to identify autoimmune conditions like celiac disease and estimate the likelihood of transplant rejection (Vlachonikola et al., 2023). Translational immunogenetics offers the potential to transform personalized therapy and enhance patient outcomes for patients with immune-related illnesses by utilizing the power of genetics and genomes (Oliveira et al., 2017). This covers the creation of vaccinations and immunotherapies based on genetic information.

9.9 Gene-environment interactions

For both preventative and therapeutic approaches, it is essential to comprehend how genetic predispositions interact with environmental variables such as nutrition, pollution, and lifestyle to impact immune function (Yang et al., 2010). Immunogenetics relies heavily on gene-environment interactions to shape immune responses and vulnerability to immunological-related illnesses. Researchers may create more focused methods for illness prevention, diagnosis, and therapy by determining the genetic and environmental components that lead to immune-related illnesses (Caspi & Moffitt, 2006).

10. Future perspective of diabetes mellitus in immunogenetics

Immunogenetics' future potential for diabetes mellitus holds great promise for expanding our knowledge of the condition, enhancing diagnostic capabilities, and creating more specialized and individualized therapies (Hajam et al., 2022).

The future of diabetes research and clinical practice is anticipated to be significantly shaped by immunogenetics in the following important areas.

10.1 Precision medicine and personalized treatment

Genetic Risk Predictionwith the development of genome sequencing and analysis methods, it will be possible to forecast a person's risk of acquiring diabetes with greater accuracy (Mujahid & Ahmad, 2023). Immunogenetic Profiling with targeted immunomodulatory therapy, such as those for patients with autoimmune forms of diabetes will be made possible by comprehensively profiling immune-related genetic variations and autoantibody profiles (Ali et al., 2022a).

10.2 Immunotherapy and disease modulation

Immunomodulation Strategies: Treatment techniques can be tailored to individuals' unique immune dysregulation patterns with the use of customized immunomodulation strategies based on individual genetic and immunological profiles (Dunn et al., 2020).

10.3 Gene editing and genetic engineering

Advancements in gene editing technologies, such CRISPR-Cas9, have the potential to alter immune cell function, halting the autoimmune damage of pancreatic beta cells and repairing genetic anomalies associated with diabetes (Willemsen et al., 2003).

Cell-Based treatments: By genetically modifying immune or stem cells, cell-based treatments for diabetes may be developed to modify immune responses or restore beta cell activity.

10.4 Integrated omics approaches

The integration of many types of data, such as genomic, transcriptomic, proteomic, and metabolomic, will offer a thorough comprehension of the molecular mechanisms behind diabetes and associated immune-related problems (Vahabi & Michailidis, 2022).

Modeling Systems Biology: To identify novel treatment targets and predictive biomarkers, systems biology techniques will be utilized to simulate intricate interactions among genetic, immunological, and environmental variables in the pathogenesis of diabetes (Thivolet, 2000).

10.5 Early detection and prevention strategies

The discovery of new biomarkers, such as immune cell signatures, autoantibodies, and genetic markers, may make it possible to identify diabetes risk and development early on and carry out preventative measures before clinical signs appear (Burek Kamenaric et al., 2020).

10.6 Patient-centered care and education

Encouraging Patients: Better genetic and immunological education and counseling will enable patients to take an active role in their individualized treatment programs, comprehend their hereditary risk factors, and make educated decisions about their health (Liu & Mardis, 2017).

10.7 Implications for ethics, law, and society (ELSI)

By addressing the ethical, legal, and social elements of genetic testing, such as privacy concerns and informed permission, the right application of genetic and immunogenetic technologies in the treatment of diabetes will be assuredand equity in access to genetic services (Sanghavi et al., 2021). In conclusion, immunogenetics' potential for diabetes mellitus presents significant opportunities for increasing our knowledge of the condition, enhancing diagnostics, and creating more specialized and individualized therapies (Greenbaum, 2013).

11. Conclusion

In conclusion, there are a number of important obstacles that the discipline of immunogenetics must overcome if we are to fully comprehend the genetic foundation of immunological responses and how they relate to both health and illness. The complexities of gene-environment interactions, the limits of existing sequencing technology, and data analysis techniques provide a number of challenges for researchers trying to unravel the genetic architecture of the immune system. Despite these difficulties, new developments in multidisciplinary partnerships, bioinformatics tools, and genomic technology provide encouraging paths forward. Through the utilization of large-scale genomic investigations, integration of multi-omics data, and application of computational techniques, we may acquire more profound understanding of the genetic factors influencing immune-related illnesses and facilitate the development of customized methods for diagnosis, treatment, and prevention.

We can speed immunogenetics research and turn scientific findings into real advantages for patients by encouraging cooperation, supporting data-sharing programs, and funding creative research techniques. As the genetic landscape of the immune system becomes more complicated and understood, we must continue to be on the lookout for new problems and chances for innovation.

In the future, we may enhance human health outcomes by deepening our understanding of immunogenetics and seizing these problems as chances for development and exploration. These open-ended inquiries serve as a reminder of the immune system's complexity and the substantial amount of work that remains to properly comprehend its genetic foundation. Advances in these fields may result in new approaches to the diagnosis, treatment, and prevention of a variety of illnesses, including cancer, autoimmune disorders, and infections. Addressing these issues will need ongoing integration of new technology, multidisciplinary research, and international cooperation.

References

Addala, V., Newell, F., Pearson, J. V., Redwood, A., Robinson, B. W., Creaney, J., & Waddell, N. (2024). Computational immunogenomic approaches to predict response to cancer immunotherapies. *Nature Reviews Clinical Oncology, 21*(1), 28–46.

Agathangelidis, A., Vlachonikola, E., Davi, F., Langerak, A. W., & Chatzidimitriou, A. (September 1, 2022). High-throughput immunogenetics for precision medicine in cancer. In *, 84. Seminars in cancer biology* (pp. 80–88). Academic Press.

Ali, S. I., Rather, M. A., Sheikh, W. M., Nabi, S. U., Ganai, A., Altaf, M., Nath, S., Ahmad, S. B., Wani, I. A., & Bashir, S. M. (2022a). Immunopharmaco-genomics: Future of clinical medicine. In *A molecular approach to immunogenetics* (pp. 347–384). Academic Press.

Ali, A., Dar, M. A., Malla, B. A., Maqbool, I., Hamdani, S. S., Bashir, S. M., & Ganie, S. A. (2022b). Understanding the immunogenetics of human viral diseases. In *Immunogenetics: A molecular and clinical overview* (pp. 131–163). Academic Press.

Al-Mayah, S. J. (March 1, 2024). Evaluation of BTLA (CD272) immune checkpoint levels related to hepatitis B virus infection in diabetes mellitus patients. *Medical Science Journal for Advance Research, 5*(1), 49–57.

Al-Rashed, M., Foshay, K., & Abedalthagafi, M. (January 8, 2020). Recent advances in meningioma immunogenetics. *Frontiers in Oncology, 9*, 1472.

Alves, C., Souza, T., Meyer, I., Toralles, M. B., & Brites, C. (2006). Immunogenetics and infectious diseases: Special reference to the mayor histocompatibility complex. *Brazilian Journal of Infectious Diseases, 10*, 122–131.

Ansari, M. A., Chauhan, W., Shoaib, S., Alyahya, S. A., Ali, M., Ashraf, H., Alomary, M. N., & Al-Suhaimi, E. A. (December 2023). Emerging therapeutic options in the management of diabetes: Recent trends, challenges and future directions. *International Journal of Obesity, 47*(12), 1179–1199.

Antonides JD. Avian immunogenetics and evolution of a passerine bird in the face of malarial parasites (Doctoral dissertation, Purdue University).

Arage LL, Deybasso HA, Gebremichael DY, Nuramo BG, Mekuria ZN. HIV/AIDS-Research and palliative care dove press.

Asgarbeik, S., Amoli, M. M., Vahidi, A., & Klashami, Z. N. (February 15, 2021). Genetic research in immunogenetics group of endocrinology and metabolism research institute. *Journal of Diabetes and Metabolic Disorders*, 1–9.

Ash, D., & Roy, T. (January 1, 2022). Immunogenetics in the diagnosis of clinical disorders. In *Immunogenetics: A molecular and clinical overview* (pp. 35–56). Academic Press.

Ashhab, A. A., Rodin, H., Campos, M., Abu-Sulb, A., Hall, J. A., Powell, J., & Debes, J. D. (August 26, 2020). Response to hepatitis B virus vaccination in individuals with chronic hepatitis C virus infection. *PLoS One, 15*(8), e0237398.

Bach, F. H., & Bach, M. L. (January 1, 1972). Fundamental Immunogenetics—their application to histocompatibility. In *, 1. Clinical immunobiology* (pp. 157–178). Elsevier.

Basler, M., & Groettrup, M. (November 2020). Recent insights how combined inhibition of immuno/proteasome subunits enables therapeutic efficacy. *Genes and Immunity, 21*(5), 273–287.

Bastin, P., Matthews, K. R., & Gull, K. (August 1, 1996). The paraflagellar rod of kinetoplastida: Solved and unsolved questions. *Parasitology Today, 12*(8), 302–307.

Baum, T. P., Pasqual, N., Thuderoz, F., Hierle, V., Chaume, D., Lefranc, M. P., Jouvin-Marche, E., Marche, P. N., & Demongeot, J. (January 1, 2004). IMGT/GeneInfo: Enhancing V (D) J recombination database accessibility. *Nucleic Acids Research, 32*(suppl_1), D51–D54.

Black, L. A., & Zorina, T. (August 1, 2020). Genetic profile considerations for induction of allogeneic chimerism as a therapeutic approach for type 1 diabetes mellitus. *Drug Discovery Today, 25*(8), 1293–1297.

Boehncke, W. H., & Brembilla, N. C. (June 3, 2018). Immunogenicity of biologic therapies: Causes and consequences. *Expert Review of Clinical Immunology, 14*(6), 513–523.

Borish, L. (May 1, 1999). Genetics of allergy and asthma. *Annals of Allergy, Asthma, & Immunology, 82*(5), 413–426.

Borysewicz-Sańczyk, H., Sawicka, B., Wawrusiewicz-Kurylonek, N., Głowińska-Olszewska, B., Kadłubiska, A., Gościk, J., Szadkowska, A., Łosiewicz, A., Młynarski, W., Kretowski, A., & Bossowski, A. (August 21, 2020). Genetic association study of IL2RA, IFIH1, and CTLA-4 polymorphisms with autoimmune thyroid diseases and type 1 diabetes. *Frontiers in Pediatrics, 8*, 481.

Bossini-Castillo, L., López-Isac, E., & Martín, J. (November 1, 2015). Immunogenetics of systemic sclerosis: Defining heritability, functional variants and shared-autoimmunity pathways. *Journal of Autoimmunity, 64*, 53–65.

Bragina, E. Y., Tiys, E. S., Freidin, M. B., Koneva, L. A., Demenkov, P. S., Ivanisenko, V. A., Kolchanov, N. A., & Puzyrev, V. P. (August 2014). Insights into pathophysiology of dystropy through the analysis of gene networks: An example of bronchial asthma and tuberculosis. *Immunogenetics, 66*, 457–465.

Burek Kamenaric, M., Ivkovic, V., Kovacevic Vojtusek, I., & Zunec, R. (December 9, 2020). The role of HLA and KIR immunogenetics in BK virus infection after kidney transplantation. *Viruses, 12*(12), 1417.

Candore, G., Balistreri, C. R., Listi, F., Grimaldi, M. P., Vasto, S., Colonna-Romano, G. I., Franceschi, C., Lio, D., Caselli, G., & Caruso, C. (November 2006). Immunogenetics, gender, and longevity. *Annals of the New York Academy of Sciences, 1089*(1), 516–537.

Cao, J., & Yan, Q. (July 1, 2020). Cancer epigenetics, tumor immunity, and immunotherapy. *Trends in Cancer, 6*(7), 580–592.

Carton, Y., & Nappi, A. J. (January 2001). Immunogenetic aspects of the cellular immune response of Drosophila against parasitoids. *Immunogenetics, 52*, 157–164.

Caruso, C., Ligotti, M. E., Accardi, G., Aiello, A., & Candore, G. (September 2, 2022). An immunologist's guide to immunosenescence and its treatment. *Expert Review of Clinical Immunology, 18*(9), 961–981.

Caspi, A., & Moffitt, T. E. (July 1, 2006). Gene–environment interactions in psychiatry: Joining forces with neuroscience. *Nature Reviews Neuroscience, 7*(7), 583–590.

Castrillo SM. reportImmunogenetics in autoimmune encephalitis and related disorders (doctoral dissertation, Université de Lyon).

Chen, L., Magliano, D. J., & Zimmet, P. Z. (April 2012). The worldwide epidemiology of type 2 diabetes mellitus—present and future perspectives. *Nature Reviews Endocrinology, 8*(4), 228–236.

Chen, A. Y., Huang, C. W., Liu, S. H., Liu, A. C., & Chaung, H. C. (August 31, 2021). Single nucleotide polymorphisms of immunity-related genes and their effects on immunophenotypes in different pig breeds. *Genes, 12*(9), 1377.

Chinniah, R., Sevak, V., Pandi, S., Ravi, P. M., Vijayan, M., Kannan, A., & Karuppiah, B. (August 2021). HLA-DRB1 genes and the expression dynamics of HLA CIITA determine the susceptibility to T2DM. *Immunogenetics, 73*(4), 291–305.

Cookson, W. (December 1, 2004). The immunogenetics of asthma and eczema: A new focus on the epithelium. *Nature Reviews Immunology, 4*(12), 978–988.

Cotet, T. S., Agrafiotis, A., Kreiner, V., Kuhn, R., Shlesinger, D., Manero-Carranza, M., Khodaverdi, K., Kladis, E., Desideri Perea, A., Maassen-Veeters, D., & Glänzer, W. (September 1, 2023). ePlatypus: An ecosystem for computational analysis of immunogenomics data. *Bioinformatics, 39*(9), btad553.

De la Fuente, J., & Contreras, M. (December 2, 2021). Vaccinomics: A future avenue for vaccine development against emerging pathogens. *Expert Review of Vaccines, 20*(12), 1561–1569.

De Miranda, N. F., & Scheeren, F. A. (April 4, 2024). Immunogenetic diversity and cancer immunotherapy disparities. *Cancer Discovery, 14*(4), 585–588.

DeGraba, T. J. (November 1, 2004). Immunogenetic susceptibility of atherosclerotic stroke: Implications on current and future treatment of vascular inflammation. *Stroke, 35*(11_Suppl. l_1), 2712–2719.

Ding, Y., Zhang, P., Deng, T., Yan, X., Zhang, M., Xie, Z., Huang, G., Wang, P., Cai, T., Zhang, X., & Xiao, X. (2024). Association of human leukocyte antigen (HLA) footprints with the comorbidity of latent autoimmune diabetes in adults (LADA) and hepatitis C virus (HCV) infection: A multicenter cross-sectional study. *Diabetes & Metabolic Syndrome: Clinical Research Reviews, 18*(1), 102939.

Dunn, G. P., Cloughesy, T. F., Maus, M. V., Prins, R. M., Reardon, D. A., & Sonabend, A. M. (October 2020). Emerging immunotherapies for malignant glioma: From immunogenomics to cell therapy. *Neuro-Oncology, 22*(10), 1425–1438.

Emam S. Cellular immuno-genomics: A systems biology approach to investigate genetic regulation of macrophage function and disease resistance of dairy cattle (Doctoral dissertation, University of Guelph).

Farid, N. R. (November 30, 1990). *The immunogenetics of autoimmune diseases.* CRC Press.

Farzan, R. (2024). Artificial intelligence in Immuno-genetics. *Bioinformation, 20*(1), 29.

Feldtkeller, E., Bruckel, J., & Khan, M. A. (July 1, 2000). Scientific contributions of ankylosing spondylitis patient advocacy groups. *Current Opinion in Rheumatology, 12*(4), 239–247.

Fernandes, A. P., Pace, A. E., Zanetti, M. L., Foss, M. C., & Donadi, E. A. (October 1, 2005). Immunogenetic factors associated with type 1 diabetes mellitus. *Revista Latino-Americana de Enfermagem, 13*(5), 743–749.

Fuggle, S. V., & Taylor, C. J. (June 6, 2012). *Histocompatibility and immunogenetics. Handbook of renal and pancreatic transplantation.*

Gao, X., Yang, J., & Chen, Y. (December 2020). Identification of a four immune-related genes signature based on an immunogenomic landscape analysis of clear cell renal cell carcinoma. *Journal of Cellular Physiology, 235*(12), 9834–9850.

Garg, A. D. (August 2023). The dynamic interface of genetics and immunity: Toward future horizons in health & disease. *Genes and Immunity, 24*(4), 155–158.

Ginter, E., & Simko, V. (2013). Type 2 diabetes mellitus, pandemic in 21st century. In *Diabetes: An old disease, a new insight.*

Giudicelli, V., Chaume, D., & Lefranc, M. P. (January 1, 2005). IMGT/GENE-DB: A comprehensive database for human and mouse immunoglobulin and T cell receptor genes. *Nucleic Acids Research, 33*(Suppl. l_1), D256–D261.

Gonzalez-Galarza, F. F., McCabe, A., Dos Santos, E. J., Jones, A. R., & Middleton, D. (July 1, 2021). A snapshot of human leukocyte antigen (HLA) diversity using data from the Allele frequency net database. *Human Immunology, 82*(7), 496–504.

Goyal, R., Singhal, M., & Jialal, I. (January 2024). Type 2 diabetes. 2023 Jun 23. In *StatPearls [Internet]. Treasure Island (FL).* StatPearls Publishing.

Gragert L. Analysis of human leukocyte antigen (HLA) immunogenetic data for hematopoietic stem cell transplantation and disease association.

Greenbaum, D. (August 16, 2013). Grand challenge: ELSI in a changing global environment. *Frontiers in Genetics, 4,* 61936.

Hadzidimitriou, A., Agathangelidis, A., Darzentas, N., Murray, F., Delfau-Larue, M. H., Pedersen, L. B., Lopez, A. N., Dagklis, A., Rombout, P., Beldjord, K., & Kolstad, A. (September 15, 2011). Is there a role for antigen selection in mantle cell lymphoma? Immunogenetic support from a series of 807 cases. *Blood, The Journal of the American Society of Hematology, 118*(11), 3088–3095.

Hajam, Y. A., Kumar, R., Bhat, R. A., Rani, R., Sharma, B., & Sharma, P. (January 1, 2022). Basics of immunogenetics: Application and future perspectives. In *A molecular approach to immunogenetics* (pp. 41–62). Academic Press.

Hajdarevic R. Immunogenetic studies in myalgic encephalomyelitis/chronic fatigue syndrome (ME/CFS).

Hao, D., Han, G., Sinjab, A., Gomez-Bolanos, L. I., Lazcano, R., Serrano, A., Hernandez, S. D., Dai, E., Cao, X., Hu, J., & Dang, M. (November 2, 2022). The single-cell immunogenomic landscape of B and plasma cells in early-stage lung adenocarcinoma. *Cancer Discovery, 12*(11), 2626–2645.

Haralambieva, I. H., Ovsyannikova, I. G., Pankratz, V. S., Kennedy, R. B., Jacobson, R. M., & Poland, G. A. (January 1, 2013). The genetic basis for interindividual immune response variation to measles vaccine: New understanding and new vaccine approaches. *Expert Review of Vaccines, 12*(1), 57–70.

Harden, J. L., Krueger, J. G., & Bowcock, A. M. (November 1, 2015). The immunogenetics of psoriasis: A comprehensive review. *Journal of Autoimmunity, 64*, 66–73.

Haznedaroglu, I. C. (November 1, 2020). Immunogenomic phases of COVID-19 and appropriate clinical management. *The Lancet Microbe, 1*(7), e278.

Hill, A. V. (2001). Immunogenetics and genomics. *The Lancet, 357*(9273), 2037–2041.

Hirayasu, K., Ohashi, J., Kashiwase, K., Hananantachai, H., Naka, I., Ogawa, A., Takanashi, M., Satake, M., Nakajima, K., Parham, P., & Arase, H. (March 8, 2012). Significant association of KIR2DL3-HLA-C1 combination with cerebral malaria and implications for co-evolution of KIR and HLA. *PLoS Pathogens, 8*(3), e1002565.

Hollenbach, J. A., & Oksenberg, J. R. (November 1, 2015). The immunogenetics of multiple sclerosis: A comprehensive review. *Journal of Autoimmunity, 64*, 13–25.

Hollenbach, J. A., Holcomb, C., Hurley, C. K., Mabdouly, A., Maiers, M., Noble, J. A., Robinson, J., Schmidt, A. H., Shi, L., Turner, V., & Yao, Y. (February 2013). Report from the immunogenomic data analysis working group (IDAWG) 16th international HLA and immunogenetics workshop (IHIW) project: Immunogenomic data-management methods. *International Journal of Immunogenetics, 40* (1), 46.

Howell, W. M. (May 1994). HLA immunogenetics and specific IgE responses to allergens. *Clinical and Experimental Allergy, 24*(5), 401–404.

Hussain, T., & Shabir, I. (January 1, 2022). Immunogenomics: A potential approach for precision medicine. In *Immunogenetics: A molecular and clinical overview* (pp. 267–277). Academic Press.

Isaghazadeh, A., & Rezaei, N. (June 19, 2019). *Introductory chapter: Immunogenetics.* IntechOpen.

Johnson, M. B., Patel, K. A., De Franco, E., Hagopian, W., Killian, M., McDonald, T. J., Tree, T. I., Domingo-Vila, C., Hudson, M., Hammersley, S., & Dobbs, R. (December 2020). Type 1 diabetes can present before the age of 6 months and is characterised by autoimmunity and rapid loss of beta cells. *Diabetologia, 63*, 2605–2615.

Kamatani, Y., & Nakamura, Y. (June 11, 2021). Genetic variations in medical research in the past, at present and in the future. *Proceedings of the Japan Academy, Series B, 97*(6), 324–335.

Kanikowska, A., Hryhorowicz, S., Rychter, A. M., Kucharski, M. A., Zawada, A., Iwanik, K., Eder, P., Słomski, R., Dobrowolska, A., & Krela-Kaźmierczak, I. (October 7, 2021). Immunogenetic, molecular and microbiotic determinants of eosinophilic Esophagitis and clinical practice—A new perspective of an old disease. *International Journal of Molecular Sciences, 22*(19), 10830.

Karan-Djurasevic, T., & Pavlovic, S. (July 2017). Somatic hypermutational status and gene repertoire of immunoglobulin rearrangements in chronic lymphocytic leukemia. *Lymphocyte Updates-Cancer, Autoimmunity and Infection, 12*, 49–78.

Kemming, J., Thimme, R., & Neumann-Haefelin, C. (August 6, 2020). Adaptive immune response against hepatitis C virus. *International Journal of Molecular Sciences, 21*(16), 5644.

Kennedy, R. B., Ovsyannikova, I. G., Palese, P., & Poland, G. A. (June 25, 2020). Current challenges in vaccinology. *Frontiers in Immunology, 11*, 541543.

Khadhraoui, C., Kaabachi, W., Tritar, F., Daghfous, H., Hamzaoui, K., & Hamzaoui, A. (December 2020). Association of BTLA rs1982809 polymorphism with lung cancer risk in Tunisian population. *International Journal of Immunogenetics, 47*(6), 554–562.

Kim, Y. C., & Jeong, B. H. (December 2020). Ethnic variation in risk genotypes based on single nucleotide polymorphisms (SNPs) of the interferon-inducible transmembrane 3 (IFITM3) gene, a susceptibility factor for pandemic 2009 H1N1 influenza A virus. *Immunogenetics, 72*(9), 447–453.

Kiyotani, K., Toyoshima, Y., & Nakamura, Y. (2021). Immunogenomics in personalized cancer treatments. *Journal of Human Genetics, 66*(9), 901–907.

Klau, J. H., Maj, C., Klinkhammer, H., Krawitz, P. M., Mayr, A., Hillmer, A. M., Schumacher, J., & Heider, D. (2023). AI-based multi-PRS models outperform classical single-PRS models. *Frontiers in Genetics, 14,* 1217860.

Krishna, C., Tervi, A., Saffern, M., Wilson, E. A., Yoo, S. K., Mars, N., Roudko, V., Cho, B. A., Jones, S. E., Vaninov, N., & Selvan, M. E. (February 23, 2024). An immunogenetic basis for lung cancer risk. *Science, 383*(6685), eadi3808.

Kristensen, B.Ø. (December 1, 1984). Aspects of immunology and immunogenetics in human essential hypertension with special reference to vascular events. *Journal of Hypertension, 2*(6), 571–579.

Kumar, A., & Meena, L. S. (2020). Dual burden of Tuberculosis (TB) and Diabetes Mellitus (DM) as the major risk factor for wide range of population. *Diabetes & Obesity International Journal, 5*(2), 000229.

Kung, P. J., Elsayed, I., Reyes-Pérez, P., & Bandres-Ciga, S. (January 1, 2022). Immunogenetic determinants of Parkinson's disease etiology. *Journal of Parkinson's Disease, 12*(s1), S13–S27.

Lamont, S. J., Dekkers, J. C., Wolc, A., & Zhou, H. (January 1, 2022). Immunogenetics and the mapping of immunological functions. *Avian immunology,* 277–297.

Langerak, A. W., Brüggemann, M., Davi, F., Darzentas, N., van Dongen, J. J., Gonzalez, D., Cazzaniga, G., Giudicelli, V., Lefranc, M. P., Giraud, M., & Macintyre, E. A. (May 15, 2017). High-throughput immunogenetics for clinical and research applications in immunohematology: Potential and challenges. *The Journal of Immunology, 198*(10), 3765–3774.

Langerak, A. W. (2022a). *Immunogenetics: Methods and protocols.* Springer Nature.

Langerak, A. W. (2022b). The advent of precision immunology: Immunogenetics at the center of immune cell analysis in health and disease. In *, 28. Immunogenetics: Methods and protocols* (pp. 1–5). New York, NY: Springer US.

Le Pendu, J., Nyström, K., & Ruvoën-Clouet, N. (August 1, 2014). Host-pathogen co-evolution and glycan interactions. *Current Opinion in Virology, 7,* 88–94.

Lee, H. J., Li, C. W., Hammerstad, S. S., Stefan, M., & Tomer, Y. (November 1, 2015). Immunogenetics of autoimmune thyroid diseases: A comprehensive review. *Journal of Autoimmunity, 64,* 82–90.

Lee, C. N., Chen, T. Y., & Wong, T. W. (March 15, 2022). The immunogenetics of photodermatoses. In *The immunogenetics of dermatologic diseases* (pp. 369–381). Cham: Springer International Publishing.

Lefranc, M. P., Giudicelli, V., Kaas, Q., Duprat, E., Jabado-Michaloud, J., Scaviner, D., Ginestoux, C., Clement, O., Chaume, D., & Lefranc, G. (January 1, 2005). IMGT, the international ImMunoGeneTics information system®. *Nucleic Acids Research, 33*(suppl_1), D593–D597.

Lefranc, M. P. (January 1, 2003). IMGT, the international ImMunoGeneTics database®. *Nucleic Acids Research, 31*(1), 307–310.

Lefranc, M. P. (December 2005). IMGT, the international ImMunoGeneTics information system®: A standardized approach for immunogenetics and immunoinformatics. *Immunome Research, 1,* 1.

Lewis, M. A., Uhrig, J. D., Adams, E. T., Brown, J. A., Sanders, A., & RTI International All of Us Innovator Team. (August 8, 2022). Engagement marketing for social good: Application to the all of us research program. *Frontiers in Genetics, 13,* 889195.

Li, Y. J., Phillips, E. J., Dellinger, A., Nicoletti, P., Schutte, R., Li, D., Ostrov, D. A., Fontana, R. J., Watkins, P. B., Stolz, A., & Daly, A. K. (January 2021). Human leukocyte antigen B* 14: 01 and B* 35: 01 are associated with trimethoprim-sulfamethoxazole induced liver injury. *Hepatology, 73*(1), 268–281.

Lian, J., Yue, Y., Yu, W., & Zhang, Y. (November 10, 2020). Immunosenescence: A key player in cancer development. *Journal of Hematology & Oncology, 13*(1), 151.

Limas, C. J., Kroupis, C., Haidaroglou, A., & Cokkinos, D. V. (February 2002). Hyperprolactinaemia in patients with heart failure: Clinical and immunogenetic correlations. *European Journal of Clinical Investigation, 32*(2), 74–78.

Lisanwork Arage, L., Deybasso, H. A., Yilma Gebremichael, D., Gintamo Nuramo, B., & Negash Mekuria, Z. (March 2021). Retracted article: Determinants of drug-induced hepatotoxicity among patients with human immunodeficiency virus taking a high dose of rifapentine plus isoniazid drugs at the all Africa leprosy tuberculosis rehabilitation and training center in Addis Ababa, Ethiopia. *HIV/AIDS-Research and Palliative Care, 16*, 307–314.

Liu, X. S., & Mardis, E. R. (February 9, 2017). Applications of immunogenomics to cancer. *Cell, 168*(4), 600–612.

Liu, C. J., Hu, F. F., Xie, G. Y., Miao, Y. R., Li, X. W., Zeng, Y., & Guo, A. Y. (January 2023). GSCA: An integrated platform for gene set cancer analysis at genomic, pharmacogenomic and immunogenomic levels. *Briefings in Bioinformatics, 24*(1), bbac558.

Lo Faro, V., Nolte, I. M., Ten Brink, J. B., Snieder, H., Jansonius, N. M., & Bergen, A. A. (December 16, 2021). Mitochondrial genome study identifies association between primary open-angle glaucoma and variants in MT-CYB, MT-ND4 genes and haplogroups. *Frontiers in Genetics, 12*, 781189.

Looi, C. K., Foong, L. C., Chung, F. F., Khoo, A. S., Loo, E. M., Leong, C. O., & Mai, C. W. (December 2023). Targeting the crosstalk of epigenetic modifications and immune evasion in nasopharyngeal cancer. *Cell Biology and Toxicology, 39*(6), 2501–2526.

Lu, T., Shi, Y., Wang, M., Liu, W., Cao, Y., Shi, L., Ma, Q., & Liu, S. (February 2024). CCR5 promoter polymorphisms associated with nonsmall cell lung cancer. *International Journal of Immunogenetics, 51*(1), 10–19.

Mack, S. J., Erlich, H. A., Feolo, M., Fernandez-Vina, M., Gourrauud, P. A., Helmberg, W., Kanga, U., Kupatawintu, P., Lancaster, A., Maiers, M., & Maldonado-Torres, H. (January 1, 2009). Idawg-the Immunogenomic data-analysis working group. *Human Immunology, 70*, S86.

Mahdi H, Ni Y. Immunogenomic signatures to predict outcome in ovarian and endometrial cancers: Potential strategies in targeting the tumor immune microenvironment to improve response to immunotherapy.

Mak, R. K., Hundhausen, C., & Nestle, F. O. (December 1, 2009). Progress in understanding the immunopathogenesis of psoriasis. *Actas Dermo-Sifiliográficas, 100*, 2–13.

Malkan, Ü. Y., et al. (October 10, 2023). Immunogenomic approach to the clinical management of COVID-19 syndrome. *Eskisehir Medical Journal, 4*(Ek sayı), 266–279.

Marcon, J., DiNatale, R. G., Sanchez, A., Kotecha, R. R., Gupta, S., Kuo, F., Makarov, V., Sandhu, A., Mano, R., Silagy, A. W., & Blum, K. A. (July 15, 2020). Comprehensive genomic analysis of translocation renal cell carcinoma reveals copy-number variations as drivers of disease progression. *Clinical Cancer Research, 26*(14), 3629–3640.

Martin, M. J., Estravís, M., García-Sánchez, A., Dávila, I., Isidoro-García, M., & Sanz, C. (April 18, 2020). Genetics and epigenetics of atopic dermatitis: An updated systematic review. *Genes, 11*(4), 442.

Maruthamuthu, S., Rajalingam, K., Kaur, N., Morvan, M. G., Soto, J., Lee, N., Kong, D., Hu, Z., Reyes, K., Ng, D., & Butte, A. J. (February 22, 2022). Individualized constellation of killer cell immunoglobulin-like receptors and cognate HLA class I ligands that controls natural killer cell antiviral immunity predisposes COVID-19. *Frontiers in Genetics, 13*, 845474.

McDonald, W. I., Batchelor, J. R., & Francis, D. A. (October 1, 1984). The immunogenetics of multiple sclerosis. *Trends in Neurosciences, 7*(10), 369–371.

Medhasi, S., & Chantratita, N. (May 26, 2022). Human leukocyte antigen (HLA) system: Genetics and association with bacterial and viral infections. *Journal of Immunology Research*, 2022.

Messemaker, T. C., Huizinga, T. W., & Kurreeman, F. (November 1, 2015). Immunogenetics of rheumatoid arthritis: Understanding functional implications. *Journal of Autoimmunity, 64*, 74–81.

Miller, F. W. (1995). Genetics of autoimmune diseases. *Immunogenetic Risk Assessment In Human Disease*, 182–190.

Mimura, G., Kida, K., Matsuura, N., Toyota, T., Kitagawa, T., Kobayashi, T., Hibi, I., Ikeda, Y., Tuchida, I., Kuzuya, H., & Aono, S. (January 1, 1990). Immunogenetics of early-onset insulin-dependent diabetes mellitus among the Japanese: HLA, Gm, BF, GLO, and organ-specific autoantibodies—the JDS study. *Diabetes Research and Clinical Practice, 8*(3), 253–262.

Minniakhmetov, I., Yalaev, B., Khusainova, R., Bondarenko, E., Melnichenko, G., Dedov, I., & Mokrysheva, N. (February 8, 2024). Genetic and epigenetic aspects of type 1 diabetes mellitus: Modern view on the problem. *Biomedicines, 12*(2), 399.

Misra, M. K., Damotte, V., & Hollenbach, J. A. (April 2018). The immunogenetics of neurological disease. *Immunology, 153*(4), 399–414.

Mlynarski, W. M., Placha, G. P., Wolkow, P. P., Bochenski, J. P., Warram, J. H., & Krolewski, A. S. (November 1, 2005). Risk of diabetic nephropathy in type 1 diabetes is associated with functional polymorphisms in rantes receptor gene (ccr5) a sex-specific effect. *Diabetes, 54*(11), 3331–3335.

Monar, G. V., Islam, H., Puttagunta, S. M., Islam, R., Kundu, S., Jha, S. B., Rivera, A. P., & Sange, I. (March 7, 2022). Association between type 1 diabetes mellitus and celiac disease: Autoimmune disorders with a shared genetic background. *Cureus, 14*(3).

Monod, M. Y., Giudicelli, V., Chaume, D., & Lefranc, M. P. (August 4, 2004). IMGT/JunctionAnalysis: The first tool for the analysis of the immunoglobulin and T cell receptor complex V–J and V–D–J JUNCTIONs. *Bioinformatics, 20*(suppl_1), i379–i385.

Morran, M. P., Vonberg, A., Khadra, A., & Pietropaolo, M. (April 1, 2015). Immunogenetics of type 1 diabetes mellitus. *Molecular Aspects of Medicine, 42*, 42–60.

Mujahid, F., & Ahmad, N. (2023). *Immunogenetics and personalized vaccines: A new era in immunization, 10* (p. 13140).

Ndong, S. C. A., Smith, D., Petersen, D. C., Schurz, H., Uren, C., & Möller, M. (June 2023). The immunogenetics of tuberculosis (TB) susceptibility. *Immunogenetics, 75*(3), 215–230.

Niedeggen, C., Singer, S., Groth, M., Petermann-Meyer, A., Röth, A., Schrezenmeier, H., Höchsmann, B., Brümmendorf, T. H., & Panse, J. (July 1, 2019). Design and development of a disease-specific quality of life tool for patients with aplastic anaemia and/or paroxysmal nocturnal haemoglobinuria (QLQ-AA/PNH)—a report on phase III. *Annals of Hematology, 98*, 1547–1559.

Noble, J. A. (November 1, 2015). Immunogenetics of type 1 diabetes: A comprehensive review. *Journal of Autoimmunity, 64*, 101–112.

Oliveira, J., Oliveira-Maia, A. J., Tamouza, R., Brown, A. S., & Leboyer, M. (October 2017). Infectious and immunogenetic factors in bipolar disorder. *Acta Psychiatrica Scandinavica, 136*(4), 409–423.

Olokoba, A. B., Obateru, O. A., & Olokoba, L. B. (July 2012). Type 2 diabetes mellitus: A review of current trends. *Oman Medical Journal, 27*(4), 269.

Onengut-Gumuscu, S., & Concannon, P. (October 1, 2006). Recent advances in the immunogenetics of human type 1 diabetes. *Current Opinion in Immunology, 18*(5), 634–638.

Osman, A. E., Brema, I., AlQurashi, A., Al-Jurayyan, A., Bradley, B., & Hamza, M. A. (April 2, 2022). Single nucleotide polymorphism rs 2070874 at Interleukin-4 is associated with increased risk of type 1 diabetes mellitus independently of human leukocyte antigens. *International Journal of Immunopathology and Pharmacology, 36*.

Ozdemir, V., Faraj, S. A., & Knoppers, B. M. (September 1, 2011). Steering vaccinomics innovations with anticipatory governance and participatory foresight. *OMICS: A Journal of Integrative Biology, 15*(9), 637–646.

Pao, S. C., Chu, M. T., & Hung, S. I. (April 15, 2022). Therapeutic vaccines targeting neoantigens to induce T-cell immunity against cancers. *Pharmaceutics, 14*(4), 867.

Peng, K., Safonova, Y., Shugay, M., Popejoy, A. B., Rodriguez, O. L., Breden, F., Brodin, P., Burkhardt, A. M., Bustamante, C., Cao-Lormeau, V. M., & Corcoran, M. M. (June 2021). Diversity in immunogenomics: The value and the challenge. *Nature Methods, 18*(6), 588–591.

Petersdorf, E. W. (October 1, 2006). Immunogenomics of unrelated hematopoietic cell transplantation. *Current Opinion in Immunology, 18*(5), 559–564.

Pichini, A., Ahmed, A., Patch, C., Bick, D., Leblond, M., Kasperaviciute, D., Deen, D., Wilde, S., Garcia Noriega, S., Matoko, C., & Tuff-Lacey, A. (May 30, 2022). Developing a national newborn genomes program: An approach driven by ethics, engagement and co-design. *Frontiers in Genetics, 13,* 866168.

Poland GA, Ovsyannikova IG, Jacobson RM. Application of pharmacogenomics to vaccines.

Potts, W. K. (February 1, 2002). Wisdom through immunogenetics. *Nature Genetics, 30*(2), 130–131.

Pouget, J. G. (August 20, 2018). The emerging immunogenetic architecture of schizophrenia. *Schizophrenia Bulletin, 44*(5), 993–1004.

Qadir, J., & Majid, S. (2022). Immunopharmacogenomics: Clinical applications, challenges, and future prospects. *A Molecular Approach to Immunogenetics, 1,* 255–276.

Qadri, H., Shah, A. H., & Mir, M. A. (January 1, 2022). Role of immunogenetics polymorphisms in infectious diseases. In *A molecular approach to immunogenetics* (pp. 169–191). Academic Press.

Rausell, A., & Telenti, A. (October 1, 2014). Genomics of host-pathogen interactions. *Current Opinion in Immunology, 30,* 32–38.

Reece, E. A., Hagay, Z., & Hobbins, J. C. (May 1, 1991). Insulin-dependent diabetes mellitus and immunogenetics: Maternal and fetal considerations. *Obstetrical and Gynecological Survey, 46*(5), 255–263.

Rehman MU, Arafah A, Ali MN, Ali S, editors. Immunogenetics: A molecular and clinical overview: Clinical applications of immunogenetics.

Ridolfi, F., Peetluk, L., Amorim, G., Turner, M., Figueiredo, M., Cordeiro-Santos, M., Cavalcante, S., Kritski, A., Durovni, B., Andrade, B., & Sterling, T. R. (February 1, 2023). Tuberculosis treatment outcomes in Brazil: Different predictors for each type of unsuccessful outcome. *Clinical Infectious Diseases, 76*(3), e930–e937.

Roederer, M., Quaye, L., Mangino, M., Beddall, M. H., Mahnke, Y., Chattopadhyay, P., Tosi, I., Napolitano, L., Barberio, M. T., Menni, C., & Villanova, F. (April 9, 2015). The genetic architecture of the human immune system: A bioresource for autoimmunity and disease pathogenesis. *Cell, 161*(2), 387–403.

Ros, J., Baraibar, I., Vivancos, A., & Rodon, J. (November 11, 2019). Review of immunogenomics and the role of tumor mutational burden as a biomarker for immunotherapy response. *Journal of Immunotherapy and Precision Oncology, 2*(4), 144–151.

Sandford, A., Weir, T., & Paré, P. (June 1996). The genetics of asthma. *American Journal of Respiratory and Critical Care Medicine, 153*(6), 1749–1765.

Sanghavi, K., Feero, W. G., Mathews, D. J., Prince, A. E., Price, L. L., Liu, E. T., Brothers, K. B., Roberts, J. S., & Lee, C. (March 17, 2021). Employees' views and ethical, legal, and social implications assessment of voluntary workplace genomic testing. *Frontiers in Genetics, 12,* 643304.

Schneeberger, E. E., Citera, G., Rodríguez Gil, G., Granel, A., Arturi, A., Rosemffet, G. M., Maldonado Cocco, J. A., Berman, A., Spindler, A., & Morales, V. H. (August 2015). Clinical and immunogenetic characterization in psoriatic arthritis patients. *Clinical Rheumatology, 34,* 1413–1418.

Sen, K., Datta, S., Ghosh, A., Jha, A., Ahad, A., Chatterjee, S., Suranjika, S., Sengupta, S., Bhattacharya, G., Shriwas, O., & Avula, K. (November 25, 2021). Single-cell immunogenomic approach identified SARS-CoV-2 protective immune signatures in asymptomatic direct contacts of COVID-19 cases. *Frontiers in Immunology, 12,* 733539.

Shah, R. K., Cygan, E., Kozlik, T., Colina, A., & Zamora, A. E. (December 12, 2023). Utilizing immunogenomic approaches to prioritize targetable neoantigens for personalized cancer immunotherapy. *Frontiers in Immunology, 14,* 1301100.

Shahrier, S., Gaydarska, H., Takashima, K., Yoshizawa, G., & Minari, J. (November 28, 2023). A conceptual analysis of public opinion regarding genome research in Japan. *Frontiers in Genetics, 14,* 1170794.

Siddique, H. R. (June 6, 2023). Genes, diseases, immunity and immunogenomics. *Frontiers in Genetics, 14*, 1218084.

Singh, A. K., Netea, M. G., & Bishai, W. R. (June 1, 2021). BCG turns 100: Its nontraditional uses against viruses, cancer, and immunologic diseases. *The Journal of Clinical Investigation, 131*(11).

Sinkora, M., Stepanova, K., Butler, J. E., Sinkora, J. M., Sinkora, S., & Sinkorova, J. (February 11, 2022). Comparative aspects of immunoglobulin gene rearrangement arrays in different species. *Frontiers in Immunology, 13*, 823145.

Soleiman-Meigooni, S., Yarahmadi, A., Kheirkhah, A. H., & Afkhami, H. (March 13, 2024). Recent advances in different interactions between toll-like receptors and hepatitis B infection: A review. *Frontiers in Immunology, 15*, 1363996.

Stewart, L. L., Field, L. L., Ross, S., & McArthur, R. G. (December 1993). Genetic risk factors in diabetic retinopathy. *Diabetologia, 36*, 1293–1298.

Su, M., Chen, Z., Zheng, J., & Chen, Y. (October 2020). Genetic variants in class II transactivator are associated with chronic hepatitis B virus infection in the Han Chinese population. *International Journal of Immunogenetics, 47*(5), 435–442.

Tam, A. A., Ozdemir, D., Bestepe, N., Dellal, F. D., Bilginer, M. C., Faki, S., Bicer, C., Ersoy, R., & Cakir, B. (June 29, 2020). Low rate of latent autoimmune diabetes in adults (LADA) in patients followed for type 2 diabetes: A single center's experience in Turkey. *Archives of Endocrinology and Metabolism, 64*, 584–590.

Tao, Y., Han, X., Liu, N., Shi, L., Shi, L., Liu, S., & Yao, Y. (June 2022). Association study of TAP and HLA-I gene combination with chronic hepatitis C virus infection in a Han population in China. *International Journal of Immunogenetics, 49*(3), 169–180.

Thivolet, C. (2000). Perspectives in early detection and management of IDDM. In *Transplantation and changing management of organ failure: Proceedings of the 32nd international conference on transplantation and changing management of organ failure* (pp. 145–149). Netherlands: Dordrecht: Springer.

Thomas, N. J., Walkey, H. C., Kaur, A., Misra, S., Oliver, N. S., Colclough, K., Weedon, M. N., Johnston, D. G., Hattersley, A. T., & Patel, K. A. (February 2023). The relationship between islet autoantibody status and the genetic risk of type 1 diabetes in adult-onset type 1 diabetes. *Diabetologia, 66*(2), 310–320.

Traherne, J. A. (June 2008). Human MHC architecture and evolution: Implications for disease association studies. *International Journal of Immunogenetics, 35*(3), 179–192.

Ünlü, B., Türsen, Ü., Rajabi, Z., Jabalameli, N., & Rajabi, F. (March 15, 2022). The immunogenetics of systemic sclerosis. In *The immunogenetics of dermatologic diseases* (pp. 259–298). Cham: Springer International Publishing.

Vahabi, N., & Michailidis, G. (March 22, 2022). Unsupervised multi-omics data integration methods: A comprehensive review. *Frontiers in Genetics, 13*, 854752.

Varzari, A., Tudor, E., Corloteanu, A., Axentii, E., Vladei, I., & Deyneko, I. V. (April 23, 2024). Association between STAT4 gene polymorphism and susceptibility to pulmonary tuberculosis in the Moldavian population. *International Journal of Immunogenetics, 51*(4), 228–234.

Vaseghi-Shanjani, M., Smith, K. L., Sara, R. J., Modi, B. P., Branch, A., Sharma, M., Lu, H. Y., James, E. L., Hildebrand, K. J., Biggs, C. M., & Turvey, S. E. (November 1, 2021). Inborn errors of immunity manifesting as atopic disorders. *Journal of Allergy and Clinical Immunology, 148*(5), 1130–1139.

Vinciguerra, M., Masotti, A., & Alisi, A. (September 15, 2020). Role of epigenetic modifications on diet-induced metabolic diseases. *Frontiers in Genetics, 11*, 540628.

Vlachonikola, E., Langerak, A. W., Rosenquist, R., & Chatzidimitriou, A. (2023). The promise of immunogenetics for precision oncology. *Frontiers in Oncology, 13*.

Walport, M. J., Ollier, W. E., & Silman, A. J. (October 1, 1992). Immunogenetics of rheumatoid arthritis and the Arthritis and Rheumatism Council's National repository. *Rheumatology, 31*(10), 701–705.

Wang, Q., Vattai, A., Vilsmaier, T., Kaltofen, T., Steger, A., Mayr, D., Mahner, S., Jeschke, U., & Heidegger, H. H. (February 28, 2021). Immunogenomic identification for predicting the prognosis of cervical cancer patients. *International Journal of Molecular Sciences, 22*(5), 2442.

Wang, Y., Jiang, Y., Wang, J., Li, S., Jia, X., Xiao, X., Sun, W., Wang, P., & Zhang, Q. (August 28, 2023). Retinopathy as an initial sign of hereditary immunological diseases: Report of six families and challenges in eye clinic. *Frontiers in Immunology, 14*, 1239886.

Willemsen, R. A., Debets, R., Chames, P., & Bolhuis, R. L. (January 1, 2003). Genetic engineering of T cell specificity for immunotherapy of cancer. *Human Immunology, 64*(1), 56–68.

Wolf, Y., & Samuels, Y. (January 1, 2018). Cancer research in the era of immunogenomics. *ESMO Open, 3* (7), e000475.

Xin, Z., You, L., Na, F., Li, J., Chen, M., Song, J., Bai, L., Chen, J., Zhou, J., & Ying, B. (May 1, 2023). Immunogenetic variations predict immune-related adverse events for PD-1/PD-L1 inhibitors. *European Journal of Cancer, 184*, 124–136.

Xu, Y., Su, G. H., Ma, D., Xiao, Y., Shao, Z. M., & Jiang, Y. Z. (August 20, 2021). Technological advances in cancer immunity: From immunogenomics to single-cell analysis and artificial intelligence. *Signal Transduction and Targeted Therapy, 6*(1), 312.

Yang, K. D., Chang, J. C., Chuang, H., Liang, H. M., Kuo, H. C., Lee, Y. S., Hsu, T. Y., & Ou, C. Y. (June 2010). Gene–gene and gene-environment interactions on IgE production in prenatal stage. *Allergy, 65* (6), 731–739.

Yang, X., Lei, G., Wang, J., Wen, Z., Ma, Z., Zhao, Y., Ren, H., & Xie, H. (2022). Integrative immunogenomic analysis reveals transcriptional and immune-related differences in hepatocellular carcinoma patients with different disease-free survival. *American Journal of Cancer Research, 12*(4), 1752.

Zhang, J., Chen, L. M., Zou, Y., Zhang, S., Xiong, F., & Wang, C. Y. (May 5, 2021). Implication of epigenetic factors in the pathogenesis of type 1 diabetes. *Chinese Medical Journal, 134*(09), 1031–1042.

Zhao, L. P., Papadopoulos, G. K., Skyler, J. S., Pugliese, A., Parikh, H. M., Kwok, W. W., Lybrand, T. P., Bondinas, G. P., Moustakas, A. K., Wang, R., & Pyo, C. W. (May 1, 2024). HLA class II (DR, DQ, DP) genes were separately associated with the progression from seroconversion to onset of type 1 diabetes among participants in two Diabetes prevention trials (DPT-1 and TN07). *Diabetes Care, 47*(5), 826–834.

Zhou, Y., Simpson, J. S., Holloway, A. F., Charlesworth, J., van der Mei, I., & Taylor, B. V. (February 2014). The potential role of epigenetic modifications in the heritability of multiple sclerosis. *Multiple Sclerosis Journal, 20*(2), 135–140.

Zhu, Q., Wang, J., Zhang, W., Zhu, W., Wu, Z., Chen, Y., Chen, M., Zheng, L., Tang, J., Zhang, S., & Wang, D. (May 12, 2022). Whole-genome/exome sequencing uncovers mutations and copy number variations in primary diffuse large B-cell lymphoma of the central nervous system. *Frontiers in Genetics, 13*, 878618.

14

Integrating immunogenetics in T2DM research and practices

Binty, Unnati Shukla, Manisha Singh, R. Rachana and Shalini Mani
CENTRE FOR EMERGING DISEASES, DEPARTMENT OF BIOTECHNOLOGY, JAYPEE INSTITUTE OF INFORMATION TECHNOLOGY, NOIDA, UTTAR PRADESH, INDIA

1. Introduction

Type 2 diabetes mellitus (T2DM) is a very complex and multifactorial metabolic disorder; earlier it was considered that T2DM is only linked with lifestyle activity such as improper diet, physical activity, and obesity, but now ongoing researches suggest that T2DM is not only a metabolic disorder but immune system components and genes also play a significant role in T2DM (Laakso & Silva, 2022). In T2DM, there is an abnormally elevated glucose level, glucose intolerance, and hyperglycemia (DeFronzo et al., 2015). T2DM involves low-grade chronic inflammation, which results in beta cell dysfunction (insulin-producing cells in the pancreas) and insulin resistance (King, 2002).

Immunogenetics is the study of how genetic variations influence immune system functions. Studies have suggested that several key genes are related to immune function in T2DM disease and its progression (Beth, 2023). A few important genes that are related to T2DM are the human inflammatory cytokine gene (IL-1β,IL-6, TNF -α), leukocyte antigen (HLA), Toll-like receptor (TLRs), and nuclear factor kappa B (NF-κB) signaling pathways (Chatterjee et al., 2017). Mutation or variations in these components lead to hyperactive immune response, increased inflammation, and poor insulin signaling, ultimately causing insulin resistance and β-cell failure. So information on these genetic influences is important for identifying the risk individuals and improving early diagnosis, risk assessments, and treatment strategies (Beth, 2023).

Immunogenetics also plays an important role in pharmacogenetics—the study of how genetic variations affect an individual response (Lai et al., 2017). Differences in genetics can influence drug metabolism, efficacy, and side effects in immune-related pathways. For example, variations in the IL-1 receptor antagonist gene (ILIRN) have been linked to different responses to IL-1β inhibitors, a class of drugs that target inflammation in T2DM (Laakso & Silva, 2022). Personalize treatment plans, ensuring that patients receive the most effective and least harmful therapies can be done by gathering knowledge about these genetic markers (Mullard, 2019).

Type 2 Diabetes Mellitus. https://doi.org/10.1016/B978-0-443-33590-7.00001-0

The integration of immunogenetics into T2DM research and clinical practice can overcome diabetes (DeFronzo et al., 2015). By identifying biomarkers that are linked to immune imbalance, researchers can develop precision medicine approaches that tailor interventions to individual patients. As research in immunogenetics advances, the focus of T2DM management will likely shift toward personalized, immune-targeted treatment rather than a common approach The ability to predict disease risk, control treatment responses, and develop new immune-based interventions could highly improve outcomes for millions of T2DM patient worldwide (Laakso & Silva, 2022).

2. Genetics of T2DM

T2DM is a complex inherited condition influenced by multiple genes, which is influenced by both genetic and environmental factors. T2DM involves multiple genetic loci, and each has a small individual effect (Kreienkamp et al., 2023). Studies have suggested that there are over 400 genetic variants that are associated with T2DM, offering an understanding of the biological mechanism driving disease progression. These genetic variants are mainly responsible for beta cell function, insulin resistance, insulin secretion, glycolytic pathway, and immune-related inflammatory responses, showing the relationship between metabolism and the immune system in T2DM pathogenesis (Lê et al., 2005).

One of the most important gene-associated risk factors for T2DM is transcription factor 7 like 2 (TCF7L2), which is responsible for insulin secretion and proliferation of beta cells. Mutation in TCF7L2 has been repeatedly linked to reduced insulin secretion and elevated risk of diabetes (Altshuler et al., 2003). Similarly, genes that regulate ATP-sensitive potassium channels in beta cells such as ATP-binding cassette subfamily C member 8 (ABCC8) and potassium inwardly rectifying channel subfamily J member 11 (KCNJ11) are responsible for normal insulin. Slight changes in these genes are responsible for disrupting glucose-stimulated insulin secretions, leading individuals to T2DM (Lyssenko et al., 2003). Another hepatocyte nuclear factor 1A and 4A1 (HNF1A and HNF4A1) performs an important role in pancreatic beta cell gene function and insulin balance (The SIGMA Type 2 Diabetes Consortium, 2014).

Insulin resistance is also an important factor behind T2DM, where our peripheral tissues do not respond effectively to insulin. Many genetic variants have a role in insulin signaling and metabolic regulations. The peroxisome proliferator–activated receptor gamma (PPARG) genes have a very important role in lipid metabolism, adipocyte differentiation, and insulin sensibility. Genetic changes in these genes cause decreased insulin sensitivity and increased diabetes (Altshuler et al., 2000). Similarly, mutation in insulin receptor substrate 1(IRS1) genes, which encode a very important protein in the insulin signaling pathway, contribute to improper glucose uptake and insulin resistance (Rahman et al., 2018). Fat mass and obesity (FTO)–associated genes responsible for obesity-driven insulin resistance are another crucial genetic factor; their mutation affects energy balance, fat storage, and metabolic efficiency (Do et al., 2008).

Now not only metabolic pathway, but also inflammation and immune system dysfunction have a very important role in T2DM development. Low-grade inflammation has a role in insulin resistance, and mutation in proinflammatory cytokine is responsible for the occurrence of the disease. IL-6 gene is responsible for an inflammatory response that causes increased systemic inflammation and insulin resistance tumor necrosis factor-alpha (TNF -α). Interfering with insulin receptors causes signaling, causing metabolic dysfunction (Mirza et al., 2011).

Genes that are responsible for glucose transport and metabolism significantly influence T2DM risk. The SLC308 (zinc transporter 8) stabilizes insulin granules within β-cells, and its mutation can affect the efficiency of insulin (Chimienti et al., 2004). Glucokinase genes, a glucose sensor in β -cells, play an important role in glucose-activated insulin secretion. Mutation in these genes can disrupt β-cell responsiveness to glucose, resulting in the development of T2DM (Coghlan, 2023).

As multiple genetic risk factors are associated with this disease, researchers have developed a Polygenic Risk Score (PRS) to check whether the individual is susceptible to T2DM or not. PRS merges multiple risk alleles to anticipate disease onset, its progression, and response to treatment. Although genetic susceptibility is not enough to dictate T2DM development, combining genetic risk evaluation with lifestyle activity such as improper diet, exercise, and other metabolic markers helps early diagnostic and prevention plans for the disease (Udler et al., 2019).

Knowing the genetics of T2DM is important for clinical implications for disease management. Pharmacogenetics is the study of how genetic changes affect individual response to drugs and play an important role in personalized treatment approaches. Few genetic markers can forecast the individual response to some diabetic drugs (such as metformin, sulfonylureas, and DPP 4 inhibitors and insulin therapy), allowing personalized treatment approaches (Tkáč & Klimčáková, 2020). Additionally, a genetic pathway that is responsible for β-cell survival, insulin resistance, and inflammation allows to development of targeted therapies that can perform better than conventional glucose-lowering medication (Brunetti et al., 2014).

3. Diabetes and immune system

T2DM is marked by chronic low-grade inflammation and immune system dysfunction. The interplay between insulin resistance, metabolic stress, and immune activation contributes to impaired glucose homeostasis. (1) Insulin resistance arises when cells in tissues such as muscles, liver, and fat adipose tissue become less responsive to insulin and excess fat tissue in obesity, especially visceral fat, becomes inflamed and produces a variety of inflammatory cytokines (Donath & Shoelson, 2011). These cytokines are released into the bloodstream, leading to systemic inflammation. Immune cells such as the T cells and macrophages enter the adipose tissue, where they exacerbate the inflammatory response. This chronic inflammation impairs insulin sensitivity, a key feature of insulin resistance, and further disrupts metabolic processes, contributing to the onset of T2DM contributing to hyperglycemia. Low-grade chronic inflammation is a key driver of resistance to insulin and is associated with various immune-mediated mechanisms. Elevated inflammatory cytokines: increased levels of inflammatory signaling molecules, including (TNF-α) tumor necrosis factor-alpha, C-reactive protein (CRP), and interleukin-6 (IL-6), disrupt insulin signaling. These cytokines inhibit insulin receptor substrate (IRS) proteins, reducing their ability to propagate insulin signaling and leading to diminished glucose uptake (Tilg & Moschen, 2008). In a healthy body, insulin-sensitive state, the insulin binding to the receptor triggers a signaling pathway that leads to the addition of phosphate group to tyrosine residues on insulin receptor substrate 1 (IRS-1), activating insulin signaling pathways downstream. Although, in insulin resistance, proinflammatory molecules activate a variety of serine kinases, including c-Jun N-terminal kinase (JNK) inhibitor of NF-κB kinase subunit β (IKK-β), extracellular signal-regulated kinase (ERK), ribosomal protein S6 kinase (S6K), protein kinase C (PKC), mammalian target of rapamycin (mTOR), and glycogen synthase kinase 3β (GSK3β). These protein kinases disrupt the signaling of insulin by adding phosphate groups to serine residues rather than the residues of tyrosine, thereby impairing the action of insulin. Free fatty acids (FFAS) and reactive oxygen species (ROS): Elevated FFAs and oxidative stress (from ROS) activate inflammatory pathways, increasing metabolic dysregulation. FFAs contribute to insulin resistance by activating protein kinase C (PKC), which disrupts insulin signaling. ROS, meanwhile, exacerbates endoplasmic reticulum (ER) stress, further chepromoting inflammation and insulin dysfunction. (2) Activation of proinflammatory pathways where the major stress-activated signaling pathway, c-Jun N-terminal kinase (JNK), adds a phosphate group to IRS-1 at serine residues, preventing it from transmitting insulin's signal effectively (Aguirre et al., 2000). This results in decreased glucose absorption and exacerbates insulin resistance. An inhibitor β (IKKβ)/NF-κB of NF-κB kinase activates NF-κB, a protein that regulates gene expression responsible for increasing the production of inflammatory cytokines. NF-κB activation leads to the breakdown of IκB enables NF-κB to move into the nucleus, stimulating the expression of inflammation-related genes. This creates a feed-forward loop, in which inflammation continuously promotes insulin resistance and metabolic dysfunction. This condition is initially compensated by increasing insulin secretion (hyperinsulinemia) (Berbudi et al., 2019). Prolonged metabolic stress and chronic inflammation eventually lead to β-cell dysfunction, exhaustion, and apoptosis (Donath & Shoelson, 2011).

β-Cell exhaustion: Persistent insulin overproduction in response to insulin resistance leads to endoplasmic reticulum (ER) stress, mitochondrial dysfunction, and oxidative stress in β-cells. Over time, this results in their functional decline and reduced insulin secretion. Inflammatory cytokine-induced β-cell apoptosis: TNF-α, IL-6, and FFAs directly induce β-cell apoptosis by activating stress pathways such as JNK, which promotes cell death. Additionally, ROS accumulation damages β-cell membranes, further impairing insulin production. Macrophage infiltration and adipose tissue inflammation: In obese individuals, adipose tissue becomes infiltrated by proinflammatory M1 macrophages (CD11c + cells), which secrete TNF-α and other cytokines. These cytokines exacerbate β-cell dysfunction and contribute to systemic insulin resistance. T cell involvement: $CD8^+$ and $CD4^+$ T cells interact with macrophages in adipose tissue (McLaughlin et al., 2014), amplifying inflammation and accelerating β-cell apoptosis. The continuous immune response further disrupts insulin homeostasis and worsens disease progression.

Once initiated, the inflammatory response in T2DM creates a self-perpetuating cycle: Insulin resistance develops due to chronic inflammation, disrupting glucose uptake. In response, pancreatic β-cells compensate by increasing insulin secretion (hyperinsulinemia), leading to metabolic stress. Inflammation and immune activation further impair β-cell function, causing apoptosis and reduced insulin production. Decreased insulin secretion worsens hyperglycemia, fueling additional metabolic dysfunction and inflammation. This cycle contributes to the progressive nature of T2DM, increasing the likelihood of developing such as complications such as heart disease, nephropathy, and neuropathy.

3.1 Dysfunctional immune response and increasing susceptibility toward infections

T2DM significantly impacts the body's defense mechanism, leading to a weakened ability to combat infections and an increased susceptibility to a variety of pathogens. One of the primary mechanisms contributing to impaired immune function in T2DM is immunosuppression. Elevated blood glucose levels and insulin deficiency disrupt the normal functioning of key immune cells, i.e., phagocytes and T cells. These cells are essential for detecting and eliminating harmful microorganisms. As a result, individuals with T2DM experience a diminished immune response, leaving them more vulnerable to infections, especially those affecting the skin, urinary tract, and respiratory system. Furthermore, chronic hyperglycemia in T2DM leads to cytokine suppression. Cytokines are signaling proteins that help regulate the body's immune response by triggering inflammation and guiding immune cells to the infection site (Schaper & Rose-John, 2015). However, in individuals with T2DM, prolonged high blood sugar levels reduce the production and effectiveness of these cytokines, thereby impairing the body's ability to mount an adequate immune response against invading pathogens.

In addition to cytokine suppression, individuals with T2DM exhibit defective phagocytosis, a process in which immune cells engulf and digest pathogens. This dysfunction in phagocytic activity further compromises the immune system's ability to neutralize infections effectively. The impaired ability of immune cells to perform this essential function results in delayed clearance of pathogens and a prolonged infection process.

3.2 Immune-related genes and role in T2DM

Many genes are involved in the immune system, which can lead to the buildup and progression of the disease. One of the genesis the HLA) Human leukocyte antigen gene. The HLA genes play a role in regulating our defense mechanism against foreign invaders and antigens. HLA gene variation can also influence how the immune system activates and regulates the immune cells. Some HLA variants are also found to be associated with T2DM, by altering the immune response that affects beta cell function and insulin sensitivity. Few other sets of genes related to T2DM are those that show inflammatory responses cytokines, i.e., IL-6, IL-1β, and TNF-ALPHA.

These cytokines are proinflammatory and are central to chronic inflammation that is seen in T2DM. This plays an intrinsic role in the onset of insulin resistance. Cytokines lead to long-term low-level inflammation, which damages insulin signaling pathways and leads to β-cell dysfunction in the pancreas, which is known to be the hallmark of T2DM.

3.3 Candidate gene-based studies

Scientists study specific genes that might be linked to T2DM based on their preexisting knowledge of the disease's pathophysiology by focusing on genes that are believed to be involved in critical metabolic processes, i.e., insulin secretion, glucose homeostasis, and insulin resistance (Lu et al., 2024). The human genome project is an extensive database that assists in the identification of single nucleotide polymorphisms (SNPs). SNPs represent the most prevalent type of genetic variation to measure their contribution to T2DM susceptibility in the human genome. The human genome project allows for the precise association between the variation of genes and the most likely outcomes of disease. The key targets of the study are genes that are responsible for insulin sensitivity, β-cell function, and metabolic pathways. In the study of T2DM, one well-known gene that gained attention is peroxisome proliferator–activated receptor gamma (PPARγ), a nuclear receptor that is a primary regulator of insulin sensitivity, adipogenesis, and inflammatory responses.

- T2DM risk and PARG-PPARG is involved in the gene expression, critical for the proper functioning of insulin-responsive tissues including certain tissues in the body such as adipose tissue, muscle, and liver. Pro12Ala (where proline is substituted with alanine at position 12) is an SNP in the PPARG gene, known to have a 20% higher risk of developing T2DM in individuals carrying it (Lu et al., 2024). This SNP is believed to promote receptors' transcriptional activity, which results in the alteration of gene expression patterns that affect fat storage and glucose metabolism.
- Effect of PPARG Pro12Ala on insulin sensitivity—The Pro12Ala variant of the PPARG gene is linked to altering the receptor's functional activity. This variant increases the transcriptional activity of the PPARG gene, which affects metabolic

pathways, especially those that respond well to insulin. The regulation of glucose metabolism can be altered with the increase in activation of PPARG by promoting insulin sensitivity in peripheral tissues. Variation may also lead to inflammatory responses, which is the main cause of insulin resistance.

The individual carrying the Pro12Ala variant may enhance blood glucose levels more efficiently under certain conditions and may experience a different insulin response. Nonetheless, the general impact on the risk of disease is context-dependent and is very complex to understand. The precise mechanism as to how β-cell function gets affected by SNP is still a research field of study. The Pro12Ala variant in individuals may contribute to the enhancement in β-cell function response against metabolic stress. PPARG-mediated modulation of lipid mechanism and inflammatory pathways are known to be impacting insulin synthesis and secretion potential and β-cell survival.

4. Immunogenetics in T2DM

Immunogenetics means shedding light on genetic determinants of immune responses, and exploring how immune system disbalance can cause T2DM. Genetic changes in immune-linked genes can cause inflammations, insulin sensitivity, and beta cell functions. Many important immune genetic factors have a role in T2DM, and knowing their association is important for the preparation of targeted therapeutic strategies (Sun et al., 2021) (Fig. 14.1).

The human leukocyte antigen (HLA) system has a very important role in maintaining immune response. HLA polymorphisms are well known for their association with autoimmune disorders such as T1DM, but now the ongoing studies suggest that HLA alleles also have their contribution in immune dysregulation of T2DM. In T2DM, HLA polymorphism is responsible for modulating inflammatory pathways, causing low-grade chronic inflammation and insulin resistance (Sun et al., 2021). Few HLA class II alleles are linked to increased chances of metabolic inflammation by supporting the presentation of self-antigens to immune cells. In return, it triggers immune activation in adipose tissues and pancreatic islets, which results in beta cell dysfunction. Studies have suggested that individuals having specific HLA-DR and HLA-DQ alleles show mutated inflammatory cytokine profiles, which can be correlated with insulin resistance and increased diabetes risk (Xiao et al., 2020).

Toll-like receptors(TLRs) are a submembers of pattern recognition receptors (PRRs) that have an important role in generalized immunity by recognition of damage-associated molecular patterns (DAMPs) and pathogen-associated molecular patterns (PAMPs). TLRs, especially TLR 2 and TLR4 have been widely studied for their role in the inflammatory mechanism of T2DM. The lipopolysaccharides secreted by gram-negative bacteria activate TLR4 and are responsible for the secretion of proinflammatory cytokines such as TNF-α, IL-6, and IL-β. The continuous activation of the immune system disturbs metabolic function by interfering with insulin signaling. Genetic variation in

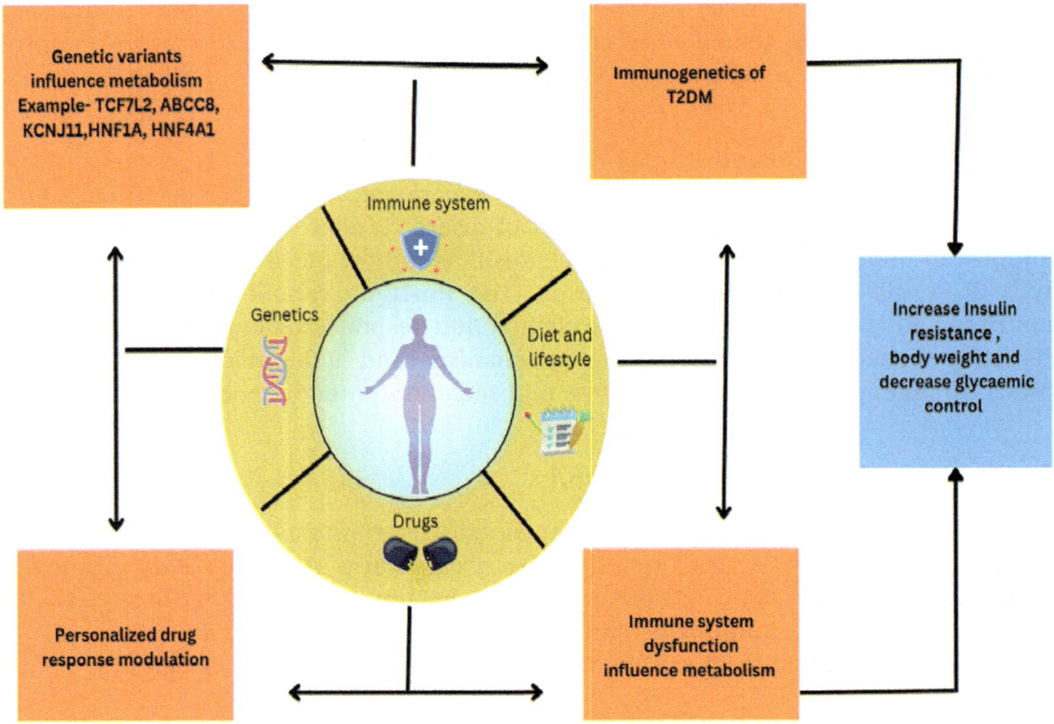

FIGURE 14.1 Complex interplay of immunogenetics of diabetes.

TLR4 causes a higher risk of systemic inflammation and obesity-induced insulin resistance. On the other hand, TLR2 has a role in T2DM development by identifying bacteria lipoproteins and endogenous molecules produced during tissue injury. Variation in TLR genes is associated with varied immune responses and increased inflammation in adipose tissues, further worsening insulin resistance (Kaur et al., 2018).

Cytokines have a very crucial role in immune response, and variations in cytokines are responsible for the modulation of inflammation and insulin sensitivity in T2DM. Proinflammatory cytokines such as TNF-α, IL-6, and IL-1β have their role in metabolic disorders. TNF-α interferes with insulin receptor substrates (IRS-1) phosphorylation and disrupts insulin signaling. Genetic variation in the TNF-α promoter region alters cytokine expression levels, which results in altered susceptibility to insulin resistance and T2DM (Akkız et al., 2017). IL-6 is also an inflammatory mediator in T2DM. Increased IL-6 levels have a role in obesity, beta cell dysfunction, and insulin resistance. Variation in the IL-6 gene promoter region is linked to increased IL-6 expressions, increased metabolic inflammation, and decreased insulin sensitivity. Another IL-1β has an important role in inflammasome activation, with genetic variation in IL-1β and its antagonist's receptor

(IL-1Rα) influencing inflammatory response in pancreatic islets, contributing to apoptosis of beta cell and impaired insulin secretion (Akkız et al., 2017).

The intracellular PRRs, i.e., nucleotide-binding oligomerization domain (NOD)–like receptors (NLRs), regulate inflammasome formation and inflammatory cytokine released. In the NLR family, NLRP3 inflammasome is important in T2DM research because of its role in metabolic inflammation and beta cell dysfunction. Metabolic stressors such as excess glucose, lipid, and relative and reactive oxygen species (ROS) activists NRP3 inflammasome, which result in release of IL-1β and IL-18, increasing inflammation and impairing insulin signaling. Genetic variation in NLRP3 genes has been linked with increased inflammasome activity and increased risk of insulin resistance and T2DM. Studies suggests that therapeutic targeting of NLRP3 inflammasomes may offer novel approaches for T2DM. Hindering inflammasome activation by small molecule inhibitors or biologics targeting IL-1β signaling has shown great results in improving insulin sensitivity and beta cell function (Masters et al., 2013).

Thus, immunogenetics provides valuable insights into the complex interplay between genetic variation and immune-mediated metabolic dysfunction in T2DM. Collectively, HLA gene TLRs, cytokine polymorphism, and NLRP3 inflammasome activation contribute to chronic inflammation that is observed in T2DM patients. Knowing these mechanisms provides new way for precision medicine, enabling personalized interventions targeting specific genetic and immunological pathways. The future research should focus on the integration of multi-omics approaches such as transcriptomics and epigenetics, to understand the immunogenetics foundation of T2DM and advance the development of innovative therapeutic strategies (Masters et al., 2013).

5. Pharmacogenetics

The concept "pharmacogenetics" was introduced by Vogel (1959) to explain why individuals react differently to the same medication. In the 1950s, clinical findings on genetic variations in treatment responses were documented for the first time, leading to the development of pharmacogenetics and later pharmacogenomics (Kalow, 2005). Pharmacogenomics now employs genome-wide methods to identify inherited variations that affect drug responses. Pharmacogenetics identifies how a single nucleotide change in the genes, which encode receptors of drugs, enzymes, and transporters, is linked with drug effectiveness and toxicity. CYP2C8, CYP2D6, and CYP2C9 are associated with the metabolism of various drugs (Rettie & Jones, 2005).

These differences in drug responses are impacted by multiple factors, for example, physical activity, ethnicity/race, hypertension, age, and gender (American Diabetes Association, 2013). Pharmacogenetic studies are focused on family-based observations of how drug response. Techniques such as the growth of candidate gene approaches, genome-wide association studies, and linkage analyses have been known to provide insights in how gene variants lead to the impact in the response to certain drugs, which allows for more personalized treatment and has significantly increased in the field of pharmacogenomics and pharmacogenetics.

The variations in immunogenetics, especially in immune regulation and cytokine signaling, can significantly influence the response of patients to commonly prescribed antidiabetic medications. By incorporating immune-genetic profiling into clinical practice, clinicians can refine treatment strategies to improve efficacy and minimize adverse effects. Key antidiabetic drugs such as metformin, DPP-4 inhibitors, GLP-1 receptor agonists, and, SGLT2 inhibitors, demonstrate how immune-genetic factors modulate their effectiveness (Table 14.1). As the first-line treatment for T2DM, metformin improves insulin sensitivity and modulates gut microbiota (American Diabetes Association, 2011). However, variations in biomarkers of inflammation such as TNF-α and IL-6 can affect the drug's efficacy, particularly in patients with heightened immune responses. Metformin, an oral hypoglycemic agent and the sole representative of the biguanide class used in clinical practice, remains the first-line treatment for T2D, according to clinical guidelines. Despite its widespread use, the precise mechanism behind its glucose-lowering effects is not fully understood. It is known that metformin reduces endogenous glucose production, particularly through a reduction in hepatic gluconeogenesis, which is thought to occur via initiation of AMP-activated protein kinase (AMPK) and direct inhibition of mitochondrial function (Viollet et al., 2012). Additionally, metformin improves insulin sensitivity and promotes glucose uptake induced by insulin in skeletal muscles. Notably, metformin is unmetabolized by the body but is eliminated unchanged through active tubular secretion in the kidneys. The excretion of metformin in urine and bile is also aided via different variants of multidrug and toxin extrusion (MATE) transporter, including (MATE1 and MATE2) (Otsuka et al., 2005). Despite its effectiveness, the blood sugar-lowering action of metformin exhibits considerable

Table 14.1 Summary of commonly used antidiabetic drugs and their targets and respective candidate genes involved.

Class	Mechanism of action	Common medical representatives	Candidate genes involved
Biguanide	Activates AMP-kinase, reduces hepatic gluconeogenesis enhances insulin sensitivity	Metformin	*SLC22A1, SLC22A2, SLC22A3, SLC47A1, SLC47A2*
Sulfonylureas	Inhibits KATP channel on β-cell membrane, stimulates insulin secretion	Glibenclamide, gliclazide, glimepiride, glipizide	*KCNJ11, ABCC8, CYP2C9, TCF7L2, IRS1, MIR4532*
DPP-4 inhibitors	Inhibits DPP-4 enzyme, affects GLP-1 receptor pathway, promotes glucose-dependent insulin secretion	Alogliptin, linagliptin, saxagliptin, sitagliptin, vildagliptin	*POSSIBLY TCF7L2, DPP4, GLP1R, KCNQ1*
SGLT-2 inhibitors	Inhibits SGLT2 transporters in the kidney	Canagliflozin, dapagliflozin, empagliflozin	*Not known yet*

interindividual variability, and its use is linked with gastrointestinal adverse effects in a substantial proportion of patients, leading to therapy discontinuation in some cases. This variability in response and side effects is likely influenced by genetic factors affecting the drug's metabolic pathways.

DPP4 inhibitors (DPP41) and GLP-1 receptor agonist (GLP1RA) are the diabetes medications that help the body release more insulin in people with T2DM or when required. The genetic variations in cytokines genes TNF-α and IL-6 may regulate the activation of the immune, thus impacting the efficacy of DPP-4 inhibitors. This highlights the significance of personalized medications for therapeutic results (Table 14.1).

Second-line glucose-lowering agents, i.e., DPP-4 inhibitors. They function by boosting an incretins pathway via hormones GLP1 and GIP that regulate pancreas to secrete insulin (Nauck & Meier, 2018), which are typically degraded by the enzyme DPP4 (Hinnen, 2015). However, due to genetic variation among individuals, medication may vary from person to person. According to American diabetes association (ADA) and the European Association for the Study of Diabetes (EASD), medications are required for individuals requiring combination therapy or in cases of adverse reactions to first-line treatment, such as metformin (Buse et al., 2020). Scientists have identified several genes that influence how people respond and the impact of the effectiveness of these medications. Among most is the GLP1R, by Sathananthan and colleagues, in the year of 2010, which codes for the GLP-1 receptor. For example, the rs6923761 variant is associated with variations in β-cell response. Homozygous carriers of the major allele in rs6923761 exhibit enhanced β-cell responsiveness to GLP-1 infusion, leading to increased insulin secretion (Table 14.1).

According to research, studies suggest that specific GLPR1 genotypes during GLPRA1 therapy are associated with a greater reduction in waist size and blood pressure, though some studies report no significant change in HbA1c levels (de Luis et al., 2015). The TCF7L2gene encodes a transcription factor essential for β-cell function and GLP1R expression, thereby influencing the efficacy of incretin-based therapies. The TCF7L2 SNP rs7903146 has been linked to reduced responsiveness to DPP-4 inhibitors. However, individuals carrying the T allele exhibit enhanced sensitivity to GLP-1 receptor agonists (GLP1RA), which suggests a differential pharmacogenetic influence on treatment outcomes. The DPP4 gene encodes the DPP-4 enzyme, the primary target of the DPP41. Genetic variants that result in increased enzymatic activity reduce the effectiveness of DPP41 therapy, potentially impacting glycemic control (Wilson et al., 2017). KCNQ1 gene, which plays a crucial role in the regulation of insulin release (Müssig et al., 2009), has been linked to the pharmacogenetics of therapies acted on the incretin pathway. The polymorphism rs163184 in KCNQ1 is associated with variability in HbA1c reduction among patients undergoing DPP-4 inhibitor treatment. Although some results supporting conflicting results, GLP1R, TCF7L2, DPP4, and KCNQ1 are the genes in understanding the genetic factors influencing individual responses to incretin based therapies. Their role highlights the importance of personalized treatment approaches in type 2 diabetes management.

SGLT2 inhibitors are medications that lower blood sugar by helping the kidneys remove excess glucose through urine (Table 14.1). In addition to lowering blood sugar levels, these medications can also help with weight loss and reducing blood pressure (Wright et al., 2011). However, differences in genes related to immune and kidney function may affect how well these drugs work and how safe they are in different people.

Metformin, a common diabetes medication for T2DM, relies on specific transporters in the Body to be absorbed, distributed, and removed. These transporters in the body are made by genes, i.e., SLC22A1, SLC22A2, SLC47AI, and SLC47A2 (Table 14.1). Variants in these genes can change how metformin is processed, leading to different responses among individuals. SLC22A1, which codes for organic cation transporter1 (OCT1), plays a role in the transportation of metformin into the liver (Shu et al., 2007). Certain genetic changes can reduce this transport by making metformin less effective. The polymorphism in this gene is rs12208357 and rs34130459, which can reduce the ability of this protein to transport metformin in which case the drug might not work as well for some people. However, different studies have shown mixed results, so more research is needed. SLC22A2 (OCT2) is involved in metformin's removal through the kidneys, and gene variations such as rs201919874 and rs145450955, may increase the metformin level in blood, with higher or lower levels of drugs in their system indicate how well it works for them (Nasykhova et al., 2020). **SLC47A1** (MAT1) is a transporter protein encoded by the SLC47A1 gene and plays a significant role in exporting metformin from liver and kidney cells into bile and urine for excretion. This process helps regulate drug levels in the body and its effective in lowering blood sugar. A common genetic variant in SLC47A1, known as rs2289669, has been linked to a slightly better response to metformin, with some studies showing greater reduction in HbA1c (Saiz-Rodríguez et al., 2023). Lastly, **SLC47A2** (MATE2), helps in removing metformin from the cells into the urine for excretion. Genetic variants such as rs562968062 and rs12943590 can affect how the metformin medication effectively functions. Although studies have shown mixed results, their impact on effectiveness varies due to genetic variations in people and respond differently to metformin (Chung et al., 2013).

Sulfonylureas are a type of medication used to treat T2DM. They work by stimulating the beta cells of the pancreas to release more insulin, which helps in lowering blood sugar levels. These drugs enhance their effects by attaching to specific protein sulfonylurea receptor 1 [SUR1] on the insulin-producing beta cells. ABCC8 gene codes for (SUR1) subunit of ATP-sensitive potassium (K_ATP) channels, essential for the secretion of insulin (Table 14.1). However, people can respond differently to these drugs because of their genes. One important factor is how the liver breaks down sulfonylurea. The process is controlled by an enzyme called CYP2C9 (cytochrome P450), which comes in different genetic versions. Many individuals have versions such as CYP2C92 and CYP2C93, which leads to decreased enzyme function. As a result, this causes the drug to remain in the body for an extended period, enhancing the blood sugar-lowering effect. These changes are linked to the pharmacokinetics of sulfonylurea. A large-scale study of approximately 1073 patients (GoDARTS64) revealed that individuals having these genetic variants were over three times (3.4-fold) more likely to achieve their optimal blood sugar targets than those with the wild-type allele (Slieker et al., 2023). The variations in genetic were associated with higher level of sulfonylurea in the blood, which leads to the differences in how patients respond to treatment. Another key gene, ABCC8, responsible for encoding the SUR1 subunit, regulates the effectiveness of how well sulfonylurea binds to insulin-producing cells. Additional genetic studies, including on those KCNJ11 E23K variant, have linked with the efficacy of sulfonylurea, especially among Caucasian individuals (Javorsky et al., 2012), The specific genetic change such as 3c—t and Thr759Thr polymorphism were found to be linked to T2DM in Caucasian populations (Weisnagel et al., 2001); however, later studies, such as one conducted in populations from south India, did not find the same association.

Genetic variations rs1801278 in the IRS1 and rs7903146 in the TCF7L2 genes are linked to reduced effectiveness of sulfonylurea treatment in Caucasian patients in T2DM (Loganadan et al., 2016). Interestingly, the impact of these genetic differences can vary across ethnic groups, meaning that a sulfonylurea medication that works well for one person might not be as effective for someone with a different genetic background. For example, rs12255372 in Indian populations has linked to how well sulfonylurea works (Dhawan & Padh, 2016), while variations in the TCF7L2 gene, such as rs7903146, are linked with T2DM in different ethnic groups (Schroner et al., 2010), which altogether underscores the significance of incorporating genetic background into clinical decision-making when selecting appropriate diabetes pharmacotherapy. In Chinese populations, specific genetic variant called rs60452575 in the MIR4532 has been found to affect the activity of the KCNJ11 gene and influence how well sulfonylurea medications work (Zeng et al., 2020). Due to these genetic differences, researchers are investigating pharmacogenetics testing as a tool to assess patients gene before prescribing antidiabetes medications. This approach aims to optimize treatment efficacy identify most effective treatment based on an individual's genetic makeup by enabling more personalized election of pharmacotherapy. Given that differences in metformin response in individuals. The inconsistent findings across different populations holds a promise for improving precision medicine and reducing the unwanted negative effects.

The integration of AI and big data in healthcare is advancing the feasibility of personalized medicine, particularly for individuals with type 2 diabetes (T2DM) and related conditions. By analyzing a patient's genetic profile, immune response, and clinical data, AI can assist clinicians in selecting the most effective treatment with minimal adverse effects, thereby optimizing therapeutic outcomes. AI can analyze an individual's genetic profile and medical history to assist clinicians in developing personalized treatment strategies. This approach enhances treatment efficacy and safety.

For instance, patients with T2DM often present with comorbid cardiovascular and kidney disease, necessitating a treatment approach that extends beyond glycemic control to include cardiorenal protection. Evidence suggests that comprehensive risk factor management can significantly enhance long-term health outcomes. Notably, SGLT2 inhibitors exemplify this strategy, as they do not only reduce blood glucose levels but also confer additional benefits, including weight reduction and renal protection.

6. Current Perspectives and future prospects

The initiative of precision medicine in T2DM in the year of 2018 shows a transformative approach toward managing diabetes by the Society of American Diabetes Association, the European Association for the Study of Diabetes, and the US National Institute of Diabetes (Chung et al., 2020). Precision medicine showed success in the treatment of monogenic diabetes by single gene mutations. Implementing this technique proves to be challenging to T2DM as the complex interplay of various genetic differences and some other environmental factors. There are several markers linked to T2DM, but the contribution is unknown to the progression of the disease due to individual variants. The biobanks show potential direction for advancing precision medicine in T2DM. Biobanks are a large collection of molecular, genetic, and clinical data that encourages in-depth analysis into the underpinnings of the disease. They are playing a vital role in identifying ethnic-specific genetic markers, especially in diverse populations such as India (Chung et al., 2020). Initiatives like this could enable deeper knowledge into the complex genetic foundation of T2DM as well as enhance the treatment strategies.

A clinical trial compared groups between standard care ($n = 188$) with multifactorial intensive therapy ($n = 207$) (Sasso et al., 2021) to focus on treating kidney disease in people with type 2 diabetes. The result indicated that the intensive therapy was addressing health risk more effectively than standard care. The intensive care prevents fatal/nonfatal vascular complications in people with diabetic nephropathy, an early usage of the treatment provided the long-term protection. Accordingly, both integrated and multifaceted approach treatments improve the prognosis of individual having diabetes. The results are crucial to share for new discoveries and insights. Databases such as Human Gene Mutation Database (Stenson et al., 2017) and ClinVar (Landrum et al., 2016) have been established to store data through data sharing.

Evidence from major clinical and real-world studies shows that SGLT2 inhibitory has exhibited positive multifaceted effects on blood pressure, body weight, and improved kidney function (eGFR) and better cardiovascular health (American Diabetes Association, 2011), which proves that antiglycemic medication can be utilized to improve health outcomes in preventing or reducing macro- and microvascular complications and plays a benefitting role. These medications particularly beneficial for diabetic patients or those susceptible to diabetes-related conditions such as health failure, cardiovascular disease, and chronic kidney disease. With this, scientists can manufacture glycemic therapies based on patients' cardiovascular health and diabetic nephropathy.

Implementing precision medicine in diabetes is important for the healthcare system with the help of electronic health records. It is vital for easy accessibility and mobility to be shared across different systems over a wide area to help improve patient care and treatment. Collaborating across multiple societies, i.e., researchers, healthcare agency, suppliers, financial sponsors, and regulatory authorities, is proved to be crucial for improving how diabetes can be diagnosed, prevented, monitored, and treated with precision medicine. It is vital to establish a dynamic network of stakeholders that incorporates patient advocates and public institutions to advance objectives and secure funding.

While precision medication for diabetes that utilizes sequencing technologies tends to be more costly than traditional treatments, precision medicine has proved to be cost-effective in cases of monogenic diabetes. Since complications arising from diabetes are the main driver of treatment costs, early detection, prevention, and intervention based on genetic variations through precision medicine may encourage acceptance. A thorough assessment of the costs versus benefits of sequencing technologies, genomics, and biomarkers is essential to promote their application in population-specific clinical guidelines. The application of technological advancements in diabetes management, such as wearable glucose-tracking devices that allow for low-invasion and continuous tracking of glucose, is strongly promoted and implemented in many healthcare facilities; this serves as a prime example of highly tailored medical treatments for diabetes (Klonoff et al., 2020).

Personalized treatment protocols and algorithms for diabetes treatment tailored to genotype should be constructed using the clinical data that has been gathered, facilitating the implementation of such evidence in clinical practice. The application of artificial intelligence in clinical-based decision-making for devising optimal treatment strategies for numerous patients will herald a revolutionary shift in the personalized medicine landscape for diabetes. Educational programs are necessary to guide and inform clinical technicians, geneticists, and other healthcare workers in the application of tailored diabetes treatment at the individual patient level and in managing possible incidental discoveries such as unexpected inherited mutations. Sufficient development for the workforce of genomic can be accomplished through securing appropriate funding for education of genomics. The involvement of regulatory agencies in the early stages of successful implementation and application of precision medicine development in diabetes is essential.

Identifying genetic variations among individuals and understanding their contribution to the predisposition and progression of T2D would significantly advance in managing the disease, enhancing medical conditions and preventing risk. In this, we have highlighted the existing understanding of genetic risk factors associated with T2DM and emphasized the benefit of studies of pharmacogenomics in establishing feasible connections between genetic predispositions and treatments in pharmacological. With personalized medicine, patients can gain more effective drug therapies with improved adherence in routine clinical practices. Monogenic forms of diabetes are currently being managed using precision diabetes medicine, including maturity-onset diabetes of the young, congenital hyperinsulinemic hypoglycemia, and neonatal diabetes. This precision medicine holds the potential for tailored therapies for individuals with various diabetes types, such as T2DM (Sirdah & Reading, 2020), which is a complex condition that involves multiple genes, and its clinical presentation that reflects the interplay of genetic as well as environmental factors, making it complex to categorize subgroups via molecular diagnostics (Florez, 2017). Approach toward precision medicine in T2DM is by categorizing patients in different groups based on their unique response to treatments and investigating the biological foundations of each group using advanced sequencing technologies and gene expression arrays (Huang & Florez, 2011). The large-scale genetic and electronic health record data from vast populations are necessary in assisting for the targeted therapy for T2DM.

The main goal of personalized treatment care in T2DM is to develop tailored management strategies that synchronize with patient's preferences and their unique characteristics, some of the risk factors, and drug metabolism profile. To improve patient adherence, individualized method aims to enhances the effectiveness of the treatment as well as reducing the side effects, Precision medicine in T2DM holds promise for optimizing glycemic control, improving overall patient outcomes, and minimizing complications. Although, further intensive research is needed to fully establish its benefits. By the help of genomic data, pharmacogenomics, and clinical insights, this strategy aims to transition from standardized treatment models to a more precise, patient-targeted approach in diabetes care.

A recent study utilizing imaging of the live cell that revealed the capacity of insulin vesicles to effectively bind with the plasma membrane, which is directly linked with secretion of insulin in islet beta cells in humans. This process plays a significant role in individuals with T2D. The study demonstrated that the secretion of defective insulin in T2D beta cells was primarily due to a substantially reduced rate of docking interactions, rather than a deficiency in the transport of insulin vesicles to the plasma membrane. In fact, docking interactions were observed to be five times more common in nondiabetic beta cells than in diabetic beta cells, while the transport of insulin vesicles attachment to the membrane remained similar between the two groups. Further expression profiling indicated the expression of key proteins involved in granule docking was downregulated in T2D beta cells. These findings suggest that in T2D, impaired molecular binding of insulin vesicles to the secretion site leads to insufficient levels of plasma insulin, contributing to hyperglycemia. Importantly, this study also suggests that the diabetic phenotype is not primarily due to intracellular insulin deficiency or a reduced number of insulin vesicles in beta cells. Thus, enhancing granule docking in islet beta cells presents a novel and promising therapeutic target for the advancement of new antidiabetic therapies designed for improving insulin secretion in individuals with T2D.

7. Clinical application of immunogenetics in T2DM

7.1 Genetic screening and risk assessment

Genetic screening of immunogenetic markers allows prerisk stratification, which allows prevention before clinical symptoms appear. Individuals with risked with increased risk HLA genotype can be closely analyzed for metabolic changes, allowing timely lifestyle or pharmacological changes to prevent or delay disease onset.

7.2 Personalized treatment strategies

Immunogenetics profiling allows making optimized treatment plans based on patients' genetic backgrounds. Few HLA alleles are linked with different responses to common anti-/diabetic medication. For example, HLA-DQ variants are responsible for differential response to metformin, the first-line therapy for T2DM. TNF-α variation influences patient response to thiazolidinediones (TZDs), which is responsible for target inflammation-related insulin resistances. By combining immunogenetics insight into treatment decisions, clinicians can make therapy regimes increasing efficacy and decrease adverse effect.

7.3 Immunomodulatory therapies

Glycemic index can be controlled by targeting inflammatory pathways influenced by genetic predisposition. Examples of potential immunogenetics-driven therapies include cytokines inhibitor (for example, anti-TNF or IL-6 blockers) to decrease systemic inflammations, T regulatory (Treg) cell therapies, which modulate immune response and may preserve pancreatic beta cell function and probiotic and microbiome associated strategies tailored to immunogenetics profiles, which influence gut-mediated immune response and metabolic regulation.

There are challenges in clinical implementation, such as cost and accessibility, because genetic testing is expensive, which limits the widespread adoption in clinical practices. There is a lack of standardization because census guidelines for integrating immunogenic marker into diagnostic and therapeutic protocols are yet not completely evolved.

8. Conclusion

The integration of immunogenetics in type 2 diabetes mellitus (T2DM) research and practice marks a positive shift in our knowledge and management of this complex metabolic disorders. Earlier it was considered that the disease is primarily driven by beta cell dysfunction and insulin resistance, but the emerging evidence shows the important role of immune dysregulation in its pathogenesis. Advances in GWAS, NGS, and disease analysis have shown key genetic variation affecting immune-mediated inflammatory pathways, insulin signaling, and glucose metabolism offering insight into disease susceptibility and progression. But challenges such as genetic heterogenicity, population specific variation, and ethical consideration in genetic testing must be addressed to improve clinical utility. Future research should focus on multi-omics approaches, artificial intelligence, and large-scale biobanks to filter risk stratification and therapeutic decision-making. By linking immunogenetics with clinical practices, we can make more personalized and effective framework for T2DM managements, ultimately making the treatment more effective and reducing the global burden of this disease.

References

Aguirre, V., Uchida, T., Yenush, L., Davis, R., & White, M. F. (2000). The c-Jun NH(2)-terminal kinase promotes insulin resistance during association with insulin receptor substrate-1 and phosphorylation of Ser(307). *The Journal of Biological Chemistry, 275*(12), 9047–9054.

Akkız, H., Bayram, S., Bekar, A., Akgöllü, E., & Ülger, Y. (2017). Functional genetic variations of IL-6 and TGF-β1 in type 2 diabetes and diabetic nephropathy. *Scientific Reports, 7*, 6897.

Altshuler, D., Hirschhorn, J. N., Klannemark, M., Lindgren, C. M., Vohl, M. C., Nemesh, J., … Groop, L. (2000). The common PPARγ Pro12Ala polymorphism is associated with decreased risk of type 2 diabetes. *Nature Genetics, 26*(1), 76–80.

Altshuler, D., Hirschhorn, J. N., Klannemark, M., Lindgren, C. M., Vohl, M. C., Nemesh, J., … Groop, L. (2003). The common PPARγ Pro12Ala polymorphism is associated with decreased risk of type 2 diabetes. *Nature Genetics, 34*(2), 131–136.

American Diabetes Association. (2011). Standards of Medical Care in Diabetes—2011. *Diabetes Care, 34* (Suppl 1), S11–S61.

American Diabetes Association. (2013). Standards of medical care in diabetes—2013. *Diabetes Care, 36* (Suppl 1), S11–S66.

Berbudi, A., Rahmadika, N., Tjahjadi, A. I., & Ruslami, R. (2019). Type 2 diabetes and its impact on the immune system. *Current Diabetes Reviews, 16*(5), 442–449.

Beth, T. (2023). Diabetes immunogenetics: Its role in genetics and genes development. *Immunogenetics: Open Access, 8*(3).

Brunetti, A., Brunetti, F. S., & Chiefari, E. (2014). Pharmacogenetics of type 2 diabetes mellitus: An example of success in clinical and translational medicine. *World Journal of Translational Medicine, 3* (3), 141–149.

Buse, J. B., Wexler, D. J., Tsapas, A., Rossing, P., Mingrone, G., Mathieu, C., D'Alessio, D. A., & Davies, M. J. (2020). 2019 Update to: Management of hyperglycemia in type 2 diabetes, 2018. A consensus report by the American Diabetes Association (ADA) and the European Association for the Study of Diabetes (EASD). *Diabetes Care, 43*(2), 487–493.

Chatterjee, S., Khunti, K., & Davies, M. J. (2017). Type 2 diabetes. *The Lancet, 389*(10085), 2239–2251.

Chimienti, F., Devergnas, S., Favier, A., & Seve, M. (2004). Identification and cloning of a cell-specific zinc transporter, ZnT-8, localized into insulin secretory granules. *Diabetes, 53*(9), 2330–2337.

Chung, J.-Y., Cho, S. K., Kim, T. H., Kim, K. H., Jang, G. H., Kim, C. O., Park, E.-M., Cho, J.-Y., Jang, I.-J., & Choi, J. H. (2013). Functional characterization of MATE2-K genetic variants and their effects on metformin pharmacokinetics. *Pharmacogenetics and Genomics, 23*(7), 365–373.

Chung, W. K., Erion, K., Florez, J. C., Hattersley, A. T., Hivert, M. F., Lee, C. G., McCarthy, M. I., Nolan, J. J. , Norris, J. M., Pearson, E. R., Philipson, L., McElvaine, A. T., Cefalu, W. T., Rich, S. S., & Franks, P. W. (2020). Precision medicine in diabetes: A consensus report from the American Diabetes Association (ADA) and the European Association for the Study of Diabetes (EASD). *Diabetes Care, 43*(7), 1617–1635.

Coghlan, M. P. (2023). Glucokinase inhibition: A novel treatment for diabetes? *Diabetes, 72*(2), 170–179.

de Luis, D. A., Diaz Soto, G., Izaola, O., & Romero, E. (2015). Evaluation of weight loss and metabolic changes in diabetic patients treated with liraglutide, effect of RS 6923761 gene variant of glucagon-like peptide 1 receptor. *Journal of Diabetes and its Complications, 29*(4), 595–598.

DeFronzo, R. A., Ferrannini, E., Groop, L., Henry, R. R., Herman, W. H., Holst, J. J., … Weiss, R. (2015). Type 2 diabetes mellitus. *Nature Reviews Disease Primers, 1*, Article 15019.

Dhawan, D., & Padh, H. (2016). Genetic variations in TCF7L2 influence therapeutic response to sulfonylureas in Indian diabetics. *Diabetes Research and Clinical Practice, 121*, 35–40.

Do, R., Bailey, S. D., Desbiens, K., Bélisle, A., Montpetit, A., Bouchard, C., Pérusse, L., Vohl, M. C., Rankinen, T., & Hudson, T. J. (2008). Genetic variants of FTO influence adiposity, insulin sensitivity, leptin levels, and resting metabolic rate in the Quebec family study. *Diabetes, 57*(4), 1147–1150.

Donath, M. Y., & Shoelson, S. E. (2011). Type 2 diabetes as an inflammatory disease. *Nature Reviews Immunology, 11*(2), 98–107.

Florez, J. C. (2017). Pharmacogenetics in type 2 diabetes: Precision medicine or discovery tool? *Diabetologia, 60*(5), 800–807.

Hinnen, D. (2015). Dipeptidyl peptidase-4 inhibitors in diverse patient populations with type 2 diabetes. The Diabetes Educator, 41(1_suppl), 19S-31S.

Huang, C., & Florez, J. C. (2011). Pharmacogenetics in type 2 diabetes: Potential implications for clinical practice. *Genome Medicine, 3*(11), 76–76.

Javorsky, M., Klimcakova, L., Schroner, Z., Zidzik, J., Babjakova, E., Fabianova, M., Kozarova, M., Tkacova, R., Salagovic, J., & Tkac, I. (2012). KCNJ11 gene E23K variant and therapeutic response to sulfonylureas. *European Journal of Internal Medicine, 23*(3), 245–249.

Kalow, W. (2005). In F. Innocenti (Ed.), *Pharmacogenomics. Methods in Molecular Biology™, 311* (pp. 3–14). Humana Press.

Kaur, C. P., Figueroa, M. S., & Badhan, R. (2018). Toll-like receptor 2 (TLR-2) gene polymorphisms in type 2 diabetes mellitus: A systematic review and meta-analysis. *World Journal of Diabetes, 9*(7), 107–131.

King, G. L. (2002). The role of inflammatory cytokines in diabetes and its complications. *Diabetologia, 45* (7), 859–870.

Klonoff, D. C., Florez, J. C., German, M., & Fleming, A. (2020). The need for precision medicine to be applied to diabetes. *Journal of Diabetes Science and Technology, 14*(6), 1122–1128.

Kreienkamp, R. J., Voight, B. F., Gloyn, A. L., & Udler, M. S. (2023). Genetics of type 2 diabetes. In J. M. Lawrence, S. S. Casagrande, W. H. Herman, et al. (Eds.), *Diabetes in America* (3rd ed.). National Institute of Diabetes and Digestive and Kidney Diseases (NIDDK).

Le, K. A., Mahurkar, S., Alderete, T. L., Hasson, R. E., Adam, T. C., Kim, J. S., Beale, E., Greenberg, A. S., & Goran, M. I. (2005). Predictors of and longitudinal changes in insulin sensitivity in overweight Latino children: A 3-year prospective study. *Diabetes, 54*(1), 166–174.

Laakso, M., & Silva, L. F. (2022). Genetics of type 2 diabetes: Past, present, and future. *Nutrients, 14*(15), 3201.

Lai, N., Jayaraman, A., & Kaestner, K. H. (2017). The transient nature of microRNAs in islets and β-cells. *Diabetologia, 60*(11), 2106–2117.

Loganadan, N. K., Huri, H. Z., Vethakkan, S. R., & Hussein, Z. (2016). Genetic markers predicting sulphonylurea treatment outcomes in type 2 diabetes patients: Current evidence and challenges for clinical implementation. *The Pharmacogenomics Journal, 16*(3), 209–219.

Lu, X., Xie, Q., Pan, X., et al. (2024). Type 2 diabetes mellitus in adults: Pathogenesis, prevention and therapy. *Signal Transduction and Targeted Therapy, 9*, 262.

Lyssenko, V., Lupi, R., Marchetti, P., Del Guerra, S., Orho-Melander, M., Almgren, P., Sjögren, M., Ling, C., Eriksson, K. F., Lethagen, Å., Melander, O., Groop, L., & Berglund, G. (2003). Large-scale association studies of variants in genes involved in pancreatic beta-cell function in relation to risk of type 2 diabetes mellitus. *Diabetes, 52*(2), 568–574.

Masters, S. L., Dunne, A., Subramanian, S. L., Hull, R. L., Tannahill, G. M., Sharp, F. A., Becker, C., Franchi, L., Yoshihara, E., Chen, Z., Mullooly, N., Mielke, L. A., Harris, J., Coll, R. C., O'Neill, L. A. J., O'Neill, R. J., Núñez, G., McLoughlin, R. M., & Martinon, F. (2013). Upregulated NLRP3 inflammasome activation in patients with type 2 diabetes. *Diabetes, 62*(1), 194–204.

Mirza, S., Hossain, M., Mathews, C., Martinez, P., Pino, P., Gay, J. L., Rentfro, A., McCormick, J. B., & Fisher-Hoch, S. P. (2011). Type 2-diabetes is associated with elevated levels of TNF-alpha, IL-6 and adiponectin and low levels of leptin in a population of Mexican American: A cross-sectional study. *Cytokine, 57*(1), 136–142.

Mullard, A. (2019). Parsing clinical success rates. *Endocrine Reviews, 40*(6), 1500–1501.

Müssig, K. M., Staiger, H., Machicao, F., Kirchhoff, K., Guthoff, M., Schäfer, S. A., Kantartzis, K., Silbernagel, G., Stefan, N., Holst, J. J., Gallwitz, B., Häring, H.-U., & Fritsche, A. (2009). Association of type 2 diabetes candidate polymorphisms in KCNQ1 with incretin and insulin secretion. *Diabetes, 58* (7), 1715–1720.

Nasykhova, Y. A., Tonyan, Z. N., Mikhailova, A. A., Danilova, M. M., & Glotov, A. S. (2020). Pharmacogenetics of type 2 diabetes-progress and prospects. *International Journal of Molecular Sciences, 21*(18), 6842.

Nauck, M. A., & Meier, J. J. (2018). Incretin hormones: Their role in health and disease. *Diabetes, Obesity & Metabolism, 20*(Suppl 1), 5–21.

Otsuka, M., Matsumoto, T., Morimoto, R., Arioka, S., Omote, H., & Moriyama, Y. (2005). A human transporter protein that mediates the final excretion step for toxic organic cations. *Proceedings of the National Academy of Sciences of the United States of America, 102*(50), 17923–17928.

Rahman, S., Islam, R., & Karim, M. R. (2018). IRS-1 genetic polymorphism (r.2963G>A) in type 2 diabetes mellitus patients during severe hyperglycemia. *Bioinformation, 14*(8), 462–468.

Saiz-Rodríguez, M., Ochoa, D., Zubiaur, P., Navares-Gómez, M., Román, M., Camargo-Mamani, P., Luquero-Bueno, S., Villapalos-García, G., Alcaraz, R., Mejía-Abril, G., Santos-Mazo, E., & Abad-Santos, F. (2023). Identification of transporter polymorphisms influencing metformin pharmacokinetics in healthy volunteers. *Journal of Personalized Medicine, 13*(3), 489.

Sasso, F. C., Pafundi, P. C., Simeon, V., et al. (2021). Efficacy and durability of multifactorial intervention on mortality and major adverse cardiovascular events in type 2 diabetic kidney disease: A randomized clinical trial. *Cardiovascular Diabetology, 20,* 145.

Schroner, Z., Javorsky, M., Tkacova, R., Klimcakova, L., Dobrikova, M., Habalova, V., Kozarova, M., Zidzik, J., Rudikova, M., & Tkac, I. (2010). Effect of sulphonylurea treatment on glycaemic control is related to TCF7L2 genotype in patients with type 2 diabetes. *Diabetes, Obesity and Metabolism, 13*(1), 89–91.

Shu, Y., Sheardown, S. A., Brown, C., Owen, R. P., Zhang, S., Castro, R. A., Ianculescu, A. G., Yue, L., Lo, J. C., Burchard, E. G., Brett, C. M., & Giacomini, K. M. (2007). Effect of genetic variation in the organic cation transporter 1 (OCT1) on metformin action. *The Journal of Clinical Investigation, 117*(5), 1422–1431.

Sirdah, M. M., & Reading, N. S. (2020). Genetic predisposition in type 2 diabetes: A promising approach toward a personalized management of diabetes. *Clinical Genetics, 98*(6), 525–547.

Slieker, R. C., Donnelly, L. A., Akalestou, E., Lopez-Noriega, L., Melhem, R., Güneş, A., Abou Azar, F., Efanov, A., Georgiadou, E., Muniangi-Muhitu, H., Sheikh, M., Giordano, G. N., Åkerlund, M., Ahlqvist, E., Ali, A., Banasik, K., Brunak, S., Barovic, M., Bouland, G. A., & Burdet, F. (2023). Identification of biomarkers for glycaemic deterioration in type 2 diabetes. *Nature Communications, 14*(1).

Stenson, P. D., Mort, M., Ball, E. V., et al. (2017). The human gene mutation database: Towards a comprehensive repository of inherited mutation data. *Human Genetics, 136*(6), 665–677.

Sun, J., Luo, J., Wang, X., & Chen, Y. (2021). Toll-like receptor 4 gene polymorphisms and susceptibility to type 2 diabetes mellitus: A meta-analysis. *Journal of Diabetes Investigation, 12*(8), 1452–1462.

Tilg, H., & Moschen, A. R. (2008). Inflammatory mechanisms in the regulation of insulin resistance. *Molecular Medicine (Cambridge, Mass.), 14*(3-4), 222–231.

Tkáč, I., & Klimčáková, L. (2020). Pharmacogenetics of type 2 diabetes: Progress and prospects. *Pharmacogenomics and Personalized Medicine, 13,* 79–92.

Udler, M. S., McCarthy, M. I., Florez, J. C., & Mahajan, A. (2019). Genetic risk scores for diabetes diagnosis and precision medicine. *Endocrine Reviews, 40*(6), 1500–1520.

Viollet, B., Guigas, B., Garcia, N. S., Leclerc, J., Foretz, M., & Andreelli, F. (2012). Cellular and molecular mechanisms of metformin: An overview. *Clinical Science (London), 122*(6), 253–270.

Vogel, F. (1959). Moderne probleme der humangenetik. In *Ergebnisse der inneren medizin und kinderheilkunde* (pp. 52–125). Springer Berlin Heidelberg.

Weisnagel, S. J., Rankinen, T., Nadeau, A., Rao, D. C., Chagnon, Y. C., Pérusse, L., & Bouchard, C. (2001). Decreased fasting and oral glucose stimulated C-peptide in nondiabetic subjects with sequence variants in the sulfonylurea receptor 1 gene. *Diabetes, 50*(3), 697–702.

Wilson, J. R., Shuey, M. M., Brown, N. J., & Devin, J. K. (2017). Hypertension and type 2 diabetes are associated with decreased inhibition of dipeptidyl peptidase-4 by sitagliptin. *Journal of the Endocrine Society, 1*(9), 1168–1178.

Wright, E. M., Loo, D. D. F., & Hirayama, B. A. (2011). Biology of human sodium glucose transporters. *Physiological Reviews, 91*(2), 733–794.

The SIGMA Type 2 Diabetes Consortium. (2014). Association of a low-frequency variant in HNF1A with type 2 diabetes in a Latino population. *JAMA, 311*(22), 2305–2314.

Xiao, X., Lao, K., Yao, Y., Zhou, X., Chen, X., Zhang, J. A., & Jiang, L. (2020). HLA class II allele analyses implicate common genetic components in type 1 and non–insulin-treated type 2 diabetes. *The Journal of Clinical Endocrinology & Metabolism, 105*(3), e245–e254.

Zeng, Z., Huang, S.-Y., & Sun, T. (2020). Pharmacogenomic studies of current antidiabetic agents and potential new drug targets for precision medicine of diabetes. *Diabetes Therapy, 11*(11), 2521–2538.

Further reading

A review of current trends with type 2 diabetes epidemiology, aetiology, pathogenesis, treatments and future perspectives. *Diabetes, Metabolic Syndrome and Obesity*, (2021).

Ahmad, E., Lim, S., Lamptey, R., Webb, D. R., & Davies, M. J. (2022). Type 2 diabetes. *The Lancet, 400* (10365), 1803–1820.

Ansari, P., Flatt, P. R., Harriott, P., & Abdel-Wahab, Y. H. A. (2021). Insulinotropic and antidiabetic properties of Eucalyptus citriodora leaves and isolation of bioactive phytomolecules. *Journal of Pharmaceutics & Pharmacology, 73*, 1049–1061.

Bashir, H., Bhat, S. A., Majid, S., Hamid, R., Koul, R. K., Rehman, M. U., Din, I., Bhat, J. A., Qadir, J., & Masood, A. (2020). Role of inflammatory mediators (TNF-α, IL-6, CRP), biochemical and hematological parameters in type 2 diabetes mellitus patients of Kashmir, India. *Medical Journal of the Islamic Republic of Iran, 34*. Article 5.

Bhattacharyya, O., Mossialos, E., & Asaria, M. (2023). Precision medicine in type 2 diabetes mellitus: Utility and limitations. *Diabetes Care, 46*(12), 2341–2352.

Buzzetti, R., Zampetti, S., & Maddaloni, E. (2015). Autoimmune aspects of type 2 diabetes mellitus. *Trends in Endocrinology and Metabolism, 26*(7), 375–386.

Cole, J. B., & Florez, J. C. (2020). Genetics of diabetes mellitus and diabetes complications. *Nature Reviews Nephrology, 16*, 377–390. https://doi.org/10.1038/s41581-020-0278-5

Ferreira, P. L., Morais, C., Pimenta, R., Ribeiro, I., Amorim, I., Alves, S. M., & Santiago, L. (2024). Knowledge about type 2 diabetes: Its impact for future management. *Frontiers in Public Health*.

Ghisi, G. L. M., Aultman, C., Konidis, R., Foster, E., Tahsinul, A., Sandison, N., et al. (2020). Effectiveness of an education intervention associated with an exercise program in improving disease-related knowledge and health behaviours among diabetes patients. *Patient Education and Counseling, 103,* 1790–1797. https://doi.org/10.1016/j.pec.2020.04.007

Kany, S., Vollrath, J. T., & Borna, R. (2019). Cytokines in inflammatory disease. *International Journal of Molecular Sciences, 20*(23), 6008.

Kudabayeva, K., Tleumagambetova, B., Bazargaliyev, Y., Kosmuratova, R., & Zhylkybekova, A. (2024). Global trends in LADA type diabetes research: A bibliometric analysis of publications from web of science and scopus, 1994–2024. *Journal of Diabetes Research, 2024*(1).

Li, J., Wang, W., Liu, F., Qiu, L., Ren, Y., Li, M., Li, W., Gao, F., & Zhang, J. (2024). Genetically predicted 1091 blood metabolites and 309 metabolite ratios in relation to risk of type 2 diabetes: A Mendelian randomization study. *Frontiers in Genetics, 15.*

Mezil, S. A., & Abed, B. A. (2021). Complication of diabetes mellitus. *Annals of Romanian Society of Cell Biology, 25,* 1546–1556.

Pei, X., Huang, D., & Li, Z. (2024). Genetic insights and emerging therapeutics in diabetic retinopathy: From molecular pathways to personalized medicine. *Frontiers in Genetics, 15.* Article 1416924.

Pokushalov, E., Ponomarenko, A., Shrainer, E., Kudlay, D., & Miller, R. (2024). Biomarker-guided dietary supplementation: A narrative review of precision in personalized nutrition. *Nutrients, 16*(23), 4033.

Raoufinia, R., Rahimi, H. R., Saburi, E., & Meysam, M. (2024). Advances and challenges of the cell-based therapies among diabetic patients. *Journal of Translational Medicine, 22*(1).

Savytska, M., Kyriienko, D., Komisarenko, I., Kovalchuk, O., Falalyeyeva, T., & Kobyliak, N. (2023). Probiotic for pancreatic β-cell function in type 2 diabetes: A randomized, double-blinded, placebo-controlled clinical trial. *Diabetes Therapy, 14*(11), 1915–1931.

Schwartz, S. S., Corkey, B. E., R Gavin, J., DeFronzo, R. A., & Herman, M. E. (2024). Advances and counterpoints in type 2 diabetes. What is ready for translation into real-world practice, ahead of the guidelines. *BMC Medicine, 22*(1).

Sharma, R., Pankaj, M., Majeed, J., & Aggarwal, G. (2024). Challenges and opportunities in precision therapy for diabetic patients. *Health Sciences Review, 12.*

Singh, S., Usman, K., & Banerjee, M. (2016). Pharmacogenetic studies update in type 2 diabetes mellitus. *World Journal of Diabetes, 7*(15).

15

Genetics and immunity: Mapping pathways in type II diabetes (T2D)

Abdullah Khan and Rudrank Moharana
C.G. BHAKTA INSTITUTE OF BIOTECHNOLOGY, UKA TARSADIA UNIVERSITY, BARDOLI, SURAT, INDIA

1. Introduction

1.1 Overview of T2D

Type II diabetes (T2D) is a non-autoimmune metabolic disease marked by insulin resistance and a gradual decline in pancreatic β-cell function, resulting in hyperglycemia (high concentrations of glucose in blood) (Blériot et al., 2023). Over 95% of individuals with diabetes have T2D, and it is a severe worldwide health problem, representing one of the major contributors to disability and premature death worldwide (Ma & Tong, 2024). T2D burden is increasing at the fastest rate in low- and middle-income nations, but developed nations continue to battle with high rates and complications. The causes include genetic predisposition, ethnicity, and age, sedentary lifestyle (decreasing levels of physical activity), unhealthy dietary factors, cigarette smoking, and psychosocial stress (Harding et al., 2024; Zheng et al., 2018). Unlike Type I diabetes, T2D generally emerges after age 45, but recent decades have seen increasing diagnoses among children, adolescents, and young adults, reflecting global patterns of rising childhood obesity and sedentary lifestyle.

1.2 Global prevalence and public health significance

The global burden of T2D has never been greater. The International Diabetes Federation (IDF) Diabetes Atlas 2025 estimates that about 11.1% of adults aged 20–79 years—roughly one in nine worldwide—are currently living with diabetes, of which more than 90% is T2D, which is induced by socio-economic, demographic, environmental, and genetic determinants (Zheng et al., 2018). This translates to roughly 589 million adults worldwide. It is important to note that 40% of these individuals remain undiagnosed, as they are unaware of this condition (Beagley et al., 2014). Its unstoppably increasing prevalence affects almost every region, yet over 80% of individuals with diabetes reside in low- and middle-income nations, highlighting ongoing disparities concerning healthcare access, education,

Type 2 Diabetes Mellitus. https://doi.org/10.1016/B978-0-443-33590-7.00011-3

and prevention programs (Dyson, 2016), contributing to substantial public health challenges and economic losses due to increased healthcare costs and reduced workforce productivity. By 2050, IDF estimates indicate that 1 in every 8 adults, about 853 million, will be living with diabetes, up by 46%.

Public health systems face mounting costs for diabetes care, ranging from medication and primary intervention to the management of disabling complications. T2D is a predominant cause of morbidity, disability, and early mortality, profoundly affecting vision, skeletal, cardiovascular, and renal health (Thomas, 2022), highlighting its significant public health impact. T2D is currently the ninth most important cause of death globally and a principal contributor to reduced quality of life, particularly for marginalized populations (Harding et al., 2024).

2. Genomic framework of type II diabetes

T2D is an excellent example of a complex, polygenic disorder in which disease risk arises from the interaction of several genetic, environmental and lifestyle variables. Unlike some monogenic variations of diabetes, in instances characterized by a single-gene mutation produce a predictable phenotype, T2D develops through the cumulative influence of hundreds to thousands of loci, each of them exerts a modest effect on risk. Large family and twin studies have consistently demonstrated substantial heritability with estimates ranging between 30% and 70%, thereby underscoring the critical role of genetic determinants in disease susceptibility (Almgren et al., 2011; Poulsen et al., 1999).

The identification of genetic contributors to T2D has been revolutionized by genome-wide association studies (GWAS), which have uncovered more than 400 loci related with disease risk across several populations (Mahajan et al., 2018). Importantly, most of these associations map not to protein-coding regions, but to the non-coding regulatory elements of the genome. This finding highlights the role of genetic variation in shaping transcriptional activity, chromatin accessibility and enhancer function within tissues central to glucose homeostasis, particularly pancreatic islet (islet of Langerhans), liver, skeletal muscle, and adipose tissue (Fuchsberger et al., 2016; Parker et al., 2013). These discoveries that shifted the focus from structural mutation to regulatory architecture, revealing that many risk variants operate by altering the transcription and translation of genes involved in insulin secretion, insulin signaling, and adipocyte biology. Although common variants account for most of the risk at the population level, each individual variant typically confers a modest effect size, with odds ratios rarely exceeding 1.3. Nevertheless, their cumulative impact can stratify individuals into markedly different levels of genetic susceptibility, as captured by polygenic risk scores. Despite steady advances, polygenic risk score currently explains only a modest fraction of the estimated heritability, indicating that additional factors, including rare variants, structural variation, epigenetic mechanisms, and gene-environment interactions, remain to be fully elucidated (Selvam et al., 2017).

Moreover, studies have revealed that ancestry-specific variants can contribute to differential susceptibility among populations. For example, alleles at KCNQ1 have been shown to confer particularly strong risk in East Asian populations, while variants in SLC16A11, enriched in Latino groups with Native American ancestry, illustrate how population history shapes the architecture of disease risk (Williams Amy et al., 2014). Such findings not only emphasize the need for inclusive, multi-ethnic studies but also demonstrate the global diversity of genetic mechanisms underlying T2D.

Taken together, the genetic architecture of T2D is characterized by its polygenic nature, substantial heritability, predominance of regulatory variation, and population-specific differences in allele frequency and effect. These insights provide a foundation for understanding the biological pathways that influence the development and progression of a diseases, while also highlighting the importance of integrating genetic data with environmental and lifestyle contexts to refine risk prediction and develop targeted interventions.

2.1 Polygenic nature and heritability of type II diabetes

T2D is a polygenic disorder as stated above, where disease susceptibility arises from the cumulative impact of numerous genetic variants, each exerting relatively minute contribution to overall risk. So, we will discuss the major genes and loci implicated in diabetes include susceptibility genes such as *TCF7L2, PPARG, KCNJ11*, and *HHEX*, as well as loci near *SLC30A8, CDKN2A/B*, and *FTO*, which influence pancreatic insulin secretion, glucose metabolism, and β-cell function, and obesity-related risk. Then we as role of common versus rare genetic variants, and Ethnic and ancestry-specific differences in genetic risk.

2.1.1 Major genes and loci implicated

The genetic landscape of T2D is defined by numerous loci across the genome, but a few genes have emerged as consistently strong contributors to disease susceptibility. These loci highlight the multifactorial biology of T2D, encompassing pancreatic β-cell function, adipose tissue differentiation, and insulin signaling. So, here are some major genes.

TCF7L2 (Transcription Factor 7-Like 2): Among all identified loci, TCF7L2 represents the most robust and reproducible genetic determinant of T2D. First ascertained through genome-wide association studies, variants in TCF7L2 particularly the intronic SNP rs7903146 show a strong association with increased risk across diverse populations (Grant et al., 2006). Mechanistic studies indicate that TCF7L2, a transcription factor within the Wnt signaling pathway, is pivotal in β-cell proliferation, insulin secretion, and incretin signaling. Risk alleles are thought to impair insulin secretion in contrast to insulin action, suggesting a primary β-cell defect as the underlying mechanism (Lyssenko et al., 2007).

PPARG (Peroxisome Proliferator-Activated Receptor Gamma): The PPARG gene encodes a nuclear receptor that controls the development of adipocytes, lipid metabolism, and insulin sensitivity. The Pro12Ala polymorphism (rs1801282) is considered part of the earliest and most widely studied variants implicated in T2D risk. Carriers of the Ala12 allele have a reduced risk of T2D and improved insulin sensitivity compared with Pro12 homozygotes (Altshuler et al., 2000). The relevance in function of this gene is further underscored by the fact that thiazolidinediones, a class of agents that increase insulin sensitivity, act as ligands of PPARG (Lehmann et al., 1995). Thus, PPARG represents a locus where genetic discovery and pharmacological evidence converge.

KCNJ11 (Potassium Inwardly Rectifying Channel, Subfamily J, Member 11): KCNJ11 encodes the Kir6.2 subunit comprising the ATP-sensitive potassium (KATP) channel in pancreatic β-cells. This channel connects intracellular metabolism to membrane depolarization and is essential for glucose-stimulated insulin release. Variants such as E23K (rs5219) have been linked to a higher risk of type II diabetes (Yorifuji et al., 2005). Functional studies suggest that risk alleles alter KATP channel activity, impairing insulin release. Importantly, this gene shares a pharmacological link: sulfonylureas, a commonly used class of antidiabetic drugs, act by closing KATP channels, thereby promoting insulin secretion (Beaudelaire Tsiaze et al., 2012).

IRS1 and IRS2 (Insulin Receptor Substrates 1 and 2): IRS1 and IRS2 encode adapter proteins that mediate the insulin receptor signaling downstream of the insulin receptor Tyrosine kinase. Variants near IRS1 have been linked to T2D risk, insulin resistance, and altered fat distribution (Rung et al., 2009). Reduced insulin sensitivity and compromised downstream signaling through the PI3K-Akt pathway are common among carriers of risk alleles. In animal models, IRS2 is essential for insulin signaling and β-cell survival, while having a weaker correlation with the prevalent risk of T2D in people (Withers et al., 1998). Together, these genes show how insulin signaling abnormalities might play a role in the pathophysiology of type II diabetes.

Thanks to extensive GWAS, sequencing, and ancestry-specific research, more genes and loci have been linked to T2D. The most significant genes are TCF7L2, PPARG, KCNJ11, and IRS1/2; however, a few other genes are constantly present in all populations.

The polygenic and heterogeneous character of T2D is demonstrated in the large number of additional genes that contribute significantly to susceptibility beyond the conventional locus. These genes cover an extensive spectrum of biological processes, encompassing insulin secretion, adipogenesis, glucose sensing, lipid metabolism, and pancreatic β-cell formation and function (Table 15.1).

2.1.2 Role of common versus rare genetic variants in type II diabetes

Both frequent small-effect variations and uncommon large-effect variants are involved in the genetic architecture of T2D. When combined, they provide light on the disease's polygenic character and provide information about the biology at play as well as possible treatment options.

Table 15.1 Other genes and loci implicated in type II diabetes.

Gene/ Locus	Key Variant(s)	Biological role	Effect on T2D risk	Key References
SLC30A8	LoF alleles- (loss of function) alleles	ZnT8 transporter in β-cells	Some alleles increase risk of T2D; but LoF variants protective	Flannick et al. (2014); Sladek et al. (2007)
KCNQ1	Multiple intronic SNPs	β-cell excitability	Strong effect in East Asians	Yasuda et al. (2008)
FTO	rs9939609	Obesity regulation	Indirect via BMI	Frayling et al. (2007)
HHEX/IDE	rs1111875	Pancreatic development, insulin degradation	Altered β-cell development	Sladek et al. (2007)
CDKAL1	rs7754840	β-cell tRNA modification	Reduced insulin secretion	Steinthorsdottir et al. (2007)
HNF1A, HNF4A, GCK	Multiple	β-cell transcription/ glucose sensing	Monogenic diabetes, influences T2D traits	Pearson (2019)
SLC16A11	Multiple	Hepatic lipid metabolism	Risk allele enriched in Mexicans	Williams Amy et al. (2014)
TBC1D4	p. Arg684Ter	Skeletal muscle insulin response	Large effect in Greenlandic inuit	Moltke et al. (2014)
PAM	rs35658696	Prohormone amidation	Incretin resistance, impaired insulin secretion	Mahajan et al. (2018)

2.1.2.1 Common variants: Small effects, large contribution

The main findings of GWAS have emerged as a prominent genetic variation, which are generally classified as those having a minor allele frequency (MAF) > 5%. More than 400 shared loci from various ancestries have been linked to T2D thus far (Mahajan et al., 2018). With odds ratios distributed between 1.05 and 1.30, these variations often have a moderate influence on disease risk when taken alone. However, they have a significant combined effect on the population. The intronic mutation rs7903146 in TCF7L2, for instance, continues to be the most potent common signal linked to T2D in a variety of populations (Grant et al., 2006). Other significant common variations include KCNJ11 E23K (linked to decreased insulin secretion) (Altshuler et al., 2000), obesity-associated loci like FTO, which indirectly raise the vulnerability to type II diabetes by body mass index elevation (Frayling et al., 2007), and PPARG Pro12Ala (where the Ala allele is protective) (Lehmann et al., 1995).

These prevalent variations demonstrate how important regulatory systems are in the development of illness. A substantial portion of signals detected by GWAS localize to non-coding areas, frequently acting as enhancers in the liver, adipose tissue, or pancreatic islets (Frayling et al., 2007). Common variations suggest routes in hepatic glucose control, adipocyte differentiation, insulin secretion, and β-cell formation. Although each mutation has a little impact, when combined through polygenic risk scores (PRS), they enable the classification of people into very distinct groups based on their genetic vulnerability (Parker et al., 2013).

2.1.2.2 Rare variants: Large effects, limited frequency

Both coding mutations and loss-of-function alleles are examples of rare variations (MAF <1%) that frequently have greater effect sizes and offer direct insight into the biology of illness. Despite being rare on their own, these variations are very instructive as they can identify the genes that are causing the problem and potential treatments.

One of the most notable examples is SLC30A8, which is responsible for encoding the β-cell zinc transporter protein ZnT8. While common variants increase T2D risk, rare loss-of-function variants in SLC30A8 actually reduce susceptibility to diabetes, suggesting that ZnT8 inhibition may represent a therapeutic strategy (Selvam et al., 2017). Similarly, variants in PAM impair incretin hormone processing and increase T2D risk, revealing a direct mechanistic link between gut hormone biology and β-cell function (Flannick et al., 2014).

Rare variations can have significant impacts in situations that are peculiar to a community. As an example of how uncommon, ancestry-specific variations can significantly influence risk, a nonsense mutation in TBC1D4 discovered in the Greenlandic Inuit causes a tenfold increase in postprandial hyperglycemia when homozygous (Moltke et al., 2014). Another illustration is SLC16A11, which has been found in Latino communities and is enriched because of Native American heritage. It influences hepatic lipid metabolism (Williams Amy et al., 2014).

2.1.3 Ethnic and ancestry-specific differences in genetic risk

T2D has a different genetic makeup in different human ethnicities. The involvement of certain genetic loci to illness risk varies among ancestry groups resulting from population-level differences in allele frequencies, linkage disequilibrium (LD) structure, and population history. Because they affect our comprehension of disease processes, the transferability of genetic risk prediction tools, and the development of population-specific therapies, these distinctions are significant from a scientific and clinical standpoint.

2.1.3.1 Population-enriched risk alleles

There are notable variations in the frequency or effect magnitude of a number of T2D-associated loci among ethnic groups:

KCNQ1: Originally discovered in East Asian populations, variations in KCNQ1 emphasize population-specific allele frequency differences by conferring a greater risk impact in Asians as opposed to Europeans (Altshuler et al., 2000). KCNQ1 affects insulin secretion and encodes a voltage-gated potassium channel predominantly expressed in pancreatic islets.

SLC16A11: Native American ancestry enriches SLC16A11 variations, which were identified by the SIGMA type II diabetes Consortium in Mexican and Latino populations (Williams Amy et al., 2014). This locus affects lipid metabolism by encoding a mono-carboxylate transporter that is expressed in the liver. There is a molecular connection

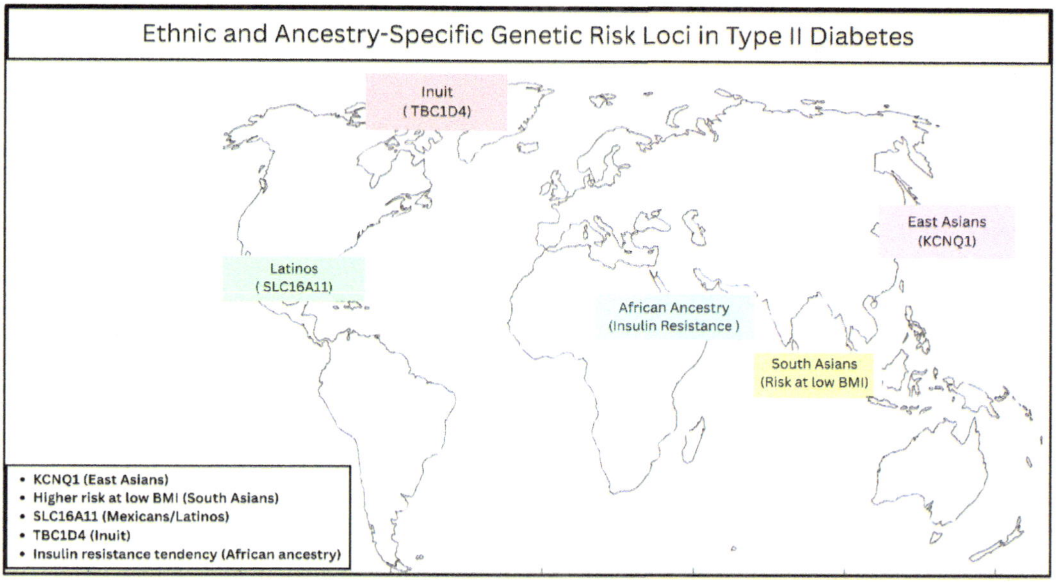

FIGURE 15.1 World map-style schematic showing ancestry-specific differences in T2D genetic risk: East Asia: *KCNQ1* risk variants strongly associated with T2D. Mexico/Latino populations: *SLC16A11* variants enriched due to Native American ancestry. Greenlandic inuit: *TBC1D4* nonsense variant conferring high postprandial diabetes risk. South Asians: Higher T2D risk at lower BMI thresholds, reflecting genetic predisposition and fat distribution. African ancestry: Greater insulin resistance tendency despite preserved insulin. *Map lines delineate study areas and do not necessarily depict accepted national boundaries.*

between insulin resistance and the risk allele's carriers' impaired hepatic triglyceride management.

TBC1D4: The Greenlandic Inuit have a nonsense mutation (p. Arg684Ter) in TBC1D4, and homozygous carriers have significantly reduced muscle postprandial glucose absorption and a considerably elevated vulnerability to type II diabetes (Moltke et al., 2014). This is an illustration of a high-impact, uncommon, population-specific variation. Although HNF1A, HNF4A, and GCK are traditionally linked to monogenic diabetes (MODY), variations in these genes can also vary in prevalence among groups, which affects how much they are involved in the genetic vulnerability to T2D (Pearson, 2019). Compared to Europeans, South Asians and East Asians are more likely to acquire type II diabetes at lower body mass index (BMI) thresholds, according to epidemiological and genetic research. A higher predisposition for visceral and hepatic fat deposition at lower BMI is partially caused by variations in the distribution of adiposity (Yoon et al., 2006). Environmental exposures and genetic predispositions most likely contribute to these phenotypic variations.

On the other hand, individuals of African ancestry frequently show higher insulin resistance but a stronger ability to secrete insulin, which can be attributed to both genetic and non-genetic factors (Adeyemo & Rotimi, 2009). However, the majority of

GWAS conducted to date have been Eurocentric, which has hampered the performance of PRS in non-European populations and decreased finding power (Martin et al., 2019) (Fig. 15.1).

2.1.3.2 Implications for polygenic risk scores and precision medicine

Variations in LD architecture and allele frequencies restrict the transferability of PRS between populations. A PRS trained on European cohorts, for instance, can significantly underperform when it comes to predicting the risk of T2D in Asian, Latino, or African populations (Duncan et al., 2019). It has been demonstrated that increasing the variety of GWAS participants enhances risk prediction and draws attention to new biology (Ingelheim et al., 2022).

Multi-ancestry studies are therefore essential for both identifying new loci that could be absent or uncommon in European cohorts and for ensuring equal treatment. The identification of TBC1D4 and SLC16A11 are excellent illustrations of how inclusive research broadens our knowledge of the biology and pathophysiology of T2D.

2.2 Family history and inheritance patterns in type II diabetes

Family history plays a significant role and is among the most reliable indicators of T2D risk. People who have first-degree relatives with type II diabetes are much more likely to get the disease, according to epidemiological research. Compared to people without a family history, the lifetime risk is roughly doubled if one parent is afflicted, and three to four times higher if both parents are affected (Swan, 2000). The increased probability of sibling recurrence emphasizes the disease's common genetic and environmental causes (Raboudi et al., 1989).

Even after controlling for lifestyle and metabolic characteristics, the Framingham Offspring Study revealed that a parent's history of diabetes was independently linked to a higher prevalence of T2D in middle-aged populations (Wilson et al., 2007). In a similar vein, family history is a low-cost risk stratification tool in clinical settings and is frequently included in prediction models along with fasting glucose, age, and body mass index (BMI) (Lyssenko et al., 2005).

2.2.1 Inheritance patterns: complex, non-mendelian

T2D has complicated, polygenic inheritance in contrast to monogenic diabetes (such as maturity-onset diabetes of the young, or MODY), which has a Mendelian inheritance pattern. Numerous common variations, uncommon variants with a greater effect, and shared family circumstances all contribute to risk. This explains why there is considerable familial clustering but no clear dominant or recessive pattern (Fuchsberger et al., 2016). This complexity is further demonstrated by the concordance rates in twin studies, which imply both substantial heredity and environmental contributions: monozygotic twins exhibit 70%–90% concordance, whereas dizygotic twins only exhibit 20%–30% (Poulsen et al., 1999). Thus, a combination of common lifestyle characteristics including eating habits, physical activity, and cultural customs, along with a shared genetic tendency, leads to family aggregation.

2.2.2 Parental transmission effects

Fascinatingly, research points to potential parent-of-origin impacts. According to some data, a mother's history of diabetes may put her children at slightly higher risk than a father's, possibly as a result of both genetic and intrauterine exposure to hyperglycemia (Knowler et al., 1981). This illustrates how inherited susceptibility is increased by developmental programming.

2.2.3 Clinical implications

Clinically speaking, family history is still a strong, affordable, and accessible method of identifying those who are more likely to be at risk. Even if improved biomarkers and genomic risk scores are developing, family history still records shared environmental exposures and known and undiscovered genetic factors. Because of this, it is extremely useful for risk assessment, patient counseling, and preventative measures (Khera et al., 2018).

2.3 Gene–environment interactions in type II diabetes

Environmental exposures and genetic vulnerability interact to cause T2D. Although a baseline tendency is defined by genetic polymorphisms, lifestyle and environmental circumstances have a significant impact on whether or not this predisposition manifests. This interplay explains why people with high genetic risk might not get sick if they lead healthy lives, whereas others with a low genetic load might have T2D if they live in unfavorable environments.

Obesity and Adiposity as Key Mediators: Obesity is a major mediator of genetic risk and the predominant environmental risk factor associated with T2D. For example, genetic variations in the FTO gene are associated with elevated body BMI, and adiposity plays a pivotal role in how they affect the risk of T2D (Frayling et al., 2007). Similar to this, a large number of GWAS-identified SNPs indirectly affect insulin resistance, adipocyte activity, or fat distribution (Voight et al., 2011). Significantly, population-specific gene–environment sensitivity to adiposity is suggested by the fact that South and East Asian populations acquire T2D at lower BMI thresholds than Europeans (Yoon et al., 2006).

Lifestyle Modifiers of Genetic Risk: Numerous studies show that genetic risk is reduced by healthy lifestyle choices. In the United States, maintaining a normal body weight, stopping smoking, eating a nutritious diet, and getting regular exercise dramatically reduced the prevalence of type II diabetes, even in those with the highest polygenic risk quartile (Li et al., 2020). In a similar vein, the Diabetes Prevention Program (DPP) demonstrated that dietary changes and increased physical activity, two lifestyle interventions, was associated with a 58% reduction in type II diabetes incidence among high-risk adults. These effects were consistent irrespective of genetic predisposition (Intervention & Metformin, 2002).

Nutrient–Gene Interactions: Genetic variations and certain dietary components may combine to affect risk. For instance, the detrimental impact of high glycemic load meals on the development of diabetes is amplified by risk alleles in TCF7L2. Additionally, PPARG variations alter insulin sensitivity through mild interactions with dietary fat consumption (Memisoglu et al., 2003). These results imply that genetically based personalized diet might improve preventative measures.

Pharmacogenetic Interactions: Drug response is another area where gene-environment interactions occur. Response to sulfonylureas is affected by variations in KCNJ11 and ABCC8, which encode KATP channel subunits, whereas TCF7L2 polymorphisms alter the efficacy of incretin-based treatments (Tk & Gotthardov, 2016). While these pharmacogenetic insights are not yet common in clinical practice, they demonstrate how genetic background might influence the effectiveness of treatments.

2.3.1 Other environmental modifiers

Gene–environment interactions in T2D are influenced by environmental factors other than nutrition and obesity.

- Insulin sensitivity is compromised by physical inactivity, which increases hereditary risk.
- Glycemic control is exacerbated by sleep loss and circadian disturbance, especially in those who are genetically susceptible (Shan et al., 2015).
- Higher prevalence of T2D is linked to smoking and air pollution, which may increase genetic vulnerability through inflammation and oxidative stress (Eze et al., 2015).

2.4 Diet, lifestyle, and environmental modifiers in type II diabetes

T2D is mostly determined by genetic susceptibility, although environmental exposures, lifestyle choices, and dietary habits all have a substantial impact on the disease's development. These variables interact with genetic risk to alter susceptibility in addition to directly affecting insulin sensitivity and β-cell activity. Crucially, even in people with a high hereditary load, lifestyle changes can significantly lower the prevalence of T2D.

Dietary Factors: Dietary composition and quality have a significant impact on the risk of type II diabetes. Protective dietary patterns: Whole grain, fruit, vegetable, legume, nut, and fiber-rich diets are consistently shown to be associated with lower susceptibility to T2D (Sylvia et al., 2016). Following the Mediterranean diet lowers chronic inflammation and increases insulin sensitivity (Esposito et al., 2014). Negative dietary factors: Consuming large amounts of processed meats, sugar-sweetened drinks, refined carbs, and saturated/trans fats raises the risk of T2D by facilitating weight gain, inducing insulin resistance, and impairing metabolic function (Pan et al., 2011). Micronutrients and bioactive substances: While deficiencies may increase risk, adequate consumption of magnesium, polyphenols, and omega-3 fatty acids has been associated with better glycemic management (Larsson & Wolk, 2007). Gene–diet interactions are highlighted by the fact that those with TCF7L2 risk alleles are more sensitive to diets with a high glycemic index/load (Cornelis et al., 2009).

Physical Activity and Sedentary Behavior: By increasing muscle glucose absorption, decreasing visceral fat deposition, and boosting insulin sensitivity, physical exercise has a positive glucose homeostasis impact. Regardless of weight change, moderate to intense exercise lowers the emergence of T2D cases (Aune et al., 2015). Even among those who satisfy exercise requirements, sedentary behavior, especially prolonged sitting is independently linked to an elevated risk (Biswas et al., 2015).

Obesity and Weight Management: The greatest modifiable risk factor for T2D is excessive adiposity. Particularly harmful is central (visceral) obesity, which causes β-cell stress and insulin resistance. Glycemic control and disease incidence are greatly improved by even small weight loss (5%–10% of body weight) (Toumillehto et al., 2013).

Gut Microbiome as a Mediator: The gut microbiota role as a mediator between host metabolism, environment, and food is becoming more well acknowledged. Reduced butyrate-producing bacteria are among the altered gut microbial compositions seen in T2D patients (Wang et al., 2012). Changes in the makeup of the microbiota brought about by nutrition might affect insulin sensitivity and glucose tolerance, indicating possible treatment options with diet, probiotics, and prebiotics.

3. Impact of genetics on disease progression

T2D is mostly caused by hereditary factors, but new research indicates that same variables also affect how the illness progresses, how well a therapy works, and how likely complications are. Knowing these genetic factors may assist guide precision medicine strategies and helps explain inter-individual variability in clinical outcomes.

Progression from Prediabetes to Diabetes: In addition to determining baseline vulnerability, genetic variations also affect how quickly prediabetes or impaired glucose tolerance (IGT) develops into overt type II diabetes. For example, because risk alleles in TCF7L2 affect insulin production and β-cell activity, they are linked to accelerated development (Lyssenko et al., 2007). Likewise, variations in CDKAL1 and SLC30A8 impact β-cell capacity, which leads to rapid β-cell loss and an earlier start of illness (Fuchsberger et al., 2016). These results imply that earlier screening and more stringent preventative actions can be advantageous for carriers of specific variations.

Glycemic Trajectories and Treatment Response: Patients' responses to various treatment approaches are influenced by their genetic background. Response to sulfonylureas, which increase insulin secretion, is changed by variations in KCNJ11 and ABCC8 (encoding KATP channel subunits) (Gloyn et al., 2004). The polymorphism in PPARG Pro12Ala alters insulin sensitivity and may affect how well thiazolidinediones (TZDs) work (Altshuler et al., 2000). By affecting the hepatic absorption of metformin, variants of SLC22A1 (encoding the organic cation transporter OCT1) change the medication's glycemic efficacy (Ningrum et al., 2022). These pharmacogenetic consequences demonstrate how genetics influences treatment outcomes and the promise of genotype-guided therapy going forward.

T2D complications: The risk of microvascular and macrovascular problems may also be influenced by genetics. For instance, particularly in Asian populations, variations in the ACE and AGT genes have been correlated with an elevated risk of diabetic nephropathy (Ruggenenti et al., 2008). Diabetic cardiovascular disease has been associated with polymorphisms in genes that control vascular function (NOS3) and lipid metabolism (APOE, LPL) (Doria et al., 2008). By maintaining hyperglycemia over time, genetic variations that worsen glycemic dysregulation (such as TCF7L2) indirectly increase the risk of complications (Grant et al., 2006).

3.1 Genetic influence on β-cell function and insulin resistance

When the amount of insulin secreted by pancreatic β-cells is inadequate to overcome insulin resistance in peripheral tissues, T2D develops. Genetic factors contribute to insulin resistance (tissue responsiveness) as well as β-cell function (insulin secretion and production). The diverse pathophysiology of type II diabetes is highlighted by the fact that different gene sets primarily impact one or the other.

3.1.1 The impact of genetics on β-cell function

The key significance of poor β-cell function in disease pathogenesis is highlighted by the fact that a significant percentage of T2D risk loci found by GWAS map to genes involved in β-cell formation, survival, and insulin production (Fuchsberger et al., 2016; Mahajan et al., 2018). The most robust and often repeated locus for type II diabetes is TCF7L2. Variants accelerate the transition from reduced glucose tolerance to diabetes by impairing β-cell insulin production and incretin signaling (Lyssenko et al., 2007). In β-cells, KCNJ11 and ABCC8 encode subunits of the ATP-sensitive K+ (KATP) channel, which connects insulin release with glucose metabolism. Insulin secretory response is decreased by risk variants (e.g., KCNJ11 E23K) (Gloyn et al., 2003). ZnT8, a zinc transporter found in insulin granules, is encoded by SLC30A8. Ironically, uncommon loss-of-function mutations offer protection against type II diabetes, whereas risk alleles decrease insulin production and crystallization (Williams Amy et al., 2014). HHEX, CDKAL1, and MTNR1B: Affect glucose-stimulated secretion, circadian insulin release regulation, and β-cell mass (Rönn et al., 2023). Although they are uncommon, monogenic diabetes genes (HNF1A, HNF4A, and GCK) offer mechanistic proof that diabetes may be caused only by β-cell abnormalities (Pearson, 2019).

3.1.2 Genetic influence on insulin resistance

A number of important genes control lipid metabolism, insulin signaling pathways, and adipose tissue biology, although fewer loci directly correlate with insulin resistance.

Variants close to IRS1 (Insulin Receptor Substrate 1) are linked to altered adipose distribution, elevated hepatic insulin resistance, and decreased insulin signaling (Rung et al., 2009). Adipogenesis's main regulator is PPARG (Peroxisome Proliferator-Activated Receptor-γ). The Ala allele offers some protection through increased insulin sensitivity, but the Pro12Ala variation modifies receptor activation (Altshuler et al., 2000). FTO: Mostly a locus for obesity. Variants raise the likelihood of T2D and insulin resistance by increasing adiposity (Frayling et al., 2007). SLC16A11: Found in Latino and Mexican communities. encodes a hepatic monocarboxylate transporter; variations contributing to an elevation in insulin resistance and hepatic triglyceride accumulation (Williams Amy et al., 2014). A Greenlandic Inuit variation known as TBC1D4 results in impaired insulin-stimulated glucose uptake in muscle, which sequentially affects peripheral insulin sensitivity (Moltke et al., 2014).

3.2 Genetic clusters and their metabolic traits in type II diabetes

Because T2D is polygenic, it is helpful to group genetic risk loci according to biological pathways and related metabolic characteristics. Integrative multi-omics analyses and extensive GWAS have demonstrated that T2D risk loci may be arranged into functionally coherent clusters, each of which makes a distinct contribution to the disease's pathogenesis. Precision subtyping is made possible by these clusters, which also shed light on the variability of T2D.

1. **Cluster of β-Cell Dysfunction:** Most of the loci are related to poor insulin secretion. Genes that decrease β-cell proliferation, insulin granule production, and incretin responsiveness include TCF7L2, CDKAL1, HHEX, MTNR1B, KCNJ11, and SLC30A8. Carriers frequently have reduced early-phase insulin release and a lower BMI (Fuchsberger et al., 2016; Mahajan et al., 2018).

2. **Cluster for Proinsulin Processing:** The conversion of proinsulin to insulin is influenced by genes such as ARAP1, MADD, and PCSK1, which results in increased proinsulin/insulin ratios and ineffective glucose control, a sign of β-cell fatigue (Strawbridge et al., 2011).

3. **The Cluster of Obesity and Adiposity:** Energy balance, appetite control, and fat partitioning are all impacted by variations in FTO, MC4R, TMEM18, and PPARG. By encouraging increased BMI, visceral obesity, and systemic insulin resistance, these genes indirectly raise the susceptibility of T2D (Frayling et al., 2007; Loos & Yeo, 2014).

4. **Cluster of Insulin Resistance:** Genes including IRS1, PPARG, KLF14, LYPLAL1, SLC16A11, and TBC1D4 either increase hepatic fat accumulation or hinder insulin

signaling and adipose tissue expandability. Typically, carriers have fatty liver, dyslipidaemia, and elevated fasting insulin (Rung et al., 2009; Strawbridge et al., 2011).

5. **Liver Cluster and Lipid Metabolism:** Dysregulation of hepatic lipid and glucose metabolism is caused by variations in GCKR, PNPLA3, PPP1R3B, and SLC16A11. This results in non-alcoholic fatty liver disease (NAFLD), a condition strongly associated with T2D, and increased triglycerides (Speliotes et al., 2010).

6. **Cluster for Incretin and Hormone Processing:** PAM variations impair the activity of GLP-1 and hinder insulin production after meals by reducing amidation of incretin peptides (Mahajan et al., 2018).

3.3 Genetic determinants of disease heterogeneity in type II diabetes

Instead of being a single illness, T2D is a diverse condition with several underlying molecular pathways, clinical subtypes, and risk profiles unique to different populations. This variation is mostly due to genetics, which affects the metabolic phenotype, complication risk, illness onset, and severity. The implementation of precision medicine in diabetes management necessitates an understanding of these factors.

3.3.1 Heterogeneity in clinical presentations

Individuals with T2D also differ in their clinical characteristics due to genetic loci.

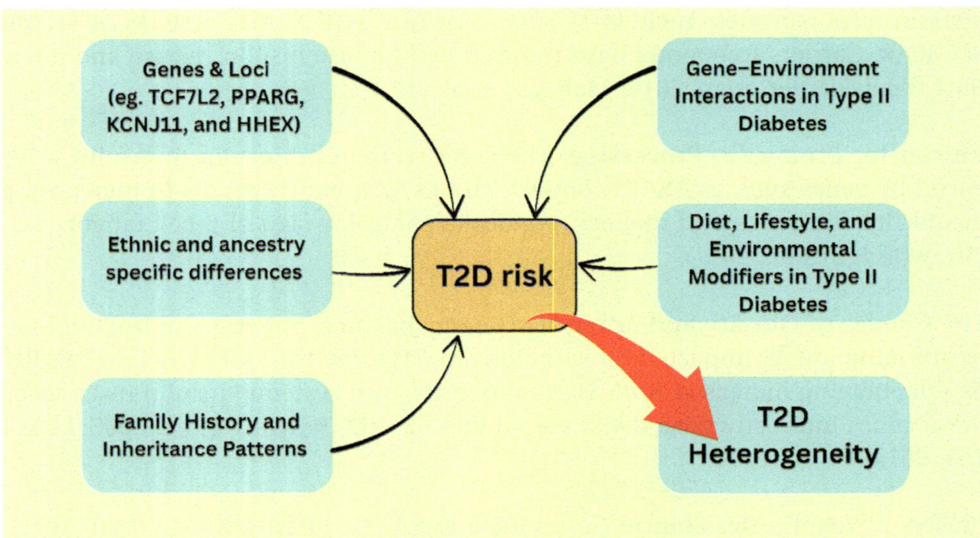

FIGURE 15.2 Cause of heterogeneity in type II diabetes. Multiple genetic, biochemical, and clinical manifestations exist, resulting in a highly diverse and complicated illness rather than a single homogeneous condition.

Lean versus obese T2D: Individuals with β-cell function-affecting genetic variations (TCF7L2, CDKAL1, SLC30A8) may have diabetes even when their BMI is relatively low, which is indicative of insufficient insulin production (Fuchsberger et al., 2016). On the other hand, those with variations in FTO, PPARG, IRS1, or SLC16A11 frequently develop diabetes in conjunction with insulin resistance and obesity (Loos & Yeo, 2014) (Fig. 15.2).

Comparing early-onset and late-onset type II diabetes: Some genetic variations make the disease more likely to start earlier by speeding up the β-cell decrease. For instance, a lower age of diagnosis and reduced early-phase insulin release are associated with risk alleles in MTNR1B (Bouatia-Naji et al., 2009).

Differential complication risk: Heterogeneity in complication patterns may be caused by variations in genes that control vascular biology (ACE, NOS3) and lipid metabolism (APOE, LPL), which may affect the risk of nephropathy, retinopathy, or the burden of cardiovascular disease among individuals with type II diabetes (Doria et al., 2008).

4. Immune components in T2D pathogenesis

4.1 The immunology of type II diabetes

T2D is no longer viewed solely as a metabolic disorder of insulin resistance and cell dysfunction; it is now recognized as a chronic, low-grade inflammatory disease (Duncan & Schmidt, 2006) in which interactions between metabolic stressors and the innate and adaptive immune system drive disease onset, progression, and complications (Hameed et al., 2015). Metabolic perturbations such as nutrient excess, lipotoxicity, hyperglycemia, and altered gut microbial metabolites produce signals known as damage-associated molecular patterns (DAMPs) that provoke immune activation within metabolic organs such as adipose tissue, liver, skeletal muscle, and pancreatic islets (Garcia-Martinez et al., 2015). These immune responses both impair insulin signaling and contribute to progressive cell dysfunction, establishing a feed-forward loop that mechanistically links metabolic processes with immune responses. Recent scientific advances have highlighted the pivotal role of immune system dysfunction in the development and progression of T2D. These stresses stimulate immune cells to produce proinflammatory rather than homeostatic responses (Golden & Simmons, 2021). Activated monocytes and macrophages infiltrate insulin-sensitive tissues and become proinflammatory in phenotype, secreting cytokines that make the insulin resistance and tissue injury worse. Increased monocyte numbers, macrophage phenotype shifts, reduced $CD4^+$ T-cells, and aberrant B-cell activity disrupt normal regulation and lead to tissue damage (Li et al., 2022). Similarly, hyperglycemia promotes the accumulation of advanced glycation end-products (AGEs) and reactive oxygen species (ROS), which activate innate immune receptors and amplify inflammation (Negre-Salvayre et al., 2009). Instead of resolving damage or injury, immune cells in T2D maintain a sustained, low-grade inflammatory state, known as "metaflammation," which plays a central role in reduced responsiveness to insulin and β-cell dysfunction (Kuryłowicz & Koźniewski, 2020).

The earliest and most reproducible immune changes in obesity-associated T2D occur in white adipose tissue (WAT). As adipocytes hypertrophy, they become hypoxic and release chemokines that recruit monocytes, which further differentiate into adipose tissue macrophages (ATMs) with a proinflammatory phenotype that interferes with insulin signaling in adipocytes and promotes systemic insulin resistance, as proved in earlier research approaches through single-cell analysis and functional studies (Cai et al., 2022).

4.2 Chronic low-grade inflammation and its mediators

A hallmark of T2D is long-term, low-grade inflammation in metabolic tissues, which contrasts with acute, protective inflammation accompanying infections. In adipose tissue, immune cells infiltrate and produce proinflammatory signals that undermine insulin sensitivity (Cai et al., 2022). Macrophages are the major mediators, changing from an antiinflammatory M2 phenotype that promotes tissue repair to a proinflammatory M1 phenotype that secretes cytokines and chemokines. These cytokines also recruit other immune cells and, locally, impair the insulin receptors' function in adipocytes and muscle tissue (Koh et al., 2018). In the pancreas, inflammation damages β-cells, reducing their ability to survive and release insulin, creating a vicious cycle of deteriorating blood sugar control (Dludla et al., 2023). The interaction between immune mediators and metabolic stress prevents the resolution of inflammation, paving the way for an enduring state that supports disease progression in T2D.

4.3 Key cytokines in T2D

Some cytokines are especially crucial in the inflammatory environment of T2D. IL-1β is a key pro-inflammatory cytokine that not only suppresses insulin secretion but also causes apoptosis in islet cells of the pancreas. A central mechanistic connection between metabolic disturbance and innate immune activation lies in the stimulation of the NLRP3 inflammasome in myeloid cells, which cleaves and activates IL-1β, which then disrupts insulin signaling and damages β-cell function, reducing insulin secretion (Gora et al., 2021). Similarly, TNF-α contributes to metabolic imbalance by directly interfering with insulin receptor signaling by activating serine kinases that inhibit insulin receptor substrate (IRS) proteins, thus promoting insulin resistance in both muscle and adipose tissues (Moller, 2000; Pei et al., 2022). IL-6 plays a dual role: while transient elevations may support glucose metabolism, sustained elevations in T2D enhance hepatic glucose production, systemic inflammation, and worsen insulin resistance (Peppler et al., 2019; Rehman et al., 2017). IL-18, another inflammasome-associated cytokine, is elevated in obesity and T2D, where it drives inflammation within adipose tissue and thereby links obesity to metabolic malfunction. Recent research studies on mouse models have found that IL-18 signaling appears to regulate adipose tissue growth and glucose homeostasis, since its deficiency in mice results in spontaneous obesity and impaired glucose tolerance (Lana et al., 2024). Together, these cytokines make up a pathological circuit that interferes with the insulin signaling network, destroys pancreatic β-cells, and maintains systemic inflammation, making them major therapeutic targets in diabetes immunology.

4.4 Immune cell dysfunction in T2D

Dysregulation of immune cells is the focus of immunopathology in T2D. The adaptive immune system is integral to the local inflammatory environment in metabolic tissues. Lymphocytes, including T-cells, demonstrate an imbalance with elevated proinflammatory $CD4^+$ subsets (Th1 and Th17) responses combined with decreased or functionally reduced regulatory T-cell (Treg) populations, which normally maintain tissue homeostasis. This shift promotes continuous cytokine release and sustained tissue inflammation, which worsens the insulin resistance (Noack & Miossec, 2014; Zi et al., 2022). B-cells also contribute by antigen presentation and secreting proinflammatory cytokines, and, in certain cases, producing autoantibodies that enhance tissue destruction and metabolic impairment (Nikolajczyk, 2010). Animal studies using B-cell depletion models have shown that reducing B-cell populations lowers inflammatory activity, improves insulin responsiveness within visceral adipose tissue (VAT), and leads to improved systemic glucose tolerance (Harmon et al., 2016). Thus, both effector and regulatory arms of the adaptive immune system modulate metabolic inflammation.

On the innate side, macrophages predominate the inflammatory environment of adipose tissue and pancreatic islets, polarize toa proinflammatory M1 phenotype. This polarization supports a chronic inflammatory state, which negatively affects both insulin responsiveness and survival of β-cells (Koh et al., 2018). Natural killer (NK) cells and innate lymphoid cells (ILCs) also shape macrophage polarization and adipocyte function (Saetang & Sangkhathat, 2017). Complement activation (King & Blom, 2021) and circulating acute-phase proteins (such as CRP and fibrinogen) correlate with cardiometabolic risk and reflect low-grade inflammation that accompanies T2D (Lubrano et al., 2025). Taken together, the abnormality of these immune cells ensures that inflammation in T2D is not self-limiting but rather becomes a stimulator of disease progression.

5. Genetic polymorphisms influencing immunity in T2D

5.1 Genetic variants in cytokine genes affect immune responses and inflammation

T2D is denoted not only by insulin resistance and impaired β-cell function but also by a persistent, but also by state of low-grade, long-standing inflammatory state. In this context, cytokines originating from adipose tissue, immune cells, and vascular endothelium collectively play crucial roles in disease progression. Single-nucleotide polymorphisms (SNPs) in cytokine genes may change transcriptional activity or protein function and consequently regulate basal and inducible cytokine production; inherited variations thus add to inter-individual variation in inflammatory tone, level of insulin resistance, and subsequent immune responses, among individuals prone to or already affected by T2D (Arora et al., 2011).

5.1.1 IL-6 (Interleukin-6)

Common functional SNP(s): −174G > C (rs1800795) is the most extensively investigated promoter variant; other SNPs (e.g., rs1800796) have also been studied. Functional and population studies demonstrate that rs1800795 varies with differences in IL-6 transcription as well as circulating IL-6 levels in certain settings. Individuals with different genotypes vary in basal IL-6 levels and inducibility, but the direction and magnitude of effect may be population-dependent (Ageeva, 2024).

Mechanistic consequence: IL-6 signals act through gp130 → JAK/STAT3 and can induce SOCS3 expression; SOCS3 suppresses insulin receptor signaling (through IRS1/IRS2), leading to peripheral insulin resistance. IL-6 also transacts with NF-κB pathways and modulates hepatic gluconeogenesis and adipocyte metabolism. Therefore, promoter variants that up- or down-regulate IL-6 expression can shift the balance between typical immune responses and chronic metabolic inflammation that foster T2D pathogenesis (Reda et al., 2018; Shi et al., 2019).

Genetic evidence: Heterogeneous results by diabetes type and ethnicity in large meta-analyses:rs1800795 C-allele has been found protective against T2D in some meta-analytic strata (especially in Asians/mixed cohorts), while other analyses report no association or contrary effects for type 1 diabetes (T1D), highlighting disease-specific and ethnicity-dependent functions. This heterogeneity suggests gene × environment interaction (e.g., BMI, diet, infection history) and calls for caution in generalizing results.

5.1.2 TNF-α (tumor necrosis factor-alpha)

Common functional SNP(s): −308G > A (rs1800629) (Ghareeb et al., 2021) and −238G > A (rs361525) (Qidwai & Khan, 2011) within the TNF promoter are well investigated. The −308 A allele has been linked in vitro with increased promoter activity and increased TNF-α expression in defined cell systems.

Mechanistic consequence: TNF-α directly impedes insulin signaling by stimulating serine residue phosphorylation of IRS1, often mediated by JNK (c-Jun N-terminal kinase), disrupting downstream signaling, altering adipocyte lipolysis, and facilitating macrophage invasion to adipose tissue; all key pathways in obesity-associated insulin resistance. Thus, promoter polymorphisms that augment TNF expression would predispose to or worsen insulin resistance and the inflammatory milieu of T2D (Guria et al., 2023).

Genetic evidence: Ethnicity-specific meta-analyses and multiple case-control studies report associations between TNF promoter SNPs and risk of T2D or severity of metabolic/inflammatory phenotypes (Enni and Mahmud, 2024); however, findings are inconsistent between populations, and effect sizes are modest.

5.1.3 IL-18 (Interleukin-18)

Common functional SNP(s): Promoter SNPs −137G > C (rs187238) and −607C > A (rs1946518). These SNPs may affect IL-18 transcriptional activity as well as circulating IL-18 levels (Hoseini et al., 2018).

Mechanistic consequence: IL-18 also induces Th1 responses and production of IFN-γ; high IL-18 levels correlate with insulin resistance, atherosclerosis, and the development of microvascular complications. Aberrant expression of IL-18 (via promoter variants) can thus contribute to metabolic inflammation and compromise host defense mechanisms (Bahrami et al., 2021).

Genetic evidence: Polymorphisms within IL-18 promoter have been linked to an increased risk of developing inflammatory disorders and, in a few cohorts, diabetes-related complications (e.g., diabetic nephropathy, cardiovascular disease) (Booker, 2013). The findings are characterized by population heterogeneity and the importance of haplotype context.

5.2 Impact on infections, complications, and clinical relevance

Genetic polymorphisms in proinflammatory cytokine genes such as IL-6, TNF, and IL-18 not only determine basal inflammatory tone in T2D but also control the host's susceptibility to infections and the development of diabetic complications. IL-6 (e.g., 174G > C), TNF (−308G > A, −238G > A), and IL-18 (−137G > C, −607C > A) polymorphisms have been shown to impact cytokine expression, thereby affecting immune cell recruitment, macrophage polarization, and wound healing responses. Dysregulated cytokine production connected to these alleles can be detrimental to neutrophil and macrophage function, leading to delayed microbial clearance and more severe diabetic foot ulcers, osteomyelitis, and other skin and soft tissue infections, with certain studies in South Indian and Turkish populations indicating correlations between these genotypes and ulcer grade, severity of infection, and risk of amputation. In addition to infection, these polymorphisms have been implicated in microvascular and macrovascular complications (Mansour et al., 2023). TNF promoter and IL-18 promoter SNPs have been associated with diabetic nephropathy and chronic kidney disease (Umapathy et al., 2018), whereas heightened IL-18 expression has been implicated in atherosclerosis and cardiovascular risk, underlining a genetic contribution to inter-individual variability in complication burden (Cavalcante et al., 2020). While associations differ across ethnic groups and study design, the biological plausibility is supported by mechanistic data, as excess TNF-α and IL-6 disrupt insulin receptor signaling and endothelial function, and IL-18 promotes proatherogenic IFN-γ–dominated immune responses (Bhat & Dhawan, 2015). Collectively, these findings suggest that cytokine gene polymorphisms, through the regulation of inflammation, may modulate both susceptibility to infections and the course of vascular complications in T2D, but their potential as predictive markers must be tested in large, multi-ethnic populations.

6. Immune alterations and clinical outcomes in type II diabetes

6.1 Impaired immune responses and increased infection risk

T2D is strongly linked with altered immune competence, leading to an enhanced risk to infections. Hyperglycemia compromises the chemotaxis, phagocytosis, superoxide formation and bactericidal action of neutrophils (Jafar et al., 2016), while macrophages show decreased antigen presentation and uncontrolled cytokine production. Adaptive immunity, too, is compromised, with T-cell proliferation and regulatory T-cell functions impaired, making host defense mechanisms weaker. This immunocompromised state translates clinically into a higher risk of respiratory and urinary tract infections, skin, soft tissue, and opportunistic fungal infections (Dropulic & Lederman, 2016). Furthermore, the increased pathogen colonization potential in hyperglycemic conditions, coupled with weakened barrier functions, increases infection risk and severity.

6.2 Effects on wound healing and chronic complications

Wound healing is unusually impaired in T2D owing to a synergistic interplay of vascular, metabolic, and immune derangements. Chronic hyperglycemia results in the development of AGEs, microvascular injury, and reduced tissue perfusion, all of which restrict the transport of oxygen and nutrients to damaged tissue sites (Levy et al., 2008). On an immunological level, prolonged and chronic inflammation caused by excessive proinflammatory cytokines, including TNF-α, IL-2, IL-6, IL-10, IL-17, and IL-1β, delays the resolution phase required for tissue healing due to the prolonged inflammatory phase. These cytokines recruit immune cells to the wound site, but their function is dysregulated in T2D. Neutrophils and macrophages in individuals with diabetes often remain in a sustained proinflammatory state, disrupting the ability of macrophages to shift their functional state, preventing the transition to proliferative and remodeling phases of healing (Nirenjen et al., 2023). Clinically, this results in long-lasting non-healing wounds, with diabetic foot ulcers representing a frequent and serious complication, which predisposes patients to recurrent infections and amputations. Beyond wound healing, chronic immune activation is also responsible for long-term complications such as atherosclerosis, nephropathy, and retinopathy, where inflammatory mediators play a central pathogenic role.

6.3 Immune markers as predictors of disease progression and therapy response

Emerging evidence points toward immune biomarkers as valuable predictors of disease progression and therapeutic response in T2D. High systemic concentrations of proinflammatory cytokines correlate with insulin resistance, inadequate regulation of blood glucose, and elevated likelihood of various cardiovascular diseases (CVDs) such as

Table 15.2 Key immunological and inflammatory markers implicated in T2D, their biological functions, and relevance to disease pathogenesis.

Marker	Function	Relevance in T2D	References
IL-1β	Induce inflammation; impairβ-cell function and its apoptosis	Elevated in T2D; correlated with poor glycemic control; contributes to insulin resistance	Venieratos et al. (2010)
IL-6	Metabolic regulation effects within the liver and skeletal muscle	Elevated in T2D; induces insulin resistance via JAK/STAT3-SOCS3 pathway; involved in adipose tissue inflammation; used in risk stratification	Gao et al. (2024); Zatterale et al. (2020)
TNF-α	Activates various inflammatory pathways and can impair insulin signaling	Elevated in T2D; inhibits insulin receptor signaling (IRS-1 phosphorylation)	Alipourfard et al. (2019)
IL-10	Helps dampen inflammation	Often found decreased in T2D	Pirola and Ferraz (2017)
IL-13	Promotes M2 macrophage polarization; opposes proinflammatory cytokines	Reflects a compensatory antiinflammatory response	Shapouri-Moghaddam et al. (2018)
CRP	Acute phase proteins, produced by liver hepatocytes, are induced by IL-6, IL-1 and are markers of systemic inflammation.	Elevated in T2D and before onset, high CRP levels are linked with the development of T2D and cardiovascular complications	Stanimirovic et al. (2022)
MCP-19 (Monocyte Chemoattractant Protein-1) or CCL2	Chemokine attracting macrophages; involved in recruitment into adipose and other tissues	Elevated in T2D; contributes to inflammation of adipose tissue; correlates with glucose intolerance	Kochumon et al. (2020)
IGF-1(Insulin-like growth Factor1)	Participate in regulating cell growth, survival, and insulin signaling crosstalk	Altered levels in T2D; low IGF-1 may be associated with a worse metabolic profile (Withers & White, 2000)	Withers and White (2000)
Humanin	Mitochondrial peptide which reduces oxidative stress; improves cell survival, insulin sensitivity	Levels are decreased in prediabetes and T2D; low humanin may reflect mitochondrial dysfunction in T2D	Ramanjaneya et al. (2019)
Globulins	Serum proteins of acute adaptive immune system	Elevated IgA, IgG, and gamma-globulin have been observed; may reflect chronic immune stimulation	Le et al. (2025)
CSF1R (Colony stimulating factor 1 receptor)	Regulates the proliferation and differentiation of macrophages; innate immune cell regulation	Identified through coexpression networks as a "hub gene" overexpressed in T2D; associated with macrophage infiltration, adipogenesis, and inflammatory signaling	Yuan et al. (2023); Zhou et al. (2022)

coronary artery disease (CAD), angina, congenital heart defects, arrhythmias, and heart attack (Abdulmuttaleb et al., 2024). Similarly, distorted innate immune cells, such as higher levels of proinflammatory M1 macrophages alongside a decline in antiinflammatory M2 macrophages, serve as markers of disease severity. Circulating biomarkers, including C-reactive protein (CRP), soluble adhesion molecules, and chemokines, provide additional prognostic information. These immune changes not only reflect disease load but can also help predict treatment responses. For example, lower IL-6 and CRP concentrations after lifestyle modification, metformin use, or GLP-1 receptor agonist therapy indicates improved metabolic and inflammatory status (Guarnotta et al., 2021). As a result, immune markers are increasingly recognized as useful tools for risk stratification, therapeutic monitoring, and guiding personalized treatment strategies in T2D (see Table 15.2).

7. Therapeutic implications

7.1 Targeting inflammatory pathways

Therapies directed at targeting proinflammatory cytokines, including the use of IL-1 receptor antagonists (e.g., anakinra), have achieved enhanced glycemic control, decreased systemic inflammation, and maintenance of pancreatic β-cell function (Peiró et al., 2017). Similarly, antiinflammatory agents, including Salsalate and TNF-α inhibitors, have proven promising in restoring insulin efficacy, albeit with results still inconsistent between populations (Esser et al., 2015). Beyond this, novel immunomodulators, like small-molecule inhibitors, monoclonal antibodies, and plant-based bioactive compounds, are also being investigated for their capacity to modulate immune responses without compromising host defense. Together, these strategies highlight the potential that controlling inflammation may complement standard glucose-lowering treatments by addressing both metabolic and immunological disturbances in T2D.

7.2 Personalized medicine: Genetic and immunological profiling in T2D management

Given the heterogeneity of T2D, patients differ significantly in the emergence and course of disease, and in determining response to therapy. Technological advancements in genomics, immunology, and systems biology now allow personalized medicine strategies to optimize treatment. Genetic profiling of cytokine gene variants (e.g., IL-6, IL-18, TNF), insulin resistance loci, and β-cell function can help predict susceptibility, progression, and therapeutic responsiveness (Banerjee, 2014). Immunological profiling, including the assessment and measurement of circulating cytokines, autoantibodies, and inflammatory signatures, may also assist in the choice of patients who are most likely to respond to immunomodulatory treatments (Laigle et al., 2023). In addition, combining multi-omics information with electronic health records is opening the door to personalized treatment regimens ranging from targeted use of antiinflammatory agents to preventive lifestyle measures in those with a genetic predisposition. Thus, personalized medicine has the potential not only to maximize glycemic control but also to minimize complications by targeting the immune and genetic basis of T2D.

8. Conclusion

Type II diabetes reflects the combined influence of genetic, immunological, and environmental factors, giving rise to its diverse clinical outcomes. Genetic studies have pinpointed risk factors linked to β-cell dysfunction, insulin resistance, obesity, lipid metabolism, and immune regulation. Even with strong heredity, family history, and lifestyle-related factors such as dietary habits, physical exercise, weight management, sleep, and stress control, they remain key predictors of when and how the disease develops. Advances in genomics have revealed widespread regulatory variation and ancestry-specific risks, while immunological findings underscore the contribution of persistent inflammation to disease progression and complications. Together, these findings underscore the need for integrated models that combine genetic, immunological, and environmental information to enhance risk assessment and therapeutic strategies. Precision medicine strategies, which utilize polygenic risk scores, immune markers, and pharmacogenetic findings, offer a path toward personalized prevention and treatment. Ultimately, addressing the dual genetic and immunological etiology of T2D may accelerate early detection, optimize treatment outcomes, and minimize the global burden of this multifactorial disease.

References

Abdulmuttaleb, N. A., Mohammed, M. Q., & Mohsein, O. A. (2024). Exploring the connection between inflammatory cytokines, hypertension, and diabetes in angina patients. *International Journal of Chemical and Biological Sciences, 6*(2), 52–62. https://doi.org/10.33545/26646765.2024.v6.i2a.103

Adeyemo, A., & Rotimi, C. (2009). Genetic variants associated with complex human diseases show wide variation across multiple populations. *Public Health Genomics, 13*(2), 72–79. https://doi.org/10.1159/000218711

Ageeva, E. S. (2024). The role of genetic factors in likelihood of type 2 diabetes mellitus. *Health Risk Analysis, 3*, 167–182. https://doi.org/10.21668/health.risk/2024.3.17.eng

Alipourfard, I., Datukishvili, N., & Mikeladze, D. (2019). TNF-α downregulation modifies insulin receptor substrate 1 (IRS-1) in metabolic signalling of diabetic insulin-resistant hepatocytes. *Mediators of Inflammation, 2019*(1), Article 3560819. https://doi.org/10.1155/2019/3560819

Almgren, P., Lehtovirta, M., Isomaa, B., Sarelin, L., Taskinen, M. R., Lyssenko, V., Tuomi, T., & Groop, L. (2011). Heritability and familiality of type 2 diabetes and related quantitative traits in the Botnia study. *Diabetologia, 54*(11), 2811–2819. https://doi.org/10.1007/s00125-011-2267-5

Altshuler, D., Hirschhorn, J. N., Klannemark, M., Lindgren, C. M., Vohl, M. C., Nemesh, J., Lane, C. R., Schaffner, S. F., Bolk, S., Brewer, C., Tuomi, T., Gaudet, D., Hudson, T. J., Daly, M., Groop, L., & Lander, E. S. (2000). The common PPARγ Pro12Ala polymorphism is associated with decreased risk of type 2 diabetes. *Nature Genetics, 26*(1), 76–80. https://doi.org/10.1038/79216

Arora, P., Garcia-Bailo, B., Dastani, Z., Brenner, D., Villegas, A., Malik, S., Spector, T. D., Richards, B., El-Sohemy, A., Karmali, M., & Badawi, A. (2011). Genetic polymorphisms of innate immunity-related inflammatory pathways and their association with factors related to type 2 diabetes. *BMC Medical Genetics, 12*(1), 95. https://doi.org/10.1186/1471-2350-12-95

Aune, D., Norat, T., Leitzmann, M., Tonstad, S., & Vatten, L. J. (2015). Physical activity and the risk of type 2 diabetes: A systematic review and dose-response meta-analysis. *European Journal of Epidemiology, 30*(7), 529–542. https://doi.org/10.1007/s10654-015-0056-z

Bahrami, A., Sathyapalan, T., & Sahebkar, A. (2021). The role of Interleukin-18 in the development and progression of atherosclerosis. *Current Medicinal Chemistry, 28*(9), 1757–1774. https://doi.org/10.2174/0929867327666200427095830

Banerjee, M. (2014). Genetic polymorphisms of cytokine genes in type 2 diabetes mellitus. *World Journal of Diabetes, 5*(4), 493. https://doi.org/10.4239/wjd.v5.i4.493

Beagley, J., Guariguata, L., Weil, C., & Motala, A. A. (2014). *Global estimates of undiagnosed diabetes in adults*. Retrieved September 11, 2025, from www.diabetesresearchclinicalpractice.com/article/S0168-8227(13)00384-7/fulltext.

Beaudelaire Tsiaze, E., Huang, Y.-C., Bombek, L. K., Yang, S.-B., Jevšek, M., Seino, S., & Slak Rupnik, M. (2012). Age-dependent changes in the exocytotic efficacy in Kir6.2 ablated mouse pancreatic β-cells. *Open Journal of Molecular and Integrative Physiology, 02*(03), 51–60. https://doi.org/10.4236/ojmip.2012.23008

Bhat, O. M., & Dhawan, V. (2015). *Role of IL-18 and its signalling in atherosclerosis.*

Biswas, A., Oh, P. I., Faulkner, G. E., Bajaj, R. R., Silver, M. A., Mitchell, M. S., & Alter, D. A. (2015). Sedentary time and its association with risk for disease incidence, mortality, and hospitalization in adults a systematic review and meta-analysis. *Annals of Internal Medicine, 162*(2), 123–132. https://doi.org/10.7326/M14-1651

Blériot, C., Dalmas, É., Ginhoux, F., & Venteclef, N. (2023). Inflammatory and immune etiology of type 2 diabetes. *Trends in Immunology, 44*(2), 101–109. https://doi.org/10.1016/j.it.2022.12.004

Booker, C. (2013). *Inflammation in type 2 diabetes and the neuroendocrine role of IL-18.*

Bouatia-Naji, N., Bonnefond, A., Cavalcanti-Proença, C., Sparsø, T., Holmkvist, J., Marchand, M., Delplanque, J., Lobbens, S., Rocheleau, G., Durand, E., De Graeve, F., Chèvre, J. C., Borch-Johnsen, K., Hartikainen, A. L., Ruokonen, A., Tichet, J., Marre, M., Weill, J., Heude, B., … Froguel, P. (2009). A variant near MTNR1B is associated with increased fasting plasma glucose levels and type 2 diabetes risk. *Nature Genetics, 41*(1), 89–94. https://doi.org/10.1038/ng.277

Cai, Z., Huang, Y., & He, B. (2022). New insights into adipose tissue macrophages in obesity and insulin resistance. *Cells, 11*(9), 1424. https://doi.org/10.3390/cells11091424

Cavalcante, J. E. A., de Sousa, E. L. H., de Oliveira Rodrigues, R., de Almeida Viana, G., Duarte Gadelha, D., de Carvalho, M. M. D., Sousa, D. L., Silva, A. J. X., Filho, R. R. B. X., Fernandes, V. O., Montenegro Júnior, R. M., de Sousa Alves, R., Meneses, G. C., Sampaio, T. L., & Queiroz, M. G. R. (2020). Interleukin-18 promoter −137 G/C polymorphism (rs187238) is associated with biochemical markers of renal function and cardiovascular disease in type 2 diabetes patients. *Clinical Biochemistry, 80*, 1–7. https://doi.org/10.1016/j.clinbiochem.2020.03.011

Cornelis, M. C., Qi, L., Kraft, P., & Hu, F. B. (2009). TCF7L2, dietary carbohydrate, and risk of type 2 diabetes in US women. *American Journal of Clinical Nutrition, 89*(4), 1256–1262. https://doi.org/10.3945/ajcn.2008.27058

Dludla, P. V., Mabhida, S. E., Ziqubu, K., Nkambule, B. B., Mazibuko-Mbeje, S. E., Hanser, S., Basson, A. K., Pheiffer, C., & Kengne, A. P. (2023). Pancreatic β-cell dysfunction in type 2 diabetes: Implications of inflammation and oxidative stress. *World Journal of Diabetes, 14*(3), 130–146. https://doi.org/10.4239/wjd.v14.i3.130

Doria, A., Patti, M. E., & Kahn, C. R. (2008). The emerging genetic architecture of type 2 diabetes. *Cell Metabolism, 8*(3), 186–200. https://doi.org/10.1016/j.cmet.2008.08.006

Dropulic, L. K., & Lederman, H. M. (2016). Overview of infections in the immunocompromised host. *Microbiology Spectrum, 4*(4), 4. https://doi.org/10.1128/microbiolspec.DMIH2-0026-2016

Duncan, B. B., & Schmidt, M. I. (2006). The epidemiology of low-grade chronic systemic inflammation and type 2 diabetes. *Diabetes Technology & Therapeutics, 8*(1), 7–17. https://doi.org/10.1089/dia.2006.8.7

Duncan, L., Shen, H., Gelaye, B., Meijsen, J., Ressler, K., Feldman, M., Peterson, R., & Domingue, B. (2019). Analysis of polygenic risk score usage and performance in diverse human populations. *Nature Communications, 10*(1). https://doi.org/10.1038/s41467-019-11112-0

Dyson, P. (2016). Prevalence, public health aspects and prevention of diabetes. In *Advanced nutrition and dietetics in diabetes* (pp. 1–8). John Wiley & Sons, Ltd. https://doi.org/10.1002/9781119121725.ch1

Enni, M. A., & Mahmud, S. (2024). A systematic review of snp polymorphism studies in south asian populations: Implications for diabetes and autoimmune disorders. *American Journal of Scholarly Research and Innovation, 03*(01), 20–51. https://doi.org/10.63125/8nvxcb96

Esposito, K., Maiorino, M. I., Petrizzo, M., Bellastella, G., & Giugliano, D. (2014). The effects of a mediterranean diet on the need for diabetes drugs and remission of newly diagnosed type 2 diabetes: Follow-up of a randomized trial. *Diabetes Care, 37*(7), 1824–1830. https://doi.org/10.2337/dc13-2899

Esser, N., Paquot, N., & Scheen, A. J. (2015). Anti-inflammatory agents to treat or prevent type 2 diabetes, metabolic syndrome and cardiovascular disease. *Expert Opinion on Investigational Drugs, 24*(3), 283–307. https://doi.org/10.1517/13543784.2015.974804

Eze, I. C., Hemkens, L. G., Bucher, H. C., Hoffmann, B., Schindler, C., Künzli, N., Schikowski, T., & Probst-Hensch, N. M. (2015). Review association between ambient air pollution and diabetes mellitus in Europe. *Environmental Health Perspectives, 123*(5), 381–389.

Flannick, J., Thorleifsson, G., Beer, N. L., Jacobs, S. B. R., Grarup, N., Burtt, N. P., Mahajan, A., Fuchsberger, C., Atzmon, G., Benediktsson, R., Blangero, J., Bowden, D. W., Brandslund, I., Brosnan, J., Burslem, F., Chambers, J., Cho, Y. S., Christensen, C., Douglas, D. A., … Altshuler, D. (2014). Loss-of-function mutations in SLC30A8 protect against type 2 diabetes. *Nature Genetics, 46*(4), 357–363. https://doi.org/10.1038/ng.2915

Frayling, T. M., Timpson, N. J., Weedon, M. N., Zeggini, E., Freathy, R. M., Lindgren, C. M., Perry, J. R. B., Elliott, K. S., Lango, H., Rayner, N. W., Shields, B., Harries, L. W., Barrett, J. C., Ellard, S., Groves, C. J., Knight, B., Patch, A. M., Ness, A. R., Ebrahim, S., … McCarthy, M. I. (2007). A common variant in the FTO gene is associated with body mass index and predisposes to childhood and adult obesity. *Science, 316*(5826), 889–894. https://doi.org/10.1126/science.1141634

Fuchsberger, C., Flannick, J., Teslovich, T. M., Mahajan, A., Agarwala, V., Gaulton, K. J., Ma, C., Fontanillas, P., Moutsianas, L., McCarthy, D. J., Rivas, M. A., Perry, J. R. B., Sim, X., Blackwell, T. W., Robertson, N. R., Rayner, N. W., Cingolani, P., Locke, A. E., Tajes, J. F., … McCarthy, M. I. (2016). The genetic architecture of type 2 diabetes. *Nature, 536*(7614), 41–47. https://doi.org/10.1038/nature18642

Gao, Q., Huan, C., Jia, Z., Cao, Q., Yuan, P., Li, X., Wang, C., Mao, Z., & Huo, W. (2024). SOCS3 methylation partially mediated the association of exposure to triclosan but not triclocarban with type 2 diabetes mellitus: A case-control study. *International Journal of Molecular Sciences, 25*(22), Article 12113. https://doi.org/10.3390/ijms252212113

Garcia-Martinez, I., Shaker, M. E., & Mehal, W. Z. (2015). Therapeutic opportunities in damage-associated molecular pattern-driven metabolic diseases. *Antioxidants and Redox Signaling, 23*(17), 1305–1315. https://doi.org/10.1089/ars.2015.6383

Ghareeb, D., Abdelazem, A. S., Hussein, E. M., & Al-Karamany, A. S. (2021). Association of TNF-α-308 G>A (rs1800629) polymorphism with susceptibility of metabolic syndrome. *Journal of Diabetes and Metabolic Disorders, 20*(1), 209–215. https://doi.org/10.1007/s40200-021-00732-3

Gloyn, A. L., Weedon, M. N., Owen, K. R., Turner, M. J., Knight, B. A., Hitman, G., Walker, M., Levy, J. C., Sampson, M., Halford, S., Mccarthy, M. I., Hattersley, A. T., & Frayling, T. M. (2003). Brief genetics report. *Diabetes, 52*(February).

Gloyn, A. L., Pearson, E. R., Antcliff, J. F., Proks, P., Bruining, G. J., Slingerland, A. S., Howard, N., Srinivasan, S., Silva, J. M. C. L., Molnes, J., Edghill, E. L., Frayling, T. M., Temple, I. K., Mackay, D., Shield, J. P. H., Sumnik, Z., van Rhijn, A., Wales, J. K. H., Clark, P., ... Hattersley, A. T. (2004). Activating mutations in the gene encoding the ATP-sensitive potassium-channel subunit Kir6.2 and permanent neonatal diabetes. *New England Journal of Medicine, 350*(18), 1838–1849. https://doi.org/10.1056/nejmoa032922

Golden, T. N., & Simmons, R. A. (2021). Immune dysfunction in developmental programming of type 2 diabetes mellitus. *Nature Reviews Endocrinology, 17*(4), 235–245. https://doi.org/10.1038/s41574-020-00464-z

Gora, I. M., Ciechanowska, A., & Ladyzynski, P. (2021). NLRP3 inflammasome at the interface of inflammation, endothelial dysfunction, and type 2 diabetes. *Cells, 10*(2), 314. https://doi.org/10.3390/cells10020314

Grant, S. F. A., Thorleifsson, G., Reynisdottir, I., Benediktsson, R., Manolescu, A., Sainz, J., Helgason, A., Stefansson, H., Emilsson, V., Helgadottir, A., Styrkarsdottir, U., Magnusson, K. P., Walters, G. B., Palsdottir, E., Jonsdottir, T., Gudmundsdottir, T., Gylfason, A., Saemundsdottir, J., Wilensky, R. L., ... Stefansson, K. (2006). Variant of transcription factor 7-like 2 (TCF7L2) gene confers risk of type 2 diabetes. *Nature Genetics, 38*(3), 320–323. https://doi.org/10.1038/ng1732

Guarnotta, V., Bianco, M. J., Vigneri, E., Panto', F., Lo Sasso, B., Ciaccio, M., Pizzolanti, G., & Giordano, C. (2021). Effects of GLP-1 receptor agonists on myokine levels and pro-inflammatory cytokines in patients with type 2 diabetes mellitus. *Nutrition, Metabolism, and Cardiovascular Diseases, 31*(11), 3193–3201. https://doi.org/10.1016/j.numecd.2021.07.015

Guria, S., Hoory, A., Das, S., Chattopadhyay, D., & Mukherjee, S. (2023). Adipose tissue macrophages and their role in obesity-associated insulin resistance: An overview of the complex dynamics at play. *Bioscience Reports, 43*(3), Article BSR20220200. https://doi.org/10.1042/BSR20220200

Hameed, I., Masoodi, S. R., Mir, S. A., Nabi, M., Ghazanfar, K., & Ganai, B. A. (2015). *Type 2 diabetes mellitus: From a metabolic disorder to an inflammatory condition.* Retrieved September 12, 2025, from https://pmc.ncbi.nlm.nih.gov/articles/PMC4434080/.

Harding, J. L., Weber, M. B., & Shaw, J. E. (2024). The global burden of diabetes. In *Textbook of diabetes* (pp. 28–40). John Wiley & Sons, Ltd. https://doi.org/10.1002/9781119697473.ch3

Harmon, D. B., Srikakulapu, P., Kaplan, J. L., Oldham, S. N., McSkimming, C., Garmey, J. C., Perry, H. M., Kirby, J. L., Prohaska, T. A., Gonen, A., Hallowell, P., Schirmer, B., Tsimikas, S., Taylor, A. M., Witztum, J. L., & McNamara, C. A. (2016). Protective role for B-1b B cells and IgM in obesity-associated inflammation, glucose intolerance, and insulin resistance. *Arteriosclerosis, Thrombosis, and Vascular Biology, 36*(4), 682–691. https://doi.org/10.1161/ATVBAHA.116.307166

Hoseini, F., Mahmazi, S., Mahmoodi, K., Ali Jafari, G., & Soltanpour, M. S. (2018). Evaluation of the role of -137G/C single nucleotide polymorphism (rs187238) and gene expression levels of the IL-18 in patients with coronary artery disease. *Oman Medical Journal, 33*(2), 118–125. https://doi.org/10.5001/omj.2018.23

Ingelheim, B., Nordisk, N., Ingelheim, B., Lilly, E., Nordisk, N., Ingelheim, B., Lilly, E., Nordisk, N., Pharmaceuticals, B., Respironics, P., Ingelheim, B., Lilly, E., Nordisk, N., Ingelheim, B., Nordisk, N., Hutchinson, F., & Hospital, G. G. (2022). *HHS Public Access, 54*(5), 560–572. https://doi.org/10.1038/s41588-022-01058-3. Users.

Intervention, L., & Metformin, O. R. (2002). Reduction of the incidence of type 2 diabetes with lifestyle intervention or metformin. *International Urology and Nephrology, 34*(1), 162–163. https://doi.org/10.1097/01.ogx.0000055759.75837.e7

Jafar, N., Edriss, H., & Nugent, K. (2016). The effect of short-term hyperglycemia on the innate immune system. Retrieved September 12, 2025, from www.amjmedsci.org/article/S0002-9629(15)00027-0/abstract.

Khera, A. V., Chaffin, M., Aragam, K. G., Haas, M. E., Roselli, C., Choi, S. H., Natarajan, P., Lander, E. S., Lubitz, S. A., Ellinor, P. T., & Kathiresan, S. (2018). Genome-wide polygenic scores for common diseases identify individuals with risk equivalent to monogenic mutations. *Nature Genetics, 50*(9), 1219–1224. https://doi.org/10.1038/s41588-018-0183-z

King, B. C., & Blom, A. M. (2021). Complement in metabolic disease: Metaflammation and a two-edged sword. *Seminars in Immunopathology, 43*(6), 829–841. https://doi.org/10.1007/s00281-021-00873-w

Knowler, W. C., Pettitt, D. J., Savage, P. J., & Bennett, P. H. (1981). Diabetes incidence in pima indians: Contributions of obesity and parental diabetes. *American Journal of Epidemiology, 113*(2), 144–156. https://doi.org/10.1093/oxfordjournals.aje.a113079

Kochumon, S., Al Madhoun, A., Al-Rashed, F., Thomas, R., Sindhu, S., Al-Ozairi, E., Al-Mulla, F., & Ahmad, R. (2020). Elevated adipose tissue associated IL-2 expression in obesity correlates with metabolic inflammation and insulin resistance. *Scientific Reports, 10*(1), Article 16364. https://doi.org/10.1038/s41598-020-73347-y

Koh, Y.-C., Yang, G., Lai, C.-S., Weerawatanakorn, M., & Pan, M.-H. (2018). Chemopreventive effects of phytochemicals and medicines on M1/M2 polarized macrophage role in inflammation-related diseases. *International Journal of Molecular Sciences, 19*(8), 2208. https://doi.org/10.3390/ijms19082208

Kuryłowicz, A., & Koźniewski, K. (2020). Anti-inflammatory strategies targeting metaflammation in type 2 diabetes. *Molecules, 25*(9), 2224. https://doi.org/10.3390/molecules25092224

Laigle, L., Chadli, L., & Moingeon, P. (2023). Biomarker-driven development of new therapies for autoimmune diseases: Current status and future promises. *Expert Review of Clinical Immunology, 19*(3), 305–314. https://doi.org/10.1080/1744666X.2023.2172404

Lana, J. P., de Oliveira, M. C., Silveira, A. L. M., Yamada, L. T. P., Costa, K. A., da Silva, S. V., de Assis-Ferreira, A., Gautier, E. L., Dussaud, S., Pinho, V., Teixeira, M. M., Marcelin, G., Clément, K., & Ferreira, A. V. M. (2024). Role of IL-18 in adipose tissue remodeling and metabolic dysfunction. *International Journal of Obesity, 48*(7), 964–972. https://doi.org/10.1038/s41366-024-01507-5

Larsson, S. C., & Wolk, A. (2007). Magnesium intake and risk of type 2 diabetes: A meta-analysis. *Journal of Internal Medicine, 262*(2), 208–214. https://doi.org/10.1111/j.1365-2796.2007.01840.x

Le, T. N., Bright, R., Truong, V.-K., Li, J., Juneja, R., & Vasilev, K. (2025). Key biomarkers in type 2 diabetes patients: A systematic review. *Diabetes, Obesity and Metabolism, 27*(1), 7–22. https://doi.org/10.1111/dom.15991

Lehmann, J. M., Moore, L. B., Smith-Oliver, T. A., Wilkison, W. O., Willson, T. M., & Kliewer, S. A. (1995). An antidiabetic thiazolidinedione is a high affinity ligand for peroxisome proliferator-activated receptor γ (PPARγ). *Journal of Biological Chemistry, 270*(22), 12953–12956. https://doi.org/10.1074/jbc.270.22.12953

Levy, B. I., Schiffrin, E. L., Mourad, J.-J., Agostini, D., Vicaut, E., Safar, M. E., & Struijker-Boudier, H. A. J. (2008). Impaired tissue perfusion. *Circulation, 118*(9), 968–976. https://doi.org/10.1161/CIRCULATIONAHA.107.763730

Li, H., Khor, C. C., Fan, J., Lv, J., Yu, C., Guo, Y., Bian, Z., Yang, L., Millwood, I. Y., Walters, R. G., Chen, Y., Yuan, J. M., Yang, Y., Hu, C., Chen, J., Chen, Z., Koh, W. P., Huang, T., & Li, L. (2020). Riesgo genético, adherencia a un estilo de vida saludable y riesgo de diabetes tipo 2 entre 550 000 adultos chinos: Resultados de 2 cohortes asiáticas independientes. *American Journal of Clinical Nutrition, 111*(3), 698–707.

Li, H., Meng, Y., He, S., Tan, X., Zhang, Y., Zhang, X., Wang, L., & Zheng, W. (2022). Macrophages, chronic inflammation, and insulin resistance. *Cells, 11*(19), 3001. https://doi.org/10.3390/cells11193001

Loos, R. J. F., & Yeo, G. S. H. (2014). The bigger picture of FTO - The first GWAS-identified obesity gene. *Nature Reviews Endocrinology, 10*(1), 51–61. https://doi.org/10.1038/nrendo.2013.227.The

Lubrano, V., Sabatino, L., Papa, A., & Balzan, S. (2025). Interleukin-6, C-Reactive protein and fibrinogen: Novel insights as inflammatory risk factors in atherosclerosis and diabetes. *Medicine and Pharmacology*. https://doi.org/10.20944/preprints202504.0133.v1

Lyssenko, V., Almgren, P., Anevski, D., Perfekt, R., Lahti, K., Nissén, M., Isomaa, B., Forsen, B., Homström, N., Saloranta, C., Taskinen, M. R., Groop, L., & Tuomi, T. (2005). Predictors of and longitudinal changes in insulin sensitivity and secretion preceding onset of type 2 diabetes. *Diabetes, 54*(1), 166–174. https://doi.org/10.2337/diabetes.54.1.166

Lyssenko, V., Lupi, R., Marchetti, P., Del Guerra, S., Orho-Melander, M., Almgren, P., Sjögren, M., Ling, C., Eriksson, K. F., Lethagen, Å. L., Mancarella, R., Berglund, G., Tuomi, T., Nilsson, P., Del Prato, S., & Groop, L. (2007). Mechanisms by which common variants in the TCF7L2 gene increase risk of type 2 diabetes. *Journal of Clinical Investigation, 117*(8), 2155–2163. https://doi.org/10.1172/JCI30706

Ma, R. C. W., & Tong, P. C. Y. (2024). Epidemiology of type 2 diabetes. In *Textbook of diabetes* (pp. 55–74). John Wiley & Sons, Ltd. https://doi.org/10.1002/9781119697473.ch5

Mahajan, A., Taliun, D., Thurner, M., Robertson, N. R., Torres, J. M., Rayner, N. W., Payne, A. J., Steinthorsdottir, V., Scott, R. A., Grarup, N., Cook, J. P., Schmidt, E. M., Wuttke, M., Sarnowski, C., Mägi, R., Nano, J., Gieger, C., Trompet, S., Lecoeur, C., ... McCarthy, M. I. (2018). Fine-mapping type 2 diabetes loci to single-variant resolution using high-density imputation and islet-specific epigenome maps. *Nature Genetics, 50*(11), 1505–1513. https://doi.org/10.1038/s41588-018-0241-6

Mansour, A., Mousa, M., Abdelmannan, D., Tay, G., Hassoun, A., & Alsafar, H. (2023). Microvascular and macrovascular complications of type 2 diabetes mellitus: Exome wide association analyses. *Frontiers in Endocrinology, 14,* Article 1143067. https://doi.org/10.3389/fendo.2023.1143067

Martin, A. R., Kanai, M., Kamatani, Y., Okada, Y., Neale, B. M., & Daly, M. J. (2019). Clinical use of current polygenic risk scores may exacerbate health disparities. *Nature Genetics, 51*(4), 584–591. https://doi.org/10.1038/s41588-019-0379-x

Memisoglu, A., Hu, F. B., Hankinson, S. E., Manson, J. A. E., De Vivo, I., Willett, W. C., & Hunter, D. J. (2003). Interaction between a peroxisome proliferator-activated receptor γ gene polymorphism and dietary fat intake in relation to body mass. *Human Molecular Genetics, 12*(22), 2923–2929. https://doi.org/10.1093/hmg/ddg318

Moller, D. E. (2000). *Potential role of TNF-α in the pathogenesis of insulin resistance and type 2 diabetes.* Retrieved September 12, 2025, from www.cell.com/trends/endocrinology-metabolism/abstract/S1043-2760(00)00272-1.

Moltke, I., Grarup, N., Jørgensen, M. E., Bjerregaard, P., Treebak, J. T., Fumagalli, M., Korneliussen, T. S., Andersen, M. A., Nielsen, T. S., Krarup, N. T., Gjesing, A. P., Zierath, J. R., Linneberg, A., Wu, X., Sun, G., Jin, X., Al-Aama, J., Wang, J., Borch-Johnsen, K., ... Hansen, T. (2014). A common Greenlandic TBC1D4 variant confers muscle insulin resistance and type 2 diabetes. *Nature, 512*(7513), 190–193. https://doi.org/10.1038/nature13425

Negre-Salvayre, A., Salvayre, R., Augé, N., Pamplona, R., & Portero-Otín, M. (2009). Hyperglycemia and glycation in diabetic complications. *Antioxidants and Redox Signaling, 11*(12), 3071–3109. https://doi.org/10.1089/ars.2009.2484

Nikolajczyk, B. S. (2010). B cells as under-appreciated mediators of non-auto-immune inflammatory disease. *Cytokine, 50*(3), 234–242. https://doi.org/10.1016/j.cyto.2010.02.022

Ningrum, V. D. A., Sadewa, A. H., Ikawati, Z., Yuliwulandari, R., Ikhsan, M. R., & Fajriyah, R. (2022). The influence of metformin transporter gene SLC22A1 and SLC47A1 variants on steady-state pharmacokinetics and glycemic response. *PLoS One, 17*(7 July), 1–12. https://doi.org/10.1371/journal.pone.0271410

Nirenjen, S., Narayanan, J., Tamilanban, T., Subramaniyan, V., Chitra, V., Fuloria, N. K., Wong, L. S., Ramachawolran, G., Sekar, M., Gupta, G., Fuloria, S., Chinni, S. V., & Selvaraj, S. (2023). Exploring the contribution of pro-inflammatory cytokines to impaired wound healing in diabetes. *Frontiers in Immunology, 14,* Article 1216321. https://doi.org/10.3389/fimmu.2023.1216321

Noack, M., & Miossec, P. (2014). Th17 and regulatory T cell balance in autoimmune and inflammatory diseases. *Autoimmunity Reviews, 13*(6), 668–677. https://doi.org/10.1016/j.autrev.2013.12.004

Pan, A., Sun, Q., Bernstein, A. M., Schulze, M. B., Manson, J. A. E., Willett, W. C., & Hu, F. B. (2011). Red meat consumption and risk of type 2 diabetes: 3 Cohorts of US adults and an updated meta-analysis. *American Journal of Clinical Nutrition, 94*(4), 1088–1096. https://doi.org/10.3945/ajcn.111.018978

Parker, S. C. J., Stitzel, M. L., Taylor, D. L., Orozco, J. M., Erdos, M. R., Akiyama, J. A., Van Bueren, K. L., Chines, P. S., Narisu, N., Black, B. L., Axel, V., Pennacchio, L. A., & Collins, F. S. (2013). Chromatin stretch enhancer states drive cell-specific gene regulation and harbor human disease risk variants. *Proceedings of the National Academy of Sciences of the United States of America, 110*(44), 17921–17926. https://doi.org/10.1073/pnas.1317023110

Pearson, E. R. (2019). Diabetes tipo 2: Una enfermedad multifacética. *Diabetologia, 62*(7), 1107–1112.

Pei, J., Wang, B., & Wang, D. (2022). Current studies on molecular mechanisms of insulin resistance. *Journal of Diabetes Research, 2022*(1), Article 1863429. https://doi.org/10.1155/2022/1863429

Peiró, C., Lorenzo, Ó., Carraro, R., & Sánchez-Ferrer, C. F. (2017). IL-1β inhibition in cardiovascular complications associated to diabetes mellitus. *Frontiers in Pharmacology, 8,* 363. https://doi.org/10.3389/fphar.2017.00363

Peppler, W. T., Townsend, L. K., Meers, G. M., Panasevich, M. R., MacPherson, R. E. K., Rector, R. S., & Wright, D. C. (2019). Acute administration of IL-6 improves indices of hepatic glucose and insulin homeostasis in lean and obese mice. *American Journal of Physiology - Gastrointestinal and Liver Physiology, 316*(1), G166–G178. https://doi.org/10.1152/ajpgi.00097.2018

Pirola, L., & Ferraz, J. C. (2017). Role of pro- and anti-inflammatory phenomena in the physiopathology of type 2 diabetes and obesity. *World Journal of Biological Chemistry, 8*(2), 120. https://doi.org/10.4331/wjbc.v8.i2.120

Poulsen, P., Ohm Kyvik, K., Vaag, A., & Beck-Nielsen, H. (1999). Heritability of type II (non-insulin-dependent) diabetes mellitus and abnormal glucose tolerance—A population-based twin study. *Diabetologia, 42*(2), 139–145. https://doi.org/10.1007/s001250051131

Qidwai, T., & Khan, F. (2011). Tumour necrosis factor gene polymorphism and disease prevalence. *Scandinavian Journal of Immunology, 74*(6), 522–547. https://doi.org/10.1111/j.1365-3083.2011.02602.x

Raboudi, S. H., Mitchell, B. D., Stern, M. P., Eifler, C. W., Haffner, S. M., Hazuda, H. P., & Frazier, M. L. (1989). Type II diabetes mellitus and polymorphism of insulin-receptor gene in Mexican Americans. *Diabetes, 38*(8), 975–980. https://doi.org/10.2337/diab.38.8.975

Ramanjaneya, M., Bettahi, I., Jerobin, J., Chandra, P., Abi Khalil, C., Skarulis, M., Atkin, S. L., & Abou-Samra, A.-B. (2019). Mitochondrial-derived peptides are Down regulated in diabetes subjects. *Frontiers in Endocrinology, 10,* 331. https://doi.org/10.3389/fendo.2019.00331

Reda, E., Hassaneen, S., & El-Abhar, H. S. (2018). Novel trajectories of bromocriptine antidiabetic action: Leptin-IL-6/JAK2/p-STAT3/SOCS3, p-IR/p-AKT/GLUT4, PPAR-γ/Adiponectin, Nrf2/PARP-1, and GLP-1. *Frontiers in Pharmacology, 9,* 771. https://doi.org/10.3389/fphar.2018.00771

Rehman, K., Akash, M. S. H., Liaqat, A., Kamal, S., Qadir, M. I., & Rasul, A. (2017). Role of Interleukin-6 in development of insulin resistance and type 2 diabetes mellitus. Retrieved September 12, 2025, from www.dl.begellhouse.com/journals/6dbf508d3b17c437,3e1db9ff199ae23c,00d983fb2791ab09.html.

Rönn, T., Ofori, J. K., Perfilyev, A., Hamilton, A., Pircs, K., Eichelmann, F., Garcia-Calzon, S., Karagiannopoulos, A., Stenlund, H., Wendt, A., Volkov, P., Schulze, M. B., Mulder, H., Eliasson, L., Ruhrmann, S., Bacos, K., & Ling, C. (2023). Genes with epigenetic alterations in human pancreatic islets impact mitochondrial function, insulin secretion, and type 2 diabetes. *Nature Communications, 14*(1). https://doi.org/10.1038/s41467-023-43719-9

Ruggenenti, P., Bettinaglio, P., Pinares, F., & Remuzzi, G. (2008). Angiotensin converting enzyme insertion/deletion polymorphism and renoprotection in diabetic and nondiabetic nephropathies.

Clinical Journal of the American Society of Nephrology, 3(5), 1511–1525. https://doi.org/10.2215/CJN.04140907

Rung, J., Cauchi, S., Albrechtsen, A., Shen, L., Rocheleau, G., Cavalcanti-Proença, C., Bacot, F., Balkau, B., Belisle, A., Borch-Johnsen, K., Charpentier, G., Dina, C., Durand, E., Elliott, P., Hadjadj, S., Järvelin, M. R., Laitinen, J., Lauritzen, T., Marre, M., … Sladek, R. (2009). Genetic variant near IRS1 is associated with type 2 diabetes, insulin resistance and hyperinsulinemia. *Nature Genetics, 41*(10), 1110–1115. https://doi.org/10.1038/ng.443

Saetang, J., & Sangkhathat, S. (2017). Role of innate lymphoid cells in obesity and metabolic disease (review). *Molecular Medicine Reports, 17*(1), 1403–1412. https://doi.org/10.3892/mmr.2017.8038

Selvam, C., Mutisyab, D., Prakashc, S., et al. (2017). 乳鼠心肌提取 HHS public access. *Physiology & Behavior, 176*(1), 139–148. https://doi.org/10.1038/s41588-018-0183-z.Genome-wide

Shan, Z., Ma, H., Xie, M., Yan, P., Guo, Y., Bao, W., Rong, Y., Jackson, C. L., Hu, F. B., & Liu, L. (2015). Sleep duration and risk of type 2 diabetes: A meta-analysis of prospective studies. *Diabetes Care, 38*(3), 529–537. https://doi.org/10.2337/dc14-2073

Shapouri-Moghaddam, A., Mohammadian, S., Vazini, H., Taghadosi, M., Esmaeili, S., Mardani, F., Seifi, B., Mohammadi, A., Afshari, J. T., & Sahebkar, A. (2018). Macrophage plasticity, polarization, and function in health and disease. *Journal of Cellular Physiology, 233*(9), 6425–6440. https://doi.org/10.1002/jcp.26429

Shi, J., Fan, J., Su, Q., & Yang, Z. (2019). Cytokines and abnormal glucose and lipid metabolism. *Frontiers in Endocrinology, 10*, 703. https://doi.org/10.3389/fendo.2019.00703

Sladek, R., Rocheleau, G., Rung, J., Dina, C., Shen, L., Serre, D., Boutin, P., Vincent, D., Belisle, A., Hadjadj, S., Balkau, B., Heude, B., Charpentier, G., Hudson, T. J., Montpetit, A., Pshezhetsky, A. V., Prentki, M., Posner, B. I., Balding, D. J., … Froguel, P. (2007). A genome-wide association study identifies novel risk loci for type 2 diabetes. *Nature, 445*(7130), 881–885. https://doi.org/10.1038/nature05616

Speliotes, E. K., Willer, C. J., Berndt, S. I., Monda, K. L., Thorleifsson, G., Jackson, A. U., Allen, H. L., Lindgren, C. M., Luan, J., Mägi, R., Randall, J. C., Vedantam, S., Winkler, T. W., Qi, L., Workalemahu, T., Heid, I., Steinthorsdottir, V., Stringham, H., Weedon, M. N., … Loos, R. J. F. (2010). Association analyses of 249,796 individuals reveal 18 new loci associated with body mass index. *Nature Genetics, 42*(11), 937–948. https://doi.org/10.1038/ng.686

Stanimirovic, J., Radovanovic, J., Banjac, K., Obradovic, M., Essack, M., Zafirovic, S., Gluvic, Z., Gojobori, T., & Isenovic, E. R. (2022). Role of C-Reactive protein in diabetic inflammation. *Mediators of Inflammation, 2022*(1), Article 3706508. https://doi.org/10.1155/2022/3706508

Steinthorsdottir, V., Thorleifsson, G., Reynisdottir, I., Benediktsson, R., Jonsdottir, T., Walters, G. B., Styrkarsdottir, U., Gretarsdottir, S., Emilsson, V., Ghosh, S., Baker, A., Snorradottir, S., Bjarnason, H., Ng, M. C. Y., Hansen, T., Bagger, Y., Wilensky, R. L., Reilly, M. P., Adeyemo, A., … Stefansson, K. (2007). A variant in CDKAL1 influences insulin response and risk of type 2 diabetes. *Nature Genetics, 39*(6), 770–775. https://doi.org/10.1038/ng2043

Sylvia, H. L., et al. (2016). *Prevention and mangement of type 2 Diabetes- dietary compnents and nut strategies. *The Lancet, 383*(9933), 1999–2007. https://doi.org/10.1016/S0140-6736(14)60613-9

Strawbridge, R. J., Dupuis, J., Prokopenko, I., Barker, A., Ahlqvist, E., Rybin, D., Petrie, J. R., Travers, M. E., Bouatia-Naji, N., Dimas, A. S., Nica, A. C., Wheeler, E., Chen, H., Voight, B. F., Taneera, J., Kanoni, S., Peden, J. F., Turrini, F., Gustafsson, S., … Florez, J. C. (2011). Genome-wide association identifies nine common variants associated with fasting proinsulin levels and provides new insights into the pathophysiology of type 2 diabetes. *Diabetes, 60*(10), 2624–2634. https://doi.org/10.2337/db11-0415

Swan, H. J. C. (2000). The Framingham offspring study: A commentary. *Journal of the American College of Cardiology, 35*(5 Suppl. B), 2201–2207. https://doi.org/10.1016/s0735-1097(00)90009-3

Thomas, M. C. (2022). The clustering of cardiovascular, renal, adipo-metabolic eye and liver disease with type 2 diabetes. *Metabolism, 128*, Article 154961. https://doi.org/10.1016/j.metabol.2021.154961

Tk, I., & Gotthardov, I. (2016). *Pharmacogenomics pharmacogenetic aspects of the treatment.*

Toumillehto, J., Lindström, J., Eriksson, J. G., Valle, T. T., & Uusitupa, M. (2013). Prevention of type 2 diabetes mellitus by changes in lifestyle among subjects with impaired glucose tolerance. *New England Journal of Medicine, 344*(18), 1343–1350.

Umapathy, D., Krishnamoorthy, E., Mariappanadar, V., Viswanathan, V., & Ramkumar, K. M. (2018). Increased levels of circulating (TNF-α) is associated with (-308G/A) promoter polymorphism of TNF-α gene in diabetic nephropathy. *International Journal of Biological Macromolecules, 107*, 2113–2121. https://doi.org/10.1016/j.ijbiomac.2017.10.078

Venieratos, P. D., Drossopoulou, G. I., Kapodistria, K. D., Tsilibary, E. C., & Kitsiou, P. V. (2010). High glucose induces suppression of insulin signalling and apoptosis via upregulation of endogenous IL-1β and suppressor of cytokine signalling-1 in mouse pancreatic beta cells. *Cellular Signalling, 22*(5), 791–800. https://doi.org/10.1016/j.cellsig.2010.01.003

Voight, B. F., Scott, L. J., Steinthorsdottir, V., Andrew, P., Aulchenko, Y. S., Thorleifsson, G., Mcculloch, L. J., & Ferreira, T. (2011). Europe PMC funders group twelve type 2 diabetes susceptibility loci identified through large-scale association analysis. *Nat. Genet., 42*(7), 579–589. https://doi.org/10.1038/ng.609

Wang, J., Qin, J., Li, Y., Cai, Z., Li, S., Zhu, J., Zhang, F., Liang, S., Zhang, W., Guan, Y., Shen, D., Peng, Y., Zhang, D., Jie, Z., Wu, W., Qin, Y., Xue, W., Li, J., Han, L., … Wang, J. (2012). A metagenome-wide association study of gut microbiota in type 2 diabetes. *Nature, 490*(7418), 55–60. https://doi.org/10.1038/nature11450

Williams Amy, A. L., Jacobs Suzanne, S. B. R., Moreno-Macías, H., Huerta-Chagoya, A., Churchhouse, C., Márquez-Luna, C., Gómez-Vázquez, M. J., Burtt Noël, N. P., Aguilar-Salinas, C. A., González-Villalpando, C., Florez, J. C., Orozco, L., Tusié-Luna, T., Altshuler, D., Ripke, S., Manning, A. K., García-Ortíz, H., Neale, B., Reich, D., … Orozco Lorena, L. (2014). Sequence variants in SLC16A11 are a common risk factor for type 2 diabetes in Mexico. *Nature, 506*(7486), 97–101. https://doi.org/10.1038/nature12828

Wilson, P. W. F., Meigs, J. B., Sullivan, L., Fox, C. S., Nathan, D. M., & D'Agostino, R. B. (2007). Prediction of incident diabetes mellitus in middle-aged adults: The framingham offspring study. *Archives of Internal Medicine, 167*(10), 1068–1074. https://doi.org/10.1001/archinte.167.10.1068

Withers, D. J., & White, M. (2000). Perspective: The insulin signalling system—A common link in the pathogenesis of type 2 diabetes. *Endocrinology, 141*(6), 1917–1921. https://doi.org/10.1210/endo.141.6.7584

Withers, D. J., Gutierrez, J. S., Towery, H., Burks, D. J., Ren, J. M., Previs, S., Zhang, Y., Bernal, D., Pons, S., Shulman, G. I., Bonner-Weir, S., & White, M. F. (1998). Disruption of IRS-2 causes type 2 diabetes in mice. *Nature, 391*(6670), 900–904. https://doi.org/10.1038/36116

Yasuda, K., Miyake, K., Horikawa, Y., Hara, K., Osawa, H., Furuta, H., Hirota, Y., Mori, H., Jonsson, A., Sato, Y., Yamagata, K., Hinokio, Y., Wang, H. Y., Tanahashi, T., Nakamura, N., Oka, Y., Iwasaki, N., Iwamoto, Y., Yamada, Y., … Kasuga, M. (2008). Variants in KCNQ1 are associated with susceptibility to type 2 diabetes mellitus. *Nature Genetics, 40*(9), 1092–1097. https://doi.org/10.1038/ng.207

Yoon, K. H., Lee, J. H., Kim, J. W., Cho, J. H., Choi, Y. H., Ko, S. H., Zimmet, P., & Son, H. Y. (2006). Epidemic obesity and type 2 diabetes in Asia. *Lancet, 368*(9548), 1681–1688. https://doi.org/10.1016/S0140-6736(06)69703-1

Yorifuji, T., Nagashima, K., Kurokawa, K., Kawai, M., Oishi, M., Akazawa, Y., Hosokawa, M., Yamada, Y., Inagaki, N., & Nakahata, T. (2005). The C42R mutation in the Kir6.2 (KCNJ11) gene as a cause of transient neonatal diabetes, childhood diabetes, or later-onset, apparently type 2 diabetes mellitus. *Journal of Clinical Endocrinology and Metabolism, 90*(6), 3174–3178. https://doi.org/10.1210/jc.2005-0096

Yuan, L., Zhang, L., Liu, X., Li, S., & Zou, J. (2023). Identification of differential immune cells and related diagnostic genes in patients with diabetic retinopathy. *Medicine, 102*(39), Article e35331. https://doi.org/10.1097/MD.0000000000035331

Zatterale, F., Longo, M., Naderi, J., Raciti, G. A., Desiderio, A., Miele, C., & Beguinot, F. (2020). Chronic adipose tissue inflammation linking obesity to insulin resistance and type 2 diabetes. *Frontiers in Physiology, 10,* 1607. https://doi.org/10.3389/fphys.2019.01607

Zheng, Y., Ley, S. H., & Hu, F. B. (2018). Global aetiology and epidemiology of type 2 diabetes mellitus and its complications. *Nature Reviews Endocrinology, 14*(2), 88–98. https://doi.org/10.1038/nrendo.2017.151

Zhou, J., Zhang, X., Ji, L., & Jiang, G. (2022). Identification of potential biomarkers of type 2 diabetes mellitus-related immune infiltration using weighted gene coexpression network analysis. *BioMed Research International, 2022*(1), Article 9920744. https://doi.org/10.1155/2022/9920744

Zi, C., He, L., Yao, H., Ren, Y., He, T., & Gao, Y. (2022). Changes of Th17 cells, regulatory T cells, Treg/Th17, IL-17 and IL-10 in patients with type 2 diabetes mellitus: A systematic review and meta-analysis. *Endocrine, 76*(2), 263–272. https://doi.org/10.1007/s12020-022-03043-6

16

Antibody-based therapies for type 2 diabetes mellitus (T2DM)

Shafat Ali[1] and Yahya F. Jamous[2]

[1]DEPARTMENT OF ZOOLOGY, HASSAN KHOYIHAMI MEMORIAL DEGREE COLLEGE, BANDIPORA, JAMMU & KASHMIR, INDIA;; [2]WELLNESS AND PREVENTIVE MEDICINE INSTITUTE, HEALTH SECTOR, KING ABDULAZIZ CITY FOR SCIENCE AND TECHNOLOGY, RIYADH, SAUDI ARABIA

1. Introduction

Type 2 diabetes mellitus (T2DM) has become a serious and rising health problem in the world. It is the most widespread form of diabetes mellitus, and it has been noted that it causes over 90% of cases that are increasing in prevalence steadily (WHO, 2025). The recent data show that the number of adults diagnosed with diabetes in the age group of 20–79 years was approximately 589 million, and the majority of the cases were T2DM (IDF, 2025). The distribution of this health crisis is uneven as approximately 80% of the patients with diabetes are residing in low-and middle-income countries, so it is a sign of inadequate healthcare facilities and resources (IDF, 2025). The prognoses are exposed, because it is projected that the adult population with diabetes will grow to 853 million in the year 2050 (IDF, 2025). This growth will be significantly contributed by such a combination of many socioeconomic, demographic, and environmental forces such as urbanization, aging population, and the emergence of physical inactivity and obesity that is on the increase (Gieroba et al., 2025). Without a check, the epidemic will cause the damage of the heart, blood vessels, eyes, kidneys, and nerves in the long run that is severe and, therefore, make the regulatory management strategies effective and innovative (WHO, 2025).

There is at least a list of nine classes of drugs that reduce glucose level, starting with metformin and sulfonylureas and ending with insulin. Nonetheless, there are a very few successful individuals with T2DM who manage to attain or sustain glycemic control in the long run. Therefore, they remain at the risk of the complications of high blood sugar as a chronic condition (Bailey, 2025). The traditional forms of treatment, which, until now, are the core of diabetes management, also have numerous problems. Among the critical issues that patients undergoing such treatments are concerned with are adverse

Type 2 Diabetes Mellitus. https://doi.org/10.1016/B978-0-443-33590-7.00016-2

effects, reduced effectiveness in the long run, and the inability to avoid hypoglycemia (Gieroba et al., 2025). Moreover, a highly heterogenous nature of the disease makes it difficult to use the same treatment option every time: T2DM advances by showing a number of different combinations of insulin resistance and pancreatic beta-cell dysfunction and, therefore, a patient would receive more benefit with an individual approach to treatment (Reyes-Medina et al., 2025). The issue is further complicated by the fact that surveys indicate that more than 40% of T2DM patients fail to bring their blood glucose levels to the desirable HbA1c levels. Along with the unavoidability of the disease, other causes of this problem include nonadherence to the treatment plan on the part of patients, change of medications by doctors, etc. (Bailey, 2025). The limitation of the existing modes of diabetes management is blaring, and it means there is still a distance to cover in the development of new approaches of managing diabetes that will serve the interests of the patients. The traditional small-molecule medications are limited, and this prompted the research to consider biologics (mAbs in particular) as the new drug of choice in treating type 2 diabetes mellitus. A series of technological advances including engineering of chimeric and humanized antibodies, phage display, and bispecific antibodies has contributed to the development of novel therapies using mAbs (Lu et al., 2025). As of 2025, FDA had authorized 144 antibody drugs, with as many as 1516 candidates under clinical trials throughout the world (Lu et al., 2025). The technology has proved highly successful in the treatment of most diseases especially cancers and has made it to the pinnacle with their availability of drugs that are highly specific and effective.

The rationale of using such a potent modality on T2DM is multifold. Firstly, there is the low-grade chronic inflammation as one of the crucial pathophysiological determinants of T2DM and insulin resistance (Gieroba et al., 2025). The proinflammatory cytokines are interleukin-6 (IL-6) and tumor necrosis factor-alpha (TNF-α) that result in insulin resistance and beta-cell apoptosis. This provides a justifiable explanation of the utilization of neutralizing antibodies toward these specific targets as was successfully applied in autoimmune disorders. Second, the antibody-based formats comprise antibody–drug conjugate (ADCs) with the potential to deliver therapeutic agents to cells or tissues in the pathophysiology of diabetes mellitus that can potentially alleviate off-target effects (Lu et al., 2025). Finally, despite the recent achievements witnessed with incretin-based peptide agonists (e.g., GLP-1 receptor agonists), there is current research that aims to utilize the antibodies and small molecules (that interact with incretin targets), which also implies a convergence between treatments (Bailey, 2025). The known efficacy of antibodies in other complicated chronic illnesses, coupled with their wide spectrum of engineering nimbleness, renders it a favorable alternative to address the ardent gaps in the administration of T2DM.

The purpose of this chapter is to research in detail the timeline and the predictable effects of antibody therapies on the treatment of T2DM. It will examine the pathophysiological mechanisms of T2DM that can be mediated by the antibodies such as inflammatory cytokines and receptors on the cells involved in insulin resistance. The chapter will include all the types of therapeutic antibodies, including naked monoclonal antibodies, bispecific antibodies, and ADCs, and assess the possibilities of these in the treatment of diabetes mellitus. In addition, it will provide an overview of the existing clinical data, an open debate on the challenges encountered by the biologic company in the chronic metabolic disease such as T2DM and prediction of future trends such as the integration of AI in designing antibodies and develop new modes of delivery. The key objective is to summarize the current experience and to promote the further development of the understanding about how the antibody-based approaches can transform the individual approach to the treatment of T2DM and, therefore, enhance the quality of life of the patient.

2. Pathophysiology of T2DM: Targets of antibodies

T2DM has a complex pathophysiology, thus making them a good disease to develop new biologic therapies that are specifically targeted. To discover the certain antigens that can be neutralized by monoclonal antibodies to stop the disease process, the primary defects of the metabolism and their molecular intermediates have to be revealed first. T2DM is characterized by two primary pathophysiological alterations including the insulin resistance in body tissues and the progressive deterioration of the secretory activity of the pancreatic beta-cells (Banday et al., 2020). Insulin resistance is a disorder in which the primary metabolic tissues, particularly, skeletal muscle, liver and adipose tissue, become less sensitive to insulin, thus leading to the reduced uptake of glucose and unrestrained hepatic glucose production (Khardori & Griffing, 2025). This disruption of metabolism forces the beta-cells of the pancreas to respond through the production of high levels of insulin, which is the so-called hyperinsulinemia that is the release of large amounts of insulin. However, in individuals who are genetically predisposed, the compensatory capacity of the beta-cells eventually leads to depletion. All the situations with beta-cell failure are now considered as a significant factor in defining the shift of the disease between prediabetes and complete T2DM (Butler et al., 2003). The pathological research performed on T2DM cases has been found to show such a radical drop in beta-cell mass to an extent of 60 in certain cases, which in turn translates to the diminution in the capacity of the pancreas to secrete insulin in response to glucose; hence, the issue starts. The various system defects cause the development of the vicious cycle: on the one hand, hyperglycemia due to insulin resistance puts a greater metabolic burden on beta-cells, and on the other hand, beta-cell failure further aggravates hyperglycemia, which causes the death of additional beta-cells via glucotoxicity (Banday et al., 2020). One of the alterations in the understanding of T2DM pathophysiology is the disillusionment regarding its definition as a long-lasting low-grade inflammatory disease (Antar et al., 2023). The primary cause of this inflammation is fatness or overweight because the increase of adipose tissue, in particular, visceral fat, which is the most unhealthy location as it is located around the stomach, becomes the greatest source of the proinflammatory cytokines and adipokines production (Antar et al., 2023). In many instances, such inflammatory mediators are able to destabilize the insulin activity at several stages including activation of inflammatory kinases that phosphorylate insulin receptor substrate proteins at the inhibitory sites, thereby inhibiting the signaling. It is not just the adipose tissue that is affected by the proinflammatory condition, but it disseminates to the entire body. The abundance of research studies indicated that repeatedly, the level of various inflammatory markers of diabetic patients is significantly higher than in the nondiabetic population. Such biomarkers are C-reactive protein (CRP), IL-6, and TNF-α (Okdahl et al., 2022). This ongoing inflammatory event holds a significant clinical meaning since it is a highly associated predictor of the onset of T2DM as well as the subsequent progression of its microvascular and macrovascular complications with cardiovascular disease being the most prominent cause of death among this group of patients (Antar et al., 2023).

It has been established that some proinflammatory cytokines are the primary T2DM pathogenesis agents and thus can be used to provide antibody-targeted therapeutic intervention. The primary cause of insulin resistance is TNF-α. When obesity occurs, TNF-α released by the fat tissue and the macrophages triggers the actions of insulin pathways and interferes with the pathways through the deactivation of insulin receptors, which facilitates lipolysis (Antar et al., 2023). TNF-α is an even stronger target therapy option as the relationship between high levels of serum TNF-α, insulin resistance, and glycemic control is further supported. IL-1β kills the pancreatic beta-cells directly, and thus they become dysfunctional and apoptotic (Marchetti et al., 2007). The cytokine initiates most of the pathological events in the beta-cells including oxidative stress, endoplasmic reticulum stress, and also facilitating aggregation of islet amyloid polypeptide (Marchetti et al., 2007). Being an essential element, which triggers the inflammatory process in the pancreatic islets, IL-1 can accelerate the deterioration of beta-cells, as well as provide some time to develop an antibody-mediated neutralization. The persistent increase of IL-6 has been observed to cause a skilled metabolic impact, but its prolonged existence is a major contributor to the danger of acquiring T2DM and its complications (Antar et al., 2023). High concentrations of cytokine-neutralizing antibodies have a big role to play in the treatment of T2DM because of their efficacy in a number of other immune-mediated diseases.

There are many other pathways that T2DM inflammatory antibodies can attack along with traditional cytokines. T2DM is a disease that involves the misfolding of human amylin and aggregation of the protein into toxic oligomers and amyloid fibrils that are usually found in most patients after death (Lutz & Meyer, 2015). The aggregates directly cause cytotoxicity to the beta-cells, and they activate apoptosis by disrupting the membrane, cellular stress through endoplasmic reticulum, and triggering inflammasomes among others (Lutz & Meyer, 2015). It is assumed that antibodies against the removal of the toxic amylin oligomers will contribute to the survival of beta-cells and consequently save the insulin secretory activity. Continuous hyperglycemia leads to the synthesis of advanced glycation end products (AGEs) that stimulate the RAGE to trigger proinflammatory and profibrotic responses (Antar et al., 2023). The mechanism contributes to a vicious cycle of oxidative stress and inflammation that is one of the key contributors of the diabetic complications. This could be inhibited through use of neutralizing antibodies against RAGE or the ligands to the receptors. Furthermore, the receptor of insulin can be developed as well; the agonist antibodies will duplicate the insulin effect; hence, the latter can exhibit superior pharmacokinetic characteristics. Moreover, the proteins involved in the insulin signaling pathways, particularly, the inflammatory kinases that block the activity of insulin receptor substrate are probably the targets of the inhibitory antibodies geared toward boosting the insulin sensitivity (Antar et al., 2023).

3. Monoclonal antibodies in T2DM: Direct targeting strategies

Being one of the most innovative and promising compounds, the application of monoclonal antibodies (mAbs) in T2DM is a radical shift since antidiabetic drugs are replaced by the interventions of the specific inflammatory and metabolic pathways (Table 16.1) involved in the development of the disease. Up to now, tremendous progress in the clinical use of mAbs in the autoimmune type 1 diabetes (T1D) sphere has been accomplished, and the future of mAbs as the treatment of metabolic type T2DM remains

Table 16.1 Therapeutic targets and their mechanism of action.

Therapeutic target	Mechanism of action	Key research findings	References
IL-1β	Cytokine neutralization aids in the protection of beta-cells and lessening of inflammation.	Good glucose level control and beta-cell function improvement have been reported in clinical studies; and it is also effective in preventing glucose-induced toxicity.	Sloan-Lancaster et al. (2013)
TNF-α	Cytokine neutralization leads to the enhancement of insulin sensitivity.	Systems biology points out, however, that it is the top hub; monoclonal antibody (mAb). treatment restores not only normal blood sugar but also insulin signaling in mice.	Lebovitz (2019)
IL-1 receptor	Blocking of the receptor is done to stop the signaling of IL-1α and IL-1β.	Anakinra enhances glycemic control and β-cell function in patients with T2DM.	Sloan-Lancaster et al. (2013)
Glucagon receptor	The receptor is antagonized to be able to cut down the amount of glucose produced by the liver.	Preclinically, there is a good promise for reversing the glucose homeostasis disorder.	Wei et al. (2025)
Asprosin	Hormone neutralization leads to lowering appetite and blood glucose level.	mAbs administered to obese mice result in lowering blood glucose, food intake, and body weight.	Ristic et al. (2025)

mostly a preclinical domain, but it has potential (Wei et al., 2025). The whole research is unraveling the primary direct targeting strategies that have been taken into account in research undertakings. The overall release of proinflammatory cytokines that jointly cause the emergence of insulin resistance and pancreatic beta-cells death is one of the basic functions of T2DM pathogenesis (Tsalamandris et al., 2019). The plan of neutralizing these cytokines by using mAbs is to prevent the destruction of the tissue due to an inflammatory mechanism. One of the main cytokines of inflammation and a known drug target in the treatment of T2DM is IL-1. In situations where the body experiences metabolic stress such as hyperglycemia, the body reacts by synthesizing this cytokine and eventually injures the cells by causing them to undergo apoptosis, restricting the insulin release, and causing the body to become resistant to insulin (Donath et al., 2019). IL-1receptor type I (IL-1RI) is the receptor to which IL-1β binds and hence the origin of inflammatory signals. Monoclonal antibody therapy such as canakinumab is aimed at targeting IL-1β and preventing its connection to its receptor, thus preventing the proinflammatory signal (Wei et al., 2025). The blockage of this blockade prevents the deterioration of the availability of the beta-cells, as well as its functionality. The clinical research of these antibodies is strengthened by the fact that monocytes of the T2DM patients can produce IL-1β to a much higher level, particularly in case they are exposed to high glucose conditions (Wei et al., 2025). It is proved that the inhibition of the effects of the IL-1RI with the help of a suitable antagonist results in the further decrease in the release of other inflammatory cytokines, such as IL-6, which provides a substantive reason why this approach should be chosen (Tsalamandris et al., 2019).

TNF-α along with other proinflammatory promoting proteins also plays an important role in the pathophysiology of insulin resistance. The presence of chronic high concentrations of TNF-α is observed in blood as well as in adipose tissues of the subjects with T2DM and having its complications (Sethi & Hotamisligil, 2021). The production of TNF-α in the circular pool has implications on the adipose and muscle tissue directly to the insulin receptor system, which results in the subsequent steps resulting to hyperglycemia. TNF-vacuolar attaches itself to its receptor and triggers a signal cascade that ends with the activation of the pathways such as nuclear factor kappa-B (NF-kB) and Jun NH2-terminal kinase (JNK) (Sethi & Hotamisligil, 2021). The two aforementioned pathways incorporate the phosphate groups on the serine residues of IRS-1 (insulin receptor substrate-1) that consequently reduce the insulin signaling pathway, and eventually, this results in insulin resistance. TNF-α antimonoclonal antibodies (e.g., infliximab, adalimumab) play the role of neutralizing soluble TNF-α, thus repairing the insulin-insensitivity. It has been an impressive occurrence to demonstrate the demonstration of the chronicles of long-term TNF-α blockade in one instance. The C-peptide levels were comparable to those before the intervention and infliximab had been administered, glycemic control was improved, and insulin use was reduced over 5 years of treatment by the child with T1D who was recently diagnosed and treated with infliximab due to colitis, thereby suggesting a protective role of the beta-cells in the pancreas (Rao et al., 2024). Moreover, a pilot RCT of etanercept in new-onset T1D also found the same C-peptide and HbA1c improvement as did the previous studies with TNF-α in combination with beta-cell death (Tsalamandris et al., 2019). The other method of a strategic approach is to attack the cytokine receptors. In this way, the inflammatory signaling one would be inhibited, which is actually a common example of such as IL-1 receptor (IL-1R) targeting. Anakinra is an IL-1 receptor antagonist (IL-1Ra), which is a biologic agent because of its competitiveness with IL-1 biologic agent in the binding site of the IL-1 receptor (Wei et al., 2025). The use of IL-1β receptor blocks IL-1α and IL-1β mediators signaling and therefore offers a broader range of antiinflammatory response compared with the effect of the use of IL-1β receptor alone. It was reported that this approach enables the glucose control and helps to preserve the survival of the beta-cells in the case of diabetic patients in experimental settings (Tsalamandris et al., 2019).

A newer generation of T2DM mAb therapy is a step further in the process of hormonal modulation and goes down to the more direct form of modulating the body metabolism by targeting the hormones governing metabolism in the body. That is what the scheme has to do, to recompensate the hormonal-based causes of fasting hyperglycemia and obesity. The glucagon makes one of the hormones that produce glucose by the liver have a significant role. The identification of the mAbs with the glucagon receptor signaling pathway finally results in the downregulation of the glucose production of the liver, which is considered to be among the primary causes of fasting hyperglycemia in the T2DM patients (Wei et al., 2025). The preclinical trials to experiment the use of anti-glucagon receptor mAbs have been fruitful thus far in their interest of putting glucose levels at a state of equilibrium. The majority of scientific studies underway are geared toward enhancing the insulin sensitivity although there are certain antibodies that have been developed as antagonists of insulin receptor (IR) purely to be resistant to insulin under study. As an example, the IR monoclonal antibody, IRAB-B has been identified as a specific antagonist of insulin receptor in mice that induces resistance to insulin and hyperglycemia through a rapid mechanism and is an agent of interest in the study of the pathogenesis of diabetic patients (Cieniewicz et al., 2017). Quite to the contrary, there is another group of the anti-IR antibodies, such as 83-7, 83-14, which do show some ability that can be defined as agonist, because they are activating the dysfunctional mutant insulin receptors, which define the severe insulin resistance syndromes, therefore rendering the concept of a totally novel form of treatment of these conditions a reality (Brierley et al., 2018).

4. Antibody-mediated modulation of insulin resistance

The invention of the new insulin resistance treatment drugs has also taken into consideration the inhibition of the pathological signals by antibodies, that is, the humanized monoclonal antibodies. This section explains the general concept of the pathological signals being prevented to be relayed using the assistance of antibodies, the precise locations of the insulin signal pathway that are being targeted in this way, and current findings of both preclinical and clinical trials, which validates this new approach. The insulin resistance is characterized by decreased response of insulin on target tissues (e.g., liver, muscle, fat). The chronic and low-grade inflammation resulting in the secretion of proinflammatory cytokines and cellular stress kinases as very powerful insulin resistance signals are one of the primary causes of this disorder (Hotamisligil, 2006; Li et al., 2022). These include TNF-α, which activates IKK2 and JNK. These kinases phosphorylate the insulin signaling intermediate, particularly the IRS proteins, at serine residues (e.g., IRS-1 Ser307). This serine phosphorylation prevents the signal transmission by tyrosine phosphorylation of the IRS proteins that is required to transmit the signal, and the insulin signal is effectively inhibited (He et al., 2009). The treatment concept is to apply a highly specific mechanism with monoclonal antibodies, which specifically seek to block these extracellular "resistance signals" (such as TNF-α) or the receptors. The whole process is aimed at preventing the repression of IRS proteins through serine phosphorylation and having the insulin signaling pathway functional once again and sensitizing cells to insulin. The insulin signaling mechanism is somehow involved by the antibodies in both the pathological autoantibodies and the case of research and therapeutic tools. The autoantibodies to the insulin receptors are produced by the human body in an unusual type B insulin resistance syndrome (Jialal & Basheer, 2022). The effect of such autoantibodies is opposite, that is, when the concentration is higher, they act like antagonists, i.e., they bind to the receptor, and the outcome is complete insulin resistance and hyperglycemia; when it is lower, they may resemble the action of insulin and provoke hypoglycemia. This situation describes the complexity of the role of antibodies. Some of the most crucial instruments to study insulin resistance include antibodies that specifically interact with phosphorylated proteins. A case in point is the IRS-1 phosphorylated at Ser307-specific antibodies applied in the determination of the level of inhibitory signaling in the cell and animal studies (Gao et al., 2023; He et al., 2009). Antisense oligonucleotide-based therapeutic agent against IRS-1 (GS-101) has demonstrated potential in preclinical models of pathological angiogenesis in blocking IRS-1 expression and its respective cellular functions (Qian et al., 2019). Concurrent signaling of a large number of proteins can be profiled using antibody-based arrays. Through this technology, the activation of the entire pathways has been mapped whereby it has been established that the agents such as phorbol ester (PMA) activate PKC, IKK2, and JNK that ultimately culminates to the classical IRS-1 Ser307 phosphorylation and cellular insulin resistance (He et al., 2009).

A broad spectrum of evidence in terms of both initial laboratory experiments and clinical observations and interventions has been particularly beneficial in showing the application of antibody-based modulation. A study on the human choroidal endothelial cells showed that incidence of IRS-1 in the form of GS-101 produced a drastic reduction of tube formation, proliferation, and migration capabilities of choroidal endothelial cells and generation of apoptosis. It, therefore, shows directly that IRS-1 is surely a subject of control of pathological neovascularization, which is a frequent complication of diabetes (Qian et al., 2019). The novel research on animal models has identified TNF-α as a significant contributor to the occurrence of insulin resistance in obesity. This was followed by further studies that investigated the effect of the TNF-α on the normalization of insulin resistance in these models thereby leading to this treatment strategy (Hotamisligil, 2006). A natural and very severe case of antibody-caused insulin resistance is the type B insulin resistance syndrome (TBIRS). The diagnostic markers are the antiinsulin receptor autoantibodies. In most cases, immunosuppressant agents including monoclonal antibody rituximab (anti-CD20 and destroys B cells) and cyclophosphamide, as well as corticosteroids, are used. The treatment aims at inhibiting the synthesis of pathogenic antibodies and inducing remission (Gao et al., 2023). With insulin autoimmune syndrome (IAS), the body makes autoantibodies that react against insulin, leading to spikes in blood glucose levels. The treatment has in the worst-case scenario involved plasmapheresis to clear the patient of the antibodies and immunosuppression (Hirano et al., 2008). Anti-TNF-α therapy has proven highly beneficial in autoimmune disorders such as rheumatoid arthritis but only had a modest effect in improving a level of insulin sensitivity among the individuals with type 2 diabetes in general. It implies that the intricate and multifactorial pathology of common insulin resistance might remain unreversed by the actions of the single cytokine (Berbudi et al., 2025; Li et al., 2022).

5. Antibody therapy: Protecting pancreatic beta-cells

It is the progressive destruction of functional pancreatic beta-cell mass that is the primary cellular mechanism of both pathogenetic processes T1D and T2DM. The ultimate pathways to failure and death of beta-cells are achieved in various ways of initial triggers. Treatments with antibodies, initially aimed at immunomodulatory, are being thought of as beta-cell lifeguards that simply protect the cells and hence prevent or even revert the insulin secretion decrease. The process of apoptosis (regulated cell death) is especially widespread in the beta-cells, due to their high metabolic rate and sheer inability to adapt to the cellular stress. The depletion of the beta-cells is realized mainly in two cross-associated processes. In T1D, autoimmune T lymphocytes and IL-1, IFN-γ, TNF-α type proinflammatory cytokines act in conjunction to destroy the beta-cells by stimulating their death receptor signaling (e.g., Fas receptor). Activation of the caspase enzymes to cause cell death program follows (Eizirik et al., 2013). T2DM is a symptom of low-grade chronic inflammation due to the adipose tissue and the islets that combine to expose the beta-cells to the cytotoxic cytokines (Donath et al., 2019). Insulin is produced in endoplasmic reticulum (ER) where it is folded correctly. The cells that produce the insulin in large quantities in the presence of glucose are the beta-cells and their ER is really good. However, under extreme conditions when the metabolic requirement becomes excessive, e.g., in the case of insulin resistance or when there is a genetic influence, the capacity of the ER to fold proteins may be surpassed. This leads to acquisition of distorted proteins, and this is termed as ER stress. The cell initiates UPR (unfolded protein response) to restore the balance. However, when the stress is indeed so bad or prolonged, the UPR turns into a death signal, primarily by activating transcription factor CHOP (C/EBP homologous protein), which subsequently contributes to the death of the beta-cell (Shrestha et al., 2021). The two processes have been closely associated as the inflammatory cytokines may also augment the ER balance, which consequently triggers a vicious cycle of beta-cell dysfunction and death. Antibody therapies are in progress of attacking the harmful apoptotic and inflammatory signals on beta-cells directly. Antibodies against the Fas receptor (CD95) or the TRAIL (tumor necrosis factor apoptosis-inducing ligand) receptor have proven to be successful in preclinical trial. The antibodies work by attaching to such receptors, thereby inhibiting the binding of their corresponding death ligands and, therefore, inhibiting the apoptosis program triggered by immune cells (Koliaki & Katsilambros, 2022). Neutralizing proinflammatory cytokines are one of the most developed interventions clinically. Through the clinical trials, it has been demonstrated that drugs such as canakinumab and gevokizumab can be of use to patients with T2DM. The neutralization of IL-1β that is carried out by these antibodies causes the removal of the local inflammatory condition that is observed in the islet, which causes the improvement of the beta cell functionality and the suppression of the apoptosis (Donath et al., 2019). Even though the glycemic effects have been minor, the clinical trials are affirming the cytokine blockage as one of the mechanisms to positively impact the human beta-cells. The situation is, however, different in the case of auto-immune illness in which the drug treatment has a direct advantage on the beta-cell survival of diabetic patients less frequently than in the research examining the involvement of TNF-α in insulin resistance and inflammation. T1D patients experience process of autoimmune attack suppression; therefore, the therapeutic use of anti-CD3 (e.g., teplizumab) antibodies has a predisposing effect to develop the impotency of the T cell in the patients with T1D that were recently diagnosed. Similarly, the immune system destroys the beta-cells at the same time as the therapies are free of side effects and, therefore, long-term survival (Wang & Sander, 2021).

The amyloid in the islets is a critical pathological characteristic of T2DM that is produced by aggregation of islet amyloid polypeptide (IAPP), or amylin. IAPP is a peptide released together with insulin by the beta-cells. In T2DM, accumulated due primarily to augmented discharge and/or genetic variations (in both human beings and cats), IAPP may misfold to structure harmful oligomers and fibrils. The most cytotoxic of them are the soluble oligomers, which damage cell membranes, cause ER stress, and trigger further inflammatory response, thereby causing cell death (Kapurniotu, 2020; Li & Zhang, 2025). A similar approach is being attempted with T2DM because the positive response of antibody-based therapy to neurodegenerative diseases such as Alzheimer has been encouraging. The strategy involves the use of monoclonal antibodies, which are specifically tailored to neutralize soluble oligomers, promote clearance, and block seeding and propagation. The high affinity of antibodies can be raised to recognize and bind the toxic and soluble oligomers of IAPP. The antibodies attaching to these oligomers neutralize their toxicity, prevent their ability to cause a rupture in beta-cell membrane, as well as prevent their proapoptotic signaling. The immunocomplexes of the antibody–IAPP may be recognized and eliminated by the phagocytic cells (such as macrophage), thus reducing the overall number of amyloid in the islet. Antibodies may block the seeding activity, whereby small aggregates cause misfolding and aggregation of increasing amounts of IAPP, therefore preventing the formation of amyloid deposition by binding to IAPP aggregates. Anti-IAPP antibodies during preclinical trials on mice and human islets have successfully prevented the occurrence of IAPP-induced beta-cell apoptosis and improved islet function, effectively making the treatment a promising disease-modifying treatment to T2DM (Roham et al., 2025).

6. Bispecific and multispecific antibodies for complex diseases

Due to the complicated character of T2DM, next-generation treatment has become a subject of study, proposing a condition of interrelationship between the phenomena of chronic inflammation, insulin resistance, and metabolic malfunctioning. Development of bispecific and multispecific antibodies has become the beginning of the new era, i.e., it is no longer required to block one disease-causing factor at a time but to engage several factors at a time on one biological agent. In T2DM, using bispecific antibodies can target the combination of two pathways—the inflammatory and the metabolic pathway—that drive the development of the disease will lead to increased efficacy. A combination of a number of cytokines, such as TNF-α, IL-1β, and IL-6, is the cause of the inflammation in T2DM (Donath & Shoelson, 2011). The inhibition of one cytokine may prove insufficient in regard to the clinical outcome due to the possibility of the other cytokines in the network to take over and continue with the inflammation (Brinkmann & Kontermann, 2017). Two most significant cytokines or the receptors could be prevented by a bispecific antibody simultaneously and thus the inflammation would be decreased to a larger scale and on a lasting longer basis. Immune cells that result in a local and systemic insulin resistance are abundant in the metabolic organs, which are adipose tissue, liver, and muscle (Lumeng & Saltiel, 2011). To generate extremely specific immunomodulatory signal and thereby reverse an unhealthy communication situation, a bispecific antibody might be made to bridge one type of immune cell (e.g., a proinflammatory macrophage) with another type of cell (e.g., an insulin-resistant adipocyte). T2DM has many therapeutic targets all over the body, and they are not only abnormal targets but also have normal functions. The undesirable effects may be brought about by the overall inhibition. The method is cellular specificity, which involves the production of a bispecific antibody with one arm interacting with a disease (e.g., TNF-α) and the other arm interacting with a cell marker (e.g., a protein very much expressed on macrophages in adipose tissue). In this way, the drug becomes safer and the rest of the tissues are spared because the action of this drug is limited to the specific cell type (Ma et al., 2021).

The engineering of bispecific antibodies to treat a complex disease such as T2DM will be based on the combination of various molecular forms and the different targeting approaches. Two large-scale inflammatory pathways that suppress the beta-cell activity and render insulin less effective could have both arms of a bispecific antibody activated against IL-12 and IL-6, respectively (Donath et al., 2019). By linking a soluble cytokine (such as TNF-α) with one arm and a cell-surface receptor (e.g., CCR2, leading monocytes to fat tissue) with the other, it may be possible to neutralize an inflammatory signal and at the same time prevent the recruitment of new inflammatory cells. On a more progressive approach, in addition to resistance in the insulin signaling pathway (e.g., insulin receptor), an inflammatory receptor (e.g., TNF receptor) can also be taken into account. Therefore, it would be desirable to amplify insulin signals and inhibit it at the same time using inflammation. The development of bispecific antibodies has resulted in the development of different forms of molecular formats that have their benefits (Table 16.2). IgG-like formats are complete antibodies that are Fc-containing and therefore have a long serum half-life and can also carry out effector functions of antibody-dependent cellular phagocytosis. Some of the platforms include Knobs-into-Holes and DuoBody technologies that are utilized to ensure the particular heterodimer pairing between the two different heavy chains (Brinkmann & Kontermann, 2017).

Table 16.2 Molecular formats with their potential benefits.

Platform/ format	Key engineering strategy	Potential advantages	Example (therapeutic area)	References
IgG-like formats	An Fc region retention for immune effector functions and longer half-life as well.	Pharmacokinetics, stability, and ability to activate Fc-mediated functions such as ADCC and ADCP are improved.	NI-1701 (CD19xCD47, B cell malignancies)	van de Donk and Zweegman (2023)
Knobs-into-Holes	Using mutations in the Fc part to help two dissimilar heavy chains bond as a heterodimer.	High yield of properly assembled antibodies.	Emicizumab (hemophilia A)	Brinkmann and Kontermann (2017)
DuoBody	When two antibodies with complementary mutations exchange their Fab arms, it is called controlled Fab-arm exchange (cFAE).	Fully functional bispecific IgGs can be created using this platform, which is versatile and widely accepted.	JNJ-61186372 (EGFRxc-MET for NSCLC)	Labrijn et al. (2013)
Non-IgG-like formats	Fc-free fragments such as BiTE, scFvs, or VHHs/HHs are non-IgG formats.	Reduced risk of adverse effects due to the small size, simple production, and no Fc molecule.	Blinatumomab (CD19xCD3 for ALL); VHH-based MYSTI	Wang et al., 2023; Ma et al., 2021
VHH-based (Nanobody)	Single-domain antibodies of camelids are used and easily linked to bispecifics.	High stability, solubility, and expression yield; excellent tissue penetration.	V56B2 (TNFαxIL-23 for IBD)	Roberts et al. (2021)

Camelid single-domain antibodies are small and stable and can be easily conjugated into multispecific molecules. They can offer improved access to the thickened, inflamed tissues on a small scale that is pancreatic islets or adipose. A bispecific nanobody can be developed oral, and it would be targeted to a gut-derived T2DM inflammatory signal, and then it would work locally in the gut (Ma et al., 2021).

Although the application of bispecific antibodies in the treatment of T2DM is only at its initial phases, substantial preclinical evidence, as well as experiments in the neighboring regions, confirms their utility. This was a strategy that was mainly applied to rheumatoid arthritis but currently can apply to T2DM widely. Scientists have developed a bispecific antibody with one end of the bispecific antibody binding TNF-α and the other end binding myeloid cell surface marker (e.g., in mice F4/80 or CD11b in humans). In such a configuration, anti-TNF action is localized to the cells that produce TNF the most and, thereby, neutralizes the cytokine at the point of origin in addition to reducing systemic immunosuppression (Wang et al., 2023). The antiinflammatory effect on adipose tissue will be attained when applied to T2DM without the threats of increasing the risk of infections. V56B2 antibody is a bispecific domain antibody (anti-TNF-α/anti-IL-23) that is developed to treat inflammatory bowel disease. It is administered orally, and it is resistant to gut proteases meaning that it can work effectively on neutralizing key inflammatory cytokines locally with minimal systemic exposure (Roberts et al., 2021). It may involve a revision of this approach to treat T2DM by targeting the gut-derived factors due to the developed gut–metabolism axis and the contribution of gut inflammation to insulin resistance. A good example of practical safety engineering is in the development of NI-1701 (anti-CD19/anti-CD47) to treat B cell malignancies. Through the selective blockage of the signaling that signals to the cells that they should not be eaten, that is the CD47, on the $CD19^+$ B cells, but not the red blood cells that are healthy, the latter has been a significant toxicity issue in the use of the monoclonal anti-CD47 therapy (van de Donk & Zweegman, 2023). The principle of the conditional activity can be readily applied to T2DM whereby we would target the harmful processes in hepatocytes, adipocytes, or the pancreatic beta-cells such that the other necessitated cell types are spared.

The activity of the antibodies can also be modified with considerable precision besides its structure. One of the approaches is affinity tuning of the binding arms. The case of T cell engaging bispecifics is one that the affinity to CD3 can be reduced to allow retention of good tumor cell killing, but the release of the inflammatory cytokines, which is the major side effect causing cytokine release syndrome, is significantly smaller (Slaga et al., 2018).

7. Antibody–drug conjugates for targeted delivery

The impact of the ADCs is enormous since it combines the precision of monoclonal antibodies and the potency of cytotoxic agents. These conjugates are primarily used in oncology, although the delivery concept is currently under trial in complex metabolic diseases, including T2DM that leads to the provision of a new method of addressing and eliminating the diseased cells or to administering the cytoprotective compounds to the stressed tissue. An ADC consists of a simple design that comprises the following elements; a monoclonal antibody that serves as a guiding device, a cytotoxic or cytomodulatory payload, and a chemical linker, binding the two (Beck et al., 2017). The treatment plan in T2DM would be to exploit the specificity of the antibody to deliver a pharmacologically active drug directly to the diseased-causing cell type, thereby reducing the concentration of drugs in the system and the pathologic effects of the drug.

The stress of beta-cells, amyloid deposition, and immune-cell presence are found in the form of islands in the pancreas in T2DM. It may seem counterintuitive, but, in fact, a highly developed ADC featuring a small cytotoxic payload could be utilized to kill a particular population of long-term chronic stressed beta-cells that is dysfunctional, either due to the production of misfolded proteins (such as toxic IAPP oligomers) or even distribution of inflammatory signals. This, theoretically, may empty the way to replication and functional betterment of the remaining healthy beta-cells. To have this process, a very specific antigen of such dysfunctional cells is required. Knock-out activated macrophages or T cells in the islet could be caused by an ADC. The antibody may bind a cell-surface antigen like CD64 (which is present on macrophages) or CD3 (which is present on T cells), therefore providing a potent immunosuppressive cargo that would initiate cell death in the local environment and cease the autoimmune and inflammatory response to the beta-cells (Kumar et al., 2024). The hepatic insulin resistance forms the main characteristic of T2DM. Another strategy of ADC could attack proinflammatory hepatocytes and hepatic stellate cells (HSCs). Perhaps several liver hepatocytes in a steatotic (fatty) liver can display the existence of some surface markers of stress and inflammation. An ADC might then deliver either an antifibrotic or an antiinflammatory drug directly to those cells. The cells that produce collagen predominately are the HSCs in the advanced disease and liver fibrosis. A potential application of an ADC is to select a molecule like PDGFR2 present on activated HSCs and therefore carry out a proapoptotic role by efficiently administering a cytotoxic payload that unfolds the reversal of fibrosis or prevents it and restores (Liu et al., 2022). The choice of a substance to be sent in will be decisive, and it will not be limited to the traditional chemotherapeutic drugs but also to the ones that are able to regulate the functioning of the cell and its survival.

Agents effective in causing apoptosis, as in microtubule inhibitor (e.g., monomethyl auristatin E- MMAE) or DNA damaging (e.g., calicheamicin), are usually called cytotoxic payloads (in the case of selective ablation). They would be used in selection of some groups of cells as discussed before. An MMAE payload in an ADC on a marker on proinflammatory macrophages in adipose tissue or pancreatic islets would eliminate these cells and therefore block the production of TNF-8 and IL-12 and alleviate insulin sensitivity (Ma et al., 2016). Dealing with high potency of a drug entails profound familiarity concerning the type of cell that is to be targeted to avoid causing too much damage. A more inventive application of metabolic disorders is cytoprotective and modulatory payloads (a novel frontier). The payload could be a molecule that would promote the survival or activity of cells as an alternative to a cytotoxic drug. A beta-cell or hepatocyte-specific ADC could deliver a conjugated GLP-1 analog directly delivering to these cells, leading to a highly localized and potent insulinotropic or insulin-sensitizing effect. It was then possible to combine up to four or five different anticancer drugs in a very low concentration by an ADC, which strongly lowers the potential of side effects. The possible solution to the issue of the ER stress in the beta-cells or hepatocytes may be the delivery of chemical chaperons, like 4-phenylbutyric acid (4-PBA), which would be directly transported to the cells with origination to these cells by an ADC, thereby promoting the appropriate folding of proteins and preventing the process of apoptosis (Engin & Hotamisligil, 2010). It is planned to attack drugs that control the mechanisms that result in cell death including caspases inhibitors into the beta-cells and protect them against the triplets of glucotoxicity, lipotoxicity, and inflammation, which are being delivered on them day in day out.

The application of ADC technology to metabolic diseases, rather than oncology, has a very distinct set of challenges and benefits. Its greatest obstacle is how to find cell-surface antigens that are not only highly specific to the pathological cell state (e.g., a dysfunctional beta-cell but not a healthy one) but are also not expressed on vital healthy tissues. An inappropriate target may easily result in the completely irreparable damage of the cell populations that are vital. The risk–benefit ratio in cancer treatment is tolerant of high levels of toxicity to an outcome of life saving. The safety requirement of ADC in T2DM is very high, as the condition is chronic and is treated with drugs, which are almost safe. The facts that chronic dosing is a serious concern and that there is a likelihood of cumulative toxicity over time are critical (Kumar et al., 2024). This phenomenon of bystander effect, i.e., the payload at least partially diffuses out of the cell to which it is delivered, could happen in cancer therapy with its extraordinary killing ability of mixed tumor cells and introduce a disadvantage in the situation of metabolism, i.e., in the case of metabolism, the death of neighboring healthy cells is induced in a structured organ such as the pancreatic islet, and hence the existing options of T2DM treatment do not prevent the disease development, only regulate one of the symptoms (hyperglycemia). An attentive ADC to kill pathological cells (such as the toxic IAPP-producing beta-cells or the profibrotic HSCs) may be a breakthrough therapy concerning all at once out of the others category, the disease-modifying ones. The affinity of the ADCs to the cells is such that it is incomparable with the small molecules and even the majority of biologics. This may enable activating or deactivating of some pathways within some types of cells, through which it would permit the arrival of therapeutic strategies that had not been possible before. One ADC molecule is capable of achieving the two functions of targeting (the antibody) and exhibiting a powerful therapeutic effect (the payload), thereby forming a synergistic agent that is not only able to reach the location of the disease, but also is a very precise intervention.

8. Clinical translation: Safety, practicality and efficacy

The mAb therapies have been developed to go far way in the preclinical application to treat the patient, assess the effectiveness and safety in addition to the practical application of the therapies. Although these drugs have found alternative ways of operation, their clearance through the clinical trials has not only shown their bright side of operation but also their dark side in the form of the hurdles they have to overcome in such a process. The most convincing evidence on research regarding mAbs in T2DM was provided by the studies that had specialized in the IL-1 pathway, which is an agent of inflammation in diabetes. The primary research that was mostly aimed at cardiovascular outcomes was the massive CANTOS trial (Canakinumab Anti-inflammatory Thrombosis Outcomes Study). Canakinumab, an extremely potent low-affinity anti-IL-1β mAb, was administered to the patients who already suffered a heart attack and had hsCRP level within the range of high sensitivity. The research that was not targeting diabetic patients still covered a large number of participants with T2DM. The results proved the instance of canakinumab that reduced the level of hsCRP and IL-6 by a large percentage and this through the effect of antiinflammatory. An analysis of post hoc showed that subjects treated with canakinumab had lower HbA1c levels than the placebo group and, therefore, required no insulin introduction in the median follow-up period of 3.7 years (Ridker et al., 2017). It was, therefore, the first clinical evidence-of-concept that anticytokine therapy could improve glycemic control. The anti-IL-1-β gevokizumab mAb (anti-IL-1-β) is an effective IL-1 -modulator that binds to the cytokine and does not reduce its activity. Gevokizumab was tolerated well, and beta-cell function, which was assessed by the proinsulin to insulin ratio, improved in a proof-of-concept study in patients with T2DM. The glycemic control improved (but not conclusively) (Cavelti-Weder et al., 2012). However, the bigger follow-up trials failed to demonstrate the primary efficacy, and so, development of gevokizumab in T2DM was dropped, which points to the challenges of attaining undermined large consistent glucose-lowering benefits.

The trials depict that the targeting of inflammation may offer a long-term advantage in the metabolic sanctions field, but the effects of this intervention on HbA1c are frequently less effective than the already-established drug therapy, such as metformin or SGLT2 inhibitors. This has resulted in being more conservative and placing mAbs as a niche among patients with high levels of inflammation as a key contributor in the disease. The major issue that decides the use of mAbs in a long-term, nonlethal disease is the safety issue, although antidrug antibody (ADA) response is one of the effects of using all therapeutic proteins. One of the manifestations in which ADAs demonstrate their presence is reduced drug efficacy (neutralizing antibodies), or they may also manifest themselves as altered pharmacokinetics. ADAs can also cause an infusion reaction or any other immune-mediated adverse event in some cases (Maneiro et al., 2013). Immunogenicity of a monoclonal antibody (mAb) is subject to the type (fully human, humanized, or chimeric). In this way, the fully human mAbs such as canakinumab as a rule have a reduced immunogenic capacity. Since the IL-1 pathway is an essential part of the innate immune system against the invasion of the pathogen, its inhibition is accompanied by the issue of increased vulnerability to infection. In CANTOS trial, the canakinumab arm experienced a much worse rate of fatal infections than the placebo arm (Ridker et al., 2017). Although the absolute risk was minimal, it remains a massive problem in its relation to the possible use of anticytokine mAbs in T2DM where the ratio of risk–benefit is to be put under a close scrutiny. The chance of being infected in the case of the drugs that attack other mAbs will depend on the particular immune pathway which is being targeted.

The patient convenience, adherence to treatment, and consumption of health resources are very significantly influenced by mode of drug delivery. Certain monoclonal antibodies (particularly first time immunomodulation (e.g., rituximab in type B insulin resistance)) or with a certain stability profile must be delivered via intravenous infusion. This will lead to the patient paying a doctor or clinic a lot of time, and it will also increase the chances of the patient experiencing adverse reactions during the infusion. It is not typically the preferred choice of a long-term treatment of a chronic disease such as T2DM. Subcutaneous route, however, is a far more viable and convenient method of treating chronic illnesses. The majority of the mAbs in preclinical development in T2DM, including canakinumab and gevokizumab, are presented as SC injections, which can be self-administered at home by the patient like insulin or GLP-1 receptor agonist. The disadvantages are only manifested in local reactions at the site of injection (such as pain, redness, etc.) and an enhanced absorption into the blood circulation. This route involves the development of high-concentration formulations to permit mAbs with big doses to employ this route (Porter et al., 2001). The cost of the mAb therapies may be discussed as the most significant barrier to its adoption in the case of T2DM. Comparing to small-molecule drugs, mAbs are truly expensive and difficult to design and manufacture in terms of research, development and production. The cost of the final product represents the cost of the process. In case a rare treatment has to be discussed as cost-effective, the price can be explained by the medical value. The dominance of the mAbs on the market is also undermined by the fact that their small HbA1c improvement is contrasted with the existence of generic medications (such as metformin) that are affordable to manage T2DM. To the poor and to the general population, these mAbs would only work in the situations where they can make a notable contribution in terms of complications prevention (Joensuu et al., 2015). This would really strain the already-stretched healthcare budgets and people would have lesser access to the treatment particularly in low- and middle-income countries where T2DM is already becoming pandemic. The mAb would be used in case the price would drop significantly, or the biosimilars would appear, or a subpopulation of T2DM patients who would benefit the most would be identified.

9. Challenges and future directions

The development of T2DM, which is based on antibodies, is a major breakthrough in treating the metabolic disorders. Even though the preclinical rationale is rather sound, making this hope a reality at the hospital will require overcoming a significant portion of the complexity of the disease, the safety issue, as well as the drug design. The way this field is going to develop will be based on the ways of making the treatment specific to the patient, enhance the properties of the drug as well as the vaccination strategy that is a completely novel one. Symptoms of T2DM patients are diverse, which is one of the primary issues in the disease treatment. As it has recently been determined, T2DM is a set of metabolic diseases whose causes vary and may overlap each other, such as insulin-producing cells death, insulin resistance, fat buildup in the belly, and inflammation (Ahlqvist et al., 2018). One of the key reasons as to why the clinical trials of anticytokine therapies have low success rates is the application of a drug, whose effects are widespread, to such a diverse group of patients. Precision medicine, i.e., identification of biomarkers to subdivide patients into subpopulations with high probability of responding to a particular treatment, is the future. To identify patients that have elevated level of "inflammatory burden" is one of the primary goals. This may be done through observing patients using a marker of biomarkers such as high-sensitivity C-reactive protein (hsCRP), IL-6, or a certain pattern of inflammatory gene expression in blood cells (Donath & Shoelson, 2011). This profile of patients would be the most appropriate to be targeted by anticytokine antibodies (e.g., anti-IL-1 2, anti-IL-6). The disease can be combined with other conditions whereby the beta-cell failure and amyloid deposition are the main factors in these patients. With the help of the biomarkers such as an elevated proinsulin-to-insulin ratio or toxic IAPP oligomers, it is possible to identify such patients who are already prepared to receive treatments with a high level of specificity compared with other patients (Kapurniotu, 2020; Li & Zhang, 2025). In their research, Ahlqvist et al. (2018) have determined, based on their data, clusters of T2DM (such as "severe autoimmune diabetes," "severe insulin-resistant diabetes"). Experiments that will be conducted on the use of antibody therapies in the years to come might take into consideration such or such classifications to demonstrate the accuracy-sensitive way of effectiveness. The immunomodulatory antibodies that are already known to be long-term safe in T2DM that is a chronic illness are a key concern and an aspect that requires regular and close attention. As opposed to short-term courses in oncology, diabetes treatment would be long-term and potentially long-life. It is not yet fully understood what the long-term effects of tampering with such crucial immune pathways as IL-1 or TNF-α signaling will be. It means that permanent control of the patients is necessary to diagnose any common or opportunistic infections that may be a side effect of the treatment. There is also a theoretical risk of some types of cancer, although the CANTOS trial did not reveal this effect with canakinumab (Ridker et al., 2017). Additionally, there is a potential for the development of new autoimmune diseases due to the imbalance in the immune system, and long-term use of the medication is one of the factors that carry the risk of ADAs formation, resulting in the loss of drug efficacy, redistribution in the body, or allergies. The identification of doll-skin prevalence will constitute one of the primary features of clinical practice, and organ-specific toxicity could be investigated (as an example, in the liver or fat), which will disclose unexpected organ-specific toxicities in the course of the long-time use of the drug.

The power, safety, and usability of monoclonal antibodies can be enhanced to meet their inherent nature. An antibody in the Fc (crystallizable fragment) region is critical in its interaction with the immune system. With the help of this area, it is possible to get various results depending on the needs. To top it all, those mutations that increase affinity to Fc receptor (FcRn) in endothelial cells may increase the serum half-life of the antibody up to 75-folds. This is due to the augmented activity of the recycling procedure composed of FcRn and cessation of the degradation procedure occurring in lysosomes. Such engineered antibody may cause a patient to return to his/her next dose after 2 or 3 months rather than every 2 weeks, so the compliance of the patient would significantly increase (Strohl, 2018). In antibodies to destroy a specific population of cells (such as proinflammatory macrophages), one can alter the Fc region to augment ADCP or ADCC. Nevertheless, in other cases of antibodies in which cell depletion is not tolerated (such as a bispecific antibody targeting a cell signaling receptor), silenced Fc domains can be formed to prevent these effector activities, effectively, and the safety is enhanced. As we have already noted, the next generation of sophistication is bispecific antibodies and ADCs, which allow simultaneous targeting or precise delivery of potent modulators to specific types of cells (Ma et al., 2021). Active immunization has replaced therapeutic antibodies, which only offer passive immunization, and one of the boldest future scenarios is to induce the immune system to permanently respond to the pathogens. The procedure will include inoculation of vaccine against the self-molecules that cause the diseases; therefore, the induction of blocking antibodies will occur without the inhibition of the entire immune system. Vaccination, which produces modified IAP, would produce antibodies that dissolve the toxic versions of IAP, which are produced by the islets, therefore, preventing the death of the beta-cells, which would otherwise develop amyloid. The T2DM mice animal trials have revealed that the anti-IAPP vaccine has the ability to improve the functioning of the beta-cells and tolerance to glucose (Roham et al., 2025). Theoretical assumption illustrates how the vaccine that has the potential to induce antibodies against self-cytokine such as TNF-α or IL-1β will develop. However, this approach would be highly difficult since it has the potential of causing a negative autoimmune response and therefore would require a significant amount of fine-tuning to create a regulated and safe response of the immune system. The overall advantage to a successful vaccine is that it may result in a lasting curative action only with few doses administered; therefore, it will be an exceptionally affordable and accessible remedy. The issue is that it involves the need to offer absolutely exceptional and safe, and consequently, no possibility to develop undesirable autoimmune reaction or immune complex disease whatsoever.

10. Conclusion

The preclinical research on the use of antibodies to treat T2DM has transformed the entire treatment process of hyperglycemia to the direct assault on the inflammatory and immunopathological processes that result in the disease. Clinical trials with the anti-IL-1β antibodies, including canakinumab, have proved the principle that the neutralization of some cytokines may result in significant, though small, changes in glycemic control and beta-cell functions. The new technological designs such as bispecific antibodies and ADCs are usually different than the straightforward blockade of the target by enabling sophisticated strategies comprising of cell-specific targeting, dual pathway suppression, and local delivery of cytoprotective or cytotoxic cargo. The precision is vital in tampering with the complex metabolic tissues, and systemic toxicity should not be one of the outcomes. Two of the methods under study are blocking of the signals that cause the occurrence of apoptosis and elimination of the toxic IAPP oligomers. Additionally, targeted immunomodulation with the help of engineered antibodies can be used as well. These two approaches together provide an opportunity not only to stop but also to reverse T2DM progression, which is marked with the death of beta-cells, a highly promising direction, indeed. Antibody therapies are not the substitutes of the first-line therapy such as metformin or SGLT2 inhibitors among the wide range of T2DM patients because of their high costs, route of delivery, and the specific action they perform. Quite on the contrary, they will become the niche of the future of precision medicine. The aforementioned therapies will mainly be directed toward the targeted disease-modifying intervention of the specific patient subphenotypes identified by the use of biomarkers. Anticytokine receptor antibodies might be considered their part of treatment to patients with the high inflammatory burden. Anti-IAPP vaccines or neutralizing antibodies can also be applied in cases of individuals with a rather clear and severe islet amyloid pathology. Very high insulin insensitivity in patients of specific types of immune cells can be considered to have bispecific antibodies that restore metabolic homeostasis.

The initial application of antibody therapies would in this case be aimed at turning an aspect of the disease in a specific group of patients, thereby potentially avoiding the death of the beta-cells and future complications that occur in conventional treatment. The shift of antibody therapy away off cancer and autoimmunity in metabolic disease is a challenging and an engaging undertaking. Significant challenges that need to be overcome are still present such as long-term safety, cost-effectiveness, and the immediate necessity of creating patient stratification biomarkers with high sensitivity. Nevertheless, theoretical premises and early clinical results are quite persuasive indeed. These emerging treatment modalities represent a novel challenge in the T2DM and reflect the current shift from a reactive strategy of glycemic management to a proactive strategy of an immune-metabolic accuracy. It is predictable that the T2DM will be approached with the combination of multiple approaches, and thus, antibodies will become the key players in the patients whose illness is provoked by the same pathological processes that the powerful biologics are intended to cure.

References

Ahlqvist, E., Storm, P., Käräjämäki, A., Martinell, M., Dorkhan, M., Carlsson, A., ... Groop, L. (2018). Novel subgroups of adult-onset diabetes and their association with outcomes: A data-driven cluster analysis of six variables. *Lancet Diabetes & Endocrinology, 6*(5), 361–369.

Antar, S. A., Ashour, N. A., Sharaky, M., Khattab, M., Ashour, N. A., Zaid, R. T., ... Al-Karmalawy, A. A. (2023). Diabetes mellitus: Classification, mediators, and complications; A gate to identify potential targets for the development of new effective treatments. *Biomedicine & Pharmacotherapy, 168,* Article 115734.

Bailey, C. J. (2025). Pharmacological therapies for type 2 diabetes: Future approaches. *Diabetologia,* 1–16.

Banday, M. Z., Sameer, A. S., & Nissar, S. (2020). Pathophysiology of diabetes: An overview. *Avicenna Journal of Medicine, 10*(04), 174–188.

Beck, A., Goetsch, L., Dumontet, C., & Corvaïa, N. (2017). Strategies and challenges for the next generation of antibody–drug conjugates. *Nature Reviews Drug Discovery, 16*(5), 315–337.

Berbudi, A., Khairani, S., & Tjahjadi, A. I. (2025). Interplay between insulin resistance and immune dysregulation in type 2 diabetes mellitus: Implications for therapeutic interventions. *ImmunoTargets and Therapy,* 359–382.

Brierley, G. V., Siddle, K., & Semple, R. K. (2018). Evaluation of anti-insulin receptor antibodies as potential novel therapies for human insulin receptoropathy using cell culture models. *Diabetologia, 61* (7), 1662–1675.

Brinkmann, U., & Kontermann, R. E. (2017). The making of bispecific antibodies. In *MAbs* (Vol. 9, pp. 182–212). Taylor & Francis, 2.

Butler, A. E., Janson, J., Bonner-Weir, S., Ritzel, R., Rizza, R. A., & Butler, P. C. (2003). β-cell deficit and increased β-cell apoptosis in humans with type 2 diabetes. *Diabetes, 52*(1), 102–110.

Cavelti-Weder, C., Babians-Brunner, A., Keller, C., Stahel, M. A., Kurz-Levin, M., Zayed, H., ... Donath, M. Y. (2012). Effects of gevokizumab on glycemia and inflammatory markers in type 2 diabetes. *Diabetes Care, 35*(8), 1654–1662.

Cieniewicz, A. M., Kirchner, T., Hinke, S. A., Nanjunda, R., D'Aquino, K., Boayke, K., ... Kihm, A. J. (2017). Novel monoclonal antibody is an allosteric insulin receptor antagonist that induces insulin resistance. *Diabetes, 66*(1), 206–217.

Donath, M. Y., Dinarello, C. A., & Mandrup-Poulsen, T. (2019). Targeting innate immune mediators in type 1 and type 2 diabetes. *Nature Reviews Immunology, 19*(12), 734–746.

Donath, M. Y., & Shoelson, S. E. (2011). Type 2 diabetes as an inflammatory disease. *Nature Reviews Immunology, 11*(2), 98–107.

Eizirik, D. L., Miani, M. I., & Cardozo, A. K. (2013). Signalling danger: Endoplasmic reticulum stress and the unfolded protein response in pancreatic islet inflammation. *Diabetologia, 56*(2), 234–241.

Engin, F., & Hotamisligil, G. S. (2010). Restoring endoplasmic reticulum function by chemical chaperones: An emerging therapeutic approach for metabolic diseases. *Diabetes, Obesity and Metabolism, 12,* 108–115.

Gao, X. K., Sheng, Z. K., Lu, Y. H., Sun, Y. T., Rao, X. S., Shi, L. J., ... Zhou, Y. T. (2023). VAPB-mediated ER-targeting stabilizes IRS-1 signalosomes to regulate insulin/IGF signaling. *Cell Discovery, 9*(1), 83.

Gieroba, B., Kryska, A., & Sroka-Bartnicka, A. (2025). Type 2 diabetes mellitus–conventional therapies and future perspectives in innovative treatment. *Biochemistry and Biophysics Reports, 42,* Article 102037.

He, H. J., Zong, Y., Bernier, M., & Wang, L. (2009). Sensing the insulin signaling pathway with an antibody array. *Proteomics - Clinical Applications, 3*(12), 1440–1450.

Hirano, M., Arima, H., & Oiso, Y. (2008). Immunological insulin resistance due to insulin antibodies developed after cessation of insulin therapy in a patient with type 2 diabetes. *Diabetes Care, 31*(11). e84-e84.

Hotamisligil, G. S. (2006). Inflammation and metabolic disorders. *Nature, 444*(7121), 860–867.

International Diabetes Federation. (2025). *IDF Diabetes Atlas* (11th ed.) Retrieved from https://diabetesatlas.org/resources/idf-diabetes-atlas-2025/.

Jialal, I., & Basheer, H. (2022). Syndromes of autoantibodies to the insulin receptor. *International Journal of Biochemistry and Molecular Biology, 13*(6), 87.

Joensuu, J. T., Huoponen, S., Aaltonen, K. J., Konttinen, Y. T., Nordström, D., & Blom, M. (2015). The cost-effectiveness of biologics for the treatment of rheumatoid arthritis: A systematic review. *PLoS One, 10* (3), Article e0119683.

Kapurniotu, A. (2020). Enlightening amyloid fibrils linked to type 2 diabetes and cross-interactions with Aβ. *Nature Structural & Molecular Biology, 27*(11), 1006–1008.

Khardori, R., & Griffing, G. T. (2025). Type 2 diabetes mellitus. *Medscape.* Retrieved from https://emedicine.medscape.com/article/117853-print.

Koliaki, C., & Katsilambros, N. (2022). Repositioning the role of tumor necrosis factor-related apoptosis-inducing ligand (TRAIL) on the TRAIL to the development of diabetes mellitus: An update of experimental and clinical evidence. *International Journal of Molecular Sciences, 23*(6), 3225.

Kumar, A., Mazumder, R., Rani, A., Pandey, P., & Khurana, N. (2024). Novel approaches for the management of type 2 diabetes mellitus: An update. *Current Diabetes Reviews, 20*(4), 45–61.

Labrijn, A. F., Meesters, J. I., de Goeij, B. E., van den Bremer, E. T., Neijssen, J., van Kampen, M. D., … Parren, P. W. (2013). Efficient generation of stable bispecific IgG1 by controlled Fab-arm exchange. *Proceedings of the National Academy of Sciences, 110*(13), 5145–5150.

Lebovitz, H. E. (2019). Thiazolidinediones: The forgotten diabetes medications. *Current Diabetes Reports, 19*(12), 151.

Li, M., Chi, X., Wang, Y., Setrerrahmane, S., Xie, W., & Xu, H. (2022). Trends in insulin resistance: Insights into mechanisms and therapeutic strategy. *Signal Transduction and Targeted Therapy, 7*(1), 216.

Li, G., & Zhang, D. (2025). Research progress on the correlation between islet amyloid peptides and type 2 diabetes mellitus. *Open Medicine, 20*(1), Article 20241124.

Liu, S., Han, D., Xu, C., Yang, F., Li, Y., Zhang, K., … Wen, W. (2022). Antibody-drug conjugates targeting CD248 inhibits liver fibrosis through specific killing on myofibroblasts. *Molecular Medicine, 28*(1), 37.

Lu, R. M., Chiang, H. L., Yuan, J. P. Y., Wang, H. H., Chen, C. Y., Panda, S. S., … Wu, H. C. (2025). Technological advancements in antibody-based therapeutics for treatment of diseases. *Journal of Biomedical Science, 32*(1), 98.

Lumeng, C. N., & Saltiel, A. R. (2011). Inflammatory links between obesity and metabolic disease. *The Journal of Clinical Investigation, 121*(6), 2111–2117.

Lutz, T. A., & Meyer, U. (2015). Amylin at the interface between metabolic and neurodegenerative disorders. *Frontiers in Neuroscience, 9*, 216.

Ma, L., Liu, T. W., Wallig, M. A., Dobrucki, I. T., Dobrucki, L. W., Nelson, E. R., … Smith, A. M. (2016). Efficient targeting of adipose tissue macrophages in obesity with polysaccharide nanocarriers. *ACS Nano, 10*(7), 6952–6962.

Ma, J., Mo, Y., Tang, M., Shen, J., Qi, Y., Zhao, W., … Qian, C. (2021). Bispecific antibodies: From research to clinical application. *Frontiers in Immunology, 12*, Article 626616.

Maneiro, J. R., Salgado, E., & Gomez-Reino, J. J. (2013). Immunogenicity of monoclonal antibodies against tumor necrosis factor used in chronic immune-mediated inflammatory conditions: Systematic review and meta-analysis. *JAMA Internal Medicine, 173*(15).

Marchetti, P., Bugliani, M., Lupi, R., Marselli, L., Masini, M., Boggi, U., … Cnop, M. (2007). The endoplasmic reticulum in pancreatic beta cells of type 2 diabetes patients. *Diabetologia, 50*(12), 2486–2494.

Okdahl, T., Wegeberg, A. M., Pociot, F., Brock, B., Størling, J., & Brock, C. (2022). Low-grade inflammation in type 2 diabetes: A cross-sectional study from a Danish diabetes outpatient clinic. *BMJ Open, 12*(12), Article e062188.

Porter, C. J. H., Edwards, G. A., & Charman, S. A. (2001). Lymphatic transport of proteins after sc injection: Implications of animal model selection. *Advanced Drug Delivery Reviews, 50*(1–2), 157–171.

Qian, Y. Y., Wu, H. Y., Liu, G. Q., Ren, C., Lu, P. R., & Zhang, X. G. (2019). Blockade of insulin receptor substrate-1 inhibits biological behavior of choroidal endothelial cells. *International Journal of Ophthalmology, 12*(9), 1386.

Rao, A., Quinn, L. M., & Narendran, P. (2024). Long-term TNF-alpha therapy for preserving beta cell function in new onset type 1 diabetes: A case report. *Clinical Diabetes and Endocrinology, 10*(1), 26.

Reyes-Medina, M. J., Cantón-Habas, V., Sánchez-Jiménez, F. J., Molina-Hurtado, E., & del Pilar Carrera-González, M. (2025). New approach to optimize therapy in type 2 diabetes mellitus: The importance of subclassification. *Frontiers in Endocrinology, 16*, Article 1710511.

Ridker, P. M., Everett, B. M., Thuren, T., MacFadyen, J. G., Chang, W. H., Ballantyne, C., … Glynn, R. J. (2017). Antiinflammatory therapy with canakinumab for atherosclerotic disease. *New England Journal of Medicine, 377*(12), 1119–1131.

Ristic, J., Kodalak, S., Peralta-Jiménez, G. A., Moura de Lima, M. F., Kovacevic, M., Masic, S., & Nikolic, T. (2025). Asprosin levels in adults with type 2 diabetes mellitus and diabetic kidney disease: A systematic review and meta-analysis. *Diabetes, Metabolic Syndrome and Obesity, 18*, 2493–2506.

Roberts, K. J., Cubitt, M. F., Carlton, T. M., Rodrigues-Duarte, L., Maggiore, L., Chai, R., … Crowe, J. S. (2021). Preclinical development of a bispecific TNFα/IL-23 neutralising domain antibody as a novel oral treatment for inflammatory bowel disease. *Scientific Reports, 11*(1), Article 19422.

Roham, P. H., Yadav, S. S., Senthilnathan, B., Potdar, P., Roy, S., & Sharma, S. (2025). Explaining type 2 diabetes with transcriptomic signatures of pancreatic β-Cell dysfunction and death induced by human islet amyloid polypeptide. *OMICS: A Journal of Integrative Biology, 29*(6), 268–282.

Sethi, J. K., & Hotamisligil, G. S. (2021). Metabolic messengers: Tumour necrosis factor. *Nature Metabolism, 3*(10), 1302–1312.

Shrestha, N., De Franco, E., Arvan, P., & Cnop, M. (2021). Pathological β-cell endoplasmic reticulum stress in type 2 diabetes: Current evidence. *Frontiers in Endocrinology, 12*, Article 650158.

Slaga, D., Ellerman, D., Lombana, T. N., Vij, R., Li, J., Hristopoulos, M., … Junttila, T. T. (2018). Avidity-based binding to HER2 results in selective killing of HER2-overexpressing cells by anti-HER2/CD3. *Science Translational Medicine, 10*(463), Article eaat5775.

Sloan-Lancaster, J., Abu-Raddad, E., Polzer, J., Miller, J. W., Scherer, J. C., De Gaetano, A., … Landschulz, W. H. (2013). Double-blind, randomized study evaluating the glycemic and anti-inflammatory effects of subcutaneous LY2189102, a neutralizing IL-1β antibody, in patients with type 2 diabetes. *Diabetes Care, 36*(8), 2239–2246.

Strohl, W. R. (2018). Current progress in innovative engineered antibodies. *Protein & Cell, 9*(1), 86–120.

Tsalamandris, S., Antonopoulos, A. S., Oikonomou, E., Papamikroulis, G. A., Vogiatzi, G., Papaioannou, S., … Tousoulis, D. (2019). The role of inflammation in diabetes: Current concepts and future perspectives. *European Cardiology Review, 14*(1), 50.

van de Donk, N. W., & Zweegman, S. (2023). T-cell-engaging bispecific antibodies in cancer. *The Lancet, 402*(10396), 142–158.

Wang, Y., He, X., Zheng, D., He, Q., Sun, L., & Jin, J. (2023). Integration of metabolomics and transcriptomics reveals major metabolic pathways and potential biomarkers involved in pulmonary tuberculosis and pulmonary tuberculosis-complicated diabetes. *Microbiology Spectrum, 11*(4), Article e00577-23.

Wang, G., & Sander, M. (2021). A multi-omics roadmap of β-cell failure in type 2 diabetes mellitus. *Nature Reviews Endocrinology, 17*(11), 641–642.

Wei, R., Jia, B., Zheng, S., Zhang, X., Wang, M., Sun, N., … Li, Q. (2025). Application of monoclonal antibodies in diabetes: A bibliometric analysis from 2004–2024. *Human Vaccines & Immunotherapeutics, 21*(1), Article 2536910.

World Health Organization. (2025). *Diabetes*. from https://www.who.int/health-topics/diabetes. (Accessed 18 November 2025).

17

Targeting inflammatory pathways in T2DM: Therapeutic interventions

Shafat Ali[1] and Yahya F. Jamous[2]

[1]DEPARTMENT OF ZOOLOGY, HASSAN KHOYIHAMI MEMORIAL DEGREE COLLEGE, BANDIPORA, JAMMU & KASHMIR, INDIA;; [2]WELLNESS AND PREVENTIVE MEDICINE INSTITUTE, HEALTH SECTOR, KING ABDULAZIZ CITY FOR SCIENCE AND TECHNOLOGY, RIYADH, SAUDI ARABIA

1. Introduction

Over the decades, the pathophysiology of type 2 diabetes mellitus (T2DM) has been mostly considered in terms of a bihormonal disproportion, insulin deficiency in the pancreatic beta cells and insulin resistance in the peripheral tissues (liver, muscle, and adipose). This paradigm resulted in a therapeutic armamentarium whose major aim was to reduce blood glucose, increase insulin secretion or insulin sensitivity (DeFronzo, 2009). Nevertheless, there has been a paradigm change in the past 20 years, in the realization that chronic, low-grade inflammation is not only the by-product but also key causative agent in the pathogenesis and pathophysiology of T2DM and its complications (Hotamisligil, 2006). T2DM as an inflammatory disease came into view, based on the findings of observed increases in the classic systemic inflammatory markers, including C-reactive protein (CRP), and white blood cells count, in victims of insulin resistance and with the prospective development of T2DM (Pradhan et al., 2001; Spranger et al., 2003). This is a low-grade, systemic (compared with the acute, high-grade inflammation that exists during infection) process involving a 2 to 3-fold rise in circulating proinflammatory cytokines. This is now realized to be a major interconnection between obesity, which is the major risk factor of T2DM and metabolic dysfunction. Overeating and excess amounts of saturated fatty acids as well as the growth of dysfunctional adipose tissue are the continuous stimuli to immune activity, forming a vicious circle that worsens the insulin signaling and functioning of the beta-cells (Donath & Shoelson, 2011).

A distinct set of cytokines and chemokines mediates metabolic inflammation. Tumor Necrosis Factor-alpha (TNF-α) is one of the earliest cytokines that has been associated with insulin resistance. TNF-α that is mainly secreted by the stimulated macrophages in fat tissues directly disrupts the insulin receptor, serine phosphorylation of insulin receptor substrate-1 (IRS-1), which makes the receptor inactive (Hotamisligil et al., 1995). One of the potent proinflammatory cytokines, interleukin-1 beta (IL-1β), is a key factor in

Type 2 Diabetes Mellitus. https://doi.org/10.1016/B978-0-443-33590-7.00003-4

the apoptosis of pancreatic beta cells and their dysfunction. The NLRP3 inflammasome in the macrophages and the β-cells themselves can be a result of high glucose and free fatty acids, which subsequently causes the IL-1β secretion, which further induces the β-cells death process and suppresses insulin secretion (Donath et al., 2019). Interleukin-6 (IL-6) has contextual behavior. Although hepatic insulin insensitivity and liver-produced CRP are observed with chronic elevation, it also exhibits antiinflammatory effects through its exercise (myokine release) (Carey et al., 2004). CRP is an acute phase protein that is generated by the liver as a reaction to IL-6. It has been used as a strong clinical biomarker of systemic inflammation and cardiovascular risk in T2DM (Ridker, 2003). Monocyte Chemoattractant Protein-1 (MCP-1/CCL2) is one of the most prominent chemokines that lead to the recruitment of the circulating monocytes into adipose tissue, where the former transforms into proinflammatory macrophages and enhances local and systemic inflammation (Kanda et al., 2006).

A pathobiological cross-talk between metabolic and immune cells mediates the inflammatory response in T2DM: In obesity, the phenotypic transition occurs toward a classical activation (M1, proinflammatory) macrophage as opposed to an alternative activation (M2, antiinflammatory) macrophage. These M1 ATMs (Adipose Tissue Macrophages) encircle dead adipocytes and develop into the major producers of TNF-α, IL-1β, and other inflammatory agents and actively generate local and systemic insulin resistance (Lumeng et al., 2007). The liver is an amplifier and target of inflammation. In nonalcoholic fatty liver disease (NAFLD), which is one of the comorbidities of T2DM, hepatocytes also express inflammatory mediators, and become insulin-resistant, resulting in uncontrolled gluconeogenesis. Acute-phase proteins such as CRP are also produced by the liver due to the effect of cytokines (Shoelson et al., 2006). Islands are not passive but active participants. β-cells are capable of generating IL-1β, which results in autocrine and paracrine destructive actions. Moreover, there is immune cell invasion into the islets (insulitis) that leads to the degradation of the mass and functioning of the β cells (Eguchi & Nagai, 2017).

Based on this basic immune-metabolic paradigm, this chapter takes a closer look at the targeted therapeutic interventions by initially dissecting the fundamental underlying intracellular signaling pathways converting nutrient excess into inflammation. It also discusses the pleiotropic antiinflammatory role the conventional antidiabetic drugs play, the clinically proven anticytokine therapies and the current agents under development. Finally, the chapter summarizes all the solutions, explains some difficulties in patient stratification and safety, and speculates on the future of antiinflammatory strategies in the personalized treatment of T2DM.

2. Foundational pathways linking inflammation to insulin resistance and β-cell dysfunction

The low-grade inflammation that becomes chronic in T2DM is not an accident, but rather coordinated by certain evolutionarily preserved intracellular signal transduction pathways. These pathways are very important sensors and transducers, transforming metabolic overload, i.e., excess nutrients, lipids, and cellular stress, into a concerted agglomeration of inflammatory response, which has a direct effect of impairing insulin action and health of the β-cells. It is important to learn these underlying pathways to come up with specific antiinflammatory interventions. One of the main intersections of the connections between inflammation and insulin resistance is the IκB kinase β/Nuclear Factor-kappa B (IKKβ/NF-κB) pathway. The cytoplasm holds the inactive NF-κB in its cytoplasmic inhibitor, IκB. The IKK complex, especially its catalytic subunit IKKβ, and metabolic stressors, which include TNF-α, IL-1β, and high levels of free fatty acids, activate the IKK complex. IKKβ phosphorylates IκB, which gets ubiquitinated and degraded in the proteasome thus releasing NF-κB (Shi et al., 2006). The released NF-κB moves to the nucleus and induces the transcription of a huge number of proinflammatory genes, such as TNF-α, IL-1β, IL-6, and MCP-1. Importantly, this pathway has a direct effect of disrupting the insulin signaling. IKKβ can cause serine phosphorylation of Insulin Receptor Substrate 1 (IRS-1) inhibiting its tyrosine phosphorylation and subsequent insulin signaling (Gao et al., 2002). Genetical and pharmacological inhibition of IKKβ in obese rodent models enhances insulin sensitivity and decreases the expression of cytokines, confirming its central role (Yuan et al., 2001). NF-κB in the β-cell of the pancreas enhances apoptosis and dysfunction in response to glucolipotoxic conditions, which is part of the decrease of β-cell mass (Eldor et al., 2006).

One key stress-response pathway is the c-Jun N-terminal Kinase (JNK) pathway, which is activated by endoplasmic reticulum (ER) stress, oxidative stress, and cytokine signaling, all of which are increased in T2DM. The activity of JNK is significantly enhanced in major metabolic organs of obesity, liver, fatty tissue, and muscle (Hirosumi et al., 2002). Similar to IKKβ, activated JNK (JNK1 in particular) phosphorylates IRS-1 on the inhibitory serine residues (Ser307), preventing its interaction with insulin receptor and signal transduction. In addition, JNK phosphorylates and activates the transcription factor Activator Protein-1 (AP-1), which is a dimer of Jun and Fos proteins. AP-1 collaborates with NF-κB to catalyze the expression of many inflammatory genes. The definitive demonstration of principle came by genetic research: mice deficient in Jnk1 are resistant to diet-induced insulin resistance, whereas β-cell-specific Jnk1 expression causes diabetes (Kaneto et al., 2004). The JNK pathway can therefore be directly termed as an intermediary of metabolic stress, inflammatory activation of genes and insulin action disruption.

The NLRP3 inflammasome is a multiprotein cytosolic complex, which is a major indicator of metabolic threat. It consists of sensor NLRP3, the adaptor ASC, and effector caspase-1. In T2DM, two-signal model drives its activation. Signal 1 (priming): NF-κB is triggered by high glucose or saturated fatty acids (e.g., palmitate) through TLRs, resulting in increased NLRP3 and pro-IL-1β transcription. Signal 2 (activation): NLRP3 inflammasome assembly is provoked by subsequent stimuli, including ceramide, islet amyloid polypeptide (IAPP), or by mitochondrial reactive oxygen species (mtROS) (Masters et al., 2010; Shi et al., 2003). This assembly results in the autocatalytic cleavage of procaspase-1 to active caspase-1, which later cleaves pro-IL-1β and pro-IL-18 into the active and secreted forms respectively. The involvement of IL-1β in the glucotoxicity and apoptosis of β-cells has been conclusively proven. The IL-1β induces Fas, stimulates the synthesis of nitric oxide, and reduces the functions of the mitochondrion, resulting in the death of β cells in the pancreas (Maedler et al., 2002). Insulin resistance in the peripheral tissues is also promoted by systemic IL-1β. Sheltering the NLRP3/IL-1β crossbreed pathway, thus, constitutes a very precise treatment approach directly based on the pathophysiology behind this pathway.

Pattern recognition receptors that are commonly recognized as TLR2 and TLR4 are the Toll-like Receptors (TLRs), which are associated with the recognition of pathogen-associated molecular pattern (PAMPs). They are triggered by endogenous damage-associated molecular pattern (DAMPs) and nutrition overload in the context of metabolic disease, also known as metabolic inflammation or metaflammation (Hotamisligil, 2017). Direct activation of TLR4 on macrophages and adipocytes by saturated fatty acids (e.g., palmitate) can trigger the downstream signaling through MyD88/IRAK/TRAF6 converting to the activation of both IKK/NF-κB and JNK/AP-1 pathways (Shi et al., 2006). In addition, obesity is also related to the DAMPs such as HMGB1 (high-mobility group box 1) and heat shock proteins, which are released by compressed or dying cells. Such molecules also interact with TLRs, which continues the inflammatory pathway. Insulin resistance, which is caused by fatty acids, is immune to TLR4 deficiency in mice (Shi et al., 2006). Activation of TLR also takes place in pancreatic islets, which contributes to local inflammation and β-cell failure. This pathway places innate immune receptors in a central position to fail to recognize nutrient overload as a threat leading to the activation of the chronic inflammatory condition of T2DM.

3. Conventional antidiabetic drugs with antiinflammatory pleiotropic effects

Although the main action of the traditional antidiabetic drugs is focused on lowering glucose levels, insulin sensitization, or insulin secretion, an increasing amount of data indicate that most of them have serious antiinflammatory effects. These pleiotropic effects probably play a role in their cardiovascular and renal effects that are not directly linked to glycemic control, and are a transition between conventional therapy and the specific antiinflammatory approaches.

3.1 Metformin

T2DM has metformin as a first-line treatment that is mainly used to reduce hepatic glucose inflation by stimulating AMP-activated protein kinase (AMPK). This activity has significant indirect antiinflammatory effects. AMPK activation suppresses the IKKβ/NF-κB pathway by fixing cellular energy balance. Metformin was found to decrease the activity of IKKβ and this results in a decrease in degradation of IκBα and consequently inhibition of the nuclear translocation of NF-κB (Hattori et al., 2006). This leads to decrease in the transcription of proinflammatory cytokines such as TNF-α and IL-6. Moreover, metformin suppresses complex I of the mitochondrial respiratory chain, causing a slight rise in AMP/ATP ratio that does not only activate AMPK but also decreases the generation of mitochondrial reactive oxygen species (mtROS), which is a major NLRP3 inflammasome activator (Foretz et al., 2019). Metformin therapy is linked to decreases in systemic inflammatory markers, including CRP, TNF-α and IL-6, in T2DM and polycystic ovary syndrome (PCOS) patients (Cameron et al., 2016). These antiinflammatory effects have become part and parcel of its therapeutic profile.

3.2 Thiazolidinediones (TZDs)

Thiazolidinedione (e.g., pioglitazone, rosiglitazone) are high-affinity ligands of the nuclear receptor Peroxisome Proliferator-Activated Receptor gamma (PPAR-γ). Their major insulin-sensitizing effect is through the positive regulation of adipocyte differentiation and the lipid storage in subcutaneous adipose tissue, which decreases the ectopic deposition of fat. Importantly, their antiinflammatory action is carried out by the adipose tissue remodeling mechanism. Activation of PPAR-γ in macrophages and adipocytes directly suppresses the expression of proinflammatory genes (e.g., TNF-α, IL-6, MCP-1) by inhibiting the action of NF-κB, AP-1 and STAT transcription factors (Pascual et al., 2005). TZDs cause a phenotypic transformation of adipose tissue macrophages (ATMs) between a proinflammatory, M1 M2 state in vivo. This is indicated by a decrease in the presence of the crown-like structures and increase in the presence of the M2 markers such as arginase-1 and IL-10 (Odegaard et al., 2007). This adipose tissue microenvironmental remodeling lowers the spillage of the inflammatory mediators into the systemic circulation, which helps in enhancing the systemic insulin sensitivity.

3.3 GLP-1 receptor agonists

GLP-1 RAs promote glucose-dependent secretion of insulin, inhibit glucagon, and slow gastric emptying. Nevertheless, GLP-1 receptors (GLP-1R) can be found on immune cells, namely macrophages, lymphocytes, and offer them a direct route of immunomodulation. GLP-1 RAs were found to suppress the NF-κB signaling in the vascular endothelial cells, hepatocytes and macrophages. Research shows that GLP-1 receptive agonists such as liraglutide and exenatide decrease the synthesis of TNF-α, IL-1β, IL-6 and CRP in animal models and in human research (Krasner et al., 2014). They are able to decrease the infiltration of macrophage in adipose tissue and alter the polarization to M2-type, such as TZDs. Moreover, in pancreatic islands, GLP-1 RAs directly have antiapoptotic and antiinflammatory activities, which can likely protect β-cell mass by inhibiting local IL-1β production (Shiraki et al., 2012). Such widespread antiinflammatory effects are thought to be at least partly responsible to their established cardiovascular outcome improvements.

3.4 SGLT2 inhibitors

The sodium-glucose cotransporter 2 inhibitors (SGLT2) reduce blood glucose by suppressing renal glucose reabsorption. Their strong cardiorenal effects seem not limited to glycosuria. One of the suggested effects is metabolic reprogramming: SGLT2 decrease plasma glucose and insulin levels leading to a fasting-like state and enhancing lipolysis and ketone body (β-hydroxybutyrate) production. Moreover, β-hydroxybutyrate is not only an effective source of energy but also an endogenous inhibitor of NLRP3 inflammasome that directly suppresses the production of IL-18 and IL-1β (Youm et al., 2015). Also, SGLT2 decrease the intracellular concentrations of sodium and later calcium through the $Na+/Ca2+$ exchanger and enhance the performance of mitochondria and oxidative stress present in cardiomyocytes, renal tubular cells, and endothelial cells (Vaduganathan et al., 2022). Decreased oxidative stress directly suppresses the stimulation of redox-sensitive inflammatory signaling (NF-κB and JNK) directly. SGLT2 therapy is also linked to large decreases in systemic inflammatory (e.g., CRP, IL-6) and fibrotic (e.g., TGF-β) markers, which are correlated with its capacity to delay the heart failure and CKD (chronic kidney disease) progression.

4. Targeted antiinflammatory therapies in clinical investigation

There are some therapeutic agents that are specifically designed to disrupt certain elements of the immune-metabolic axis in T2DM. These focused strategies constitute a bench to bedside translational bridge providing not only the proof-of-concept validation but also an important lesson on the difficulty of immunomodulation of chronic metabolic disease. The most clinically proven inflammatory approach to T2DM is to target the IL-1β pathway, which directly converts the pathophysiological impact of the NLRP3 inflammasome into therapeutics. Anakinra is a recombinant version of endogenous human IL-1Ra. It acts as a competitive inhibitor, and competes strongly with the IL-1 type I receptor (IL-1RI) so blocking signal transduction by IL-1α and IL-1β. Anakinra was tested in a definitive proof-of-concept randomized controlled trial that investigated 100 mg/day as the subcutaneous dose of anakinra versus placebo (Larsen et al., 2007). The therapy produced substantial systemic inflammatory response, as shown by a substantial reduction of CRP and IL-6. More importantly, it enhanced the pancreatic β-cell activity as evidenced by a 40% rise in the C-peptide response during hyperglycemic clamp and a considerable decline in the proinsulin-to-insulin ratio, an indicator of β-cell stress. This was accompanied by statistically significant decrease in glycated hemoglobin (HbA1c) by 0.46% in comparison with placebo. Nonetheless, the researchers have no significant change in insulin sensitivity using the euglycemic-hyperinsulinemic clamp, highlighting the fact that IL-1β blockage could selectively act on β-cell dysfunction rather than peripheral insulin resistance. The short half-life of anakinra in T2DM (it needs to be injected every day, which limits its use clinically), the presence of frequent injection-site reactions, and moderate but significant risk of infections are factors that limit its clinical utility.

Canakinumab is a human monoclonal IgG1/κ neutralizing antibody with specific and high affinity that neutralizes IL-1β, without blocking IL-1α or the endogenous IL-1Ra. The most important findings are based on the CANTOS trial (Canakinumab Antiinflammatory Thrombosis Outcome Study), which represents a cardiovascular outcomes trial that included 10,061 patients who had a history of myocardial infarction and tended toward persistent inflammatory phenotype (hs-CRP ≥2 mg/L) (Ridker et al., 2017). Although the main goal was to evaluate the reduction of atherosclerotic events, prespecified analysis resulted in landmark data on T2DM. Canakinumab (150 mg, injected subcutaneously after every 3 months) reduced cardiovascular events in the big subgroup of diabetes patients (n = 4000), and caused large, dose-dependent changes in HbA1c (by around 0.15%–0.25%, the median follow-up was 3.7 years) and in fasting plasma glucose (Everett et al., 2018). This trial furnished large-scale randomized evidence that during selective IL-1β neutralization, there are durable and clinically significant glucoregulatory effects. But CANTOS came up with an unappetizing safety alarm as well: a serious rise in fatal infections, which pointed to the extreme danger of immunosuppression despite a specific cytokine block in an older population with comorbidity.

TNF-α is a prototype of proinflammatory cytokines and a key contributor to insulin resistance. It has been widely investigated as an inhibitor in autoimmune disorders where it is common to have metabolic comorbidity. The primary options in the treatment of rheumatoid arthritis (RA) are etanercept (solvable TNF receptor-Fc fusion protein), and infliximab (chimeric anti-TNF-α monoclonal antibody). Another consistent finding in observational and interventional studies on RA patients with comorbid T2DM are that metabolic parameters are improved with anti-TNF therapy. Indicatively, RA patients receiving infliximab were found to exhibit a significant increase in insulin sensitivity, measured by the Homeostasis Model Assessment of Insulin Resistance (HOMA-IR), in only 2 weeks of the initial infusion regardless of the changes in disease activity, corticosteroid dose, and body weight (Gonzalez-Gay et al., 2006). This quick enhancement confirms a direct pharmacological impact of TNF-α blockade on insulin signaling probably by reversing the TNF-α-induced serine phosphorylation of IRS-1 on skeletal muscle and adipose tissue. Although TNF-α inhibitors have strong biological justification and encourage positive signals in comorbid groups, the use of TNF-α as a T2DM mono-therapy is not discussed as a viable therapy because of the poor risk-benefit profile. These agents are also associated with high risks, such as sharp rise in serious bacterial, fungal, and opportunistic infections (especially reactivation of latent tuberculosis), possible exacerbation or development of congestive heart failure, the emergence of autoantibodies (e.g., antinuclear antibodies) and, uncommonly, demyelinating diseases (Tracey et al., 2008). The overall rise in the risk of infection, and the presence of safer and more effective glucose-lowering agents makes systemic TNF-α inhibition inappropriate in the T2DM population in general, but forms an important therapy in individuals with comorbid severe inflammatory arthritis.

The glycosuria has unscientifically been reported to decrease with high-dose salicylates over a 100 years ago. Their action was also explained by the fact that they are direct inhibitors of IκB kinase β (IKK β), which is the central activator of the NF-κB pathway (Yuan et al., 2001). In the modern TINSAL-T2D (Targeting Inflammation with Salsalate in Type 2 Diabetes) program, salsalate, which is a dimeric, nonacetylated salicylate, has been tested. Salsalate (3.5–4.5 g/day) has been shown to reduce the HbA1c by around 0.5% and notable reductions in a variety of inflammatory markers such as adiponectin (an antiinflammatory adipokine) in a 48-week, placebo controlled trial (Goldfine et al., 2010). This gave good clinical evidence-of-concept of IKKβ/NF-κB inhibition. Nonetheless, there were also alarming off-target effects that were linked to treatment: a minor yet significant rise in the urinary albumin excretion (which is indicative of possible renal stress), an increase in LDL cholesterol, and an increase in the occurrence of tinnitus. Such side effects, and the large doses needed, eventually stalled its development as a general T2DM treatment, but it is still a paradigm of drug repositioning in relation to pathway biology.

The chemokine system and especially the C–C chemokine receptor type 2 (CCR2) and its ligand the MCP-1 (CCL2) are involved in the process of recruiting inflammatory monocytes out of circulation into growing adipose tissue. The genetic loss of CCR2 in obese mice or pharmacological inhibition of this receptor lowers the adipose tissue macrophage (ATM) infiltration, the systemic inflammation, and enhances insulin sensitivity (Weisberg et al., 2006). Early-stage clinical trials of small-molecule CCR2 antagonists (e.g., MK-0812, PF-04634817) in patients with T2DM or at cardiovascular risk demonstrated a slight decrease in inflammatory biomarkers, such as hs-CRP. Nevertheless, these effects have mostly been irregular and even no large-scale outcomes trial has shown unequivocal metabolic or cardiovascular benefit in T2DM. Examples of problems are functional redundancy to the chemokine system (e.g., functions of CCR5), the inability to achieve adequate receptor blockade in human adipose tissue compartments, and possible disconnection between changes in biomarkers and hard clinical outcomes. Therefore, mechanistically CCR2 antagonism has not provided a successful therapeutic to T2DM.

5. Novel and emerging pharmacological strategies

Whereas the clinically tested agents offer important proof-of-concept, the search of safer and more effective antiinflammatory treatments of T2DM goes on (Table 17.1). The present frontier concerns the creation of much more specific inhibitors, which are able to target upstream sensors or even individual inflammatory pathways in a more precise manner to achieve a maximum benefit on metabolism without causing overall immunosuppression of the system.

5.1 NLRP3 inflammasome inhibitors

A logical development of cytokine blockade (e.g., anti-IL-1β) is direct pharmacological inhibition of the NLRP3 inflammasome. MCC950 (CRID3 or CP-456,773) is a powerful

Table 17.1 New and developing pharmacological approaches to type 2 diabetes (T2DM).

Strategy/ Drug class	Mechanism of action	Potential advantages	Examples (development stage)	References
Dual and Triple Incretin Agonists	These medications work by stimulating GLP-1, GIP and glucagon receptors at the same time. By doing so, they increase the secretion of insulin, decrease the secretion of glucagon, promote feelings of satiety and increase energy expenditure.	Compared with selective GLP-1 agonists, dual and triple incretin agonists have shown to result in better glycemic control and greater weight reduction. In addition, the triple agonists may also provide benefits to lipids and energy expenditure.	Tirzepatide (GLP-1/GIP Approved) Retatrutide (GLP-1/GIP/ Glucagon, Phase III) Cagrilintide/Semaglutide (Amylin/GLP-1 Phase II)	(Frias et al., 2021, Rosenstock et al., 2023, Bossart et al., 2022)
Oral GLP-1 Receptor Agonists	The GLP-1 Receptor Agonists are orally-administered small-molecule agonists that stimulate the GLP-1 receptors in the same way as the injectable versions of GLP-1 RA drugs.	The elimination of the need for injections will improve patient adherence and increase access to the drug. The reduction in HbA1c levels and the loss of weight are positive outcomes of this therapy.	Oral Semaglutide (Approved) Danuglipron (Phase II)	(Rodbard et al., 2019, Saxena et al., 2021)
Glucokinase Activators (GKAs)	Stimulate the hepatic and pancreatic glucokinase, which is the glucose sensor in the body. Enhances the uptake of glucose in liver and the insulin secretion of glucose-dependent type.	Attacks two major malfunctions (liver production, insulin release) through an insulin-independent process.	Dorzagliatin (Phase III) TTP399 (Phase II)	(Matschinsky & Wilson, 2019, Diao et al., 2021)
AMPK Activators	Activate AMP-activated protein kinase (AMPK), a global cellular energy sensor. Enhances insulin sensitivity, uptake of glucose and decreases hepatic gluconeogenesis.	General metabolic effects: enhances lipid metabolism, inflammation, and can prevent vasculature damage.	O304 (Phase II), PXL770 (Phase II) Berberine (Natural product)	(Coughlan et al., 2014, Steinberg & Carling, 2019)
GPCR Targets (FFAR1/ GPR40, GPR119)	Stimulate nutrient-sensing GPCRs. FFAR1 provokes secretion of insulin, which is dependent on glucose. GPR119 provokes the release of GLP-1 and GIP.	Insulin secretion is triggered by glucose-dependency to reduce the risk of hypoglycemia. Potential of combining with other agents.	Fasiglifam (Canceled, hepatotoxicity) Next-gen FFAR1/GPR119 agonist in discovery.	(Mancini & Poitout, 2013, Harada et al., 2018)
SGLT1 Inhibitors (Intestinal)	Mainly antagonize SGLT1 within the gastrointestinal tract, postponing the uptake of glucose and galactose. Modest effect on renal SGLT1/2.	Lowers the levels of postprandial glucose through a nonhormonal, complementary mechanism. May be used together with SGLT2 inhibitors.	**Sotagliflozin** (Approved for HF, T2DM indication sought - dual SGLT1/2) **Mizagliflozin** (Phase II - selective SGLT1)	(Dobbins et al., 2015, Sands et al., 2015)

Continued

Table 17.1 New and developing pharmacological approaches to type 2 diabetes (T2DM).—cont'd

Strategy/ Drug class	Mechanism of action	Potential advantages	Examples (development stage)	References
Glucagon Receptor Antagonists	Inhibit the signal of the hepatic glucagon receptor, which produces glucose. Lessens glucose excess production in the hepatic hepatocytes.	Potent glucose- Potent glucose-lowering. May be perfect in fixed-dose combinations to overcome hyperglucagonemia of other medications.	**REMD-477** (Phase II) **Volagidemab** (Phase I)	(Kulina, & Rayfield, 2016, Petersen & Sullivan, 2001)
Metabolic Inhibitors (11β-HSD1)	Block 11β-hydroxysteroid dehydrogenase type 1 and minimize the production of active cortisol in liver tissue, fatty tissue, as well as in brain tissue.	Reduces local cortisol activities to increase insulin sensitivity, can reduce hepatic fat and enhance thinking.	AZD4017 (Phase II) RO-5093151 (Phase I, discontinued)	(Kupczyk et al., 2022, Anagnostis et al., 2013)
Gene-and-Cell-Based Approaches	Gene-Based Therapy: Uses viral vectors to provide a long-lasting source for expressing either insulin or incretin hormones. Cell-Based Therapy: Transplantation (replacing) with functional glucose responsive (making more/less) insulin producing cells (islets grown from stem cells).	The potential for long term durable control of blood sugars or functional cure. Reduces or eliminates the requirement of daily insulin therapy.	VX-880 (islet cells grown from stem cells, being studied in Phase I/II clinical trials). G-LIPS (Gene therapy that creates a GLP-1 hormone, in preclinical stage).	(Bottino et al., 2018, Melton, 2021)
AI-Generated Drugs & Digital Health Therapies	AI - Identifies new drug targets and designs drug molecules or predicts combination drug therapies. Digital - Utilizes behavioral health therapies through digital media to manage patients' diets and levels of physical activity and to assist them in taking their medications.	Assists in speeding up the development of mechanistic drug action. Digital tools provide personalized and scalable forms of adjunctive therapy.	INS018_055 represents an example of an AI-generated antifibrotic drug for patients with Type 2 Diabetes Mellitus's (T2D's) comorbidity (currently in phase 1 clinical trials). Digital Cognitive Behavioral Therapy (CBT) programs available for use on the US market that have received FDA clearance or approval.	(Zhavoronkov et al., 2019, Rashid et al., 2022)

selective, small-molecule, NLRP3 inhibitor that prevents NLRP3 activation and caspase-1 cleavage and release of IL-1β/IL-18. It interferes with the ASC oligomerization of NLRP3, which is a crucial step in inflammasome, but does not impact other inflammasomes such as AIM2 or NLRC4 (Coll et al., 2019). MCC950 treatment in preclinical models of T2DM and nonalcoholic steatohepatitis (NASH) resulted in reduced systemic and hepatic inflammation, increased insulin and reduced pancreatic β-cell dysfunction and steatosis in the liver (Mridha et al., 2017). It is a very promising candidate because of its ability to prevent a point of convergence of several metabolic stresses (lipotoxicity, glucotoxicity, ER stress). Nevertheless, the development of MCC950 as a drug was itself terminated because of liver toxicity in early-phase trials. This has led to the design of next generation, structurally different NLRP3 inhibitors (e.g., NT-0796, dapansutrile) having possibly better safety profiles, some of which are currently in clinical trials in inflammatory diseases with metabolic components.

5.2 IKKβ and JNK inhibitors

JNK and IKKβ/NF-κB pathways are the central controllers of inflammatory gene expression and insulin resistance. The safe and selective inhibitors have however been highly challenging to develop with the widespread physiological functions of these kinases. Whereas salicylates such as salsalate are nonspecific competitive inhibitors of IKKβ, it has not been easy to design ATP competitive inhibitors with high specificity. IKKβ is engaged in intrinsic immunity, cell survival and tissue homeostasis. Systemic inhibition provokes the issues of immunosuppression, host defense reduction, and hepatotoxicity. Ways of avoiding this would be to make allosteric inhibitors or compounds that have limited tissue distribution. As of now, there has been no highly specific IKKβ inhibitor, which has been successfully developed in clinical development and used to treat T2DM, highlighting the toxicity challenges of this node of the central node. In the same manner, three stress-responsive, apoptotic, and developmental JNK isoforms (JNK1-3) are present. JNK1 is the major isoform that is involved in metabolic disease. Initial peptide-based inhibitors (e.g., JNK-inhibitory peptide, JIP) demonstrated efficacy in rodents with diabetes (Kaneto et al., 2004), but their translation was hampered by poor pharmacokinetics. Other indications showed that small-molecule ATP-competitive JNK inhibitors have experienced serious off-target effects and toxicity in clinical trials, which is mostly attributed to the preserved structure of the kinase ATP-binding pocket. Recent studies are looking at creating isoform-selective inhibitors (JNK1 over JNK2/3) or the use of antisense oligonucleotides (ASOs) to selectively silence hepatic JNK1 expression to induce metabolic benefit with reduced systemic toxicity.

5.3 Modulators of sphingolipid pathway

Bioactive lipids that include sphingolipids especially ceramide, accumulate in tissues during nutrient excess, and have a direct role in mediating lipotoxicity, insulin resistance and inflammation. Ceramide is capable of defining protein phosphatase 2A (PP2A) and protein kinase C zeta (PKCζ), which suppress Akt/PKB a pivotal point in the insulin signaling pathway. Besides, ceramide enhances the dysfunction of the mitochondria and the production of ROS, which may trigger the activation of the NLRP3 inflammasome (Chaurasia & Summers, 2015). Pharmacological mechanisms are meant to inhibit the production of ceramides, or speed up their breakdown. Myriocin and its analogs inhibit the first and rate-limiting enzyme in de novo ceramide synthesis. Myriocin enhances insulin sensitivity and inflammation in the case of the obese rodent models. Nevertheless, worldwide blockage of the production of sphingolipids may be very harmful as they form the parts of the cell membranes and signaling. Better still are isoform-selective CerS inhibitors. As an example, the CerS6 is involved in insulin resistance by palmitate. Selective inhibition may have tissue or pathway advantages. LCL-521 and similar compounds, which increase the activity of acid ceramidase, the enzyme that breaks ceramide down to sphingosine, have demonstrated effectiveness in ceramide levels, glucose tolerance and reducing inflammation in adipose tissues in preclinical models. Sphingolipid pathway provides a distinct target at the point where metabolism and inflammation meet yet clinical translation will need an agent of high specificity to prevent interference with the regulation of fundamental lipid biology.

5.4 Galectin-3 inhibitors

Galectin-3 is a lectin binding to β-galactoside, released by activated macrophages and other cells. It is not a typical cytokine and acts as a damage-associated molecular pattern (DAMP) and an effective initiator of inflammation, fibrosis, and tissue remodeling. Galactin-3 is increased in T2DM and is associated with insulin resistance, heart failure, and development of renal diseases. Galectin-3 facilitates the occurrence of inflammation by maintaining the activation of NLRP3 inflammasomes, macrophage polarization to M1, and the activation of profibrotic pathways such as TGF-β (Pugliese et al., 2015). Inhibitors of galactose-recognition domain modified citrus pectin (MCP) and stronger, synthetically engineered carbohydrate analogs (e.g., TD139, GB1211) are galactose-recognition domain inhibitors. Galactin-3 inhibition can decrease the macrophage invasion, inhibit fibrosis, and enhance both cardiac and renal function in preclinical stages of diabetic cardiomyopathy and nephropathy. It is an amplifier of preexisting inflammatory and fibrotic pathways and therefore is of interest as a target of combating the end-organ complications of T2DM, but not hyperglycemia per se. A number of galectin-3 inhibitors are undergoing early clinical trials in pulmonary fibrosis and NASH, and may also be extended unambiguously to diabetic complications.

6. Antiinflammatory agents: Nonpharmacological and lifestyle interventions

In addition to pharmacology, lifestyle change is the core element of T2DM management and prevention with strong and direct antiinflammatory actions (Table 17.2). These are the interventions aimed at the underlying factors of metaflammation, which are excess of nutrients and sedentarism, and they tend to offer advantages that do not merely follow what is enumerated by weight loss by itself. The main regulators of systemic inflammation are dietary composition and energy

Table 17.2 Nonpharmacological and lifestyle antiinflammatory interventions.

Intervention	Specific modality	Antiinflammatory mechanism	Key clinical/Research findings	References
Dietary Patterns	Mediterranean Diet	High in monounsaturated fatty acids (as found in olive oil), fiber, polyphenols, omega-3 fatty acids and causes the reduction in proinflammatory eicosanoids and adhesion molecule expression.	Consistently reduce the blood levels of CRP, IL-6 and TNF-α and lower the risk of Cardiovascular Disease.	Schwingshackl et al. (2020)
	Antiinflammatory/ Polyphenol-Rich Diets	High in colorful fruits and vegetables (berries, leafy greens), spices (turmeric, ginger), dark chocolate, and tea Modulating the NF-κB and Nrf2 signaling pathways.	Lessens the systemic inflammatory biomarkers. Related to better endothelial performance and metabolic condition.	Rickards et al. (2021)
	Fasting and Caloric Restriction	Lowers oxidative and metabolic stress, increases autophagy, and modifies gut microbiome and circadian biology.	Reduces leukocyte count, IL-6, and CRP. Enhances insulin sensitivity and may lessen inflammation associated with aging ("inflammaging").	de Cabo and Mattson (2019)
Nutritional Components and Supplements	Omega-3 Fatty Acids (EPA/DHA)	Integrated into cellular membranes, resulting in the synthesis of proinflammatory mediators (resolvins, protectins) that are weaker than those derived from omega-6 fatty acids.	CRP, TNF-α, and IL-6 are decreased significantly with high-dose supplementation (2–4 g/day) especially in patients who have high levels of inflammation at baseline.	Calder (2017)
	Vitamin D	Regulates natural and adaptive immunity by activating the vitamin D receptor on immune cells to induce antiinflammatory Treg-like phenotype and inhibit Th17 responses	Adequate serum concentrations (>30 ng/mL) are associated with a reduced CRP and IL-6. Deficiency should be corrected to decrease the autoimmune and metabolic disease-related inflammation	Aranow (2011)
	Curcumin	Strong suppressor of inflammatory cytokines (TNF-α, IL-1β, and IL-6), COX-2, and NF-κB. Increases the capability for antioxidants	Several meta-analysis studies show that patients suffering from chronic inflammatory conditions such as metabolic syndrome/arthritis have been shown to reversibly decrease serum levels of the proinflammatory markers CRP, IL-6 and TNF-α	Hewlings and Kalman (2017)

Continued

Table 17.2 Nonpharmacological and lifestyle antiinflammatory interventions.—cont'd

Intervention	Specific modality	Antiinflammatory mechanism	Key clinical/Research findings	References
	Probiotics and Prebiotics	Alter the makeup of the microbiota of the gut, strengthen the intestinal barrier, lower levels of endotoxemia (LPS), and encourage the synthesis of short-chain fatty acids (SCFAs) that have anti-inflammatory effects.	Certain strains, including Lactobacillus and Bifidobacterium, lower proinflammatory cytokines and hs-CRP. Diets rich in fiber raise SCFAs.	Moludi et al. (2021)
Physical Activity and Exercise	Regular Aerobic Exercise	Causes the production of hormetic, and anti-inflammatory myokines generated from muscles, such as IL-6, IL-10, and IL-1ra. Decreases visceral adipose tissue, which is a significant source of cytokines.	IL-6 is temporarily elevated by acute exercise, while baseline CRP, TNF-α, and IL-18 are subsequently reduced over time. There is an inverse relationship between inflammation and cardiorespiratory fitness.	Pedersen and Saltin (2015)
	Resistance Training	Add to amount of muscle, a metabolically active tissue sequestering the precursors of inflammation and enhancing glucose metabolism. Aerobic activity releases myokines in a similar way.	Lowers IL-6 and CRP levels without weight reduction. Especially advantageous for older and sarcopenic groups.	Sardeli et al. (2018)
Stress and Mind-Body Interventions	Mindfulness and Meditation	Decrease inflammation caused by cortisol and norepinephrine. Downregulating the activity of sympathetic nervous system (SNS) and the hypothalamic-pituitary-adrenal (HPA) axis.	Frequent practice is linked to lower CRP, increased expression of antiviral genes, and NF-κB activity.	Black and Slavich (2016)
	Cognitive Behavioral Therapy (CBT)	Modifies coping strategies and stress assessments, which reduces the production of proinflammatory cytokine and the activation of the SNS and HPA axis.	Efficient in lowering inflammation in ailments including sleeplessness, rheumatoid arthritis, and depression.	Shields et al. (2020)
	Sleep Hygiene and Optimization	Inadequate sleep triggers NF-κB activation and disrupts the circadian rhythm of cortisol and inflammatory cytokines, such as IL-6 and TNF-α, which peak at night.	Insufficient sleep and poor quality are connected to increased CRP, IL-6, and TNF-α levels. Sleeping longer reduces inflammation.	Irwin (2019)

Table 17.2 Nonpharmacological and lifestyle antiinflammatory interventions.—cont'd

Intervention	Specific modality	Antiinflammatory mechanism	Key clinical/Research findings	References
Avoidance and Mitigation	Smoking Cessation	Removes oxidants and nicotine, which activate NF-κB and harm endothelium cells.	Within weeks of quitting, inflammatory indicators (such as CRP and WBC count) drastically decrease and eventually approach values of never-smokers.	Arnson et al. (2010)
	Reduction of Environmental Toxins	Reduces exposure to heavy metals, endocrine disruptors (BPA, phthalates), and air pollutants (PM2.5), all of which can cause inflammation and oxidative stress in the body.	Reduced exposure decreases systemic inflammation and risk of inflammatory illnesses.	Pekince and Baccioglu (2022)
	Alcohol Moderation	Evades the proinflammatory consequences of excessive or binge drinking, including as increased hepatic inflammation, endotoxemia, and intestinal permeability, while the likely antiinflammatory effects of light to moderate consumption are debatable.	CRP and IL-6 are significantly elevated by heavy intake. There is disagreement about the J-curve theory for light intake, with current recommendations favoring decrease.	Imhof et al. (2001)

balance. A long-term deficiency in the energy consumption, despite the short-term absence of weight loss, quickly transforms the inflammatory condition. Caloric Restriction (CR) lowers the mass of adipose tissue, lowering the production of proinflammatory adipokines and the ability to stimulate macrophage invasion. More directly, it reduces circulating concentrations of proinflammatory nutrients such as free fatty acids and glucose, which are TLR ligands and NLRP3 inflammasome activators. Human intervention studies confirm that the CR (usually 20%–30% decrease) has a significant effect on the TNF-α, IL-6, CRP, and MCP-1 levels in the bloodstream, which drop considerably and adiponectin, which is an antiinflammatory adipokine, is elevated (Fontana et al., 2007). These alterations take place in a few days to weeks, usually before weight loss, which implies a direct metabolic control of inflammation. The Mediterranean Diet (MedDiet) is antiinflammatory and is not controlled by caloric intake, as it is characterized by large intake of monounsaturated fats (olive oil), polyphenols (fruits, vegetables, red wine), fiber, and omega-3 fatty acids (fish). Extra virgin olive oil, which contains a lot of oleic acid and phenols such as oleocanthal, does not only prevent COX enzymes (similarly ibuprofen) but also weaken the activation of NF-kB (Lopez-Miranda et al., 2010). Fruits and vegetables contain polyphenols that are antioxidants and regulate gut microbiota to enhance the generation of antiinflammatory short-chain fatty acids. Long-term randomized controlled trials including PREDIMED have demonstrated that MedDiet combined with nuts or olive oil can significantly lower the incidence of T2DM and cardiovascular events, which is associated with significant decreases in IL-6, TNF-α, and CRP (Estruch et al., 2018).

During contraction skeletal muscle itself is an endocrine organ, releasing cytokines and peptides, the so-called myokines, which produce strong systemic antiinflammatory activities. In comparison with its proinflammatory effect in conditions of chronic elevation of adipose tissue, a sharp and acute rise of IL-6 during and after exercise is one of the primary agents of metabolic advantage. The IL-6 produced by muscle increases hepatic glucose, lipolysis in adipose tissue, and has an antiinflammatory effect (stimulates IL-10 and IL-1Ra) and inhibits TNF-α production (Pedersen & Febbraio, 2008). IL-10 is an effective antiinflammatory cytokine that is released in response to exercise and suppresses NF-kB signaling, TNF-α and IL-1β. This is an exercise-induced myokine that is cleaved off a protein on the membrane of FNDC5. Irisin facilitates the browning of white adipose tissue (elevating its energy expenditure) and was demonstrated to inhibit NF-κB signaling and the expression of TNF-α and MCP-1 in the macrophages and endothelial cells and directly connects muscle activity to tissue inflammation reduction (Xin et al., 2016). Regular exercise therefore creates a temporary, positive inflammatory environment that overcomes chronic low-grade inflammation to enhance insulin sensitivity regardless of weight gain.

The most extreme case of inflammation resolution in T2DM is bariatric or metabolic surgery (e.g., Roux-en-Y gastric bypass, sleeve gastrectomy). Amazingly, there is a marked enhancement of glucose homeostasis and inflammatory biomarkers usually within days after surgery, before any significant weight loss. The severe decrease in caloric intake and the uptake of macronutrients (in particular, fat) instantly decreases the influx of proinflammatory substrates. To be more exact, the alterations in the secretion of gut hormones play a vital role. The rapid delivery of the nutrients to the distal intestine, with the acceleration of the postprandial secretion of the glucagon-like peptides-1 (GLP-1) and peptide YY (PYY), which exhibit direct antiinflammatory and insulin-sensitizing effects, is dramatic. After surgery, adipose tissue undergoes a massive restructuring in the weeks and months after surgery. This consists of decreased adipocyte hypertrophy, macrophages polarization to M2 rather than M1 phenotype, and TNF-α, IL-6, and MCP-1 production (Frikke-Schmidt et al., 2016). It is worth noting that alterations in bile acid composition and flux after surgery are capable of stimulating receptors such as TGR5 and FXR that have direct antiinflammatory actions in adipose tissue and liver. In the long-term, the maintained weight reduction and the better state of gut microbiota sustain low levels of systemic inflammation. Research demonstrates significant and sustained decreases in CRP, IL-6, and leptin, and adiponectin and cardiovascular risk decreases, associated with T2DM remission and cardiovascular risk reduction. This renders bariatric surgery an effective natural experiment to show how metabolic inflammation can be reversed.

7. Integrative perspectives, challenges, and future directions

Antiinflammatory strategies have to overcome a complex terrain to be translated into clinical reality in T2DM that was initially promising in the laboratory. The success depends on the ability to incorporate these new approaches in current paradigms and solve major scientific and practical issues. One of the most essential shortcomings of the initial clinical trials is the heterogeneity of T2DM. The use of a single antiinflammatory strategy is not likely to work as the role of inflammation in the pathophysiology of each individual varies. Precision phenotyping is the future, and it would help to select the most likely-to-benefit subgroup of patients, the high inflammatory. This involves the shift away of the classical measures such as HbA1c. Potential stratification biomarkers include high-sensitivity CRP (hsCRP) (used in CANTOS) persistent elevation (>2 mg/L), which is a high-risk inflammatory phenotype in response to blockage of IL-1β (Ridker et al., 2017). Specific inflammatory endotypes might be characterized by multianalyte profiling (i.e., of IL-1β, IL-6, TNF-α, MCP-1) or other methods. Therapy could be guided by MRI to measure the amount of visceral fat (a major source of inflammation) or examination of adipose tissue biopsy gene expression signature. Genetic variation in genes of inflammatory pathways (e.g., IL1RN, TNF) can be used to predict response to therapy. The aim is to align the drug (e.g., an NLRP3 inhibitor) and the patient who has evident signs of pathway dysregulation. One of the major obstacles to systemic anticytokine therapy is elevated chances of immunosuppression. The CANTOS study was a clear indication that even selective IL-1β-blocking has a stimulating effect on fatal infections (Ridker et al., 2017). In case of TNF-α inhibitors, the risk of serious infection and possible malignancy (e.g., lymphoma, skin cancer) is properly known. These risks are most important to mitigate and inform future development: Formulations designed to ablate inflamed metabolic tissues (e.g., liver, adipose) without immunizing the system. Investigating the possible association of metabolic advantages of immunosuppression (i.e., pulsatile vs. lower-dose therapy). By attacking upstream sensors (e.g., NLRP3) or use of specific intracellular kinases, a more favorable safety paradigm can be achieved as opposed to neutralizing general acting cytokines such as TNF-α, which play a crucial role in host defense. Patients with latent infection (e.g., TB) and recurrent and high malignancy risk are not to be included in clinical trials and subsequent treatment.

Because of the overlapping and redundancy of the inflammatory networks, monotherapy might not be sufficient. Rational combination approaches hold a potential of increased effectiveness with reduced and safer dosing. Combining multiple nodes within the same pathway (e.g., an NLRP3 inhibitor + a low dose IL-1 receptor antagonist) to block the pathway more completely. Blocking compensatory activation by means of parallel pathways inhibition (e.g., a JNK inhibitor + an IKKβ inhibitor). One of the options is the combination of a new antiinflammatory agent with an existing one such as metformin or a GLP-1 RA, which act on different mechanisms and are already safe.

Integrating pharma-therapy and intense lifestyle change (diet/exercise) to optimally lower the inflammatory stimulus and improve the response to treatment. Exercise and dietary change can reduce drug doses depending on the antiinflammatory effects that they have. A number of crucial areas need targeted research so as to develop the field: There is need to go beyond fixed cytokine levels into biomarkers that are indicative of the real-time pathway activity (e.g., phospho-proteomics on immune cells) or that can be used to predict the response to treatment a priori. The area of hyperglycemia has received much of the research effort, yet inflammation is one of the main causes of complications. Future trials ought to focus on outcome such as heart failure, reduce renal functionality and neuropathy and test agents such as galactin-3 inhibitors. The intestinal microbiome is a powerful systemic inflammatory modulator. The study of pre/probiotics, postbiotics (e.g., particular short-chain fatty acids), and interventions aimed at restoring gut barrier integrity is one of the key directions (Cani et al., 2019). In addition to inhibiting the proinflammatory signaling, an alternate paradigm that can prevent immunosuppressive side effects is the active resolution of inflammation, through specialized proresolving mediators (SPMs) such as resolvins and protectins (Serhan, 2017). Delivery of antiinflammatory payloads to metabolically activated macrophages or stressed β-cells with nanotechnology or with antibody-drug conjugates or tissue-specific promoters. Finally, antiinflammatory therapy will need to be proven in T2DM control not only to be glycemically effective, but net benefit on both hard cardiovascular and renal outcome, to shift the paradigm of the field not just to pathogenetic understanding, but to transformative clinical practice.

8. Conclusion

The study of the inflammation in T2DM has developed as a new concept into a clear pathogenic pillar, and there are particular, drug-gable targets. The best target is the IL-1β pathway, confirmed by anakinra and canakinumab clinical success and is directly associated with the NLRP3 inflammasome activation to β-cell dysfunction and systemic inflammation. The IKKβ/NF-kB axis is a master regulator but has been challenging to inhibit safely as shown by the salsalate shortcomings. There is mechanistic interest in strategies aimed at immune cell recruitment (e.g., CCR2 inhibition) though such have to date not been clinically translated successfully. Conversely, the pleiotropic antiinflammatory properties of the currently available classes of drugs, in particular, GLP-1 receptor agonists and SGLT2 inhibitors, have offered a clinically immediate and safe option of utilizing this biology, which adds to their cardiorenal advantages. The future of the antiinflammatory treatment in T2DM is not a complete substitute of the existing care, but rather a careful combination. The paradigm is changing to have a more holistic approach toward T2DM as a cardiometabolic-immune disorder. This will entail a stratified method. In most cases, the antiinflammatory effects of lifestyle change, metformin, GLP-1 RAs, and SGLT2 inhibitors will create a background of an antiinflammatory background. In a selected group of patients with high inflammatory load, which can be detected with biomarkers such as high levels of hsCRP, specific cytokine or pathway inhibition (e.g., with next-generation NLRP3 inhibitors) can become a precision adjunctive therapy, especially to preserve β-cells and prevent progressive complications. The final objective is to individualize therapy according to the prevailing pathophysiological drivers of an individual, and beautifully integrate antiinflammatory measures into the mainstream repertoire, to not only reduce glucose, but to fundamentally change the course of the disease, and its disastrous outcome.

References

Anagnostis, P., Katsiki, N., Adamidou, F., Athyros, V. G., Karagiannis, A., Kita, M., & Mikhailidis, D. P. (2013). 11beta-Hydroxysteroid dehydrogenase type 1 inhibitors: Novel agents for the treatment of metabolic syndrome and obesity-related disorders? *Metabolism, 62*(1), 21–33.

Aranow, C. (2011). Vitamin D and the immune system. *Journal of Investigative Medicine, 59*(6), 881–886.

Arnson, Y., Shoenfeld, Y., & Amital, H. (2010). Effects of tobacco smoke on immunity, inflammation and autoimmunity. *Journal of Autoimmunity, 34*(3), J258–J265.

Black, D. S., & Slavich, G. M. (2016). Mindfulness meditation and the immune system: A systematic review of randomized controlled trials. *Annals of the New York Academy of Sciences, 1373*(1), 13–24.

Bossart, M., Wagner, M., Elvert, R., Evers, A., Hübschle, T., Kloeckener, T., … Konkar, A. (2022). Effects on weight loss and glycemic control with SAR441255, a potent unimolecular peptide GLP-1/GIP/GCG receptor triagonist. *Cell Metabolism, 34*(1), 59–74.

Bottino, R., Knoll, M. F., Knoll, C. A., Bertera, S., & Trucco, M. M. (2018). The future of islet transplantation is now. *Frontiers of Medicine, 5*, 202.

Calder, P. C. (2017). Omega-3 fatty acids and inflammatory processes: From molecules to man. *Biochemical Society Transactions, 45*(5), 1105–1115.

Cameron, A. R., Morrison, V. L., Levin, D., Mohan, M., Forteath, C., Beall, C., … Rena, G. (2016). Anti-inflammatory effects of metformin irrespective of diabetes status. *Circulation Research, 119*(5), 652–665.

Cani, P. D., Van Hul, M., Lefort, C., Depommier, C., Rastelli, M., & Everard, A. (2019). Microbial regulation of organismal energy homeostasis. *Nature Metabolism, 1*(1), 34–46.

Carey, A. L., Bruce, C. R., Sacchetti, M., Anderson, M. J., Olsen, D. B., Saltin, B., … Febbraio, M. A. (2004). Interleukin-6 and tumor necrosis factor-α are not increased in patients with type 2 diabetes: Evidence that plasma interleukin-6 is related to fat mass and not insulin responsiveness. *Diabetologia, 47*(6), 1029–1037.

Chaurasia, B., & Summers, S. A. (2015). Ceramides–lipotoxic inducers of metabolic disorders. *Trends in Endocrinology and Metabolism, 26*(10), 538–550.

Coll, R. C., Hill, J. R., Day, C. J., Zamoshnikova, A., Boucher, D., Massey, N. L., … Schroder, K. (2019). MCC950 directly targets the NLRP3 ATP-hydrolysis motif for inflammasome inhibition. *Nature Chemical Biology, 15*(6), 556–559.

Coughlan, K. A., Valentine, R. J., Ruderman, N. B., & Saha, A. K. (2014). AMPK activation: A therapeutic target for type 2 diabetes? *Diabetes, Metabolic Syndrome and Obesity: Targets and Therapy*, 241–253.

De Cabo, R., & Mattson, M. P. (2019). Effects of intermittent fasting on health, aging, and disease. *New England Journal of Medicine, 381*(26), 2541–2551.

DeFronzo, R. A. (2009). From the triumvirate to the ominous octet: A new paradigm for the treatment of type 2 diabetes mellitus. *Diabetes, 58*(4), 773–795.

Diao, H., Yu, X., Li, C., Guo, Y., Shen, B., & Zhao, W. (2021). The effects and safety of activators of glucokinase versus placebo in patients with type 2 diabetes mellitus: A systematic review and meta-analysis. *Endocrine Journal, 68*(2), 189–194.

Dobbins, R. L., Greenway, F. L., Chen, L., Liu, Y., Breed, S. L., Andrews, S. M., ... Smith, C. D. (2015). Selective sodium-dependent glucose transporter 1 inhibitors block glucose absorption and impair glucose-dependent insulinotropic peptide release. *American Journal of Physiology - Gastrointestinal and Liver Physiology, 308*(11), G946–G954.

Donath, M. Y., Dinarello, C. A., & Mandrup-Poulsen, T. (2019). Targeting innate immune mediators in type 1 and type 2 diabetes. *Nature Reviews Immunology, 19*(12), 734–746.

Donath, M. Y., & Shoelson, S. E. (2011). Type 2 diabetes as an inflammatory disease. *Nature Reviews Immunology, 11*(2), 98–107.

Eguchi, K., & Nagai, R. (2017). Islet inflammation in type 2 diabetes and physiology. *The Journal of Clinical Investigation, 127*(1), 14–23.

Eldor, R., Yeffet, A., Baum, K., Doviner, V., Amar, D., Ben-Neriah, Y., ... Melloul, D. (2006). Conditional and specific NF-κB blockade protects pancreatic beta cells from diabetogenic agents. *Proceedings of the National Academy of Sciences, 103*(13), 5072–5077.

Estruch, R., Ros, E., Salas-Salvadó, J., Covas, M. I., Corella, D., Arós, F., ... Martínez-González, M. A. (2018). Primary prevention of cardiovascular disease with a Mediterranean diet supplemented with extra-virgin olive oil or nuts. *New England Journal of Medicine, 378*(25), Article e34.

Everett, B. M., Donath, M. Y., Pradhan, A. D., Thuren, T., Pais, P., Nicolau, J. C., ... Ridker, P. M. (2018). Anti-inflammatory therapy with canakinumab for the prevention and management of diabetes. *Journal of the American College of Cardiology, 71*(21), 2392–2401.

Fontana, L., Eagon, J. C., Trujillo, M. E., Scherer, P. E., & Klein, S. (2007). Visceral fat adipokine secretion is associated with systemic inflammation in obese humans. *Diabetes, 56*(4), 1010–1013.

Foretz, M., Guigas, B., & Viollet, B. (2019). Understanding the glucoregulatory mechanisms of metformin in type 2 diabetes mellitus. *Nature Reviews Endocrinology, 15*(10), 569–589.

Frías, J. P., Davies, M. J., Rosenstock, J., Pérez Manghi, F. C., Fernández Landó, L., Bergman, B. K., ... Brown, K. (2021). Tirzepatide versus semaglutide once weekly in patients with type 2 diabetes. *New England Journal of Medicine, 385*(6), 503–515.

Frikke-Schmidt, H., O'Rourke, R. W., Lumeng, C. N., Sandoval, D. A., & Seeley, R. J. (2016). Does bariatric surgery improve adipose tissue function? *Obesity Reviews, 17*(9), 795–809.

Gao, Z., Hwang, D., Bataille, F., Lefevre, M., York, D., Quon, M. J., & Ye, J. (2002). Serine phosphorylation of insulin receptor substrate 1 by inhibitor κB kinase complex. *Journal of Biological Chemistry, 277* (50), 48115–48121.

Goldfine, A. B., Fonseca, V., Jablonski, K. A., Pyle, L., Staten, M. A., Shoelson, S. E., & TINSAL-T2D (Targeting Inflammation Using Salsalate in Type 2 Diabetes) Study Team*. (2010). The effects of salsalate on glycemic control in patients with type 2 diabetes: A randomized trial. *Annals of Internal Medicine, 152*(6), 346–357.

Gonzalez-Gay, M. A., De Matias, J. M., Gonzalez-Juanatey, C., Garcia-Porrua, C., Sanchez-Andrade, A., Martin, J., & Llorca, J. (2006). Anti-tumor necrosis factor-alpha blockade improves insulin resistance in patients with rheumatoid arthritis. *Clinical & Experimental Rheumatology, 24*(1), 83.

Harada, K., Mizukami, J., Kadowaki, S., Matsuda, I., Watanabe, T., Oe, Y., ... Inaba, T. (2018). Design and synthesis of novel and potent GPR119 agonists with a spirocyclic structure. *Bioorganic & Medicinal Chemistry Letters, 28*(7), 1228–1233.

Hattori, Y., Suzuki, K., Hattori, S., & Kasai, K. (2006). Metformin inhibits cytokine-induced nuclear factor κB activation via AMP-activated protein kinase activation in vascular endothelial cells. *Hypertension, 47*(6), 1183–1188.

Hewlings, S. J., & Kalman, D. S. (2017). Curcumin: A review of its effects on human health. *Foods, 6*(10), 92.

Hirosumi, J., Tuncman, G., Chang, L., Görgün, C. Z., Uysal, K. T., Maeda, K., ... Hotamisligil, G. S. (2002). A central role for JNK in obesity and insulin resistance. *Nature, 420*(6913), 333–336.

Hotamisligil, G. S. (2006). Inflammation and metabolic disorders. *Nature, 444*(7121), 860–867.

Hotamisligil, G. S. (2017). Foundations of immunometabolism and implications for metabolic health and disease. *Immunity, 47*(3), 406–420.

Hotamisligil, G. S., Arner, P., Caro, J. F., Atkinson, R. L., & Spiegelman, B. M. (1995). Increased adipose tissue expression of tumor necrosis factor-alpha in human obesity and insulin resistance. *The Journal of Clinical Investigation, 95*(5), 2409–2415.

Imhof, A., Froehlich, M., Brenner, H., Boeing, H., Pepys, M. B., & Koenig, W. (2001). Effect of alcohol consumption on systemic markers of inflammation. *The Lancet, 357*(9258), 763–767.

Irwin, M. R. (2019). Sleep and inflammation: Partners in sickness and in health. *Nature Reviews Immunology, 19*(11), 702–715.

Kanda, H., Tateya, S., Tamori, Y., Kotani, K., Hiasa, K. I., Kitazawa, R., ... Kasuga, M. (2006). MCP-1 contributes to macrophage infiltration into adipose tissue, insulin resistance, and hepatic steatosis in obesity. *The Journal of Clinical Investigation, 116*(6), 1494–1505.

Kaneto, H., Nakatani, Y., Miyatsuka, T., Kawamori, D., Matsuoka, T. A., Matsuhisa, M., ... Hori, M. (2004). Possible novel therapy for diabetes with cell-permeable JNK-inhibitory peptide. *Nature Medicine, 10*(10), 1128–1132.

Krasner, N. M., Ido, Y., Ruderman, N. B., & Cacicedo, J. M. (2014). Glucagon-like peptide-1 (GLP-1) analog liraglutide inhibits endothelial cell inflammation through a calcium and AMPK dependent mechanism. *PLoS One, 9*(5), Article e97554.

Kulina, G. R., & Rayfield, E. J. (2016). The role of glucagon in the pathophysiology and management of diabetes. *Endocrine Practice, 22*(5), 612–621.

Kupczyk, D., Bilski, R., Kozakiewicz, M., Studzińska, R., Kędziora-Kornatowska, K., Kosmalski, T., ... Głowacka, M. (2022). 11β-HSD as a new target in pharmacotherapy of metabolic diseases. *International Journal of Molecular Sciences, 23*(16), 8984.

López-Miranda, J., Pérez-Jiménez, F., Ros, E., De Caterina, R., Badimón, L., Covas, M. I., ... Yiannakouris, N. (2010). Olive oil and health: Summary of the II international conference on olive oil and health consensus report, Jaén and Córdoba (Spain) 2008. *Nutrition, Metabolism, and Cardiovascular Diseases, 20*(4), 284–294.

Larsen, C. M., Faulenbach, M., Vaag, A., Vølund, A., Ehses, J. A., Seifert, B., ... Donath, M. Y. (2007). Interleukin-1–receptor antagonist in type 2 diabetes mellitus. *New England Journal of Medicine, 356*(15), 1517–1526.

Lumeng, C. N., Bodzin, J. L., & Saltiel, A. R. (2007). Obesity induces a phenotypic switch in adipose tissue macrophage polarization. *The Journal of Clinical Investigation, 117*(1), 175–184.

Maedler, K., Sergeev, P., Ris, F., Oberholzer, J., Joller-Jemelka, H. I., Spinas, G. A., ... Donath, M. Y. (2002). Glucose-induced β cell production of IL-1β contributes to glucotoxicity in human pancreatic islets. *The Journal of Clinical Investigation, 110*(6), 851–860.

Mancini, A. D., & Poitout, V. (2013). The fatty acid receptor FFA1/GPR40 a decade later: How much do we know? *Trends in Endocrinology and Metabolism, 24*(8), 398–407.

Masters, S. L., Dunne, A., Subramanian, S. L., Hull, R. L., Tannahill, G. M., Sharp, F. A., ... O'neill, L. A. (2010). Activation of the NLRP3 inflammasome by islet amyloid polypeptide provides a mechanism for enhanced IL-1β in type 2 diabetes. *Nature Immunology, 11*(10), 897–904.

Matschinsky, F. M., & Wilson, D. F. (2019). The central role of glucokinase in glucose homeostasis: A perspective 50 years after demonstrating the presence of the enzyme in islets of Langerhans. *Frontiers in Physiology, 10,* 148.

Melton, D. (2021). The promise of stem cell-derived islet replacement therapy. *Diabetologia, 64*(5), 1030–1036.

Moludi, J., Khedmatgozar, H., Saiedi, S., Razmi, H., Alizadeh, M., & Ebrahimi, B. (2021). Probiotic supplementation improves clinical outcomes and quality of life indicators in patients with plaque psoriasis: A randomized double-blind clinical trial. *Clinical Nutrition ESPEN, 46,* 33–39.

Mridha, A. R., Wree, A., Robertson, A. A., Yeh, M. M., Johnson, C. D., Van Rooyen, D. M., ... Farrell, G. C. (2017). NLRP3 inflammasome blockade reduces liver inflammation and fibrosis in experimental NASH in mice. *Journal of Hepatology, 66*(5), 1037–1046.

Odegaard, J. I., Ricardo-Gonzalez, R. R., Goforth, M. H., Morel, C. R., Subramanian, V., Mukundan, L., , ... Ferrante, A. W., & Macrophage-specific PPARgamma controls alternative activation and improves insulin resistance. (2007). Macrophage-specific PPARgamma controls alternative activation and improves insulin resistance. *Nature, 447*(7148), 1116–1120.

Pascual, G., Fong, A. L., Ogawa, S., Gamliel, A., Li, A. C., Perissi, V., ... Glass, C. K. (2005). A SUMOylation-dependent pathway mediates transrepression of inflammatory response genes by PPAR-γ. *Nature, 437*(7059), 759–763.

Pedersen, B. K., & Febbraio, M. A. (2008). Muscle as an endocrine organ: Focus on muscle-derived interleukin-6. *Physiological Reviews, 88*(4), 1379–1406.

Pedersen, B. K., & Saltin, B. (2015). Exercise as medicine–evidence for prescribing exercise as therapy in 26 different chronic diseases. *Scandinavian Journal of Medicine & Science in Sports, 25,* 1–72.

Pekince, md, B., & Baccioglu, md, A. (2022). Allergic and non-allergic asthma phenotypes and exposure to air pollution. *Journal of Asthma, 59*(8), 1509–1520.

Petersen, K. F., & Sullivan, J. T. (2001). Effects of a novel glucagon receptor antagonist (Bay 27–9955) on glucagon-stimulated glucose production in humans. *Diabetologia, 44*(11), 2018–2024.

Pradhan, A. D., Manson, J. E., Rifai, N., Buring, J. E., & Ridker, P. M. (2001). C-reactive protein, interleukin 6, and risk of developing type 2 diabetes mellitus. *Jama, 286*(3), 327–334.

Pugliese, G., Iacobini, C., Pesce, C. M., & Menini, S. (2015). Galectin-3: An emerging all-out player in metabolic disorders and their complications. *Glycobiology, 25*(2), 136–150.

Rashid, M. M., Askari, M. R., Chen, C., Liang, Y., Shu, K., & Cinar, A. (2022). Artificial intelligence algorithms for treatment of diabetes. *Algorithms, 15*(9), 299.

Rickards, L., Lynn, A., Harrop, D., Barker, M. E., Russell, M., & Ranchordas, M. K. (2021). Effect of polyphenol-rich foods, juices, and concentrates on recovery from exercise induced muscle damage: A systematic review and meta-analysis. *Nutrients, 13*(9), 2988.

Ridker, P. M. (2003). Clinical application of C-reactive protein for cardiovascular disease detection and prevention. *Circulation, 107*(3), 363–369.

Ridker, P. M., Everett, B. M., Thuren, T., MacFadyen, J. G., Chang, W. H., Ballantyne, C., ... Glynn, R. J. (2017). Antiinflammatory therapy with canakinumab for atherosclerotic disease. *New England Journal of Medicine, 377*(12), 1119–1131.

Rodbard, H. W., Rosenstock, J., Canani, L. H., Deerochanawong, C., Gumprecht, J., Lindberg, S.Ø., ... Montanya, E. (2019). Oral semaglutide versus empagliflozin in patients with type 2 diabetes uncontrolled on metformin: The PIONEER 2 trial. *Diabetes Care, 42*(12), 2272–2281.

Rosenstock, J., Frias, J., Jastreboff, A. M., Du, Y., Lou, J., Gurbuz, S., … Coskun, T. (2023). Retatrutide, a GIP, GLP-1 and glucagon receptor agonist, for people with type 2 diabetes: A randomised, double-blind, placebo and active-controlled, parallel-group, phase 2 trial conducted in the USA. *The Lancet, 402*(10401), 529–544.

Sands, A. T., Zambrowicz, B. P., Rosenstock, J., Lapuerta, P., Bode, B. W., Garg, S. K., … Strumph, P. (2015). Sotagliflozin, a dual SGLT1 and SGLT2 inhibitor, as adjunct therapy to insulin in type 1 diabetes. *Diabetes Care, 38*(7), 1181–1188.

Sardeli, A. V., Tomeleri, C. M., Cyrino, E. S., Fernhall, B., Cavaglieri, C. R., & Chacon-Mikahil, M. P. T. (2018). Effect of resistance training on inflammatory markers of older adults: A meta-analysis. *Experimental Gerontology, 111*, 188–196.

Saxena, A. R., Gorman, D. N., Esquejo, R. M., Bergman, A., Chidsey, K., Buckeridge, C., … Kim, A. M. (2021). Danuglipron (PF-06882961) in type 2 diabetes: A randomized, placebo-controlled, multiple ascending-dose phase 1 trial. *Nature Medicine, 27*(6), 1079–1087.

Schwingshackl, L., Morze, J., & Hoffmann, G. (2020). Mediterranean diet and health status: Active ingredients and pharmacological mechanisms. *British Journal of Pharmacology, 177*(6), 1241–1257.

Serhan, C. N. (2017). Discovery of specialized pro-resolving mediators marks the dawn of resolution physiology and pharmacology. *Molecular Aspects of Medicine, 58*, 1–11.

Shi, Y., Evans, J. E., & Rock, K. L. (2003). Molecular identification of a danger signal that alerts the immune system to dying cells. *Nature, 425*(6957), 516–521.

Shi, H., Kokoeva, M. V., Inouye, K., Tzameli, I., Yin, H., & Flier, J. S. (2006). TLR4 links innate immunity and fatty acid–induced insulin resistance. *The Journal of Clinical Investigation, 116*(11), 3015–3025.

Shields, G. S., Spahr, C. M., & Slavich, G. M. (2020). Psychosocial interventions and immune system function: A systematic review and meta-analysis of randomized clinical trials. *JAMA Psychiatry, 77* (10), 1031–1043.

Shiraki, A., Oyama, J. I., Komoda, H., Asaka, M., Komatsu, A., Sakuma, M., … Node, K. (2012). The glucagon-like peptide 1 analog liraglutide reduces TNF-α-induced oxidative stress and inflammation in endothelial cells. *Atherosclerosis, 221*(2), 375–382.

Shoelson, S. E., Lee, J., & Goldfine, A. B. (2006). Inflammation and insulin resistance. *The Journal of Clinical Investigation, 116*(7), 1793–1801.

Spranger, J., Kroke, A., Mohlig, M., Hoffmann, K., Bergmann, M. M., Ristow, M., … Pfeiffer, A. F. (2003). Inflammatory cytokines and the risk to develop type 2 diabetes: Results of the prospective population-based European Prospective Investigation into Cancer and Nutrition (EPIC)-Potsdam Study. *Diabetes, 52*(3), 812–817.

Steinberg, G. R., & Carling, D. (2019). AMP-activated protein kinase: The current landscape for drug development. *Nature Reviews Drug Discovery, 18*(7), 527–551.

Tracey, D., Klareskog, L., Sasso, E. H., Salfeld, J. G., & Tak, P. P. (2008). Tumor necrosis factor antagonist mechanisms of action: A comprehensive review. *Pharmacology & Therapeutics, 117*(2), 244–279.

Vaduganathan, M., Docherty, K. F., Claggett, B. L., Jhund, P. S., de Boer, R. A., Hernandez, A. F., … Solomon, S. D. (2022). SGLT2 inhibitors in patients with heart failure: A comprehensive meta-analysis of five randomised controlled trials. *The Lancet, 400*(10354), 757–767.

Weisberg, S. P., Hunter, D., Huber, R., Lemieux, J., Slaymaker, S., Vaddi, K., … Ferrante Jr, A. W. (2006). CCR2 modulates inflammatory and metabolic effects of high-fat feeding. *The Journal of Clinical Investigation, 116*(1), 115–124.

Xin, C., Liu, J., Zhang, J., Zhu, D., Wang, H., Xiong, L., … Tao, L. (2016). Irisin improves fatty acid oxidation and glucose utilization in type 2 diabetes by regulating the AMPK signaling pathway. *International Journal of Obesity, 40*(3), 443–451.

Youm, Y. H., Nguyen, K. Y., Grant, R. W., Goldberg, E. L., Bodogai, M., Kim, D., … Dixit, V. D. (2015). The ketone metabolite β-hydroxybutyrate blocks NLRP3 inflammasome–mediated inflammatory disease. *Nature Medicine, 21*(3), 263–269.

Yuan, M., Konstantopoulos, N., Lee, J., Hansen, L., Li, Z. W., Karin, M., & Shoelson, S. E. (2001). Reversal of obesity-and diet-induced insulin resistance with salicylates or targeted disruption of Ikkβ. *Science, 293*(5535), 1673–1677.

Zhavoronkov, A., Ivanenkov, Y. A., Aliper, A., Veselov, M. S., Aladinskiy, V. A., Aladinskaya, A. V., … Aspuru-Guzik, A. (2019). Deep learning enables rapid identification of potent DDR1 kinase inhibitors. *Nature Biotechnology, 37*(9), 1038–1040.

Index

Note: Page numbers followed by "*f*" indicate figures and "*t*" indicate tables.

J

K

U

V

W

Z

Printed and bound by CPI Group (UK) Ltd, Croydon, CR0 4YY
02/07/2026
02155142-0001